DISASTER MEDICINE

DISASTER MEDICINE

Editors

DAVID E. HOGAN, D.O., F.A.C.E.P.

Affiliate Faculty
Department of Emergency Medicine
Oklahoma State University;
Research Director
Emergency Medicine Residency Programs
St. Michael and Integris Southwest Medical Center
Oklahoma City, Oklahoma

JONATHAN L. BURSTEIN, M.D., F.A.C.E.P.

Director of Disaster Medicine
Beth Israel Deaconess Medical Center;
Assistant Professor of Emergency Medicine
Harvard Medical School
Boston, Massachusetts

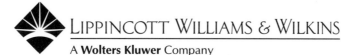

LIPPINCOTT WILLIAMS & WILKINS
A **Wolters Kluwer** Company
Philadelphia · Baltimore · New York · London
Buenos Aires · Hong Kong · Sydney · Tokyo

Acquisitions Editor: Anne M. Sydor
Developmental Editors: Kristen Kirchner
Production Editor: Christiana Sahl
Manufacturing Manager: Timothy Reynolds
Cover Designer: Christine Jenny
Compositor: Lippincott Williams & Wilkins Desktop Division
Printer: Maple Press

Library of Congress Cataloging-in-Publication Data
Disaster medicine / editors, David E. Hogan, Johanthan L. Burstein.
    p. ; cm.
    Includes bibliographical references and index.
    ISBN 0-7817-2625-5
    1. Disaster medicine. 2. Emergency medical services. 3. Terrorism. 4. Medical
emergencies. I. Hogan, David E. II. Burstein, Jonathan L.
    [DNLM: 1. Disasters. 2. Emergency Medical Services. 3. Disaster Planning.
4. Emergencies. 5. Terrorism.
WB 105 D6108 2002]
RA645.5 .D565 2002
362.18—dc21   2002016183

Care has been taken to confirm the accuracy of the information presented and to
describe generally accepted practices. However, the authors, editors, and publisher are
not responsible for errors or omissions or for any consequences from application of the
information in this book and make no warranty, expressed or implied, with respect to
the currency, completeness, or accuracy of the contents of the publication. Application of
this information in a particular situation remains the professional responsibility of the
practitioner.

The authors, editors, and publisher have exerted every effort to ensure that drug
selection and dosage set forth in this text are in accordance with current
recommendations and practice at the time of publication. However, in view of ongoing
research, changes in government regulations, and the constant flow of information
relating to drug therapy and drug reactions, the reader is urged to check the package
insert for each drug for any change in indications and dosage and for added warnings
and precautions. This is particularly important when the recommended agent is a new or
infrequently employed drug.

Some drugs and medical devices presented in this publication have Food and Drug
Administration (FDA) clearance for limited use in restricted research settings. It is the
responsibility of the health care provider to ascertain the FDA status of each drug or
device planned for use in their clinical practice.

10 9 8 7 6 5 4 3 2 1

Dedicated to the victims of September 11 and all other terrorist acts
And to the billions who have suffered from disasters throughout history.
You are not forgotten.

And to those who have responded to the call and who will again:
"Take up our quarrel with the foe:
To you from failing hands we throw
The torch; be yours to hold it high."

Quotation from "In Flanders' Field"
by John McCrae

To my father and mother,
who showed me the right path.
To my four brothers,
who helped keep me on that path.
To my wife Aimee, a woman of valor,
who gives me the love and strength to face each day.

—Jonathan L. Burstein

To all who have suffered and fought disaster from the beginning of civilization
because we are all one against the foe.
To those who seek to know this foe to defeat it.
To those who fight the human disaster of terrorism.

If in a million years the remains of our civilization are found by some curious minds,
they will know that good dwelt amidst the evil and that we did pass this way.

—David E. Hogan

CONTENTS

CONTRIBUTING AUTHORS

Erik Auf der Heide, M.D., M.P.H., F.A.C.E.P. Disaster Planning and Training Specialist, Agency for Toxic Substances and Disease Registry, United States Department of Health and Human Services, Atlanta, Georgia

S. Brent Barnes, M.D. Assistant Clinical Professor, Department of Surgery, University of Oklahoma; Emergency Physician, Oklahoma University Medical Center–Presbyterian Hospital, Oklahoma City, Oklahoma

Sharon Bradley, R.N. Vice President, University Health Systems, Greenville, North Carolina

Frederick M. Burkle, Jr., M.D., M.P.H., F.A.A.P., F.A.C.E.P. Senior Scholar, Scientist, and Visiting Professor, Center for International Emergency Disaster and Refugee Studies, Schools of Public Health and Medicine, Johns Hopkins University Medical Institutions, Baltimore, Maryland

Jonathan L. Burstein, M.D., F.A.C.E.P. Assistant Professor, Department of Emergency Medicine, Harvard Medical School; Director of Disaster Medicine, Department of Emergency Medicine, Beth Israel Deaconess Medical Center, Boston, Massachusetts

Michael Chamales, M.D. Assistant Professor, Department of Surgery, Texas Tech University Health Sciences Center; Attending Physician, Emergency Department, University Medical Center, Lubbock, Texas

Daniel J. Dire, M.D., F.A.C.E.P., F.A.A.E.M. Associate Professor, Department of Emergency Medicine; Director of Operational Medicine, Center for Disaster Preparedness, University of Alabama–Birmingham, Birmingham, Alabama

Constance J. Doyle, M.D. Clinical Instructor, Department of Emergency Medicine, University of Michigan; Core Faculty, Department of Emergency Medicine, St. Joseph Mercy Hospital, Ann Arbor, Michigan

Edward M. Eitzen, Jr., M.D., M.P.H. Adjunct Associate Professor, Department of Military and Emergency Medicine, Uniformed Services University of the Health Sciences, Bethseda, Maryland; Commander, United States Army Medical Research Institute of Infectious Diseases Academy, Fort Detrick, Maryland

Nathan J. Elder, M.D. Department of Emergency Medicine, University of Massachusetts Medical Center, Worcester, Massachusetts

Kim D. Floyd, D.O., F.A.C.E.P. Associate Faculty, Department of Emergency Medicine, Oklahoma State University College of Medicine and Surgery; Staff, Department of Emergency Medicine, Hillcrest Health Center, Oklahoma City, Oklahoma

Fun H. Fong, Jr., M.D., F.A.C.E.P. Staff Emergency Physician, Emory–Adventist Hospital, Smyrna, Georgia

Ralph Ford, M.D.

Robert R. Frantz, M.D. Affiliate faculty, Department of Emergency Medicine, Oklahoma State University; Attending Physician, Department of Emergency Medicine, Morningstar Emergency Physicians Integris Southwest, Oklahoma City, Oklahoma

Victoria Garshnek, M.S., Ph.D. Research Scientist, Center of Excellence in Disaster Management and Humanitarian Assistance, Tripler Army Medical Center, Hawaii

Cloyd B. Gatrell, M.D., F.A.C.E.P. Director, Medical Services Systems, Department of Command, Leadership, and Management, United States Army War College, Carlisle Barracks, Pennsylvania; Staff Emergency Physician, Emergency Department, Hanover Hospital, Hanover, Pennsylvania

Carl S. Goodman, D.O. Attending Physician and Emergency Medical Services Coordinator, Department of Emergency Medicine, Brookhaven Memorial Hospital Medical Center, Patchogue, New York

P. Gregg Greenough, M.D., M.P.H. Assistant Professor, Department of Emergency Medicine, Center for International Emergency Disaster and Refugee Studies, Johns Hopkins University School of Medicine, Baltimore, Maryland

Theodore E. Harrison, M.D., M.B.A. President, Maritime Medical Systems, Ltd., Nassau, Bahamas; Attending Physician, Department of Emergency Medicine, St. Agnes Hospital, Baltimore, Maryland

Aden Hogan, Jr., B.B.A, M.P.A.   Town Administrator, Parker, Colorado; Adjunct Professor, Department of Political Science, Graduate School of Public Affairs, University of Colorado, Denver, Colorado

David E. Hogan, D.O., F.A.C.E.P.   Affiliate faculty, Department of Emergency Medicine, Oklahoma State University; Research Director, Emergency Medicine Residency Programs, St. Michael and Integris Southwest Medical Center; President, Oklahoma Chapter of the American College of Emergency Physicians; Attending Physician, Morningstar Emergency Physicians, Oklahoma City, Oklahoma

Mark Keim, M.D.   Medical Officer, International Emergency and Refugee Health, Centers for Disease Control and Prevention, Atlanta, Georgia

Mark G. Kortepeter, M.D., M.P.H., F.A.C.P.   Adjunct Assistant Professor, Department of Pathology, F. Edward Hebert School of Medicine, Uniformed Services University of the Health Sciences, Bethseda, Maryland; Chief, Medical Division, United States Army Medical Research Institute of Infectious Diseases Academy, Fort Detrick, Maryland

Elizabeth Lacy, D.O., R.P.H.   Attending Physician, Las Colinas Medical Center, Irving, Texas

Julio Lairet, D.O., N.R.E.M.T.-P.   Captain, United States Air Force; Resident, Department of Emergency Medicine, San Antonio Uniformed Health Education Consortium —Emergency Medicine Residency Program (SAUSHEC EMRP), Brooke Army Medical Center, Wilford Hall Medical Center, San Antonio, Texas

Howard W. Levitin, M.D., F.A.C.E.P.   Clinical Assistant Professor, Department of Medicine, Indiana University School of Medicine, Indianapolis, Indiana; Staff Physician, Emergency Department, St. Francis Hospital & Health Centers, Beech Grove, Indiana

David L. McCarty, M.D., F.A.C.E.P.   Department of Emergency Medicine, University of Oklahoma Health Sciences Center, Oklahoma City, Oklahoma; Staff Physician, Department of Emergency Medicine, Comanche County Memorial Hospital, Lawton, Oklahoma

John T. Meredith, M.D., F.A.C.E.P.   Assistant Professor, Department of Emergency Medicine, Brody School of Medicine, East Carolina University; Disaster Medicine Chief, Department of Emergency Medicine, University Health Systems, Pitt County Memorial Hospital, Greenville, North Carolina

Michael F. Murphy, E.M.T.-P., B.S.   Director, Metropolitan Medical Response System, Oklahoma City/Tulsa, Emergency Medical Services Authority, Oklahoma City, Oklahoma

Neill S. Oster, M.D.   Assistant Professor, Department of Emergency Medicine, Mount Sinai School of Medicine, New York, New York; Associate Attending Physician, Department of Emergency Medicine, Elmhurst Hospital Center, Elmhurst, New York

Steven Parrillo, D.O.   Assistant Professor, Department of Emergency Medicine, Thomas Jefferson University; Associate Professor, Department of Emergency Medicine, Philadelphia College of Osteopathic Medicine; Senior Faculty, Department of Emergency Medicine, Albert Einstein Medical Center, Philadelphia, Pennsylvania

Reuben G. Pinkson, Jr., M.A.Ed.   Area Emergency Manager, Department of Veterans Administration, Emergency Management Strategic Healthcare Group, Oklahoma City VA Medical Center, Oklahoma City, Oklahoma

Gary Quick, M.D., F.A.C.E.P.   Attending Emergency Physician and Ultrasound Coordinator, Department of Emergency Medicine, Midwest Regional Medical Center, Midwest City, Oklahoma; Attending Emergency Physician, Department of Emergency Medicine, Muskogee Regional Medical Center, Muskogee, Oklahoma

John R. Rowe, M.D., M.P.H.   Chief, Occupational Medicine; Command Surgeon, United States Army Materiel Command, Alexandria, Virginia; Aerospace Medicine Specialist, Aviation Medicine, DeWitt Army Community Hospital, Ft. Belvoir, Virginia

Carl H. Schultz, M.D.   Clinical Professor, Department of Emergency Medicine, University of California–Irvine College of Medicine, Irvine, California; Director, Emergency Medical Services and Disaster Medicine Fellowship, Department of Emergency Medicine, University of California–Irvine Medical Center, Orange, California

Henry J. Siegelson, M.D., F.A.C.E.P   Clinical Assistant Professor, Department of Emergency Medicine, Emory University, Atlanta, Georgia; Staff Emergency Physician, Department of Emergency Medicine, WellStar Cobb Hospital and Medical Center, Austell, Georgia

Thomas M. Stein, M.D., F.A.C.E.P.   Assistant Professor, Department of Emergency Medicine, MCP-Hahnemann School of Medicine, Philadelphia, Pennsylvania; Medical Director of Emergency Medical Services and Lifeflight, Department of Emergency Medicine, Allegheny General Hospital, Pittsburgh, Pennsylvania

Joshua S. Vayer, M.D.   Director, Casualty Care Research Center; Research Assistant Professor, Department of Military and Emergency Medicine, Uniformed Services University of the Health Sciences, Bethesda, Maryland

James S. Walker, D.O., F.A.C.E.P., F.A.C.O.E.P.   Professor, Department of Emergency Medicine, University of Oklahoma Health Sciences Center; Medical Student Coordinator, Department of Emergency Medicine, University Hospital, Oklahoma City, Oklahoma

Arthur G. Wallace, Jr., D.O., M.P.H.   Clinical Assistant Professor, Department of Emergency Medicine, Oklahoma State University, College of Osteopathic Medicine; Director, Emergency Department, Tulsa Regional Medical Center, Tulsa, Oklahoma

PREFACE

Civilization begins with order, grows with liberty, and dies with chaos.

Will Durant

The universe is not a safe place to live. This truth has been experienced countless times by species on this planet. Life on Earth clings tightly to a complex ecosystem wrapped in a thin envelope of atmosphere. Mass extinctions have visited the planet on a regular basis, rearranging the order of life, oblivious to the activities of individual species.

Human beings are relative newcomers to the biologic equation of this planet. Of much more recent development are the fragile civilized constructs of this species. As late as 10,000 B.C. human beings are believed to have first begun to change from disorganized hunter–gatherer groups to a highly organized and interdependent civilization. The current global community, and perhaps humanity itself, could be swept from existence by natural hazards within this new century. Human beings, in their ingenuity, have created new technologic hazards that also threaten their own existence. Moreover, mankind continues to perpetrate acts of violence against each other on a regular basis, using increasingly sophisticated methods.

Humanity is perhaps the first species on Earth to realize its own vulnerability to disasters. With this understanding of vulnerability comes a responsibility to study the nature of the hazards that result in disasters and threaten societies. The knowledge gained in such study must then be used by health care providers to decrease the frequency and impact of disasters and to provide medical care, assistance, and education to communities impacted by disasters. Finally, we have a responsibility to apply these principles in order to protect civilization on a global scale.

We have begun to discover the concepts and develop the tools that may preserve our civilization from eventual extinction. A portion of this process involves the study of, response to, and mitigation of events that cause mass suffering. This, in part, is the definition of *Disaster Medicine*. The universe grants no species the *right* to survive. However, the practice of disaster medicine, in the true tradition of medicine, may suggest that humanity has a *reason* to survive.

This book represents a germinal attempt to collect information about the nature of various types of disasters and the associated planning and response procedures. The editors and authors have taken a clinical approach that stems from the point of view of the practicing emergency health care provider. Planning and response to disasters should be based on valid assumptions. Therefore, the chapters in this book have been based on scientific studies and reports when such information was available. Much more research, however, is needed to understand these events fully. The editors welcome constructive comments regarding the content of this text.

—*David E. Hogan*
—*Jonathan L. Burstein*

ACKNOWLEDGMENTS

Numerous people have helped and supported me in my endeavors. Most especially, I must thank Joseph Waeckerle, my mentor and guide to the world of disaster medicine and medical writing and a Good Man in the truest sense. Thanks, of course, are also extended to my coauthor Dave Hogan, who kept me on track through the long struggle.

I would also like to particularly thank Lenward T. Smith for introducing me to emergency medical care, Lester Kallus for introducing me to disaster medicine, and Peter Viccellio and Fred Schiavone for turning a lost intern into a (hopefully) competent emergency physician.

Furthermore I wish to thank Richard Wolfe and Jonathan Edlow at Beth Israel Deaconess Medical Center for enabling me to work on this book and Jennifer Leaning for inspiring me to see the vast scope of, and need for, disaster medical care; for helping me to make sense of it, and for giving me the opportunity to learn while teaching her students.

And to the citizens and emergency responders of New York City, thank you for allowing me to help you in your time of need and for being so giving and caring to a single stranger as your world was falling apart.

—*Jonathan L. Burstein*

Thanks go to my family for reminding me why this project was so important to complete.

I also acknowledge Dr. David Munter and Dr. Tom Stein for showing me what an Emergency Physician is and for giving me models to follow; Dr. Dan Dire for showing me the path for learning through investigation; Dr. Erik Noji and Dr. Scott Lillibridge for introducing me to the science and methods to carry out those investigations; Dr. Richard Aghababian for demonstrating leadership and compassion in a chaotic world; and Dr. Frederick (Skip) Burkle for demonstrating courage, valor, and a passion for making a difference.

Finally, I thank Dr. Joseph Waeckerle for his patience, compassion, and perseverance in teaching me how to write it down.

—*David E. Hogan*

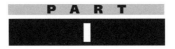

PART

I

GENERAL CONCEPTS

1

BASIC PHYSICS OF DISASTERS

DAVID E. HOGAN
JONATHAN L. BURSTEIN

Knowledge comes, but wisdom lingers.

–Alfred Lord Tennyson

Worldwide, over 3.4 million lives were lost due to disasters over the past quarter century. Hundreds of millions of people endured diverse suffering caused by these events, and tens of billions of dollars helped repair the damage and reconstruct those lives. Although many societies reached out to others in need in the past, not until the latter part of the last century have highly organized efforts been created to assist with disaster response.

In order to call an event a disaster, people must be affected. The risk of disasters producing mass casualties worldwide is increasing, in large part because of the increase in world population (1). The world population reached an estimated 6 billion on November 16, 1999. With a steady growth of approximately 1.33% (78 million people each year), current projections are that the population will be 8.9 billion by the year 2050 (2). The majority of these individuals are living in areas of the earth that are prone to hurricanes, earthquakes, floods, and drought. As such, the potential for human impact from these natural hazards is growing accordingly.

The rate of occurrence of hazardous events on earth may be increasing; this is possibly due to regular variation in natural cycles such as solar maxima, earthquakes, and volcanic activity. In addition, the earth is warming, which, at a minimum, is projected to increase severe storm activity in some areas and to cause drought in others. The technologic development of human society has resulted in the creation of an entirely new set of hazards, such as industrial waste and radiation and chemical disasters. Tons of hazardous wastes are transported through dense population areas each day, with each ton representing a latent disaster. Increasing development and dependence on an industrial-technologic complex present new possibilities for disaster.

Humankind continues to be its own worst enemy. Will Rogers said it this way in his autobiography, "You can't say civilization don't advance . . . in every war they kill you in a new way" (3). With wars both great and small occurring at regular frequency on Earth, ample opportunity is found for 'advancement'. These activities create, both directly and indirectly, numerous casualties that require medical care and public health management. The creation of weapons of mass destruction and the real and the potential use of these devices against human populations represent a new and complex problem for emergency health care providers.

DISASTER IN PERSPECTIVE

Disasters are generally considered "low probability—high impact" events. In fact, only a few disasters in the United States have resulted in over 1,000 casualties (4). When disaster does strike, only 10 to 15 disasters a year result in more than 40 casualties. These statistics are often used to defer funding for disaster-planning efforts in lieu of other projects. However, in fact, the impact of disaster in the United States and worldwide is much more significant than these narrow statistics imply.

For instance, although Hurricane Andrew killed only 44 individuals directly, it affected the lives of almost 3 million people, caused over 3 billion dollars damage, and involved significant national resources for rescue and recovery efforts. The disruption of the normal lives of the population measures the true impact of a disaster. Medical infrastructures may be totally disrupted during a disaster, thus requiring time to reestablish normal function. Recovery efforts to repair a disaster-stricken community and the psychoemotional damage may last for years.

DEFINING A DISASTER

The definition of a disaster is as broad as the number of people studying these events. Examples of disaster definitions are found in various sources. Usually each definition reflects the nature and focus of the organization or individuals defining it. The World Health Organization (WHO) defines a disaster as "a sudden ecological phenomenon of sufficient magnitude to require external assistance" (5). This broad focus definition may exclude some events that result in mass casualties. A more focused definition by practitioners of emergency medicine is when ". . . the number of patients presenting within a given time period are such that the emergency department cannot provide care for them without external assistance." This definition excludes events, such as aircraft crashes, that result in mass death but place little or no stress on the medical system (6). Others define disasters as an imbalance in the availability of medical care and a maldistribution of medical resources versus casualties within a community. Most emergency health care providers have some definition in mind regarding disasters, but more commonly the response is simply that they "know a disaster when they see one."

Disasters are not defined by a specific number of casualties but rather by the event itself and the venue in which it occurs. A motor vehicle crash with five victims in a metropolitan area will likely go unnoticed except as a footnote in the evening paper. The same crash victims presenting to a rural community emergency department will probably require activation of the hospital disaster plan. In all definitions, disasters are something outside the normal experience of daily life that requires a change from daily management style and thinking.

DISASTER MEDICINE

Disaster medicine is a system of study and medical practice associated primarily with the disciplines of emergency medicine and public health. Disaster medicine is concerned with the health and medical and emotional issues of disaster victims. To provide care efficiently, however, the health care provider must be familiar with several elements of disaster management, including planning, mitigation, assessment, response, and recovery. Disasters may destroy or disable the medical infrastructure of a given area, making access to routine health care impossible for victims. Infectious diseases endemic to the population may increase in frequency, mandating the deployment of epidemiologic surveillance and intervention programs. Nutritional problems that necessitate evaluation and intervention can surface, particularly during long-duration complex disasters. Long-term and short-term emotional and psychiatric conditions may plague the disaster-stricken community, requiring counseling and well-planned support systems.

When using the broad definition of disaster medicine, one must realize that no individual can be facile in all elements of this topic. Finding any true experts in disaster medicine is difficult. Analogous to the observation of World War II correspondent Ernie Pyle that, to the individual soldier, the war was rarely bigger than 100 yards on either side (7), those in disaster medicine would acknowledge that, while each may become skilled in his or her 100 yards of a disaster, he or she needs a larger view to improve planning and response significantly.

EMERGENCY MEDICINE ROLE IN DISASTER MEDICINE

Emergency physicians, nurses, and paramedics in the United States have commonly been drawn to disaster med-

icine. These health care providers usually represent the first line of medical defense in a community, and they often are the first to know of a disaster impact. The American College of Emergency Physicians (ACEP) states that "emergency physicians should assume a primary role in the medical aspects of disaster planning, management and patient care." Additionally ACEP believes that emergency physicians should ". . . pursue training that will enable them to fulfill this responsibility" (8–10).

DISASTER BASIC PHYSICS

As the title of this chapter suggests, a set of repeating elements occurs during most disasters and makes up the disaster process. These elements have been variously described, and they may constitute a set of basic physics on which one's understanding of disasters may build. In addition, recurrent problems are consistently seen with communications, personnel, and supplies (11). These events represent a set of human behaviors that are quite persistent. Some disaster plans have sought to prevent these behaviors from occurring during a disaster and have met with variable success. A more reasonable approach might be to start by more fully understanding these behaviors. Once they are understood, planning may take the form of channeling these behaviors into activities that are more constructive, rather than opposing the strong force of mass human will. The following reviews briefly of some of the common elements of disasters.

The Disaster Cycle

Each disaster follows a general pattern in its development. This pattern is often repeated throughout nature and is demonstrated in Fig. 1.1. The phases of disasters have been variously defined and described. All the divisions of the life of a disaster are artificial as one phase of a disaster merges with another. However, dividing disasters into phases is useful from both a response and research point of view (5,12,13). Disaster planning, response, and research may be simplified by using the disaster cycle as a model for these complex events.

Initially, a quiescent level or interdisaster period is seen during which the combinations of events that will eventually lead to the disaster are occurring. Although the disaster in the making may not be obvious, the underlying cause of the disaster may be readily apparent. Disaster risk assessment techniques may be of benefit during this period in predicting what types of local hazards may result in a disaster.

A prodrome or warning phase develops next and lasts a variable amount of time depending on the disaster type. The warning period represents a time during which a particular event (e.g., a hurricane, volcanic eruption, or armed conflict) clearly is likely to occur. Steps may be taken during the warning period to mitigate the effects of the event.

General Phases of the
Disaster Life Cycle

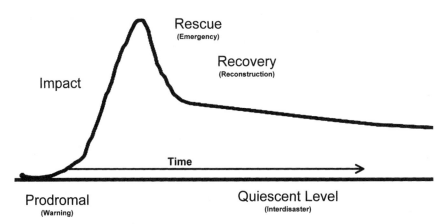

FIGURE 1.1. The disaster cycle.

During this phase, public warnings and protective action, such as sheltering and evacuation, may occur.

The impact phase coincides with the occurrence of the event. This phase may be short, as in an earthquake, or prolonged, as in famine. Usually, little can be done to decrease the impact of the disaster on human populations if prior steps have not been taken. Even protective behaviors, such as sheltering during a tornado, require previous education and warning programs. Proper planning and reasonable preemptive actions will have the greatest effect in decreasing the impact of the actual disaster-causing event.

The rescue phase (also known as the emergency, the relief, or the isolation phase) represents a time during which immediate assistance can save lives. During this time, people may be salvaged by first responder actions, search and rescue, and basic and advanced life support methods. This period often depends on bystander rescue as the local search and rescue agencies (if they exist) may be overwhelmed or incapacitated.

The recovery or reconstruction phase has been variously subdivided, but it can be considered as a single entity. This phase consists of all the required actions and elements (e.g., emergency medical services, public health, engineering, social services) needed to return the population back to a functional society. This period may last months or years, and it resolves with the community returning to the quiescent or interdisaster phase.

The Geographic Effect

A well-known truism for disasters in most regions of the world is that the closest health care facilities to the disaster site will be the ones most significantly impacted by casualties. This is of clinical and statistical significance, and it is illustrated in Fig. 1.2 from the casualty distribution of the Oklahoma City bombing (14). The geographic effect results from a number of factors. Casualties capable of self-

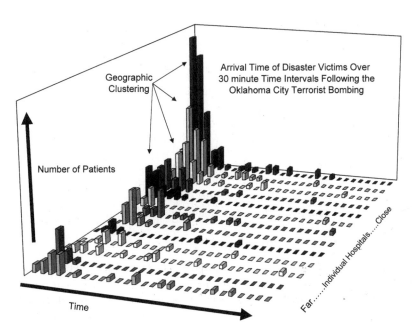

FIGURE 1.2. Geographic clustering by distance and time from the blast site after the Oklahoma City terrorist bombing. (From Hogan DE. *Oklahoma City MMRS study guide.* Oklahoma City, OK: MorningStar Emergency Physicians, 2001, with permission.)

extrication and transport usually travel to the closest facility for care by whatever means is available. Laypersons assisting nonambulatory victims will usually transport them to the closest facility. Some casualties go to the closest facility out of hospital loyalty or for financial reasons.

Prehospital personnel contribute to the geographic effect. In the process of triage by first responders, victims are commonly brought to the Emergency Medical Services (EMS) triage field location by laypersons. These victims may already be loaded in the back of pickup trucks or other vehicles. If the victim is stable and a lack of immediate EMS transport exists, the layperson drivers are often directed to take the victims to the closest facility (15). In addition, after triage and initial treatment, prehospital personnel often transport casualties to the closest facility because of concerns about patient stability, familiarity with the local emergency department (ED), and hopes of achieving a short turnaround time.

The geographic effect may result in a substantial maldistribution of casualties throughout the community. The closer facilities may be overwhelmed with victims, while other facilities are almost idle. Most disaster plans for EMS contain mechanisms to decrease the impact of the geographic effect, such as transporting some critical casualties to farther facilities or putting priority three casualties on buses and taking them to more distant EDs for treatment. Such actions have met with limited success, probably because they go against human nature. How many, after losing their home and means of transport, are going to be willing to be placed on a bus and taken to an unfamiliar hospital on the other side of town? Further research into the causes of the geographic effect may lead to innovative plans to blunt its impact by accepting these acts of human nature and planning for them.

The Dual Wave Phenomenon

Casualties generally arrive for care at emergency departments after a disaster in two waves (11,16). The first wave of patients usually begins appearing within 15 to 30 minutes of the impact of the disaster. It is comprised primarily of the walking wounded or priority three victims due to the fact that they were able to self-extricate and walk or drive to the ED. Then, within a variable time (on average, 30–60 minutes), a second wave of casualties begins to arrive. These casualties are typically unable to get to the ED by themselves because of the need for extrication or transport and the severity of their injuries. This second wave consists mostly of priority one and priority two victims. This effect seems to be more pronounced at facilities that have been more heavily impacted by the geographic effect (14). The danger is in overloading an ED with priority three and priority two victims from the first wave before the arrival of the more critical cases in the second wave. Adherence to good triage principles can decrease the impact of the dual-wave phenomenon on a facility.

The Babel Effect

The most common problem associated with any disaster is a failure in communications (11). This breakdown is due to the sudden increase in the volume and the need to communicate for the victims, responders, and witnesses of a disaster. Land telephone lines are not capable of managing high percentages of users at one time. The result is a rapid saturation of the available circuits and a jamming of the telephone lines. Cellular telephones suffer from a similar fate as the available cells are quickly engaged with high volume traffic. In addition, land line facilities and cellular towers may be destroyed. Disaster communication plans that rely on cellular or land line telephones alone have high risk for failure.

Radio communication technology is commonly employed by emergency and disaster response agencies. However, with this technology, the increased volume of radio traffic also overwhelms the limited number of frequencies available to emergency responders. In addition, local radio equipment specifically set aside for disasters usually has not been maintained. Therefore, dead batteries and electronic component deterioration are a common problem. Moreover, the personnel who suddenly need to use the radio equipment are often not properly trained. Afteraction reports of disasters often note a lack of the ability to communicate between various agencies due to the absence of shared frequencies (4). Despite these reports, many agencies never correct this problem before the next disaster.

Another common problem is the lack of clear speaking during a disaster. Most agencies rely on various codes during radio transmissions to shorten the duration of the call and to specify complex meanings. Unfortunately, radio codes often vary from region to region and from agency to agency. During the 1995 Oklahoma City bombing, an EMS inquiry as to the status of one hospital brought the reply "We are on Code Black!" The EMS dispatch understood this to mean the hospital could take no more patients and advised all EMS units to divert from this facility. In reality, "Code Black" was the term used locally at this hospital to indicate that it was ready to receive multiple patients (17). This simple misunderstanding resulted in a temporary overload of a neighboring hospital with EMS-transported victims. Code talking should be avoided during a disaster in favor of clear speaking, in accordance with the old adage "Say what you mean and mean what you say."

Communications is one area where new technology may have a profound impact on the ability to respond to a disaster. Once the human behaviors and system needs behind disaster communication problems are understood, new adaptive technologies may be created to minimize obstacles.

The Federation Effect

The helping response of individuals to victims of disasters is impressive. Like the mythical Federation of Star Trek, humans are a species of "Captain Kirks and Kathryn Janeways" with an innate urge to assist others in immediate need. The initial response to the scene of a disaster is usually by laypersons residing within the local area. Often the majority of uncomplicated search and rescue is completed by laypersons who arrive at the disaster site shortly after the event before the arrival of professional responders. Many disaster response plans call for these laypersons to be removed from the disaster zone. However, this may prove difficult because it goes against the human drive to assist those in need. Most laypersons involved in a disaster behave in a logical and organized manner (4) and are usually willing to follow the directions of a professional prehospital care provider. They may be organized into a useful corps of searchers or litter bearers. However, if laypersons are used in this manner, care must be taken not to expose them to known hazards of the disaster site. Some communities have initiated training programs for laypersons in areas at high risk for specific disasters such as earthquake (18). The aim of such training is to protect the public by educating them about the hazards of specific disasters and to provide organization and safety protocols for the activities these people will be doing anyway. When properly educated and deployed, layperson responders may provide a substantial augmentation to professional prehospital responders.

Voluntary medical personnel responding to a disaster scene present additional problems. These individuals usually respond to the scene out of altruism, or they are called to the scene by requests of the news media (17). Because these individuals responding to the scene have some degree of medical expertise, they may be both a blessing and a curse. Most health care providers, particularly physicians, are accustomed to a substantial degree of control of their practice environment, and most are unfamiliar with prehospital protocols or capabilities. Such medical practice attitudes do not translate well into the chaotic environment of a disaster. In addition, most volunteer health care providers responding to a disaster are not aware of the dangers at the disaster site. Recently, this resulted in the death of at least one volunteer responder (16). Moreover, due to the austere conditions at the disaster site, physicians and nurses usually cannot provide care that is any more sophisticated than that given by paramedics (19–21). Some reports have indicated that physicians and nurses responding to the scene of a disaster have no significant impact on the eventual morbidity and mortality of victims (22,23). Occasionally, volunteer medical responders have even been disruptive to the search and rescue and triage activities of prehospital personnel (17). In general, during a disaster, medical personnel should report to their local hospital in accordance with their hospital disaster plan. They should not report to the disaster site unless they are a part of a special disaster response team that has been organized by and that trains regularly with the municipal search and rescue. Occasionally, the medical incident commander may request that specific individuals with specialized training, such as confined space medicine or surgical expertise, report to the scene.

Disaster Supplies

The following two basic problems exist regarding materials needed for a disaster response: the organization of available supplies and the organization of donations. The initial 24 hours of any disaster response usually rely on the available resources within the disaster-stricken community. An organized approach for sorting and distributing supplies to the disaster responders is essential to prevent either waste or want. Various strategies exist for accomplishing this task, and they should be an integral part of all disaster response plans.

Disasters also result in massive donation programs. Although funding is usually the most critical need of a disaster area, massive amounts of materials ranging from blankets to medications usually arrive. The amount and nature of these donations can be so significant as to constitute a second disaster (24). Staffing and resources must be allocated to manage the flow of such materials in an effort to organize and use needed items and to prevent the waste of the less useful materials.

Tetanophobia

The most common immunization given in most disasters is tetanus toxoid (16,25). Volunteer and public health services often organize community outreach programs to provide tetanus shots and other services to a disaster-stricken population. The incidence of tetanus in the United States has decreased significantly in the past 40 years, primarily due to improved wound care techniques and tetanus prophylaxis (26). Although a real risk for tetanus exists due to wounds suffered during the impact and recovery phase of a disaster, these immunizations are not without risk; thus, they should be given after intelligent consideration.

The most common adverse reaction to tetanus toxoid immunization is local swelling, pain, erythema, and edema at the site of injection. This most frequently occurs in the hyperimmune patient, and it is associated with the deposition of immune complexes from the serum into the tissue around the injection site (27). This usually occurs because of a tetanus booster that is given too soon (<5 years) after the previous booster. These patients present to the emergency department or their primary care physician's office with a red, hot, swollen arm, often with a central pustulous-appearing structure. Usually this represents an Arthus reaction, but the temptation to treat it as a cellulitis with antibiotics is often too strong to resist. The resulting scenario is that of a recovery worker who received a tetanus shot from an agency that did not take a proper history of immunizations. An Arthus reaction (fever, myalgias, pain) develops in the worker (who is working hard in the heat); the worker then reports to the local ED where he or she is given an antibiotic that causes enteric upset and further dehydration and misery. This effect of tetanophobia may be diminished by adherence to strict immunization protocols and education while still providing the responders and victims with important and needed protection.

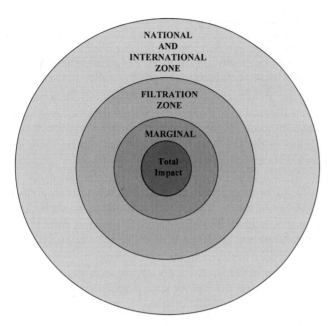

FIGURE 1.3. Spatial zones of a disaster.

aster. Both zones have variable levels of structural ruin and casualties depending on the type and severity of the disaster. Usually sufficient confusion exists within these zones so that rescue workers and victims may not have a good concept of the overall impact of the disaster. This can result in rescue efforts and supplies being diverted to the marginal zone first, rather than to the total impact zone where they are most needed.

The zone of filtration represents a region that is not directly affected by the disaster. Within this zone, however, refugees from the total and marginal impact zones may be found following a migration to this area in an attempt to escape the shock of the heavily damaged regions. This may put stress on the local facilities for health care, sanitation, and nutrition resources.

The zone of national and international aid represents the collection and coordination zone for the arrival of various levels of relief supplies and personnel. Proper disaster assessment procedures can help ensure that such relief efforts are coordinated within the various other zones of the disaster.

Disaster Zones

Early work by Wallace and others has defined a set of concentric zones surrounding most disasters (28). These zones, which have been used to conceptualize the impact and response to disasters, are depicted in Fig. 1.3.

The zone of total impact and the zone of marginal impact represent areas that are directly damaged by the dis-

Injury Control Principles in Disasters

The application of injury control methods to include the chronology of injury patterns described by Haddon has been utilized for disasters (12,29). This method divides complex events such as disasters into discrete phases and factors within a matrix as Fig. 1.4 demonstrates. Using the matrix, one may more clearly identify areas of need for planning and resource allocation and may focus injury prevention strategies.

	Human	Structure Technology	Physical Environment	Socioeconomic
Prodrome				
Impact				
Recovery				

FIGURE 1.4. The Haddon Matrix applied to disasters. (From Noji EK, Siverston KT. Injury prevention in natural disasters. A theoretical framework. *Disasters* 1987;11:290–296, with permission.)

SUMMARY

Disasters are highly complex events resulting in immediate medical problems, as well as longer-term public health and psychoemotional disruptions. Responding to disasters effectively requires an understanding of the causative reasons for disasters and of the common responses of human populations in a disaster situation. Disasters often share a set of common events and recurrent problems. Organization of thinking about disasters into phases and causes can assist in understanding these chaotic events.

REFERENCES

1. Noji EK. Progress in disaster management. *Lancet* 1994;343:1239.
2. World Health Organization. Statistical Information System page. Available at: http://www.who.int/whosis. Accessed March 12, 2002.
3. Day D. *The autobiography of Will Rogers.* Boston: Houghton Mifflin, 1949.
4. Auf Der Heide E. *Disaster response: the principles of preparation and coordination.* St. Louis: CV Mosby, 1989.
5. Noji EK. *The public health consequences of disasters.* New York: Oxford University Press, 1997.
6. Callun JR, Dinerman NM. Disaster preparedness. In: Sheecy S, ed. *Emergency nursing: principles and practice*, 3rd ed. St. Louis: CV Mosby, 1992:28–39.
7. Tobin J. *Ernie Pyle's war: America's eyewitness to World War II.* Wichita, Kansas: University Press, 1998.
8. American College of Emergency Physicians. The role of the emergency physician in mass casualty/disaster management. *JACEP* 1976;5:901.
9. American College of Emergency Physicians Practice Management Committee. Definition of emergency medicine and the emergency physician. *Ann Emerg Med* 1986;15:1240.
10. American College of Emergency Physicians Disaster Committee. Disaster medical services. *Ann Emerg Med* 1985;14:1026.
11. Waeckerle JF. Disaster planning and response. *N Engl J Med* 1991;324:815–821.
12. Noji EK, Siverston KT. Injury prevention in natural disasters. A theoretical framework. *Disasters* 1987;11:290–296.
13. Cuny FC. Introduction to disaster management, lesson 5: technologies of disaster management. *Prehospital Disaster Med* 1993;6:372–374.
14. Hogan DE. *Oklahoma City MMRS study guide.* Oklahoma City, OK: MorningStar Emergency Physicians, 2001.
15. The Learning Channel. *Paramedics: force five.* Bethesda, MD: Discovery Communications, 2000.
16. Hogan DE, Lillibridge SR, Waeckerle J, et al. Emergency department impact of the Oklahoma City terrorist bombing. *Ann Emerg Med* 1999;34:160–167.
17. Hogan DE. The Oklahoma City terrorist blast: a case study in disaster. In: Landsman LY, ed. *Emergency preparedness in health care organizations.* Oak Brook, IL: Joint Commission on Accreditation of Health Care Organizations, 1996:1–16.
18. Abrams JI, Pretto EA, Angus D, et al. Guidelines for rescue training of the lay public. *Prehospital Disaster Med* 1993;8:151–156.
19. Mahoney LE, Reutershan TP. Catastrophic disasters in the design of disaster medical care systems. *Ann Emerg Med* 1987;16:1085–1091.
20. Feldstein BD, Gallery ME, Sanner PH, et al. Disaster training for emergency physicians in the United States: a systems approach. *Ann Emerg Med* 1985;14:36–40.
21. Bern AI. Disaster medical services. In: Roush WR, Aranosian R, Blair T, et al., eds. *Principles of EMS system: a comprehensive text for physicians.* Dallas: American College of Emergency Physicians, 1989:77–93.
22. Marr J. Kalamazoo medics say 'fantastic'! to health personnel response after tornadoes. *Mich Med* 1980;79:374–376.
23. Morris BAP, Armstrong TM. Medical response to a natural disaster: the Barrie tornado. *CMAJ* 1986;134:767–769.
24. Quarantelli EL. *Delivery of emergency medical services in disasters: assumptions and realities.* New York: Irvington 1985.
25. May BM, Hogan DE, Feighner K. Impact of a tornado on a community hospital. *Journal of the American Osteopathic Association* 2002;102:225–228.
26. Centers for Disease Control. CDC Tetanus–United States, 1987 and 1988. *MMWR* 1990;39:37–41.
27. Cohen SH, Hoeprich PD. Immunoprophylaxis of infectious diseases. In: Hoeprich PD, Jordan MC, Ronald AR, eds. *Infectious diseases: a treatise of infectious processes.* Philadelphia: JB Lippincott, 1994:323–324.
28. de Ville de Goyet C, Lechat MF. Health aspects of natural disasters. *Trop Doctor* 1976;6:152–157.
29. Haddon W. Options for the prevention of motor vehicle crash injury. *Israel J Med Sci* 1980;16:45–68.

2

TRIAGE

DAVID E. HOGAN
JULIO LAIRET

I have measured out my life with coffee spoons.

—*T.S. Eliot*

The three major phases of initial mass casualty and disaster care are as follows: triage, evacuation, and definitive medical management (1). Triage is the keystone of good disaster medical management (2). The performance of accurate triage provides disaster responders with the best opportunity to do the greatest good for the greatest number of casualties. Performing triage in a disaster setting requires a paradigm shift on the part of those performers, and it is highly dependent on experience. No single book chapter or training program can provide sufficient information for training a triage officer. This chapter will, however, attempt to provide a perspective of triage based on the personal views of individuals who have performed disaster triage, as well as on the available scientific data on the topic.

HISTORICAL PERSPECTIVE

The word *triage* is derived from the French word *trier*, which means "to sort." The way that patients are triaged or sorted for care has evolved throughout history. The origin of modern triage can be traced back to the Napoleonic era where Baron Dominique Jean Larrey (1766–1842), a surgeon in Napoleon's army, developed and implemented a system in which the soldiers requiring the most urgent care were attended to first regardless of rank (3). His system also instituted initial treatment of the wounded while still on the battlefield, prior to being transported to hospitals located in the rear. Before Larrey, all of the wounded would remain in the battlefield until the battle was complete, after which they would be gathered and transported to the hospitals where care was initiated. This delay of care often resulted in unnecessarily poor outcomes.

In 1846, John Wilson introduced the next major contribution to current triage philosophies. He noted that, for lifesaving surgery to be effective, it must be initiated for the patients in most need, while simultaneously withholding care both from patients whose injuries would likely prove fatal and also from those patients whose care could be deferred until a later time.

World Wars I and II brought advances to the approach and treatment of acutely injured patients. During World War I, patients were triaged at central casualty collection points from where they would be directed to the appropriate receiving facility. World War II introduced a tiered approach to triage in which casualties were first treated in the field by medics and then were passed down the line to higher levels of care as dictated by the level of injury. This approach was responsible for saving more lives, especially in soldiers with abdominal wounds, than any other factor during World War II (3).

During the Korean War, the aeromedical evacuation of patients after initial triage became common, greatly improving the survival of casualties. This system was further refined during the Vietnam conflict, where rapid triage and advanced resuscitation in the field were coupled with helicopter evacuation. These triage and evacuation techniques resulted in a reduction in mortality rates from 4.7% in World War II to 1% during the Vietnam conflict (3). As the art of triage has further evolved, patient outcomes have improved. One variable aiding this has been a decrease in the time from injury to definitive care. During World War II, the average time lapse from injury to definitive care was 12 to 18 hours; this time span was decreased during the Vietnam conflict to less than 2 hours (4).

TRIAGE PHILOSOPHY

Multiple approaches to triage are found in the literature and in practice. Most triage methodology is focused on the prehospital sorting and distribution of patients, as no consistent approach for teaching or performing triage after the prehospital encounter has been established. One model for understanding disaster triage divides the process into the following five conceptual categories: daily triage, incident triage, disaster triage, tactical-military triage, and special condition triage.

Daily triage is performed on a routine basis in the emergency care system. Triage categories vary from institution to institution, but their overall goal is to identify the sickest patients in order to supply early evaluation and treatment. In addition, the highest intensity of care is provided to the most seriously ill patients, even if those patients have a low probability of survival.

Incident or mass casualty incident (MCI) triage is a continuum of the triage philosophy that comes into place when the local emergency care system becomes more stressed but is not overwhelmed. During this type of triage, the highest intensity of care is still provided to the most critically ill victims. Additional resources may be used (on-call and backup personnel), but disaster plans may not be activated. The minimal or delayed cases may wait for longer periods than they might during daily triage function, but they will eventually receive care.

Disaster triage is employed when the local resources are unable to provide immediate care on a timely basis to all victims needing such care. The philosophy of the health care provider changes from providing high intensity care to the sickest victims to doing the greatest good for the greatest number. With the limited availability of resources to care for the number of patients arriving, resource management considerations come into play. The focus shifts to the identification of injured victims who have a good chance of survival with immediate medical interventions and resources. This is approached by the identification of victims at the extremes of injury, a concept depicted in Fig. 2.1 (1). The initial goal is to sort victims into those who are lightly injured and who can wait for care without risk and those who are so hopelessly injured that they will not survive. When this has been done, a central cadre of victims will be identifiable–those with serious and critical injuries. The next task is to prioritize this set of victims for transportation and treatment based on their level of injury and the available resources. Victims with hopeless injuries and little chance of survival may receive only compassion, pain relief, and monitoring.

Tactical and military triage are quite similar to other forms of triage. The unique characteristic however, is the addition of an overall mission-oriented perspective. Some triage decisions may be based primarily on mission objectives rather than on following usual medical guidelines. In essence, this philosophy still follows the greatest good approach because failure to achieve a mission objective may have profoundly adverse results on the health and well being of a much greater population.

Special condition triage may be used when additional factors are present in the population of victims. Examples of these include incidents involving weapons of mass destruction (WMD) with radiation, biologic, or chemical contaminants. These victims may suffer from the additive effects of such agents (e.g., increased mortality in radiation-contaminated trauma cases). Additionally, decontamination may be needed, and protective equipment may be required for health care providers.

The concepts of undertriage and overtriage must be understood. Undertriage is associated with triage sensitivity in identifying patients needing critical care interventions. It results when triage activities underestimate the severity of injury and send the patient to a noncritical area for care. This has an obvious impact on the morbidity and mortality of the individual patient. Because no triage system is perfect, acceptable undertriage rates have been defined as 5% or less (5).

Overtriage occurs when a noncritical patient is triaged to a critical care area. Rates of overtriage of up to 50% have been defined as acceptable in an effort to reduce undertriage (6). However, overtriage has the less obvious effect of overburdening the critical care system with noncritical patients. High levels of overtriage have been demonstrated to increase the morbidity and mortality of critical patients within the system (7).

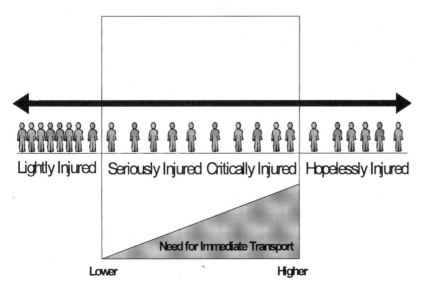

FIGURE 2.1. The focus of triage at extremes of care.

TRIAGE SYSTEMS AND ORGANIZATION

Over the years, many different triage systems have emerged. Although various nomenclatures and systems are in common use throughout the world, commonalities do exist. Most systems of triage sort patients into four major categories designated by colors. The deployment of prehospital triage resources and organization of personnel are discussed in the chapter on EMS in disasters.

A priority one or immediate (RED) patient is classified as one whose injury is critical but who can be cared for with only minimal time or resources and who after treatment would have a good prognosis for survival. Examples include a patient with a massive hemorrhage that could be controlled with a simple operative procedure or one with a tension pneumothorax who needs only a needle thoracostomy and chest tube for stabilization.

Priority two or delayed (YELLOW) patients include patients whose injuries are significant but who are able to tolerate a delay in care without the risk of substantial morbidity. A patient with an isolated simple femur or humerus fracture would be placed in this category.

Priority three, minimal, or nonurgent (GREEN) patients are those whose injuries are minor enough that they can wait for treatment (also known as the walking wounded). These patients' injuries can be addressed after caring for patients with more serious injuries. Examples include isolated abrasions, contusions, sprains, minor fractures, or an isolated laceration with bleeding that has been controlled without the loss of a significant amount of blood.

Expectant patients (BLACK) include those whose injuries are so severe that they have only a minimal chance of survival even if significant resources are expended. Examples of expectant patients are those with massive head injuries or a 95% coverage with third-degree burns.

Some have discussed adding a further category (BLUE) to include patients who will probably not survive but who should be transported and treated after priority one patients but before priority two patients (3,8). The logic behind this is that most priority two cases are able to wait and that some of the cases that are triaged as expectant fall into this category. This would relieve prehospital personnel from making some of the decisions regarding expectant cases. In addition, if resources are available, these cases can receive interventions as indicated. The addition of a further category is, however, not generally accepted at this time.

In addition, patients who are unresponsive, pulseless, and breathless when they are encountered are triaged as dead. In a disaster situation, resuscitative attempts should not be initiated. Dead victims should be tagged for record only and should be moved to a separate location far from living casualties as soon as possible.

PERFORMANCE OF TRIAGE

Although training may provide a framework for a triage officer, field experience is probably the only true teacher (9). The complex process of accurately deciding which patients need what care and resources and in what order they need them is a daunting task. Despite the difficulties, disaster triage can be highly accurate in identification of casualty injuries (10). Although actual experience is the best teacher, it is not necessarily the only teacher. Clinical experience in a busy trauma center or an austere environment provides a good background. The thorough knowledge of emergency medicine, trauma, and the principles of surgery, coupled with clinical experience in the rapid assessment of critical patients, is essential. Burkle, in the first disaster medicine text, outlined the essential elements of a good triage officer based on disaster and warfare experience, and these still hold true today. They are listed in Table 2.1.

The application of trauma scoring during triage by the acquisition of anatomic and physiologic data has been attempted during mass care events (9). However, reliance on trauma scoring methods alone risks a low sensitivity during initial triage, thus increasing the undertriage rate. Scoring systems have been noted to predict the likelihood of mortality after trauma, but they are less sensitive in assisting in prioritizing patients for transport and care (11). The experienced triage officer must be able to combine multiple sensory clues with the physiologic and anatomic information to obtain an overall picture of the casualty (9,12). In a study of triage methods during the Persian Gulf War, Burkle et al. indicated a set of anatomic and physiologic parameters that may assist the triage officer in improving triage sensitivity. These are depicted in Table 2.2.

During a disaster situation, health care providers encounter a number of obstacles that are not seen on a routine basis. The number of victims arriving per unit of time may be overwhelming. In addition, the availability of initial resources will often be extremely limited. Patients may require extrication and evacuation that result in delays in patient transport. Experience has resulted in the formula-

TABLE 2.1. TRAITS OF A GOOD TRIAGE OFFICER

Clinically experienced
Well recognized
Good judgment and leadership
Cool under stress
Decisive
Knowledgeable regarding available resources
Sense of humor
Imaginative and creative in problem solving
Available
Knowledgeable regarding anticipated casualties

Modified from Burkle FM, ed. *Disaster medicine: application for the immediate management and triage of civilian and military disaster victims.* New Hyde Park, NY: Medical Examination Publishing, 1984.

TABLE 2.2. CLUES TO IMPROVE TRIAGE SENSITIVITY

Physiologic clues
  Altered mental status
    Anxious
    Apprehensive
  Pulse examination
    Soft
    Nonexpansive
Anatomic clues
  Body region injury
    Chest
    Abdomen
    Amputation
Specific measurements
  Resting tachycardia
  Systolic pressure <100 mm Hg
  Pulse pressure <30 mm Hg
  Resting tachypnea

Modified from Burkle FM, Newland C, Orebaugh S, et al. Emergency medicine in the Persian Gulf War—part 2: triage methodology and lessons learned. *Ann Emerg Med* 1994;23:748–754.

tion of some basic principles, which are listed in Table 2.3, for performing disaster triage.

Triage is not a static activity. After the initial categorization of patients by the triage officer, patients remaining in the area are retriaged on a constant basis. Stabilization actions (e.g., oxygen, intravenous lines, dressings) are carried out on the patients awaiting transport or definitive treatment. The triage officer or initial treatment officer directs the application of these stabilization procedures with an emphasis on treating shock, correcting mechanical defects, instituting early wound care procedures, and monitoring for changes in the patient's condition (1). Triage categorization of a casualty may change based on changes in the patient's condition and in available resources. Retagging of the casualty may be required.

TABLE 2.3. SUCCESSFUL DISASTER TRIAGE PRINCIPLES

Never move a casualty backward (against the flow)
Never hold a critical patient (immediate) for further care
Salvage life over limb
Triage officers do not stop to treat patients
Never move patients before triaged except in cases of:
  Risks due to bad weather
  Impending darkness or darkness has fallen
  A continued risk of injury
  A triage facility that is immediately available
  The tactical situation that dictates movement

Modified from Burkle FM, Newland C, Orebaugh S, et al. Emergency medicine in the Persian Gulf War—part 2: triage methodology and lessons learned. *Ann Emerg Med* 1994;23:748–754.

DOCUMENTATION OF TRIAGE ACTIVITIES

After patients are triaged, they should be methodically tagged to designate the order that they should be cared for in the treatment area. The only information available to the emergency department personnel initially may be what is written down on these triage tags. Many different commercial tags are available, and they all have unique benefits and problems. Communities should agree on a single triage tag type, and they should become familiar with its use. One community has initiated Triage Tuesday on the first Tuesday of each month based on recommendations to improve the education regarding triage (13). During Triage Tuesday, all patients arriving at emergency departments via Emergency Medical Services are accompanied not only by the usual run sheets but also by the standard triage tag. Such activities are low cost, and they promote familiarity with the triage tag system.

The perfect triage tag has not yet been created, but the tag used should have several characteristics. It should be easy to write on and weatherproof, and it should be able to be secured directly to the patient, not to the patient's clothing. In addition, it should contain, at a minimum, patient identification (name and number) and gender, the main injury or problem, the interventions performed and the time(s), the prehospital provider identification, the Emergency Medical Services unit number, and the triage category. Space for other information or checklists should be provided based on the emergency care system of each individual community. Above all, the tag must be easy to understand and use, or it will remain simply a colorful accouterment to the victim's person.

The current state of documentation of triage activities, despite a proliferation of triage tag and paperless digital systems, remains poor. This makes research into the actual performance of triage difficult because only the results of triage decisions are evaluated with any accuracy (14). Improvements in the current mechanisms of triage will occur only with a deeper understanding of what is currently done. As such, efforts to document triage activities must be improved so that these actions may be evaluated by researchers.

PREHOSPITAL TRIAGE

Prehospital providers are usually well trained in the art of triage. They encounter on a daily basis situations in which they use these skills. When a disaster occurs, prehospital personnel are the first on the scene, and they usually establish the triage and treatment areas. For this reason, a continued emphasis is placed on triage training for prehospital personnel. A system titled Simple Triage and Rapid Treatment (START) that has emerged in recent years has gained popularity (8). This system takes into account the respiratory status, the perfusion, and the mental status of the patient. START has many positive aspects, such as the ease of teach-

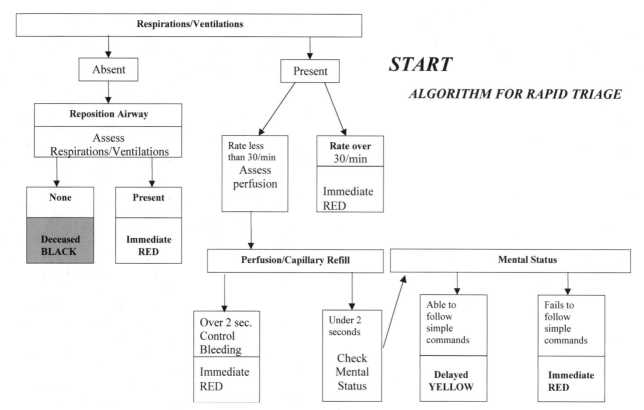

FIGURE 2.2. The Simple Triage and Rapid Treatment (START) triage algorithm. (From Super G. *START: a triage training module.* Newport Beach, CA: Hoag Memorial Hospital Presbyterian, 1984, with permission.)

ing and the simplicity of utilization in the field. The flow diagram for START is depicted in Fig. 2.2. Initially, all patients who can walk are asked to move away from the incident area to a specific location. These patients are classified as priority three or minimal (GREEN), and they will be reassessed after the more immediately critical patients are evaluated. The patients who remain are then assessed. After the patient's respiratory rate, pulse, and ability to follow commands are evaluated, they are classified as one of the three remaining categories–priority one (RED), priority two (YELLOW), and expectant (BLACK). When this system is used, the only initial treatments that are performed include opening an airway and holding direct pressure to external hemorrhage. START triage results in a substantial overtriage rate. However, this excess overtriage is offset by the ease of application over a wide range of health care providers.

SUMMARY

Triage is the first activity of mass casualty incident and disaster response. The decisions made during this phase of care have a significant impact on the health and well being of the community at large. Triage has evolved substantially over the past century, and it will continue to do so as the under-

standing of medicine and the technology progress. Performing triage during a disaster situation requires a paradigm shift in thinking on the part of health care providers with regard to transport and treatment priorities. Although experience is the best teacher, training can ease the transition from daily triage to disaster triage activities.

REFERENCES

1. Burkle FM, ed. *Disaster medicine: application for the immediate management and triage of civilian and military disaster victims.* New Hyde Park, NY: Medical Examination Publishing Co., 1984.
2. Auf Der Heide E. *Disaster response: principles of preparation and coordination.* St. Louis, MO: CV Mosby, 1989.
3. Kennedy K, Aghababian R, Gans L, et al. Triage: techniques and applications in decision making. *Ann Emerg Med* 1996;28: 136–144.
4. Eiseman B. Combat casualty management in Vietnam. *J Trauma* 1967;7:53–63.
5. Wesson DE, Scorpio R. Field triage: help or hindrance? *Can J Surg* 1992;35:19–21.
6. American College of Surgeons Committee on Trauma. Field categorization of trauma victims. *Bull Am Coll Surg* 1986;71:17–21.
7. Frykberg ER, Tepas JJ. Terrorist bombings: lessons learned from Belfast to Beirut. *Ann Surg* 1988;208:569–576.
8. Super G. *START: a triage training module.* Newport Beach, CA: Hoag Memorial Hospital Presbyterian, 1984.

9. Burkle FM, Newland C, Orebaugh S, et al. Emergency medicine in the Persian Gulf War. Part 2: triage methodology and lessons learned. *Ann Emerg Med* 1994,23:748–754.

10. Pepe PE, Kvetan V. Field management and critical care in mass disasters. *Crit Care Clin North Am* 1991;7:401–420.

11. Baxt WG, Berry C, Epperson M, et al. Failure of prehospital trauma prediction rules to classify trauma patients accurately. *Ann Emerg Med* 1989;18:1–8.

12. Esposito TJ, Offner PJ, Jurkovich GJ, et al. Do prehospital trauma center triage criteria identify major trauma victims? *Arch Surg* 1995;130:171–176.

13. Vayer JS, Ten Eych RP, Cowen ML. New concepts in triage. *Ann Emerg Med* 1986;15:927–930.

14. Hogan DE, Waeckerle JF, Dire DJ, et al. Emergency department impact of the Oklahoma City terrorist bombing. *Ann Emerg Med* 1999;34:160-167.

3

PEDIATRIC CONSIDERATIONS IN DISASTERS

KIM D. FLOYD

Whom unmerciful disaster followed fast and followed faster.
—*The Raven*

Disasters affect persons of all ages, from the very young to the very old. While no single disaster has specifically singled out the pediatric population, history illustrates the fact that any disaster can include a significant number of children. Meeting the needs of the pediatric population requires special consideration and planning before a disaster response. Recent examples of the impact of disasters on children include the tornado of May 3, 1999 in Oklahoma in which 642 individuals were injured or killed. Of these 642 victims, 122 (19%) were under 14 years of age (1). The bombing of the Murrah Building on April 19, 1995 in Oklahoma City resulted in 168 deaths, 19 (11.3%) of which were children. In addition, 47 children were injured severely enough to be taken to emergency departments (ED) (2). Hurricane Hugo took 35 lives when it struck South Carolina in 1989; of these, seven were children (3). The sad but real chain of school and church shootings has created and continues to create young victims with an alarming frequency. These disasters result in a substantially larger number and a greater severity of pediatric cases than usual and require management at the same time by prehospital, ED, and hospital services (4,5).

Terrorism is an ever-growing threat worldwide. Over 5,000 individuals were injured when sarin was intentionally released in a Tokyo subway in 1995, resulting in 12 deaths. Sixteen of the surviving victims were children less then 14 years of age, and five were pregnant women (6). Weapons of mass destruction that involve chemical and biologic agents may be more detrimental to the pediatric population, and, thus, this population requires more planning than the adult population. Most chemical warfare agents are volatile, and they have a vapor density that is greater than that of water. Therefore, these agents layer close to the ground at the level of a child's airway (6).

PHYSICAL CONSIDERATIONS

The pediatric population is a distinct entity with many differences that separate it from the adult counterpart. Because of the physiology that allows children to tolerate some insults better than adults, children are also at risk for a variety of injuries that differ from adults in onset, patterns of injuries, and susceptibility to physical forces. Because of their more rapid respiratory rates, children may be more susceptible to aerosolized toxins than adults (6). Their disproportionate body surface area-to-weight ratio places children at risk for more rapid contamination via the skin absorption of chemical agents. This same mechanism puts children at risk for rapid changes in body temperature caused by changes in environmental temperatures. Patterns of trauma in the pediatric population differ from those in the adult population for several reasons. Weight and size differences are obvious, but simple things like chest wall compliance allow for a variety of injuries in children that differ from adults.

Head Injury

Children's heads are disproportionately weighted and sized when compared to an adult's head. If a child experiences traumatic forces or becomes airborne, the odds that a child will suffer a head injury when compared to an adult are greater. In the Oklahoma City bombing in 1995, 19 children were killed. Of those 19, 90% had suffered head injuries. Of the 47 children with nonfatal injuries, four of the seven (57.1%) requiring hospitalization were admitted for head injuries (2). The severity of the head injury is often the primary determinant in the pediatric patient's outcome (3). Children under the age of 3 years have a less optimistic prognosis than older children, although children in general tend to have better outcomes than adults after sustaining a head injury (7). However, children are at greater risk for damage from secondary brain injury, and they should therefore be treated somewhat more aggressively than adults from the onset (8).

Chest Injury

Because of the increased compliance of the chest wall, energy transfer to internal organs is more substantial. As a result, an increased risk exists for pulmonary and myocardial contusions and for vascular injury without bony findings when compared to the adult cohort. Flail chest injuries are less common in children than adults; however, the greater pliability of the child's chest makes it more sensitive to flail segments or tension pneumothorax if they do occur. The presence of rib fractures suggests a substantially greater risk for intrathoracic injury in the pediatric population than in the adult segment (9).

Musculoskeletal Injury

Long bone fractures are less common in children than in adults receiving the same level of traumatic energy (3,10) due to the compliance of the long bones in children, which resist fracture to a greater extent. Pediatric musculoskeletal injuries are complicated by the growing physis of the bones and the lack of mineralization surrounding these regions. Fractures and dislocations in these regions may be less obvious, and they may disrupt or arrest bone growth.

Cervical Spine and Spinal Cord Injury

Spine and spinal cord injury are less common in children than in adults in a general sense. However, the child has greater flexibility and mobility of the cervical spine, which may result in spinal cord injury without radiographic abnormality. This should be suspected in a child with signs or symptoms of spinal cord injury even without associated radiologic findings. Aggressive treatment should be initiated in this setting using the methylprednisolone protocol recommended by the National Institutes of Health (11). Spinal immobilization should be maintained if any question of spinal cord or vertebral injury exists.

Thermal Considerations

Children are at a higher risk for hypothermia and hyperthermic injuries than adults due to, in part, their weight-to-body surface area ratio, which allows for more rapid heat transfer than that which occurs in adults. Heat loss is also greater because of the pediatric patient's increased head-to-body surface area ratio. Direct energy transfers (e.g., a downed child on cool pavement) can rapidly decrease body temperature. A child without adult supervision may not seek shelter from temperature extremes. Care should be taken to maintain thermal balance during the evaluation and treatment of pediatric disaster victims.

Burns

As was said above, the pediatric patient has a disproportionate body surface area-to-weight ratio compared to adults, placing children at risk for a higher percent of skin damage. The burned child is at even more substantial risk of thermal regulatory problems. Therapy should be initiated as soon as possible using standard burn protocols.

Volume Depletion

Volume depletion may be a substantial issue with the pediatric population. Children may tolerate more volume loss per kilogram than corresponding adults. However, when decompensation occurs, it may occur rapidly and it can be difficult to reverse. Direct fluid loss or poor oral intake may contribute to volume depletion in the pediatric patient. Aggressive fluid resuscitation should be instituted in the volume-depleted child. Crystalloids, which are the first line of fluids, should be administered in 20 mL per kg body weight boluses. If blood loss is an issue, then transfusions should begin as soon as possible. Colloid boluses are given at 10 mL per kg body weight.

PEDIATRIC GLASGOW SCORE AND TRAUMA SCORE

Many ways of evaluating injured patients are found; however, the simplest and most concise are generally preferred. Also of vital importance is the ability to articulate that information to another caretaker. Having fixed criteria for assessing, documenting, and comparing is valuable. Various scoring systems have been developed to assist in triage and in projecting prognosis in injured patients. These scores require modification when used in the pediatric population, and the limitations and strengths of the scoring systems must be understood. The Glasgow coma score is useful in assessing the mental status of a disaster victim, monitoring mental status trends, and prognosticating outcomes. The standard Glasgow coma scale used in the adult population requires modification for use in children. This adaptation is depicted in Table 3.1.

The Pediatric Trauma Score is another tool utilized in pediatric centers worldwide (Table 3.2). With this information, health care workers can convey patient status, monitor trends, and predict the prognosis. This information is also important when one is researching trauma and disaster-related questions because it provides a standardized set of data elements.

TABLE 3.1. THE PEDIATRIC MODIFICATION OF THE GLASGOW COMA SCALE

Activity	Score	Infants	Children and adults
Eye opening	4	Spontaneous	Spontaneous
	3	To speech or sound	To speech
	2	To painful stimuli	To painful stimuli
	1	None	None
Verbal	5	Appropriate words or sounds, social smile, fixes and follows	Oriented
	4	Cries, but is consolable	Confused
	3	Persistently irritable	Inappropriate words
	2	Restless, agitated	Incomprehensible sounds
	1	None	None
Motor	6	Spontaneous movement	Obeys commands
	5	Localizes to pain	Localizes to pain
	4	Withdraws to pain	Withdraws to pain
	3	Abnormal flexion (decorticate)	Abnormal flexion (decorticate)
	2	Abnormal extension (decerebrate)	Abnormal extension (decerebrate)
	1	None	None

TABLE 3.2. THE PEDIATRIC TRAUMA SCORE

Components	+2	+1	−1	Score
Weight	>20 kg (44 lbs)	10–20 kg (22–44 lbs)	<10 kg (22 lbs)	
Airway	Patent*	Maintainable†	Unmaintainable‡	
Systolic B/P	>90 mm Hg	50–90 mm Hg	<50 mm Hg	
Pulses	Radial	Carotid	Nonpalpable	
CNS	Awake	+ LOC§	Unresponsive	
Fractures	None	Closed or suspected	Multiple closed or open	
Wounds	None	Minor‖	Major, penetrating or burns#	
Total score				−6–12: decreases with severity of condition
				9–12: Minor trauma
				6–8: Potentially life-threatening
				0–5: Life-threatening
				<0: Usually fatal

*No assistance required.
†Protected by patient, but requires continuous monitoring for changes; may require positioning.
‡Requires airway adjuncts NPA, OPA, and ET or suctioning.
§Responds to voice or pain or temporary loss of consciousness noted.
‖Abrasions, minor lacerations, burns <10% and not involving hands, face, feet, or genitalia.
#Penetrating, major avulsions, lacerations, burns >10% or involving hands, face, feet, or genitalia.
Abbreviations: B/P, blood pressure; CNS, central nervous system; ET, endotracheal tube; LOC, loss of consciousness; NPA, nasal pharyngeal airway; OPA, oral pharyngeal airway.

NUTRITIONAL CONSIDERATIONS

Children, particularly those that are younger, depend on adults to make many decisions for them. Adults make decisions regarding the safety, diet, and the choice of shelter appropriate to the environmental concerns at hand for children. Nutritional concerns in most disasters in developed nations are of minimal concern due to the short duration of the event. However, some reports demonstrate links between disaster events and nutritional developmental problems, such as neural tube defects, in children born after disasters (12). The evaluation of 5-year-old children has been used to assess the nutritional status of a disaster-stricken population. Various height and weight ratios, as well as the mid upper arm circumference, have been used to evaluate nutritional disorders and to guide feeding programs (13).

PSYCHOSOCIAL CONSIDERATIONS

Children's Issues

Pediatric victims suffer psychosocial, as well as physical, trauma from all types of disasters. Children have been found to suffer from disaster due to direct involvement, as well as via media exposure, such as news reporting of a disaster. The effects of the explosion of the Challenger spaceship in 1986 were far-reaching among children (14).

Terr breaks psychosocial traumas into two types as follws: type I, which is a single traumatic event, such as a fire or a rape episode, and type II, which includes repeated, prolonged trauma, such as extensive child abuse. According to this concept, these two types of trauma result in different coping styles. Children with type I trauma receive support from family and friends, and they usually remember the traumatic event. Individuals with type II trauma are more likely to have severe post traumatic stress disorder (PTSD) symptoms, such as psychic numbing and dissociation. Type II trauma is often kept a secret, and support from family and friends may be absent (15).

The traumatized child should be watched for unusual behaviors or mannerisms. Not only may the child voice concerns about the future, but he or she may also make unusual comments, experience sleep disturbances, or enact repetitive fantasy play (16). Children who are having serious problems with grief and loss may show one or more of the following signs: an extended period of depression in which they lose interest in daily activities and events, inability to sleep, loss of appetite, prolonged fear of being alone, acting much younger than their age for an extended period, excessively imitating the dead person, repeated statements of wanting to join the dead person, withdrawal from friends, a sharp drop in school performance, or a refusal to attend school (17).

Age is important in the presentation of psychologic stress. The younger child, for example, may refuse to attend school, while the older child may minimize his or her feelings but still may show deterioration in grades and even in dealings with family members. PTSD is defined as psychologic damage resulting from experiencing, witnessing, or participating in an overwhelmingly traumatic (frightening) event. PTSD rarely appears during the trauma itself. Although its symptoms can occur soon after the event, the disorder often surfaces several months or even years later. Changes in the child's behavior, mannerisms, sleep patterns, and play activities can alert the parent to the need for psychosocial counseling (18). When helping a child understand the death and trauma associated with disasters, the discussion should be age appropriate, as should all dealings with children in the emergency setting (19).

Parental Issues

Children do not live in a vacuum in a disaster. Parenting issues must be addressed in the face of the dynamics of a given disaster. Finding shelter and clothing for the family involved in a disaster may introduce discord for the parent because of his or her own need to deal with the personal issues resulting from the stressors of that disaster. The parent's ability to cope affects the dynamics of the entire family. A parent who is at maximal stress levels may need counseling, as well as the child.

PARENTAL EDUCATION

Parents are the primary source of stability and strength during a disaster, and they should be educated on what to do in the event of a disaster. This education should continue during and after the initial impact. Safe water and food supplies should be provided for children. If possible, medications should be available. Clothing, diapers, books, and toys should accompany the children in the event of an evacuation. Parents should understand that the frequency of toxic ingestions from items such as cleaning agents and insecticides is increased in the postdisaster period. Open wounds also occur more frequently from nails, grills, open space heaters, and construction tools.

In the event of an emergency evacuation during school or church, a specific community-wide plan should be in place. The parents should be notified, and the children should be evacuated to a prearranged pickup point, if possible, to insure their safety. Ancillary service and support groups include, but are not limited to, the American Red Cross, counselors, teachers, school administrators, occupational and physical therapists, religious organizations, and other disaster relief programs.

IMPACT OF DISASTER ON PEDIATRIC EMERGENCY MEDICAL SERVICES

Prehospital

Emergency medical care providers must be adequately trained in the triage and management of the ill and/or injured child. Protocols should exist to govern the transportation of children to certain facilities, particularly when certain facilities are designated for children. The American Academy of Pediatrics recognizes Emergency Medical Services for Children (EMS-C). With this nationwide project, prehospital care for children will hopefully be improved (see below) (20–22).

Children's special needs complicate the field provider's rescue work. Extrication prolongs the time to treatment for this particularly vulnerable group of patients. Attention to volume repletion and thermoregulation should be instituted early and aggressively. Triage to the appropriate facilities is ideal, and the development and implementation of a mass casualty plan is imperative in order to avoid overloading one local facility when possible.

A community or locale should have designated facilities for the referral of critically injured pediatric patients. Referral patterns, as well as designated alternatives in the event of a disaster, should be firmly in place.

Education and training in pediatric disaster response are needed throughout the prehospital and emergency response tier. Some data indicate that the triage and initial therapy of pediatric disaster victims may be less than optimal. Van Amerongen et al., in a study of the prehospital care during the Avianca plane crash, indicated that problems existed with the triage and transport of pediatric victims (23). Five major reasons were cited for these problems as follows:

1. Unique problems associated with pediatric disaster rescue;
2. Limited training of prehospital personnel in pediatric methods;
3. Disaster plan deficiencies for pediatric response;
4. No consistent use of pediatric tertiary care centers;
5. No required use of pediatric trauma or referral centers.

Emergency Departments

EDs should have a functioning plan for dealing with any of a number of mass casualty disasters that may affect their locale. While some regions are not prone to certain disasters, history has shown that no one region is immune to the potential for disaster offered by natural phenomena or that caused by industrial or human sources. Therefore, specific plans for the triage and treatment of pediatric victims are vital. Patients and emergency medical services (EMS) will not respect "Children only" or "Adult only" EDs during a

disaster. Each facility must be able to care for and at least initially stabilize both children and adults.

While the EMS system will attempt to triage in the field, their work only affects a small portion of those seeking medical care. In the 1995 release of sarin gas into a Japanese subway, as many as 46% of the hospital staff experienced symptoms through improper handling of victims. Less than 10% of the more than 5,000 victims came to hospitals via ambulance; the remainder of victims arrived unexpectedly via taxi or automobile or on foot (24). In the bombing in Oklahoma City in 1995, as well as in the May 3, 1999 tornado, hospitals nearest the disaster zone were impacted most heavily by victims arriving in cars, vans, pickups, and police cars, thus following the geographic effect (25,26).

The ED staff and EMS providers should be educated in the care of injured and sick children. Many continuing medical education programs, such as Pediatric Advanced Life support (PALS), Advanced Pediatric Life Support (APLS), and Neonatal Resuscitation courses, are available through the American Heart Association and the American College of Emergency Physicians. The maintenance of pediatric skills may vary from institution to institution, but it should be encouraged. Many charts, tapes, and cards that are available through a variety of resources can aid in weight and drug-dosing calculations as well.

The ED should be prepared for a potential overburden of pediatric patients, and it should be able to stabilize those that are critical and to make appropriate dispositions and transfers. The American College of Emergency Physicians (ACEP) states, "It is imperative that all hospital EDs and EMS agencies have the appropriate equipment, staff, and policies to provide high quality care for children.... to facilitate, after stabilization, timely transfer to a facility with specialized pediatric services when appropriate" (27). Both ACEP and the National EMS-C Resource Alliance have publications with recommendations for proper equipment for the care of the pediatric patient. These recommendations may be modified in the event of a disaster (27,28).

Not only should the medical needs of the pediatric population be anticipated, but the EDs and hospitals should have some mechanism that enables them to provide shelter, clothing, and entertainment for these children. This may be prearranged through the hospital's ministerial or social services. Children, moreover, should be protected from the imminent onslaught of media in the critical period immediately following a disaster. They should be given time to reconcile the changes in their world before having to deal with the stress caused by others such as the news media.

DISEASE CONSIDERATIONS

Infectious disease outbreaks generally are a myth associated with disasters. If proper public health measures are used,

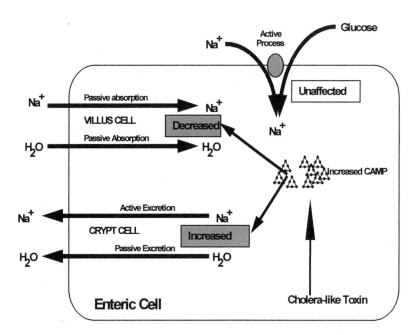

FIGURE 3.1. Enteric function and oral rehydration. (From Hogan DE. The emergency department approach to diarrhea. *Emerg Med Clin North Am* 1993;12:673–694, with permission.)

outbreaks are, in actuality, quite rare. Although the usual childhood disease rates may increase due to overcrowding, nonendemic diseases will not be a problem unless they are physically brought into the disaster area.

Enteric illnesses are the most common cause of death after a disaster in most underdeveloped nations worldwide. Most of these outbreaks are waterborne. Children have less ability than adults to maintain fluid and electrolyte balance when infected. Volume depletion occurs more quickly and it is much more devastating than in adults. However, children are much more resilient than adults, and, thus, they generally may be rehydrated by oral methods if these are instituted in a timely fashion after the onset of symptoms. Using oral rehydration solutions containing glucose and balanced electrolytes (especially sodium) takes advantage of the active sodium-glucose absorption mechanism of the gut. This active mechanism generally is unaffected by most diarrhea syndromes, and it results in the passive absorption of water as Fig. 3.1. demonstrates (29). The use of oral rehydration methods literally may save the lives of children in disaster-stricken regions. Numerous formulas for oral solutions may be found, but the one recommended by the World Health Organization is as follows: to 1 L of water, add glucose, 20 g, or sucrose, 40 g; 3.5 g NaCl; 2.5 g NaHCO$_3$; 1.5 g KCl; stir or shake well (30).

SUMMARY

The pediatric population involved in disaster has unique patterns of injury, needs, and problems. These can be minimized with the proper education of EMS and ED personnel. Patient care can be optimized with adequate and appropriate

equipment and supplies. By efficiently meeting the demands of the pediatric population that result from the impact of a disaster, morbidity and mortality may be minimized.

REFERENCES

1. Oklahoma State Health Department. *Injury update: investigation of deaths and injuries resulting from the May 3, 1999 tornadoes.* Oklahoma City, OK: Injury Prevention Service of the Oklahoma State Health Department, July 21, 2000.
2. Quintana DA, Parker JR, Jordan FB, et al. The spectrum of pediatric injuries after a bomb blast. *J Pediatr Surg* 1997;32:307–310.
3. Holbrook PR. Pediatric disaster medicine. *Crit Care Clin* 1991;7:463–470.
4. Attia WM. The blizzard of 1996: a pediatric emergency department. *Prehospital Emerg Care* 1998;24:285–288.
5. Simon HK, Stegelman M, Batton J. A prospective evaluation of pediatric emergency care during the 1996 Summer Olympic Games in Atlanta, Georgia. *Pediatr Emerg Care* 1998;14:1–3.
6. American Academy of Pediatrics Committee on Environmental Health. Chemical–biological terrorism and its impact on children: a subject review. *Pediatrics* 2000;105:662–670.
7. Bruce D. Outcome following severe head injuries in children. *J Neurosurg* 1978;48:697.
8. Chestnut RM, Marshall LF, Klauber MR, et al. The role of secondary brain injury in determining outcome from severe head injury. *J Trauma* 1993;43:216–222.
9. Garcia VF, Gotschall CS, Eichelberger MR, et al. Rib fractures in children: a marker of severe trauma. *J Trauma* 1990;30:695–700.
10. Nakayama DK, Ramenofsky ML, Rowe MI. Chest injuries in childhood. *Ann Surg* 1989;210:770–775.
11. Bracken MB, Shepard MJ, Hellenbrand KG, et al. A randomized, controlled trial of methylprednisolone or naloxone in the treatment of acute spinal-cord injury. Results of the Second National Acute Spinal Cord Injury Study. *N Engl J Med* 1990;17: 1405–1411.

12. Duff EM, Cooper ES. Neural tube defects in Jamaica following Hurricane Gilbert. *Am J Public Health* 1994;84:473–476.

13. Centers for Disease Control. Rapid nutrition evaluation in drought-affected regions of Somalia–1987. *MMWR* 1988;259: 1927,1929.

14. McKeown LA. Challenger explosion may have had lasting effects on young children. WebMD interview with Lenore Terr, M.D.. Available at: http://webmd.lycos.com/content/article/1728.50330. Accessed August 1, 2001.

15. Terr L. *Unchained memories*. New York: Harper Collins, 1994: 11,30.

16. Oklahoma State University. Parenting made easier. Available at: http://www.fcs.okstate.edu/parenting/. Accessed August 1, 2001.

17. American Academy of Child and Adolescent Psychiatry. *Children in grief.* Fact sheet no. 8, revised November 1998.

18. American Academy of Child and Adolescent Psychiatry. *Helping children after a disaster.* Fact sheet no. 36, revised May 2000.

19. Rongé LJ. Child deaths hit communities hard. Disasters demand psychological triage. *AAP News* May 1998;14:1,8.

20. Emergency Medical Services for Children. Available at: http://www.ems-c.org/index.htm. Accessed August 1, 2001.

21. American Academy of Pediatrics. How pediatricians can respond to the psychosocial implications of disasters. *Pediatrics* 1999;103: 521–523.

22. Durch JS, Lohr KN, eds. *Emergency services for children.* Washington, D.C.: National Academy Press, 1993.

23. Van Amerogen RH, Fine JS, Tunik MG, et al. The Avianca plane crash: an emergency medical systems response to pediatric survivors of the disaster. *Pediatrics* 1993;92:105–110.

24. Okumura T, Suzuki K, Fukuda A, et al. The Tokyo subway sarin attack: disaster management, part 1: community emergency response. *Acad Emerg Med* 1998;5:613–617.

25. Hogan DE, Waeckerle JF, Dire DJ, et al. Emergency department impact of the Oklahoma City terrorist bombing. *Ann Emerg Med* 1999;34:160–167.

26. Hogan DE, Askins DC, Osburn AE. The May 3, 1999, tornado in Oklahoma City. *Ann Emerg Med* 1999;34:225–226

27. American College of Emergency Physicians. *Care of children in the ED: guidelines for preparedness.* ACEP Policy Statement, ACEP policy no. 400300. Approved December 2000

28. Committee on Pediatric Equipment and Supplies for Emergency Departments, National EMS-C Resource Alliance. Guidelines for pediatric equipment and supplies for emergency departments. *Ann Emerg Med* 1998;31:54–57.

29. Hogan DE. The emergency department approach to diarrhea. *Emerg Med Clin North Am* 1993;12:673–694.

30. Meyers A. Modern management of acute diarrhea and dehydration in children. *Am Fam Physicians* 1995;51:1103–1118.

4

INFECTIOUS DISEASES AND DISASTERS

P. GREGG GREENOUGH

GENERAL CONCEPTS

As the field of disaster medicine has grown and the study of the discipline among academic centers, policy makers, humanitarian aid organizations, and governments has become more rigorous, a focus on infectious diseases as a consequence of disasters has received more intense scrutiny as well. One benefit has been clarifying the risks of the specific infectious diseases associated with certain disasters and putting to rest a number of misconceptions regarding the relationship between disasters and infectious disease epidemics.

In general, the risks of large-scale epidemics are low immediately following acute natural disasters, particularly in the developed world. In fact, disease surveillance of relief camps in the emergency phase indicates that increased disease transmission is more critical than epidemic outbreaks (1). Infectious disease outbreaks usually occur in the postimpact and recovery phases and not during the acute phase (2). The risks of epidemics increase, however, if drought, famine, and large displacements of people are involved. In these events, which have a greater degree of chronicity and which tend to last well into postdisaster and recovery phases, crude mortality rates from infectious diseases in the developing world may be 20 to 30 times higher than normal (1). The term *complex emergencies* has evolved to define better the disruption of civil societies and community structures from civil war and other causes that often generate refugee movements, thus placing millions at risk for infectious disease outbreaks. Such manmade disasters—the so-called ethnic cleansings in the Balkans and the post-Cold War, post-colonial insurgencies in Africa—is where the highest mortality rates from infectious diseases in recent history have occurred. However, these risks are decreased when potable water; safe food; sanitation services, including human and animal waste removal; adequate personal hygiene; vector control; maintenance of routine immunization programs; sufficient ventilation and space in shelters and temporary housing; and the isolation of patients with communicable diseases are provided.

Another confusing notion that is not supported by the disaster literature is the possibility that disasters might spawn new diseases. Unless an organism or vector is brought into the disaster area, the outbreaks that occur are almost always from diseases and vectors endemic to the disaster-affected area. Where infectious diseases have led directly to high mortality rates, an increase in the incidence of the endemic conditions has been observed (3). For instance, flooding may lead to increased infectious diseases, but the underlying epidemiologic conditions—the endemicity of given diseases and the public health infrastructure of the affected area before the flood, for instance—determine the extent of this risk, not the intensity of the flood itself (4). Where conditions exist that promote the increased transmission of endemic diseases, epidemics may occur. Such conditions traditionally have involved a large population of displaced people, a disruption of safe water supplies, the destruction of sanitation facilities, and interruption of health services. Thus, successful planning for potential outbreaks demands that public health and medical officers be knowledgeable of the diseases endemic to the disaster area. These include organisms that have caused disease previously but that have been controlled by local public health measures, as such diseases can reemerge following a disaster (2). Diseases that are unusual in the United States, except perhaps in travelers, such as malaria, visceral leishmaniasis, and trypanosomiasis, could surface as epidemics in places such as sub-Saharan Africa where they are endemic (5). Increased travel and intercontinental trade and development, as well as the international scope of aid workers, theoretically could introduce new organisms into a nonimmune population. To date, little evidence shows that this has occurred to any significant degree.

Although the following is not always the perception of the media and the general public, large numbers of dead bodies do not pose an infectious disease risk because the dead are victims of the disaster event itself and not of any communicable disease. Although they are physically unpleasant to disaster survivors, corpses do not need to be buried quickly for purposes of minimizing infectious disease risk. Rather, the victims should be identified first and should be given a burial appropriate for the culture and religious beliefs of the affected population. This can diminish the additional psychologic stress for their friends and families without increasing the risk of infectious disease outbreaks for the general population.

As the study of disaster medicine has evolved, not only have the misconceptions of infectious diseases in the aftermath of disasters been clarified, but the risk factors for the development of postdisaster outbreaks and how best to prevent them have been able to be pinpointed better. In general, measles, diarrheal disease, and respiratory infections, all of which are preventable diseases, constitute the vast majority of deaths following both natural disasters and complex emergencies. For example, of the nearly 350 deaths in the 12 weeks following the Mount Pinatubo eruption in the Philippines in 1992, 31% were from measles, 29% were from diarrheal illness, and 22% were from respiratory infections (6). Diseases such as typhoid, cholera, and meningitis have occurred in postdisaster environments but usually only in developing world refugee camps. Even within these settings, the overall mortality is low from these diseases (1). In reality, the displacement of large numbers of disaster survivors packed into crowded unsanitary living conditions has historically produced the most significant postdisaster infectious disease epidemics, particularly in large refugee camps and in populations affected by food shortages (7).

RISK FACTORS FOR INFECTIOUS DISEASE OUTBREAKS FROM DISASTERS

In general, any natural or manmade disaster that compromises or disrupts one or more parts of the public health infrastructure, including the sanitation systems, potable water supplies, food and nutrition stores, primary health care access (including routine vaccination programs), vector control programs, and established systematic surveillance mechanisms, can trigger infectious disease outbreaks (2). Successful intervention requires rapid assessment to determine where the breakdown points of infrastructure have occurred. Disaster managers, public health specialists, and health care providers should pay specific attention to the degree to which infection control measures have been affected during the acute disaster phase and should repair those defects and treat the cases that have surfaced. How well the likely points of breakdown are targeted in advance and how thorough the response planning has been will determine the success in minimizing the potentially devastating effects of infectious disease outbreaks from the disaster. Honing in on the weak links of the predisaster public health infrastructure and identifying the points of disruption in the immediate phase mean that useful supplies can be acquired and that valuable resources can be directed appro-

priately over the longer postimpact phase when epidemics are more likely to occur. When Hurricane Andrew destroyed 25,000 homes and left 200,000 homeless in late August 1992, the Florida Department of Health and Rehabilitative Services and the United States Army established an active surveillance system based at 43 temporary care sites and eight emergency departments for 1 month following the disaster. Looking at six index conditions, five of which would indicate a possible infectious disease outbreak (e.g., rash, diarrhea, cough, animal bite, and other infection), they concluded that no change occurred in the proportional morbidity (the total number of patient visits per total number of visits) for diarrhea than what would be expected under normal conditions and that cough had a higher proportional morbidity that was not sufficient enough, however, to be considered an epidemic. Aggressive surveillance pinpointed possible disease outbreaks for amelioration despite the fact that the electrical power supply had been disturbed, the routine disease surveillance mechanism had been disrupted, and the water generally was not potable (8).

Breaks in the public health infrastructure lead to outbreaks from the increased modes of transmission of infectious diseases, the increased susceptibility to endemic organisms among the disaster survivors, and, rarely, the introduction of new organisms into the environment by outsiders providing aid. Modes of transmission occur via airborne, waterborne, or vector-borne mechanisms that are often enhanced during a natural or manmade disaster. Increased susceptibility occurs through malnutrition, the migration of large populations, the inaccessibility of medications for disaster victims with underlying chronic disease, associated injuries such as wounds, psychologic stresses, and exposure to extreme heat and cold.

Increased Modes of Transmission

Overcrowding

Disaster survivors who lose their housing often are crowded into temporary shelters or camps that increase their risk for airborne disease transmission, especially measles, upper respiratory infections, meningitis, and tuberculosis. Increased mortality in refugee camps has been particularly linked to measles and upper respiratory infections (9). Before the 1990s, measles outbreaks after natural disasters were a more common occurrence; however, due to mass immunization in the predisaster phase and improved attention to vitamin A deficiency, such outbreaks have become less frequent, especially in the developed world. The last outbreak with high incidence rates was the Mount Pinatubo eruption cited previously. Following that disaster, over 100,000 people were housed in evacuation camps. Measles cases numbered 18,000 over the 3 months following the disaster. The disease accounted for nearly one quarter of all clinic visits and 22% of all deaths. The predisaster vaccination rates were extremely low, and they likely contributed to the high incidence (10). Measles continues to be a problem in refugee populations generated by complex emergencies, as evidenced in Somalia (1992), Nepal (Bhutanese refugees, 1992), Zimbabwe (1992), and Sudan (1985, 1993) and most recently among the East Timorese (1999).

Neisseria meningitis remains the most feared epidemic because of its rapid, fulminant course. Again, the highest at-risk populations include those living in crowded conditions associated with poor hygiene. Although bacterial meningitis is rare, it has been documented in overpopulated developing world refugee camps, notably Thailand (1980) and sub-Saharan Africa, especially Sudan (1985 and 1988), where group A meningococcal disease is endemic (11).

Upper respiratory infections contribute significantly to mortality rates in children less than 5 years of age. The incidence of upper respiratory infections following Hurricane Georges in the Dominican Republic in 1998 was 60% in surveyed households. Upper respiratory infections were more common in shelter or migrant settlements than in nonsheltered households (12).

Although tuberculosis is not a direct result of a natural disaster, the overcrowded living conditions of displaced victims and the disruption of treatment programs may lead to an increased incidence of cases or to a recurrence of cases in the prolonged postdisaster phase. Directly observed therapy programs or the medication supply may be disturbed for lengthy periods. Such disruption may have caused the fourfold increase in tuberculosis cases during the Bosnian conflict in 1992 (13). The level of malnutrition among the displaced and lowered immunity may also enhance the spread of tuberculosis following a disaster. In disaster areas where human immunodeficiency virus (HIV) infection rates are high, one may expect the high prevalence rates of tuberculosis due to coinfectivity.

Factors Contributing to Increases in Disease Vectors

Disasters that result in large areas of standing water potentially lend themselves to increased rates of vector-borne disease. Although vector-borne disease epidemics rarely occur following natural disasters, a theoretical risk exists if flooding provides more breeding sites and if extensive damage to homes allows increased exposure. The largest known malaria epidemic following a disaster occurred in Haiti in the aftermath of Hurricane Flora in October 1963. Over 75,000 cases of malaria emerged 2 to 3 months after the storm's devastation. The epidemic was attributed to the fact that over 200,000 people were homeless, and, thus, the exposure potential was greater. The combination of the storm, which generated heavy flooding and fallen trees, and the carted debris, which caused the inadvertent damming of rivers, led to more areas of standing water, creating a huge increase in mosquito breeding sites. Moreover, this area already had a large reservoir of gametocyte carriers. Although heavy rains were probably less of a factor, they also washed away layers of insecticide that had been sprayed on roofs and walls (14).

Changes in climate, especially warming of the environment, produce a greater frequency of extreme weather events (15). Such natural disasters, including more periods of heavier precipitation and more storms with higher wind speeds, increase the rate of production of stagnant pools of water. Extreme heavy rainfalls were linked to vector-borne diseases, such as the Murray Valley encephalitis and the Ross River virus outbreaks in Australia, eastern equine encephalitis in the United States, West Nile fever in southern Africa, and the cyclical epidemics of malaria in Argentina and Pakistan (16). Insect vectors may not be the only climate-linked vector problem. In the Four Corners region of the United States (border area of Colorado, Utah, Arizona, and New Mexico), 6 years of drought, followed by the El Niño Southern Oscillation, generated unusually heavy rains in May 1993, leading to an increase in the local population of deer mice, the reservoir for hantavirus. This outbreak of the flulike illness with its rapid progression to acute respiratory distress syndrome—hantavirus pulmonary syndrome—caused the rapid death of several people and created a panic among the area population during the time of year when influenza typically had high prevalence rates. Brillman et al. (17) note that an infectious disease or the threat of an outbreak can overwhelm the emergency care system and can be considered a disaster in itself. The disruption in environmental conditions can favor the increased breeding of vectors or the dispersal of diseases of low endemicity. Following a prolonged period of heavy rainfall and resultant flooding from El Niño in northeast Kenya from September 1997 until January 1998, large areas of land remained under stagnant water. Most of the area's population were nomadic pastoralists who were forced to move through the flooded region to higher ground. One humanitarian organization noted high rates of *Plasmodium falciparum* in this population, which has a low immunity to malaria (18). Malaria-specific mortality rates are high when people from areas of low endemicity are forced to flee into areas of high endemicity. Vector-borne diseases are not the only environmentally generated maladies. The Northridge, California earthquake of January 1994 caused thousands of landslides that generated dense dust clouds in nearby eastern Ventura County. Arthrospores of the fungal disease coccidioidomycosis, normally found in the Southern California soil, were carried along in these dust clouds, resulting in a threefold risk of developing the pulmonary disease. Of 203 cases, three were fatal (19).

General warming of the climate may change the endemicity of certain vector-borne diseases such as malaria, dengue fever, yellow fever, and a number of viral encephalitides, making the likelihood of these diseases emerging from a disaster a realistic threat. The increasing temperatures shorten incubation periods and increase vector breeding and bite rates, further enhancing the transmission of infection. For instance, outbreaks of St. Louis encephalitis correlated with a period of extreme heat in California in 1984 (16).

Disruption of vector control programs may lead to increased rates of vector-borne diseases, particularly in developing countries where such programs can be tenuous even in the absence of a disaster. If programs of insect control are disrupted, for instance, breeding sites will be allowed to flourish, even in urbanized areas where roofs, outdoor pots, and garbage dumps can serve as surrogate reservoirs for standing water. Where insect control has been well established in the predisaster phase and is easily restored in the disaster phase, vector-borne disease usually is not significant. Following the Midwest floods of 1993 and Hurricane Andrew in 1992, no increased incidence of malaria, St. Louis encephalitis, or dengue fever was observed despite the increased rates of mosquito biting.

Disruption in Water Supplies and Waste Management Systems

Vibrio cholerae, Shigella dysenteria; and, rarely, hepatitis A and E, leptospirosis, and *Salmonella typhi* constitute the waterborne infectious diseases that appear following disasters and complex emergencies. Diarrheal illness remains the most lethal infectious disease involving refugees and population displacements (7). Cholera, although rare in the developed world following natural disasters, has appeared in refugee camps in Bangladesh, Iraq, Malawi, Nepal, Turkey, Swaziland, and Zimbabwe (20,21). For all diarrheal illness, watery diarrhea is more common than dysentery or mucoid diarrhea. Following the Bangladeshi floods of 1988, watery diarrhea comprised 47% of all diarrheas; mucoid, 42%; and the more lethal bloody diarrheas, 11% (22). In general, children, particularly those younger than 5 years of age, tend to be more adversely affected and to have higher mortality rates (21,23).

The vulnerability of victims to waterborne diseases depends to a great extent on the preexisting levels of personal hygiene and sanitation (24). The fact that no major diarrheal epidemic occurred following South Florida's Hurricane Andrew in 1992 can be attributed to the fact that the population had an adequate supply of water, although it was nonpotable, and that the sewage system remained intact (8). By comparison, only 41% of the African population has easy access to safe water, and approximately 484 million people live in areas prone to flooding (5). Not surprisingly, the major waterborne outbreaks have occurred in regions where large populations have been displaced; where ample water for drinking, cooking, and personal hygiene has been inadequate; where water sources have become easily contaminated; and where establishment and maintenance of sanitation systems have been difficult or nonexistent.

The most drastic episode of waterborne disease mortality in recent history was that which occurred following the genocide in Rwanda in 1994. Between 500,000 and 1 million refugees suddenly flooded into the neighboring country of Zaire (now Democratic Republic of Congo) to create makeshift camps on the hard volcanic rock of the northern shore of Lake Kivu. With such a rapid influx into a poorly accommodating environment, no easy way was found for quickly purifying or transporting a large supply of water or for digging latrine pits. Thus, most refugees drank untreated water and secondarily contaminated the available surface water supply with fecal material. The rapid influx of large numbers of refugees coupled with a limited water supply meant that only 1 L of purified water was available per person per day (the recommended supply is 15 to 20 L per person per day). Over the course of the first month in Zaire, between 6% and 10% of the refugee population died, a crude mortality rate of 20 to 35 per 10,000 per day; of this, roughly 45% was from watery diarrhea, and 40% was from the bloody diarrhea that followed soon after. *V. cholerae* 01, biotype El Tor, and *S. dysenteriae* type 1 accounted for the watery and bloody diarrheas, respectively (25).

This devastating event highlights all the factors leading to a waterborne epidemic—lack of chlorination for untreated water sources, as well as the unavailability of other purification mechanisms; the lack of protection of water sources; the lack of designated areas for defecation; and inadequate water supply. The most significant factor in the magnitude of diarrheal outbreaks following disasters may be the large population displacement (7). This was the case for half a million Kurds who quickly fled Northern Iraq for Turkey in March 1991. They were forced into cold, rocky mountain passes where water, shelter, and food were scarce. Diarrheal illness accounted for more than 70% of the deaths, particularly for children under 5 years of age. In fact, two-thirds of the victims were children under 5 years of age; half of those were infants under 12 months of age. Despite the previously good health care, the diarrheal mortality was high due to the poor living conditions, including overcrowding, poor sanitation, and inadequate water supplies (23).

Damage to public water supplies and sewage systems can lead to the cross-contamination of water lines from sewage pipes if the two systems run in parallel, a scenario that could easily occur in an earthquake. Such breaks lead to a loss of water pressure that creates a vacuum into which pathogens from the broken sewer line can be drawn in. Over 2,800 cases of typhoid in Dushanbe, Tajikistan, were attributed to such a situation in early 1997 (26).

Well contamination caused watery diarrhea outbreaks in Khartoum, Sudan, during the floods of 1988. Following a flood in April 1994, nearly one-half of the population of a municipality in Finland was affected by Norwalk and rotavirus gastroenteritis from the backflow of a polluted river through a forgotten drainage pipe and into a groundwater well that served as a source of drinking water (27–29). Counties in Iowa where water facilities were affected during the Midwest floods of 1993 had an outbreak of acanthamoeba keratitis. Households that depended on well water had a protective odds ratio when compared to those who depended on municipal water sources (30). Leptospirosis, however, is the only well-documented disease that is directly transmitted through flood waters as opposed to contaminated water supplies (7).

Although waterborne diseases more typical occur after hurricanes, flooding, earthquakes, and complex emergencies, they may also be precipitated by volcanic disasters. In mid-June through early August of 1980, an outbreak of *Giardia lamblia* occurred in Red Lodge, Montana. Approximately 780 persons were affected, with an attack rate of 33%. The eruption of Mount St. Helen's in Washington in May of that year had blanketed the surrounding snow-covered mountains of Red Lodge, the source for the town's water supply, with a layer of heavy ash. The heat from the ash blanket along with a spell of warm weather caused a large water runoff from this unprotected watershed, which was known to harbor *G. lamblia,* that eventually found its way untreated and unfiltered into the town's water system (31).

As animal farming grows and requires more land area, the risk of an additional source of fecal contamination must be considered in the postdisaster phase. In 1999, Hurricane Floyd killed more than 2 million poultry and hogs in North Carolina. The state is home to industrial farming, in which large numbers of animals are kept in close quarters and their waste is kept in cesspools. Heavy rainfall and flooding overwhelmed the waste pits, causing the animal feces and urine to soak into the ground and flow into nearby rivers. In one rural county, 9% of the private wells were contaminated with fecal coliforms (32). Similarly, an outbreak of balantidiasis on the Pacific Island of Truk occurred from groundwater contaminated by pig feces following a 1971 typhoon (7).

Disruption in Other Public Health Programs and Infrastructure

Disruption in a region's routine vaccination programs could theoretically lead to a number of infectious disease outbreaks, including measles, polio, diphtheria, tuberculosis, and pertussis, particularly in areas where large numbers of displaced persons are crowded together. The elderly and immunocompromised may be at risk for pneumococcal disease where vaccination programs have been affected (33). Some African countries have lost 70% of their health network to civil war and armed conflict, and with this loss, the advances in controlling diseases and providing basic services have been virtually eliminated (5). Following 20 years of

civil war, Angola remains one of the few remaining polio reservoirs in the world. By 1999, nearly 90% of the polio victims in Angola were unvaccinated or only partially vaccinated internally displaced or refugee children (34).

That higher rates of infectious diseases are seen when routine preventive health services are disrupted is well known. Public health programs for the prevention of HIV and other sexually transmitted diseases (STDs) could be affected by disasters. A number of factors contribute to an increased HIV and STD risk, with an increase in the latter often being associated with an increase in the former. In refugee camps, prostitution often becomes a source of economy, particularly in prolonged conflicts. Camps have also been associated with higher rates of sexual assault, where rape has been increasingly used as a tool of warfare, as is evidenced in the Bosnia, Rwanda, and Kosovo conflicts. In the developing world, testing of blood products for HIV and hepatitis B may be inadequate due to the lack of reagent supplies, which increases the risks for transmission during conflicts or natural disasters where blood may be needed for transfusion (33). These are theoretical risks because transmission within displaced populations has not been well documented. Moreover, the lack of personal hygiene education can lead to outbreaks of trachoma, conjunctivitis, lice, tinea, pinworm, and scabies.

Direct Disaster-Induced Injuries

Injuries from the disaster itself can promote infection. Soft-tissue injuries from flying debris during tornadoes and hurricanes have led to secondary wound infections from a variety of organisms. Fermenting gram-negative bacilli, as well as anaerobes, *Staphylococcus, Pseudomonas,* and clostridia, have been noted (35).

Increases in Susceptibility to Endemic Organisms

Malnutrition

Malnutrition is associated with higher mortality rates from diarrheal illness, measles, malaria, and acute respiratory illness. On the other hand, measles and diarrheal illness can lead to malnutrition. This vicious cycle of infectious disease and malnutrition results in higher case fatality rates for these infectious diseases. In a survey of Rwandan refugee children in Goma, Zaire in 1994, 36% of children with dysentery were malnourished versus 12% of the children without recent dysentery for a relative risk of 2.89 (25).

Famine and decreased per-capita food production in general can result from natural disasters (e.g., extensive flooding, prolonged drought, or gradual change in climate) or armed conflicts. In fact, in conflict arenas such as Somalia, food procurement and distribution have been used as a weapon of war. In Africa, drought permanently threatens 460 million people (5). Such food scarcity leads to malnutrition, mass migration, and the consequential risk of such populations living for prolonged periods in refugee camps (36). During the conflict in Somalia in 1992, which occurred on the heels of a famine in 1991, measles, diarrhea and *Shigella* dysentery accounted for more than 80% of the deaths in one displaced persons camp, largely due to a breakdown in public health measures coupled with malnutrition. Acute malnutrition prevalence rates in displaced Somali children at that time ranged from 47% to 75% (37). Malnutrition and the contamination of scarce food supplies in camps place their populations at risk for diarrheal disease, especially the children who tend to have higher mortality rates than adults (38). Leftover millet gruel with curdled milk in several drought-affected villages in Mali resulted in over 1,700 cases of cholera in 1984 (39). Crude mortality rates of 20 to 30 times normal have occurred in refugee camps in the developing world (36). The widely accepted belief is that malnutrition enhances disease transmission, thus inflating crude mortality rates. For instance, among Kurdish refugee children from 12 to 23 months of age, a 13.5% rate of malnutrition was associated with a high incidence of diarrheal disease, particularly in that age group (20,23).

Effects of Mass Migration

Mass population movement is due primarily to war, famine, drought, or a combination of these factors. As was previously noted, such migration predisposes large numbers to overcrowding, inadequate sanitation, malnutrition, and diseases for which they may not be immune. The highest morbidity and mortality rates occur in the mass displacements of populations into areas of limited resources during the acute phase of a disaster. Measles, diarrheal illness, and acute upper respiratory infections have emerged as the most common causes of infectious disease–related deaths among refugee and internally displaced populations in the 1990s. Somalia and Rwanda provide the most poignant examples of large-scale mortality rates from infectious diseases in mass population displacements. In cases such as these, the crude death rate is inevitably higher in the refugee population than the baseline crude death rate of the host population. As was alluded to previously, children younger than 5 years of age have a disproportionately higher crude mortality rate from infectious diseases than older children and adults among displaced persons.

When groups with low disease-specific endemicity relocate to areas of high disease-specific endemicity, they put themselves at risk for diseases to which they are not immune. Leishmaniasis broke out in a southern Sudanese population when civil war caused them to relocate to areas around Khartoum, the capital (36). A similar episode in the same population occurred in 1994 when food shortages forced them northward again (40).

Disruption in Supply of Medications for Chronic Diseases

Disasters may interrupt treatment regimens in patients with diabetes mellitus, heart disease, renal disease, pulmonary disease, or immunocompromising diseases, leading to acute exacerbations of these ailments and further stressing the health care system. The Northridge, California, earthquake of 1994 disrupted the ambulatory care services in several hospitals and clinics. That, coupled with the fact that tens of thousands of residents were living outside their homes or in city parks and were unable to get to services, resulted in 15% of the surveyed households being unable to obtain necessary medications for chronic conditions (41).

Other Predisposing Factors

Any disaster-related event that may further compromise immune function adds to the risks of infectious diseases. Associated injuries, such as burns, cold exposures, crush injuries, and chemical or radiation exposures, can affect the immune system. Psychologic stress, moreover, can predispose the person to infectious diseases well into the recovery phase.

Introduction of New Organisms into the Disaster Environment

With the globalization of travel and the international nature of relief work, a theoretical risk exists for relief workers bringing infectious agents into the theater of operations. Such was the case of a malaria outbreak following the Colombia earthquake of 1983, in which the malaria was thought to be brought in from outside the area (33).

FIELD MANAGEMENT OF INFECTIOUS DISEASES

In assessing the risks of infectious disease susceptibility, Aghababian et al. break down the associated variables of risk into environmental and geographic considerations; endemic organisms; population characteristics; disaster type and magnitude; and the amount of resources available before, during, and after the disaster (33). Environmental considerations include the climate at the time of the year of the disaster and the degree of geographic isolation. The presence of certain organisms or vectors may vary, depending on the season of the disaster. During cold seasons or in cold climates, displaced persons may crowd together for warmth, thus increasing the risks of airborne diseases. Characteristics of the population may determine risk—if the affected population is composed of more elderly or the very young, a greater likelihood of infectious diseases is seen. The nature of the disaster itself may help determine the types of infectious diseases occurring. Because earthquakes have a risk of crush injury, soft-tissue infections may follow. Floods cause the disruptions of water and sanitation systems, and, therefore, they are more likely to lead to waterborne and vector-borne outbreaks. Famines and refugee-generating armed conflicts lend themselves to airborne and waterborne diseases. Finally, the availability and accessibility of resources help determine infectious disease risk. Are medical facilities disrupted? Are supply lines and transportation mechanisms intact? Is the health care system familiar with the World Health Organization essential medication list, and are medications, water, sanitary facilities, and personal items stockpiled? Is the facility storing supplies still intact? Are local, in-country trained personnel available to instruct survivors on hygiene, utilization of potable water supplies, and the maintenance of sanitary facilities? Answers to these questions will help provide an overview of what is needed during the acute phase of the disaster to prevent outbreaks.

Prevention

The first priorities in preventing infectious disease outbreaks should be repairing the point of breakdown in the public health infrastructure, conducting a rapid needs assessment, and establishing an active surveillance mechanism. Relief providers should focus on adequate shelter, water, sanitation, food, and surveillance. Some international and non-governmental relief agencies have published field manuals that are useful in establishing relief priorities.

Surveillance

In the aftermath of the November 1980 earthquake that measured 6.8 on the Richter scale and killed 3,000, injured 8,000, and left 270,000 homeless in the southern Italian regions of Campania and Basilicata, health officials rapidly established a national epidemiologic surveillance system. Despite extensive damage to the water supply and sewage facilities, no significant increase in deaths from gastroenteric or respiratory causes occurred versus the same time in a nondisaster year; this was attributable in part to a system that had been established to recognize such cases (42). By definition, surveillance is the "ongoing, systematic collection, analysis, and interpretation of health data" (43). Such a system is effective if it is achieved in a timely, simple, universally understood, accurate, and sustainable way.

Surveillance is useful when the need for rapid investigation and confirmation of a disease exists. Such data help guide resources to specific locations and for specific dis-

eases, thereby preventing the waste of resources on programs, medications, and equipment that may not be needed. Surveillance of the host and vectors of certain diseases may be helpful in deciding whether massive public health undertakings are warranted in the postdisaster phase. One such example was the Midwest floods of 1993. Although the postflood environmental conditions favored an increase in the population of the St. Louis encephalitis vector *Culex pipiens,* a mosquito endemic to the area, no increase was noted. Investigators monitoring the wild bird and mosquito population were able to call off an expensive and potentially environmentally damaging insecticide spraying program (44). Documenting diseases that do not occur, as well as those that do, can also be of benefit, especially for dispelling rumors and fears of disease outbreak generated in the media or among health care providers.

Surveillance should be coordinated by a single agency whose primary responsibility is the regular collation and feedback of data from all agencies participating in the relief effort, including state, federal, non-governmental, or international organizations. Data and/or records at points of contact with patients in the field should be routinely collected, shared, collated, and disseminated at regular meetings among various relief organizations to discuss potential outbreaks based on surveillance methods. All agencies should use a standardized form and should report cases based on simple symptom-oriented case definitions (discussed below). Knowledge of the endemic diseases and vectors of the surrounding area in which the disaster or complex emergency takes place provides a baseline for the evaluation of the effectiveness of surveillance measures in the shelter or refugee camp. This includes the knowledge of local predisaster epidemiologic statistics, such as crude mortality rates, under age 5 mortality rates, cause-specific fatality rates, and case fatality rates, as well as the overall population of the disaster-affected area, shelter, or refugee camp. Surveyors should be aware that deaths tend to be underreported and that the population size is often exaggerated, thus underestimating mortality rates in general (9). Once an epidemic has been identified by a surveillance mechanism, a method for communicating the appropriate public health measures should be instituted. Surveillance should last well into the postdisaster phase as outbreaks may be more likely to occur then (45).

Vaccines

Vaccination programs should be coordinated with the local Expanded Program on Immunizations, a World Health Organization program usually administered by a country's health ministry. In general, vaccines give more protection at lower costs. In the acute emergency phase, a measles immunization is the only vaccine necessary, especially for young children in areas with low baseline immunization rates. For children older than 9 months, vitamin A should be given simultaneously, because it can decrease mortality by 30% to 50% (43). Measles vaccines should be provided with cold chain equipment, training protocols, and management manuals. If surveillance reveals a laboratory-confirmed case of meningococcal meningitis, particularly in areas where such epidemics have occurred, a vaccination program is warranted at the onset of the epidemic, especially for family and close community contacts. For diseases like typhoid and cholera that require multiple vaccinations to provide adequate immunity, a mass vaccination program is not warranted because the period of greatest danger of contracting the disease would occur well before the serial injections could be given. Tetanus is a concern in disasters that produce fractures and lacerations, such as earthquakes and floods. Routine tetanus vaccination for those with such injuries would be expected. However, no need exists for a mass vaccination program; rather, vaccination should be given to those with injuries. Tetanus immune globulin should be given to those without a history of vaccination, as well as to those with highly contaminated wounds.

Shelters

Flooding in the northern Chinese province of Heilongjiang in 1998 left more than 1 million homeless. A United Nations Disaster Assessment and Coordination Team credited the lack of an epidemic to the fact that no more than 400 displaced persons were living together in any one location (4).

In the 1980 southern Italian earthquake mentioned previously, the displaced population was dispersed to encampments, both abroad and elsewhere in Italy, which likely diminished the infectious disease risk (42). A positive correlation has been shown between child mortality rates and the size of a refugee camp (12,46). Therefore, the reasonable conclusion is that limiting the sizes of refugee camps or a shelter population could be beneficial in reducing the spread of person-to-person disease.

Water and Sanitation

Time and again the shortage of water for drinking, cooking, and hygiene has been shown to be more significant for disease development than the presence of contamination. In other words, the quantity of water may be more significant than the quality in determining the risk for diarrheal disease outbreaks. When the water supply to Sarajevo was reduced to 5 L per person per day during the seige of 1994, increases in hepatitis A, diarrhea, and dysentery were noted. (7).

An inadequate supply of water leads to poor personal hygiene. The United Nations High Commissioner for Refugees recommends 20 L per person per day, although no scientific study has proven the value of this figure. Potable supplies should be obtained as soon as possible with the chlorination of untreated sources and the protection of existing clean sources. Protected water supplies and closed latrines were instrumental in decreasing cholera rates in Bangladeshi refugee camps (47).

Providing latrines is the most important environmental intervention for reducing the incidence of diarrhea and thus limiting the under-5-years-of-age and infant mortality rates (26). Various options exist for managing human excreta. Defecation fields, although they are the most primitive means, can be constructed quickly. Latrines for communal use are better, especially if enough latrines are provided for group or individual family use. Education on the use and maintenance of sanitary facilities is crucial for disease prevention. Children in particular must be taught how to use latrine facilities.

The ongoing evaluation and surveillance of water supply and sanitation facilities should be emphasized. In the Northern China floods of 1998, central and provincial governments were constantly monitoring the quality of drinking water, and no diarrheal outbreaks occurred. Moving to areas more amenable for accessing potable water and making an allowance for effective means of sanitation decreased the diarrheal mortality rate among the Kurdish population in 1991 (23).

Other Public Health Concerns

Breastfeeding should be encouraged during disaster periods to provide enhanced immunity for infants. Food and nutrition programs, ongoing tuberculosis therapies (directly observed therapy), and vector control should be restarted as early as possible, although this may be difficult during prolonged courses of armed conflict. Vector control should be aimed at those disease vectors endemic in the disaster area. Preventing malnutrition by providing a minimum of 1,200 to 1,500 calories daily with sufficient amounts of protein will also help prevent epidemics.

Diagnosis and Management

Toole et al. recommend that, if an outbreak is suspected, a logical chain of events must ensue. First, immediate investigation and confirmation of cases using case definitions should occur, followed by the identification of the mode of transmission, active case finding and treatment, and implementation of control measures (3).

Standardized Case Definitions

In general, health providers should recognize syndromes or a cluster of symptoms unique to measles, upper respiratory infections, diarrheal illnesses, meningitis, and malaria. Fever, cough, mouth sores, and rash could raise the suspicion of measles in an endemic area with poor immunization levels; rice-water stools with or without vomiting in a child under 5 years of age may signify cholera in an area where an epidemic is present. *Shigella* should be suspected with painful bloody stools and fever. Cough with fever indicates an upper respiratory infection and possible pneumonia. Signs of meningeal irritation with fever, especially in the presence of a purpuric rash, signal meningitis.

Field Laboratories

Laboratory confirmation of every case is not always necessary, especially if the case load is high and the resources are limited. In such situations, laboratory tests should be used to establish the presence of the disease of interest and to monitor its control, while relying on the standardized case definitions to make the diagnoses for all others. Meningitis, malaria, cholera, bacillary dysentery, and typhoid should all have laboratory confirmation at least of sentinel cases.

Deployable field laboratories can generally perform blood smears, gram stains, bacterial antigen detection, cultures, and antibiotic sensitivities. Blood samples may be sent to the Centers for Disease Control and Prevention for serologic confirmation. Routine laboratory tests, such as a complete blood cell count, are not useful in a field setting when attempting to diagnose an infectious disease. Traditionally, cultures have been the test of choice, although latex agglutination has been found to be better than a gram stain and as effective as culture for meningitis (48).

Principles of Treatment

Standardized treatment protocols should be given to health care providers along with a demographic questionnaire that highlights the historical and clinical data of individual cases.

Oral rehydration therapy is the mainstay of treatment for diarrheal illness, with intravenous hydration being used for severe cases or for those unable to take oral rehydration. Despite the fact that *S. dysenteriae* type 1 and *V. cholerae* are endemic to coastal Bangladesh, an aggressive program of oral rehydration therapy education probably kept inpatient hospital admissions for diarrheal diseases low following the devastating cyclone of April 1991 (39). Patients often need encouragement to rehydrate; in the field, designated rehydration tents or wards can be set up. The focus particularly should be on children in whom early recognition and therapy can be lifesaving. In the face of increasing resistance to sulfonamides, bacillary dysenteries should be treated with fluoroquinolones and cholera, with doxycycline (adults) or trimethoprim/sulfamethoxazole (children). An outbreak of diarrheal illness should prompt the early chlorination of water supplies.

Measles outbreaks should prompt health care providers to assess the levels of nutrition, vitamin A supplementation, and immunization coverage. Cases should be observed for the development of laryngotracheobronchitis, pneumonia, and dehydration.

Because chemotherapy resistance for malaria is variable across the world, the treatment should be based on local chemosensitivity. Emphasis should be on prevention for populations that are exposed to mosquitos, including long-sleeved shirts, long pants, insect repellents, bednets, and chemoprophylaxis. Complications include cerebral malaria, renal failure, and hemolysis.

Meningitis, which is considered an epidemic when 15 cases per 100,000 persons per week are seen, remains the most feared outbreak in a disaster population. Cases should be treated empirically in separate, specialized wards, if necessary. In displaced populations where the entire shelter or camp is in close contact with others, mass chemoprophylaxis is not feasible. In such environments, mass immunization may be the most effective means of prevention, but this is indicated only if an epidemic is impending and either group A or C serotypes is identified. With vaccinations, however, the immunity duration is short, particularly in young children, and it does not prevent the transmission of the organism by carrier individuals. Household contacts of confirmed cases should be checked for immunity, and they should be given a vaccination as necessary. Recovering patients and household contacts of a confirmed case should be given rifampicin to eliminate carriage and to prevent transmission, respectively.

Other diseases requiring antimicrobials include the pneumonias, STDs, skin infections, and tuberculosis, with the latter requiring at least 12 months of undisrupted therapy, which potentially is a problem in a disaster or conflict setting.

ROLE OF EMERGENCY DEPARTMENTS

Emergency departments (EDs) and clinics that survive the initial disaster can act as surveillance mechanisms because they are on the front line for presentations that hint at possible infectious disease epidemics and they may be the only surviving source of health care. EDs can readily keep records of outpatient visits, presenting complaints, and inpatient admissions. Data on age, sex, location, suspected diagnosis, number of admissions, and bed utilization can be useful. These records can be compiled weekly and can then be analyzed by a simple statistical program such as EPI-INFO.

Clinicians, EMS personnel, and nurses should be familiar with symptom complexes that define disaster-related illness and should be prepared for outbreaks by mobilizing equipment and familiarizing themselves with treatment protocols and protective measures. Transfer mechanisms to predesignated higher levels of care should be in place.

SPECIAL CONSIDERATIONS

Iraq's alleged use of biologic weapons against the Kurds following the Persian Gulf War in 1991 brought the specter of biologic weapons to the forefront of planning for federal management agencies and emergency personnel. Anthrax, botulinum toxin, plague, and smallpox are the most likely agents to be used, according to some bioweapons experts (49).

Most first-line physicians would not be able to rapidly make a diagnosis of infection with these agents since they are easily confused with other more common viral syndromes. Anthrax, for instance, presents with nonspecific symptoms such as fever, cough, and headache; smallpox, with fevers and myalgias. Emergency physicians should familiarize themselves with biologic agents and the symptoms associated with exposure to them (see Chapter 34 for a discussion on biowarfare agents).

REFERENCES

1. Disaster epidemiology. *Lancet* 1990;336:845.
2. Howard MJ, Brillman JC, Burkle FM. Infectious disease emergencies in disasters. *Emerg Med Clin North Am* 1996;14: 413–428.
3. Toole MJ. Communicable disease epidemiology following disasters. *Ann Emerg Med* 1992;21:418–420.
4. Beach M. China's problems persist after the flood. *Lancet* 1998;352:1203.
5. Loretti A, Tegegn Y. Disasters in Africa: old and new hazards and growing vulnerability. *World Health Stat Q* 1996;49:179.
6. Surmieda MR, Lopez JM, Abad-Viola G, et al. Surveillance in evacuation camps after the eruption of Mt. Pinatubo, Philippines. *MMWR* 1992;41:9.
7. Toole MJ. Communicable diseases and disease control. In: Noji EK, ed. *The public health consequences of disasters*. New York: Oxford University Press, 1997:79.
8. Lee LE, Fonseca V, Brett KM, et al. Active morbidity surveillance after Hurricane Andrew—Florida, 1992. *JAMA* 1993;270: 591–594.
9. Toole MJ, Waldman RJ. Prevention of excess mortality in refugee and displaced populations in developing countries. *JAMA* 1990; 263:3296–3302.
10. Centers for Disease Control. Surveillance in evacuation camps after the eruption of Mount Pinatubo, Philippines. *MMWR* 1992;41:9.
11. Moore PS, Toole MJ, Nieburg P, et al. Surveillance and control of meningococcal meningitis epidemics in refugee populations. *Bull World Health Organ* 1990;68:587.
12. Cosgrave J. Refugee density and dependence: practical implications of camp size. *Disasters* 1996;20:261–270.
13. Toole MJ, Galson S, Brady W. Are war and public health compatible? *Lancet* 1993;341:1193–1196.
14. Mason J, Cavalie P. Malaria epidemic in Haiti following a hurricane. *Am J Trop Med Hyg* 1965;14:533.
15. Woodward A. Doctoring the planet: health effects of global change. *Aust N Z J Med* 1995;25:46–53.
16. Patz JA, Epstein PR, Burke TA, et al. Global climate change and emerging infectious diseases. *JAMA* 1996;275:217–223.
17. Brillman JC, Sklar DP, Davis KD, et al. Hantavirus: emergency department response to a disaster from an emerging pathogen. *Ann Emerg Med* 1994;24:429–436.
18. Allan R, Nam S, Doull L. MERLIN and malaria epidemic in northeast Kenya. *Lancet* 1998;351:1966–1967.
19. Schneider E, Hajjeh RA, Spiegel RA, et al. A coccidioidomycosis outbreak following the Northridge, California earthquake. *JAMA* 1997;277:904–908.
20. Toole MJ, Waldman RJ. Refugees and displaced persons: war, hunger, and public health. *JAMA* 1993;270:600–605.
21. Swerdlow DL, Malenga G, Begkoyian G, et al. Epidemic cholera among refugees in Malawi, Africa: treatment and transmission. *Epidemiol Infect* 1997;118:207–214.
22. Siddique AK, Baqui AH, Eusof A, et al. 1988 floods in Bangladesh: patterns of illness and causes of death. *J Diarrhoeal Dis Res* 1991;9:310–314.
23. Yip R, Sharp TW. Acute malnutrition and high childhood mortality related to diarrhea: lessons from the 1991 Kurdish refugee crisis. *JAMA* 1993;270:587–590.
24. World Health Organization. The risk of disease outbreaks after natural disasters. *WHO Chronicle* 1979;33:214–216.
25. Goma Epidemiology Group. Public health impact of Rwandan refugee crisis: what happened in Goma, Zaire, in July, 1994? *Lancet* 1995;345:339–344.
26. Roberts L. Personal correspondence. January, 1998.
27. Kukkula M, Arstila P, Klossner ML, et al. Waterborne outbreak of viral gastroenteritis. *Scand J Inf Dis* 1997;29:415–418.
28. Crytpo
29. Kukkula M, Arstila P, Klossner ML, et al. Waterborne outbreak of viral gastroenteritis. *Scand J Inf Dis* 1997;29:415.
30. Meier PA, Mathers WD, Sutphin JE, et al. An epidemic of presumed acanthamoeba keratitis that followed regional flooding: results of a case-control investigation. *Arch Ophthalmol* 1998; 116:1090–1094.
31. Weniger BG, Blaser MJ, Gedrose J, et al. An outbreak of waterborne Giardiasis associated with heavy water runoff due to warm weather and volcanic ashfall. *Am J Pub Health* 1983; 73:868–872.
32. Kilborn PT. Storm highlights flaws in farm law in North Carolina. *New York Times* October 17, 1999.
33. Aghababian RV, Teuscher J. Infectious diseases following major disasters. *Ann Emerg Med* 1992;21:362–367.
34. International Medical Corps survey, 1999.
35. Brenner SA, Noji EK. Wound infections after tornados [Letter]. *J Trauma* 1992;33:643.
36. Shears P. Epidemiology and infection in famine and disasters. *Epidemiol Infect* 1991;107:241–251.
37. Moore PS, Marfin AA, Quenemoen LE, et al. Mortality rates in displaced and resident populations of central Somalia during 1992 famine. *Lancet* 1993;341:935–938.
38. Centers for Disease Control. Famine affected, refugee, and displaced populations: recommendations for public health issues. *MMWR* 1992;41:1.
39. Tauxe RV, Holmberg SD, Dodin A, et al. Epidemic cholera in Mali: high mortality and multiple routes of transmission in a famine area. *Epidemiol Infect* 1988;100:279–289.
40. Mercer A, Seaman J, Sondorp E. Kala azar in eastern upper Nile province, southern Sudan. *Lancet* 1995;345:187–188.
41. Frankel DH. Public health assessment after earthquake. *Lancet* 1994;343:347.
42. Alexander D. Disease epidemiology and earthquake disaster: the example of southern Italy after the 23 November, 1980 earthquake. *Soc Sci Med* 1982;16:1959–1969.

43. The Center of Excellence in Disaster Management and Humanitarian Assistance. *Combined Humanitarian Assistance Response Training*. Honolulu, February 2000.

44. Cotton P. Health threat from mosquitoes rises as flood of the century finally recedes. *JAMA* 1993;270:685–686.

45. Bissell RA. Delayed-impact infectious disease after a natural disaster. *J Emerg Med* 1983;1:59–66.

46. Mercer A. Mortality and morbidity in refugee camps in Eastern Sudan: 1985-1990. *Disasters* 1992;16:28.

47. Khan MU, Shahidullah MD. Role of water and sanitation in the incidence of cholera in refugee camps. *Trans R Soc Trop Med Hyg* 1982;76:373–377.

48. Heyman SN, Ginosar Y, Niel L, et al. Meningococcal meningitis among Rwandan refugees: diagnosis, management, and outcome in a field hospital. *Int J Infect Dis* 1998;2:137–142.

49. Henderson, DA. The looming threat of bioterrorism. *Science* 1999;283:1279–1282.

50. Toole MJ, Steketee RW, Waldman RJ, et al. Measles prevention and control in emergency settings. *Bull World Health Organ* 1989;67:381–388.

51. de Ville de Goyet C, Lechat MF. Health aspects in natural disasters. *Trop Doct* 1976;6:152–157.

52. Bennish ML, Ronsman C. Health and nutritional consequences of the 1991 Bangladesh cyclone. *Nutr Rev* 1992;50:102–105.

PHARMACEUTICALS IN DISASTERS

ELIZABETH LACY

Pharmaceutical supplies are essential in the medical care of disaster victims. Relatively little prospective information addresses the medication needs, uses, and problems in disasters. However, reports in the literature do demonstrate recurrent trends regarding pharmaceutical supplies during disaster response (1). Experiences after hurricanes, earthquakes, and volcanoes, as well as those with large relief efforts in Eastern Europe, the former Soviet Union, Africa, and South America, consistently identify recurring needs and problems. Those problems suggest the need for guidelines for pharmaceutical agents in disaster relief. As more research into disasters is done, patterns that have the ability to predict more precisely pharmaceutical needs and utilization will be detected. This data may be used to develop models to guide effective disaster planning and relief efforts (2–5).

A comparison of the requested supplies with the lists of needs from previous disasters will assist in the verification of needs and the coordination of response. These lists are available from relief agencies such as The Red Cross and Red Crescent societies. In addition, the World Health Organization (WHO) and donor countries have compiled essential drug lists (6). An example of the essential drug list developed by WHO is provided in Appendix A. Predeployment disaster assessment leads to a time lag in receiving supplies, but it does result in more efficient cost control and better quality of the overall relief effort (5,7,8). As improved methods of rapid, systematic, and accurate disaster assessment are developed, a targeted supply distribution will enhance disaster response and will improve morbidity and mortality (4,5).

MANAGEMENT OF PHARMACEUTICAL DONATIONS

Pharmaceutical agents are a key part of any disaster response; however, management of these agents can occupy a significant number of disaster response personnel. Recurrent problems have been identified, and solutions have been outlined. Therefore, general guidelines for pharmaceutical donations have been identified by WHO, and these are presented in Table 5.1.

Volume of Pharmaceutical Agents

The massive scale on which pharmaceutical donations arrive is staggering, and it commonly overwhelms relief workers. Sixteen days following the 1976 Guatemalan earthquake, over 100 tons of supplies in 7,000 cartons of various sizes arrived. This required 40 students, supervised by three pharmacists, to spend an estimated 1,120 hours sorting and classifying drugs; meanwhile, more shipments continued to arrive (7).

In the aftermath of the Armenian earthquake on December 7, 1988, over 5,000 tons of drugs and medical supplies were donated to the region. The local storage capacity was quickly overwhelmed. Even with the erection of 32 new warehouses, only 70% of the donations could be regionally housed. By January 1989, donated supplies were being shipped to Moscow for storage. Fifty people took over 6 months to review the drugs before they were able to gain a reasonable idea of what was sent to Armenia after the earthquake (9). From 1992 to mid 1996, between 27,800 and 34,800 metric tons of drugs and medical supplies were donated to Bosnia and Herzegovina; from 50% to 60% or 13,900 to 20,900 tons of these drugs were considered inappropriate (10).

TABLE 5.1. PHARMACEUTICAL DONATION GUIDELINES

No drug should be sent without a specific request or prior clearance by the receiving nation.

No drug should be sent that is not on the list of essential drugs of the receiving nation (or if not available) on the WHO list of essential drugs.

No drug should arrive with a future life (before expiration date) of less than 1 yr.

Labeling of the drug should be in the appropriate language(s) and should contain the generic name, strength, name of the manufacturer, and expiration date.

Labeling on the outside of the package should contain the same information as above, plus the total quantity of drugs in the package.

Abbreviation: WHO, World Health Organization.

The overwhelming quantity of donations, which are often unsolicited and unsorted, may become such a problem that it has been referred to as the second disaster (8). Recent trends suggest that donation response to international disasters may be on the rise, with donated supplies reaching 100 tons after the 1976 Guatemala earthquake, 383 tons following the 1985 Mexico City earthquake, and over 5,000 tons for the 1988 Armenian earthquake. This trend makes disaster assessment increasingly important for efficient relief efforts.

Sorted and Unsorted Agents

Drugs brought into disaster zones arrive as either sorted or unsorted donations. Sorted drugs are those that are marked in a manner that makes them immediately identifiable. These include those arriving in cartons containing multiple contents or single-use items. Unsorted donations contain a mixture of items without a label identifying the contents (7). They represent a significant problem for disaster relief workers. In the early medical relief efforts after the Armenian earthquake, health care providers spent nearly two-thirds of their time looking for and properly identifying useful medications. Only 20% of drugs arriving were sorted and identifiable (9). Following the 1976 Guatemala earthquake, only about 10% of donated drugs were sorted. By the 1988 Armenian earthquake, up to 70% of donations were sorted (7,9). Even with a decrease in the percentage of unsorted donations, the presence of random items severely impairs relief efforts. Unsorted donations consume personnel resources that may already be in short supply following a disaster. They interfere with disaster relief by competing for resources that are better directed toward more critical activities.

Drug Dumping

Publicity following major disasters leads to a frenzy of donation activity that is often inappropriate and that creates many secondary problems for recipients on scene. In part, this phenomenon is fueled by the idea that any supply or drug is better than none. In addition, most donors believe these donations will find a use in a disaster zone, no matter what is sent. Most donations are well intended; however, in some circumstances, donors have been accused of drug dumping.

Drug dumping is the donation of useless or unusable medicines. The volume of these drugs can be impressive and can impose new problems on the recipients. From 1983 to 1987, Sudan dealt with an estimated 8 million tablets of expired chloroquine and 500,000 tablets of piperazine. One unannounced shipment to Georgia in 1994 contained 20 tons of expired silver sulfadiazine ointment that took months to incinerate (11). Other examples of this continued practice are found in Bosnia and Herzegovina; these included army medical supplies from World War II, plaster tapes dated 1961, and dapsone for leprosy treatment, a disease not found in the region (10).

Benefits to the dumpers can be substantial; they include decreased risks and costs associated with storage, substantial tax deductions, and the avoidance of destruction cost, which is estimated at $2,000 United States dollars per ton. Bosnia and Herzegovina received an estimated 17,000 tons of unusable medication. Even after deductions for transport cost to the region, the donors may have saved $25.5 million, while creating a problem that cost the recipients $34 million for the destruction of the agents (10).

Recipients must deal with costs of health and environmental hazards, storage, handling, sorting, managing, and destruction of useless medicines (10). In addition, they may have to deal with the ramifications of having banned, illegal, or nonregistered substances in their country. Donors following the WHO guidelines in Bosnia-Herzegovina were found to have a lower percentage of donations that were perceived as inappropriate (5%) than did the other donors (10).

Logistics

The packaging and transport of donations can become a problem, even with solicited, sorted supplies. Pharmaceutical agents are often shipped in packages weighing hundreds of pounds that are too large to be easily handled. This difficulty may be particularly important during a disaster when transportation routes and handling equipment may be suboptimal (8). Small packages that can be transported by one or two persons are recommended (9). The WHO guidelines for drug donations specify 50 kg as the upper limit for individual carton weight (6). Donations of transportable storage facilities and logistical equipment are another important consideration during a large-scale response because local resources may be rapidly saturated (9).

Drugs may be delivered as prepackaged kits, such as those based on the WHO model list of essential drugs, or as loose individual products. Recent reports from experiences with these kits from Bosnia-Herzegovina and Croatia are conflicting. A WHO evaluation concluded that recipients in this region preferred the kits, while another study of hospitals found that only 14% preferred kits and 70% preferred loose supplies (12). Comments from this survey regarding kits addressed the issue of discrepancy between the contents and the quantities of kits meeting actual needs. Some kit items were not needed, and thus they had to be stockpiled or wasted, while others were not adequately supplied. The benefits of kits included the ability to prepackage and store kits for multiple uses, the easier operational handling, and the lower expenses than those associated with custom-tailored deliveries (12).

Packaging

Poorly packaged and improperly labeled shipments may be contaminated or ruined. Pharmaceutical packages should be labeled with field conditions in mind. Supplies may have to endure the elements, and they may not be stored in the controlled conditions recommended. Weather-resistant labels in the local language, generic names, dosage form, quantities, expiration date, batch number, and special storage conditions should be listed. International coding (green for medical supplies and equipment, red for food, blue for clothing) should be used whenever possible (6,9,18). WHO guidelines state that drug packages should not be intermingled with other supplies (6). Occasionally, overpackaging is a problem. Hammers and screwdrivers should be adequate tools for opening packages; otherwise, the contents may be impervious to use (8).

Expiration of Pharmaceutical Agents

Expired or soon-to-expire drugs are repeatedly seen in large international relief missions (7,9). Several problems exist when considering the use of outdated drugs. Some drugs are not safe when expired. One notable drug in this category is tetracycline, which may result in nephrotoxicity. Expired products are widely regarded as therapeutically useless and possibly dangerous, and they create a sorting and disposal problem for people on scene at disaster sites.

In Armenia, 8% (40 tons) of the medications donated were past their expiration dates. One estimate found 12 tons of unnecessary or expired donations warehoused in Georgia. Nine tons expired before or within 3 months of arrival (11). United States pharmacists are taught that most drugs are safe and only slightly less potent beyond their expiration dates. The percentage of active compound remaining per unit of time beyond the expiration date is information that is not commonly available from pharmaceutical manufacturers. If this information were more commonly available, standard procedures could be developed for the use of donated pharmaceutical agents during disasters. Current WHO and Pan American Health Organization (PAHO) guidelines forbid the sending of expired or soon-to-expire pharmaceutical agents to a disaster zone.

Pharmaceutical Storage

Drug stability and storage requirements are issues that need to be addressed when considering drugs for use in disasters. Donated supplies often must endure the elements, and they generally are not stored in the recommended climate-controlled conditions (8). After the Armenian earthquake, an estimated 4% of pharmaceutical agents, mostly intravenous fluids, vaccines, and injectables, were improperly deemed spoiled by the local health care providers upon arrival because of freezing in transport (9). No detailed information regarding the types of pharmaceutical agents destroyed in Armenia was available. While frozen storage with thawing before use is commonly practiced with certain pharmaceutical agents in United States hospitals, multiple freeze-thaw cycles are unacceptable for many drugs. Frozen stability information is readily available. Perhaps with more education or more easily available information, some of these materials could have been salvaged.

The extreme humidity of tropical countries may alter pharmaceutical stability. Packing with desiccants is recommended for shipments bound for these regions (8). Biologic products, such as insulin and some vaccines, do not tolerate temperature extremes or vigorous shaking motions without decomposition. Pharmaceutical stability should be considered by disaster planners and donors.

Identification of Pharmaceutical Agents

The identification of drugs is essential to their usefulness in a disaster. Proper packaging will help ensure that the labels remain on the items and that they are not defaced or damaged beyond recognition. Language can be a common barrier in identifying what drugs are on hand. Drug shipments labeled in French, which was not a locally spoken language, that arrived in Sudan caused sorting difficulties (13). After the Armenian earthquake, none of the boxes of donated medical supplies were written in the local language, and very few were even written in Russian. Antibiotics with at least 238 different names labeled in 21 languages were on hand. Only one-third were legible with the inclusion of the generic names (9). Moreover, 70% of the items were labeled with the brand or trade name only. Trade names for the same chemical entities often vary by country. Identifying a medication and its usage, among the thousands of products available, each with multiple names, was a tremendously difficult task that was further compounded by the fact that untrained persons did much of the sorting (9).

Donations should be labeled and sorted according to the category of use (7). Pharmaceutical textbooks such as the *Martindale cross-referencing international trade names* were invaluable in Armenia, and they will help to facilitate the usage of international donations in future disasters as well (9). The identification of proper drug indications is essential for appropriate use, and, when it is lacking, patients may be harmed. For example, a donated veterinary anti-helmintic medication was mistaken for an endometriosis treatment, and 11 Lithuanian woman were temporarily blinded in 1992 (6). In Bangladesh, following a cyclone in 1991, the oversupply of metronidazole was thought to contribute to its use for the widespread, inappropriate treatment of some diarrheal illnesses (14). Appropriate references or readable product package inserts should accompany international donations. Some agencies have advocated that reference works, such as the *AHFS drug information*, which is updated annually, be included in each box of pharmaceutical supplies, especially in packages bound for areas that may not be as familiar with Western products and terminology (15). Pharmaceutical agents cannot be used to help the intended disaster victims if they cannot be accurately identified in a timely manner.

DETERMINING PHARMACEUTICAL NEEDS

Several factors influence the pharmaceutical needs of a disaster-stricken area. The type and phase of the disaster often dictate what medicines are needed. Epidemiologic patterns of diseases of the region in crisis and common sense as to the relevance of pharmaceutical supplies being sent to a disaster must also be considered to meet needs while avoiding waste. The local level of health care and standard treatments should be considered. Conditions influencing or enhancing communicable diseases are also important considerations. Any assessment data or requests from the recipient regarding needs should be strongly considered. The combination of the previous factors in decision-making will lead to improved response and relief efforts.

Hazardous materials are a potential problem during disasters. Hazardous material teams may be a valuable resource for planning, decontamination, and treatment in such situations. Ideally, known antidotes, treatments, and protective agents should be stockpiled in advance. This need for advance placement was demonstrated during the 1979 accident at the Metropolitan Edison nuclear generating station at Three Mile Island. The threat of a large volume release of highly radioactive fission products, including iodine-131, sent federal agencies scrambling to provide emergency assistance. Providing enough potassium iodide for a 10-day supply for 250,000 families in the area took 72 hours, over $400,000, the Food and Drug Administration's (FDA) Bureau of Drugs, two midwestern drug companies, an east coast bottle dropper manufacturer, two state police forces, the Pennsylvania Health Department, the Nuclear Regulatory Commission, and Department of Defense (16).

Immediately following the impact of a disaster, each city must depend on its own resources. International or large-scale domestic relief takes a minimum of 24 to 72 hours for organization, transport, and distribution to the disaster site. Usually drugs sent for the rescue phase of a disaster do not arrive until days to months after the recovery period begins (7–9). Blood and plasma products from outside sources usually arrive too late (7). Even very rapid aid from outside the disaster zone will have a minimal effect on early deaths and casualties (5). The local or regional area must supply the pharmaceutical agents that are used for the rescue phase of most disasters. Disasters in more populated, developed regions usually do not overwhelm the regional supplies for the rescue phase. In fact, no country in either of the American hemispheres is likely to run short of all essential pharmaceutical agents early in a disaster response. However, assessment, communications, and distribution logistics are still barriers to immediate medical care. When disasters are large enough to require outside assistance, the needs are usually for primary care medicines (17).

In the recovery phase of a disaster, victims may have difficulty accessing physicians and pharmaceutical services for ongoing medical care due to the loss of the medical infrastructure. At the same time, pharmacists and physicians may not have access to patients' medical records. Primary care of acute and chronic conditions is the mainstay of health care relief efforts during the recovery phase of any type of disaster (17–19). Endemic illnesses unique to each region should be considered when planning or requesting pharmaceutical agents (7). Epidemiologic surveillance programs will assist in fine-tuning the need for specific pharmaceutical agents. Such a survey 2 months after Hurricane Georges in the Dominican Republic resulted in improved nutritional support and medical treatment for persons in shelters (20).

Examples of drugs being sent to the stricken region even though they are epidemiologically inappropriate are common. Chloroquine and metrifonate were sent to Armenia in 1988 following the earthquake, even though malaria is not endemic to this region. Eleven percent (550 tons) of medicines sent to Armenia were found to be useless, while another 21% (1,050 tons) were not useful for the recovery phase (9).

Often, the drugs sent are not indicated for the particular medical problems generated by the disaster. Pharmaceutical agents that are often found to be unnecessary in disaster response include vitamin preparations, inappropriate immunizations, and nasal sprays. X-ray preparations were shipped to the southern part of Sudan in spite of the fact that x-ray machines are not available. Monoamine oxidase inhibitors sent to the same region interact with the staple diet in Sudan, which includes various beans and fermented maize; and few there had any use for contact lens solution. Antihyperlipidemics and appetite stimulants were not applicable to the starving victims' needs (6,13). General medical and chronic care pharmaceutical agents are the mainstay of such relief efforts (17–19).

Most disasters are not followed by an increased incidence of infectious diseases. Experience has shown that public health measures are more effective than massive postdisaster immunization in limiting disease (5,21). In general, infectious diseases are not likely during the initial stage of sudden impact disasters, such as tornado or earthquake; but they are likely when a disaster leads to overcrowding and a break in public health practices (4). For example, decreased compliance with health regulations and quarantines following the 1907 San Francisco fire led to a plague outbreak.

Crowding and water contamination have led to documented increases in influenza, malaria, salmonella carriers, typhoid, hepatitis, gastroenteritis, measles, and respiratory infections following disasters in the 20th century (5,21).

Massive vaccination efforts following disasters, particularly typhoid immunizations, have been a popular disaster relief response. These efforts have been criticized as a waste of resources by several authors (5,21). The effectiveness of mass typhoid immunization programs has not been studied (5). Generally, current thinking is that large-scale vaccination programs after disasters are not warranted. Instead, immunization programs should be targeted to certain high-risk groups, such as the elderly and chronically ill in crowded conditions. These groups may require measels, influenza, pneumococcus, and *Haemophilus influenza* vaccinations. Groups exposed to outbreaks of known communicable diseases, such as *Neisseria meningitis*, may also benefit from immunization. Children and adults suffering from malnutrition, particularly those with vitamin A deficiency in refugee camps, are at risk for increased susceptibility to measles outbreaks; they should be vaccinated under these circumstances (22). Maintenance of routine vaccination programs in place before disaster is important, and efforts should be made to supply these programs (21). Refugee populations in underdeveloped nations are deficient in immunizations for measles, diphtheria, pertussis, tetanus, and polio (14).

Another group needing consideration for vaccinations are the relief workers themselves. Workers should have appropriate vaccinations before arrival in the region, as well as chemoprophylaxis for malaria in endemic regions. Immunization guidelines are available from WHO and the Centers for Disease Control and Prevention (CDC). The CDC provides weekly updates of recommended vaccinations based on predominate endemic agents, and current recommendations should be followed before departure when possible (21).

Pathogens expected in a region after disaster are generally the same as those before the disaster as new organisms rarely emerge (4,21). A population may be more susceptible to the usual pathogens after disaster due to factors such as malnutrition, environmental stress, injuries, interruption of treatment of chronic diseases, contamination of water supply and food storage facilities, and crowding leading to increased exposure to respiratory pathogens. However, new pathogens have been introduced to regions by relief workers following disasters. For example, 35 cases of malaria in Colombia following the 1983 earthquake were thought to have been a result of the organism having been brought in by a relief worker (21). Good health and appropriate chemical and immunologic prophylaxis of the relief workers before departure will help to protect both the disaster victims from imported pathogens and the rescuers from endemic diseases.

Soft-tissue injuries are a prominant complaint following many disasters. Many of these injuries occur during recovery operations. Diphtheria and tetanus vaccines are in high demand, and the local stocks are often quickly depleted. This was one of the most commonly used pharmaceutical items on St. Croix following Hurricane Hugo and in Oklahoma City following the bombing (23,24).

Antimicrobial agents considered as first line agents include penicillin, macrolides, first-generation cephalosporins, and trimethoprim/sulfamethoxazole (21). Following Hurricane Hugo's destruction of St. Croix in September 1989, disaster medical assistance teams found dicloxacillin to be the most commonly prescribed outpatient antibiotic, and parenteral cephalosporin was the most commonly prescribed inpatient antibiotic (23). Antibiotics were the most frequently mentioned supply problem during the Bosnia and Croatia conflict in 1994 to 1995, with cephalosporins being mentioned most often (12). Intramuscular administration is preferred because intravenous infusion requires equipment that is not always available (21).

PHARMACEUTICAL SUPPLY REQUIREMENTS

Sudden reductions in available medical resources commonly occur after disasters. Following Hurricane Andrew, one report of 1,500 patient encounters in a field hospital found that all supplies of tetanus toxoid, antibiotics, and insulin were depleted within 24 hours. Replacement of basic pharmaceutical supplies and refill medications were the most pressing medical care problems (18). Of 1,544 patient encounters seen at this Homestead field hospital, only five were injuries resulting directly from the hurricane; 285 cases were injuries associated with clean-up, and 1,254 visits provided routine care (18). After Hurricane Iniki struck Kauai, Hawaii in September 1992, disaster medical assistance teams found that 99% of their patients were ambulatory with minor injuries (40.4%) and illnesses (38.6%) or preventive service (9%) needs. Only 5.4% of these patients were referred to fixed facilities; most patients had non–life-threatening conditions. The conclusions were that, in this setting, teams need to be prepared for the provision of primary health care extending beyond the impact phase of a hurricane (17). Similar patterns have been reported following Hurricanes Frederick, Elena, Gloria, Hugo, Andrew, and George (17,20). The need for basic medical care after any type of disaster that reduces local medical resources or destroys the medical infrastructure is the mainstay of medical disaster relief efforts (23). The disaster itself may lead to only a modest increase in direct injuries. Pharmaceutical inventories of relief supplies should be directed toward meeting this goal of provision of primary care.

Disasters may require the mass evacuation of people from their home region, thus denying victims medical care and leaving them dependent on relief help. During Operation Fiery Vigil, more than 20,000 military dependents were evacuated from Clark Air Base in the Philippines to Guam following the eruption of Mount Pinatubo. Of the 20,000 evacuees, approximately 2,500 needed medical care during the evacuation. Some medical problems, such as sunburn, dehydration, and motion sickness, were associated with the evacuation operation. However, the majority of pharmaceutical agents dispensed were for routine and chronic medical diagnoses (25).

Large-scale civil unrest may also result in the sudden disruption of the available basic medical resources to a population. After the Los Angeles riots in April 1992, many inhabitants of the region had difficulty obtaining or maintaining primary health care needs. Over 5 days of civil disorder, 53 people died, 2,325 were injured, and 248 were admitted to hospitals. At least 38 private medical and dental offices, 15 county health centers, 45 pharmacies, 20 drug and alcohol centers, and multiple Women, Infants, and Children (WIC) program vouchering sites were destroyed or disabled as a result of the riots (26). Although regional medical resources were not overwhelmed and hospitals remained open, many persons suffered the loss of basic health care services. An estimated 20,000 patients lost services and records. Most pharmacies and health care providers in the riot area did not reopen. County health authorities intervened by offering relocated facilities to house private care providers; they also filled prescriptions and maintained methadone supplies where needed. Public health agencies were recommended to include the provision of basic pharmaceutical agents in their disaster-planning activities (26).

Pharmaceutical agents used in disasters vary between countries and disasters. Using drugs that are familiar to the local providers is important for providing optimal care and preventing medication errors. While the individual agents used may vary by international location, the same therapeutic categories are repeatedly found to be useful. Antibiotics, tetanus toxoid, insulin, analgesics, cardiac medications, anticonvulsants, rehydration fluids, cold preparations, and contraceptives are commonly mentioned. Additional therapeutic categories of disaster medical assistance team formularies include advance cardiac life support, antidiarrheal agents, antiemetics, antihypertensives, antiinflammatory agents, bronchodilators, intravenous solutions, oral electrolyte solutions, baby formula, muscle relaxants, and steroids (23). Sending complex drugs to disaster zones should be avoided. Local physicians are not familiar with their use, and, thus, they cannot be maintained after relief workers leave (7). Pharmaceutical manufacturers and wholesalers in many countries have readily available lists of the several hundred, top-selling drugs dispensed in various regions. These lists may assist in tailoring supplies of locally familiar drugs from each therapeutic category needed.

DISPENSING PHARMACEUTICAL AGENTS

Some difficulties in dispensing medications following a disaster are unavoidable. Three problems typically seen in regions struck by natural disaster are the lack of electrical power, appropriate stocks of medications, and narcotic security (19). The lack of electricity and telephone service will put a modern pharmacy out of normal operation. Pharmacists may be unable to contact physicians to authorize prescriptions or to access patient records to refill current medications. The state Boards of Pharmacy should have plans to communicate to pharmacists what they may legally do to serve the public needs during disasters.

In previous domestic disasters, such as floods, hurricanes, and tornadoes, pharmacists have used professional judgment to dispense sufficient quantities of medication to patients until the records and prescribers could be accessed. Lists of medications dispensed should be kept, compared, and added to patient records as soon as possible. Narcotics dispensing should be kept to a minimum. When pharmacies are physically damaged or are in temporary locations, narcotics need to be relocated to secure areas during nonoperating hours (19).

The relocation of a pharmacy to a temporary site or the deployment of a pharmacy with a field unit within the United States requires compliance with state laws. Such requirements should be part of the planning procedure for each organization. The physical requirements for a pharmacy during a disaster (such as running water and temperature control) need to be addressed by each state Board of Pharmacy. Packaging and labeling requirements may also be difficult to meet after a disaster. Small zipper-lock plastic bags with label slips that can be written on with pen or pencil are helpful for dispensing individual prescriptions. These bags are easy to pack and transport, they are lightweight, and they occupy less space than traditional prescription vials (1).

Countries in need of international disaster relief should make provisions for and clarify the status of licensure requirements within their borders during disaster to encourage assistance from international relief providers (8). Pharmacists have adapted well to working in field situations as a constructive part of the health care relief effort. After Hurricane Andrew, seven clinical pharmacists worked in temporary medical sites with pharmacy stock consisting of donated drugs. The pharmacists played an integral role in providing information to physicians regarding the limited pharmaceutical agents available, therapeutic substitutions, dosage conversions, and new medications. Prescriptions were frequently dispensed only with verbal orders. In addition, instructions to patients were commonly verbal. In some cases, language barriers provided significant obstacles to communications and patient counseling (27).

PERSONNEL CONSIDERATIONS

Personnel available during disasters will vary significantly between countries and disasters. Individuals with pharmacy or medical training may facilitate the sorting of donated pharmaceuticals in large disaster relief efforts. In Armenia, many medical personnel had been killed and the sorting of massive quantities of inadequately labeled pharmaceutical donations was slowed by the use of completely untrained persons (9). In other disasters, such as the Guatemala earthquake and Operation Fiery Vigil, the expanded use of pharmacy students and technicians helped to provide faster sorting and dispensing of supplies (7,25). In domestic disasters such as Hurricane Andrew and in the aftermath of tornadoes and floods, using pharmacists with the legal flexibility to use professional judgment and provide needed medications, as well as lifting the requirements for written labels, is recommended (18,19,27). Pharmacy personnel have proven to be a valuable resource, and they should continue to be included in disaster planning and response.

SUMMARY

Pharmaceutical supply and donation remain critical elements of disaster medical relief. Historically, disasters attract large pharmaceutical donations, both solicited and unsolicited, often in proportion to media coverage of the event. Difficulties with drug donations are frequently encountered, including massive quantities and improperly labeled, packaged, expired and unsorted pharmaceutical agents. Serious problems of identification, sorting, and logistics are often encountered. Items are often inappropriate for the type or phase of the disaster and the endemic diseases of the region. Local health care providers may have no knowledge of the appropriate uses for many of the donated pharmaceutical agents. Many of the agents may not be replaceable when relief supplies are exhausted. Narcotics handling and dispensing may be problematic. Education regarding these problems and solutions of pharmaceutical agents during disasters should be a standard part of the disaster physician's curriculum. Better anticipation of needs based on epidemiologic data of experiences and improved field disaster assessment will provide enhanced medical care during future disasters.

REFERENCES

1. Lesho EP. Planning a medical relief mission. *JAOA* 1995;95: 37–44.
2. Noji E. Disaster epidemiology: challenges for public health action. *J Public Health Policy* 1992;13:332–340.
3. Noji E. Disaster epidemiology. *Emerg Med Clin North Am* 1996; 14:289–300.
4. Lillibridge SR, Noji EK, Burkle FM Jr. Disaster assessment: the emergency health evaluation of a population affected by disaster. *Ann Emerg Med* 1993;22:1715–1720.
5. Lechat MF. Accident and disaster epidemiology. *Public Health Rev* 1993/1994;21:243–253.
6. Hogerzeil HV, Couper MR, Gray R. Guidelines for drug donations. *BMJ* 1997;1082:737–740.
7. de Ville De Goyet C, Lechat MF, Boucquey C. Drugs and supplies for disaster relief. *Trop Doct* 1976;6:168–170.
8. Pan American Health Organization. *Medical supply management after natural disaster.* Washington, D.C.: Pan American Health Organization Scientific Publication no. 438, 1983.
9. Autier P. Drug supply in the aftermath of the 1988 Armenian earthquake. *Lancet* 1990;335:1388–1390..
10. Berckmans P, Dawans V, Schmets G, et al. Inappropriate drug donations in Bosnia and Herzegovina, 1992 to 1996. *N Engl J Med* 1997;18:1842–1845.
11. Schouten E. Drug donations must be strictly regulated. Georgia has tight guidelines. *BMJ* 1995;311:684.
12. Michael M. Medical supplies donated to hospitals in Bosnia and Croatia, 1994-1995. Report of a survey evaluating humanitarian aid in war. *JAMA* 1996;7:364–368.
13. Cohen S. Drug donations to Sudan. *Lancet* 1990;22:745.
14. Rahaman MO, Bennish M. Health related response to natural disaster: the case of the Bangladesh cyclone of 1991. *Soc Sci Med* 1993;36:903–914.
15. Musulin M. Help the republics of the former Soviet Union. *Am J Hosp Pharm* 1992;49:1112–1113.
16. Sholz J. American politics: hostages of each other: the transformation of the nuclear power industry after Three Mile Island. *Am Political Sci Rev* 1995;89.
17. Henderson AK, Lillibridge SR, Graves RW, et al. Disaster medical assistance teams: providing health care to a community struck by Hurricane Iniki. *Ann Emerg Med* 1994;23:726–730.
18. Alson R, Alexander D, Leonard RD. Analysis of medical treatment at a field hospital following Hurricane Andrew, 1992. *Ann Emerg Med* 1993;22:1721–1728.
19. Scott S, Constantine LM. When natural disaster strikes with careful planning, pharmacist can continue to provide essential services to survivors in the aftermath of a disaster. *Am Pharm* 1990;11:651.
20. Centers for Disease Control. Needs assessment following hurricane Georges–Dominican Republic 1998. *MMWR* 1999;48: 93–95.
21. Aghababian RV, Teuscher J. Infectious diseases following major disaster. *Ann Emerg Med* 1992;21:362–367.
22. Shears P, Berry AM, Murphy R, et al. Epidemiological assessment of the health and nutrition of Ethiopia refugees in emergency camps in Sudan, 1985. *BMJ* 1987;295:314–318.
23. Roth PB, Vogel A, Key G, et al. The St. Croix disaster and the national disaster medical system. *Ann Emerg Med* 1991;20: 329–335.
24. Hogan DE, Waeckerle JF, Dire DJ, et al. Emergency department impact of the Oklahoma City terrorist bombing. *Ann Emerg Med* 1999;34:160–170.
25. Shalita EA, Samford JE. Pharmaceutical services to evacuated U.S. military dependents. *Am J Hosp Pharm* 1992;49:2474–2476.
26. Evans CA. Public health impact of the 1992 Los Angeles civil unrest. *Public Health Rep* 1993;108:265–272.
27. Nestor A, Aviles AI, Kummerle DR, et al. Pharmaceutical services at a medical site after Hurricane Andrew. *Am J Hosp Pharm* 1993;50:1896–1898.

CRITICAL INCIDENT STRESS

NEILL S. OSTER
CONSTANCE J. DOYLE

When sorrows come, they come not as single spies, but in battalions!
—Shakespeare, *Hamlet*, Act IV

Long after the physical injuries from a disaster have mended, each community continues deal with the psychoemotional problems of the event. These problems are much longer lasting, and they may affect individuals for the remainder of their lives. Critical incident stress (CIS) problems are often worse than the physical injuries because they affect essentially 100% of the population at risk. These problems may be difficult to distinguish from physical ailments. The focus of medical disaster planning is usually on the immediate surgical and medical needs of the victims. Little attention may be paid in planning to emotional and psychiatric support. Emergency medical services (EMS) is a trauma-oriented system in which fewer than 3 to 5 hours of training in the average EMS training program is devoted to mental health issues. Current triage systems fail to discriminate for patients with high risk for or evidence of CIS early in the response phase.

Each disaster creates emotional trauma victims. Victims do not need to be physically present at the time of the disaster in order to be affected significantly by the event. Some authors have divided victims into the following three categories based on the likelihood of CIS: primary, secondary, and tertiary. Primary victims are those who suffered at the site of the disaster. These individuals may have both physical and emotional injury from the event. Secondary victims are the noninjured rescue workers in whom symptoms may develop and who are often at high risk for emotional trauma. Tertiary victims are the relatives, friends, and witnesses to the event who have not suffered physical trauma themselves. The degree of involvement of an individual in a traumatic event stratifies their level of risk for the development of CIS. Critical incidents disrupt the victims' sense of control, as they suddenly or unexpectedly change their daily standard operating procedures. Emotional devastation may replace the calm of everyday life, while basic values and freedoms may be irrevocably altered.

DISASTER PHASES IN MENTAL HEALTH

Disasters have a series of phases that have been well described. The nature of the emotional response exhibited by the population exposed to a disaster can be correlated with that life cycle. Not all disasters have well-defined preimpact or warning phases. Of those that do, specific stresses and emotional responses may be observed. During the preimpact phase, the primary stress is worry about the upcoming event. In most individuals, some degree of anxiety will develop. Others will proceed with a level of denial that is consistent with their ability to cope. The warning phase starts with the notice that the disaster is impending. Anticipation of the upcoming stress increases significantly during this time. Some individuals will take varying degrees of protective action while others will still operate under denial. The impact phase begins when maximal and unavoidable direct physical stress occurs. According to various studies, up to 25% of individuals will remain calm and functional, 75% may be temporarily stunned into inaction, and from 12% to 25% may exhibit inappropriate behavior such as confusion, anxiety, or hysteria (1). During the recoil phase, the stress subsides. Over 90% of the victims will have a return of awareness. They may become conscious of recent events and may start to express emotions verbally for the first time. As time passes and the disaster moves into the postimpact or recovery phase, individuals experience stress from the primary and residual effects of the disaster. Grief, depression, post traumatic stress disorder (PTSD), psychosomatic complaints, and other varied responses become manifest. Conflict-related disasters with repeated periods of impact cause much higher levels of stress and dysfunction. In addition, although panic is relatively uncommon during disasters, it may be provoked in circumstances such as crowded subways, buildings, and train stations and during acts of terrorism.

CRITICAL INCIDENT STRESS

The most significant risk factor for the development of CIS, which can be alternatively referred to as the human stress reaction, is involvement, directly or indirectly, with a traumatizing event (2). A critical incident is defined by the *Diagnostic and statistical manual of mental disorders*, 4th edition, (DSM-IV) as any significant emotional event that has the ability to produce unusual distress in a normal healthy person (3). CIS is a normal reaction to an abnormal event. By virtue of the uniqueness of their professions, rescue workers, emergency medical technicians, firefighters, law enforcement officers, nurses, and physicians are at high risk for the development of CIS. Studies have looked at the increased stress levels in these high-risk groups (4–6). These studies consistently report increased cardiovascular disease; increased levels of stress and stress-related disorders; and higher rates of divorce, alcoholism, and suicide when compared to the general population.

Essentially, everyone involved with the disaster will develop an emotional response. The majority of persons will recover from their symptoms spontaneously with little more than a sympathetic listener. The population suffering from a disaster may be considered to be under massive collective stress. This stress will result in specific types of symptoms. Although some authors indicate that problems associated with this stress are really an adaptive failure on the part of the individual under stress, others state that such an approach detracts from the individual's need for assistance (1). A number of factors influence the degree to which symptoms will develop after a disaster. People with proactive, problem-solving personalities generally do better (5). Some studies have suggested that elderly victims suffer significantly more, but a more recent investigation has cast some doubt on this finding and in fact suggests that the elderly may do somewhat better than some age groups (1). The life experiences of a person also will influence their response. Prior exposure to disasters will modify the emotional response to disaster stress. In addition, the degree of community awareness and support, as well as of family support, has a great impact on the degree of reaction expressed by the victim.

CRITICAL INCIDENT STRESS MANAGEMENT

The rescue and recovery phases of the World Trade Center bombing in New York, the Alfred Murrah Building bombing in Oklahoma, and the TWA flight 800 disaster on Long Island have employed a mechanism for understanding and decompressing the traumatic psychologic effects that followed these devastating events. This mechanism is known collectively as critical incident stress management (CISM), and it has been used over 400 times in the past decade (7). CISM assesses the large picture surrounding a critical incident by observing and noting what the event entailed and how people were affected. It is a comprehensive look at the emotional and psychologic status of the survivors, witnesses, and first responders. CISM attempts to expedite

recovery in a population suffering from the psychologic effects of acute critical incidents. It has been shown to shorten the recovery process from acute stress, to decrease associated health disorders, and ultimately to improve job satisfaction and performance (8–10).

CRITICAL INCIDENT STRESS DEBRIEFING

Critical incident stress debriefing (CISD) is a formal process of trying to resolve the emotional content of an incident in order to prevent PTSD. In all models of CISM, the systems designed involve facilitators with formal training in crisis interventions, often utilizing those with expertise from the emergency and disaster services. The focus in CISD is on normal people with normal reactions to an abnormal situation, rather than on abnormal psychology (11).

CISD teams often include at least one mental health professional. In some models for CISD teams, peer counselors are used either as a sole facilitator of the process or they work in conjunction with a mental health professional (11). Peer counselors consist of formally trained peers of emergency responders. Mitchell (5) proposes that the use of peers promotes a better rapport between the debriefers and the victims because they have an intimate understanding of the work conditions experienced by the responders. In Mitchell's model, the team comes from outside the area or institution that is holding the debriefing (11). Those from the same institution are believed to be too involved to debrief friends and coworkers. Small critical incident groups may require only one individual to debrief the event successfully; larger events, however, may require several mental health providers, with or without peer counselors, to debrief all who were involved effectively.

Phases to a Formal Debriefing

Six phases are present in a formal debriefing. In the introductory phase, a facilitator makes the appropriate introductions and explains the purpose and goals for the debriefing. During the fact phase, participants introduce themselves and describe what their role in the event was. Emphasis is on description only, not on a critique of performance. Multiple responders will have performed various tasks and will have participated at different locations; therefore, recall and descriptions of the event will vary depending on the individual's role. This process can help all participants gain insight into the big picture of the event. In the feeling phase, group participants discuss their feelings about the event; this is followed by the symptom phase, where participants are asked about their physical and mental symptoms and they analyze their stress response reaction. In the teaching phase, the facilitator describes what symptoms the group should look for both in themselves and when they are evaluating others. The formal debriefing ends with the reentry phase, during which time the facilitator gives members final assurances and a follow-up plan, including when to meet again and possible referrals for individual therapy.

Data have demonstrated that early intervention in CISM has decreased the emergence of PTSD. Studies on firefighters revealed that 17% experienced PTSD symptoms versus a 3% prevalence in the general population (12). Firefighters who were involved in four critical incidents a year were at 150 times higher risk for the development of PTSD. Conversely, the same firefighters were 40% less likely to experience psychiatric disorders if family, peer, or supervisory support networks were available.

Critical Incident Defusing

Following a critical incident, some individuals may suffer severe emotional distress as a direct result of that incident. Such individuals need urgent or emergent assistance; for them, waiting 24 to 48 hours would be inappropriate. Critical incident defusing is an abbreviated version of CISD, and it takes place as soon as possible after the critical incident is finished. The process typically lasts less than 1 hour, and it is designed either to eliminate the need for a formal CISD or to enhance the CISD if one is to take place. The following three components make up the critical incident defusing process: introduction, exploration, and information. The leader may be a peer support person or a professional support person from the CIS team.

Demobilization

After a disaster or a large-scale mass casualty incident, interventions should be provided to bridge the transition from the traumatic event back to the day-to-day world. These interventions typically last approximately 10 minutes; during this time, discussions of critical stress and signs and symptoms take place, and suggestions for coping are given.

DEVELOPING A CRITICAL INCIDENT STRESS DEBRIEFING TEAM

CISD teams are developed and maintained by a variety of institutions and jurisdictions. Teams are generally staffed by volunteers, although the expenses are often charged to the entities requesting debriefings. A mobilized team that is not part of the involved system will usually require support, such as office space, bookkeeping, and recordkeeping; some form of dispatch; and a communications network. Work-release agreements with employers are usually discussed in advance in case work time is needed. Planning for emergency operations at a disaster site, tactics to handle the media, communications strategies, and death notification protocol must be established in advance.

Team meetings are set up periodically to plan activities, to discuss strategies, and to provide training and educational updates. Team members need training in the CISD or other CISM processes. Periodic training courses in both basic and advanced CISD methods are available around the country. Training includes education on stress recognition and management, debriefing guidelines, group dynamics, and the formal processes of a CISD. The team must also research community resources and referrals for those who need more in-depth debriefing and therapy. Each team functions independently. Formally trained CISD teams generally follow the guidelines of the program developed by Mitchell. Although other forms of critical incident debriefing exist, they are loosely organized and they are not as well accepted as Mitchell's procedures. The International Critical Incident Stress Foundation serves as a resource for both formal CISD groups and for others involved in debriefings.

Continuous Quality Improvement in Team Development

A critique is held after each debriefing by the team members who are involved in the debriefing. Teams are expected to do some follow-up on group members to assure that the basic goals have been met. Follow-up is loosely arranged, and it may vary from team to team. Worksite visits, telephone calls, referrals, meetings, and educational programs are acceptable follow-up. To date, no formal continuous quality improvement or outside peer review of teamwork exists. Data are not collected from these sessions nor are they independently reviewed, partly because of confidentiality concerns. Those who participate in the group debriefing sessions are cautioned that all of the session is confidential and that the privacy of the individuals who attend must be protected by all. Indeed, in some cases of crises, managers may want to use material to critique a participant's performance at the crisis—hence, the need for confidentiality. Some discussions regarding methods and results during recent disaster debriefing sessions are conducted in a general manner at the annual meeting of the International Critical Incident Stress Foundation. This allows members to learn from past events.

Process

Formal training in CIS includes course work in basic and advanced CISD concepts, crisis intervention, and normal psychology (11). An introduction is made to the characteristics of disaster and emergency services and the demands and stresses of working at a critical incident site. Training includes team formation and evaluation, the formal processes in debriefing techniques, public health issues, and physical and emotional reactions to stress.

Deployment of a CISD team occurs at the request of the entity or institution that is involved in a critical incident. Groups to be debriefed may vary from victims of the crisis, families or friends, and rescue workers, including some who may not have been on scene, such as dispatchers. On a local level, emergency departments or other locations in a health care facility may need debriefing after unusually intense events. Some thought has been given recently to the periodic debriefing of emergency personnel because of the repeated small traumas and the large number of verbal and other assaults that they endure.

Organizing a Stress Management Program

If organizations such as hospitals and EMS systems are committed to prevention programs, orientation and in-service teaching time can be dedicated to these important issues. Programs endorsed by the administration send a strong message to the staff on the importance of stress management. If expectations for employee and professional wellness are set from day one, job satisfaction and attrition rates are lower. Some professional organizations have embraced wellness concepts and have included stress management and critical incident stress programs as part of their professional curricula. The costs of employee hiring and training and attrition of trained personnel must be weighed when considering these programs.

POST TRAUMATIC STRESS DISORDER

In the late 1800s, Janet (13) described a breakdown of normal adaptation, information processing, and action that resulted from overwhelming trauma. This breakdown was also noted to occur with reexposure through thought or dreams that were termed automatic emotional and physical fixation to the trauma. Pavlov demonstrated the chronic changes in the autonomic nervous system that occurred in response to repeated traumatic exposure (13,14). Soldiers in World War I developed an autonomic syndrome known as soldier's heart. The term shell shock was given to the soldiers to describe the effect of repetitive bombings and the ensuing neurotrauma (13,14). Today, these symptoms are termed as post traumatic syndrome disorder (PTSD). The DSM-IV lists PTSD under anxiety disorders with a definition of "...when a person experiences, witnesses or is otherwise confronted by an event threatening death or serious injury to self or another person; and when the response involves intense fear, helplessness or horror" (3). Predictors of PTSD include the severity of the event, on-scene involvement, prior traumatic exposures, prior psychiatric disorders, and a lack of CISM. These risk factors are summarized in Table 6.1. PTSD is known to be comorbid with other disorders, such as anxiety, mood, substance abuse, depression, and possibly psychotic symptoms (15–17).

TABLE 6.1. RISK FACTORS FOR POST TRAUMATIC STRESS DISORDER DEVELOPMENT AFTER DISASTERS

Intense exposure to death and injury
Exposure of survivors to dead bodies
Overwhelming life-threatening danger
Unexpected or first exposure to disaster
Intense initial phase (prolonged stress)
Manmade disaster with no warning
High impact ratios
Dependence on outside agencies
Exposure to prolonged stress

Time Course

The development of PTSD may be delayed from 1 week to 30 years, and it is divided into three stages. Stage 1 is associated with an adrenergic surge that occurs acutely, but persons rarely dwell long term on the incident. It may last up to 1 month, and, if symptoms last more than 6 weeks, the patient is considered to have entered stage 2. Stage 2 is characterized by a sense of helplessness and a loss of self-control. Autonomic and somatic manifestations dominate. Moreover, it is accompanied by lifestyle and personality changes. Stage 3 is characterized by profound despondency and demoralization.

Prognosis

Overall, the majority (70% to 90%) of patients with PTSD do well (18). Thirty percent recover rapidly, 40% manifest mild symptoms, 20% manifest moderate symptoms, and 10% do not recover or get worse. Patients with a good prognosis are those with a rapid onset and a short duration of symptoms. These people usually have a strong social support network, and they also usually have participated in one form of CISD. Sixty percent of the victims (an estimated 5,500 people) from the Tokyo subway sarin disaster claim that they suffer ongoing effects (19). The main reason cited is the lack of support of and education given for the physical and mental disorders they experienced.

Treatment

Mental health professionals, including psychiatrists and psychologists, are regarded as the gold standard providers of care to the PTSD patient. Psychotherapy and behavior therapy are generally thought necessary, and they have yielded good results; in addition, some patients may benefit from psychotropic medications (15,19). When managing these patients, initially maintaining a broad-based differential diagnosis is necessary in order to avoid the pitfall of biasing the approach to the patient's complaint.

CHILDREN IN DISASTERS

The true degree of emotional trauma among children is usually underestimated after a disaster. Multiple reasons for this exist. Most studies on the subject to date have had significant methodologic flaws. Parents are either unaware or unwilling to admit to any inability to protect their children from stress, and therefore they underreport it. The extrapolation of emotional status from nondisaster events to disasters may also give a false evaluation of the level of symptoms in children. Most of the childhood emotional effects of disaster are age-related. The impact of disaster on children should be thought of in terms of their developmental age and not their chronologic age. Preschoolers are still experiencing some normal separation anxiety. Disasters will increase these normal feelings. Increased arousal, sleep disturbances, clinging, and fear of being alone all become manifest. School-age children tend to be less dependent on their parents. As such, their response to the stress of a disaster may be less consistent. They may exhibit reckless behavior and may experience more psychosomatic complaints. Adolescents, who are more independent, often become involved in productive activities, such as rescue and recovery work. Some however, may regress and may display withdrawn functioning under significant denial. Normal adolescent anxiety may be increased particularly if they identify with the victims. Factors contributing to an increased emotional trauma in children are listed in Table 6.2.

THE ELDERLY IN DISASTERS

Prior studies have stated that the elderly are at a greater risk for emotional trauma following a disaster than younger adults. In reality, this assumption may be exaggerated. The elderly are indeed at an increased risk for physical injury in some circumstances, but they are not necessarily at an increased risk for psychoemotional disorders. However, the impact of the loss of a spouse, relative, or even a pet may be greater in the elderly. Another factor is the loss of self-reliance. In some cases, the disruption of normal routines

and living environment may result in confusion and aberrant behavior. However, the life experiences of the elderly may be a valuable resource during the recovery phase of the disaster. They often have more realistic expectations of what their recovery needs are.

RESCUE WORKERS IN DISASTERS

Rescue workers are not immune to the effects of a disaster. The most common secondary victims of a disaster are those providing care to the victims. These include not only search and rescue personnel but also physicians, nurses, and other hospital staff. The stress reactions seen in nonprofessionals involved in disaster response resemble the symptoms seen in primary victims. Many professional responders also report serious symptoms following a disaster. Rescue workers will have more intense emotional trauma if they are involved in a failed rescue attempt (especially if children are involved). However, up to 90% of the professionals involved will have good coping skills. The major symptoms reported by professionals are outlined in Table 6.3. These reported symptoms obviously could adversely impact an ongoing recovery effort. Some specific factors that can decrease the frequency and severity of symptoms in professionals are listed in Table 6.4.

The most serious reactions occur among rescue workers involved with body handling. These are due in part to the profound sensory stimulation experienced by these personnel. Inexperienced body handlers have significantly more symptoms than those with prior experience. Symptoms can also be correlated with the number of bodies encountered by the rescue worker. Several methods have been noted for

TABLE 6.3. ADDITIONAL SYMPTOMS OF POST TRAUMATIC STRESS DISORDER IN PROFESSIONAL DISASTER WORKERS

Decreased ability to judge risk
Decreased leadership ability
Decreased work efficiency
Decreased ability to work cooperatively

TABLE 6.2. RISK FACTORS FOR POST TRAUMATIC STRESS DISORDER IN CHILDREN AFTER DISASTERS

High intensity event
Injury to the child
Loss of parent or significant person
Fear of death
Fear of separation
Fear of recurrence of the disaster

TABLE 6.4. FACTORS FOR DECREASING POST TRAUMATIC STRESS DISORDER SYMPTOMS IN DISASTER WORKERS

Prior disaster training
Specific disaster education
Maturity
Experience with prior disasters
Leadership type

TABLE 6.5. COPING METHODS FOR DISASTER RECOVERY WORKERS

Avoid humanization of the bodies
Do not look at the faces
Do not learn the names of the victims
Concentrate on the tasks at hand
Concentrate on the benefit to society

helping those working with the bodies cope with the stress; these are outlined in Table 6.5.

SUMMARY

Each disaster presents a slightly different profile of emotional trauma. However, some trends are predictable. All persons involved with a disaster will suffer to some degree from the emotional trauma. Human-created disasters seem to cause a more intense reaction than those of natural occurrence. The most consistent positive predictor of significant symptoms is the degree of direct involvement in the disaster. Methods such as CISD are beneficial in decreasing the long-term impact of disasters on victims and disaster workers. Planning for disaster response should include CIS management protocols.

Contact Phone Numbers for Workshops and Reference

Acute Trauma Stress Management Office	631-385-7551
American Academy of Experts in Traumatic Stress	631-543-2217
International Critical Incident Stress Foundation, Inc.	410-313-2473
National Institute of Mental Health	301-443-2403
National Society for Post-traumatic Stress Disorder	802-296-5132
Ray Shelton, PH.D., A.E.M.T. (workshops)	516-681-3976
United States Veterans Administration (Readjustment Counseling)	202-233-3317

REFERENCES

1. Burkle FM. Acute-phase mental health consequences of disasters: implication for triage and Emergency Medical Services. *Ann Emerg Med* 1996;28:119–128.
2. Lewis GW. *Critical incident stress and trauma in the workplace.* Bristol, PA: Accelerated Development, 1994.
3. *Diagnostic and statistical manual of mental disorders,* 4th ed. Washington, D.C.: American Psychiatric Association, 1994.
4. Cerne F. Hospitals not immune to high cost of stress. *Hospital* 1988;62;69.
5. Mitchell JT. When disaster strikes: the critical incident stress debriefing process. *JEMS* 1983;8:36–39.
6. Oster NS, Wong R, Horowitz S, et al. Anomalies of cardiac rate and rhythm in emergency medicine residents while on duty. *Ann Emerg Med* 1998;314:537.
7. Everly GS. *Innovations in disaster and trauma psychology,* Vol. 1. Ellicott City, MD: Chevron Publishing ,1995.
8. Dyregrov A. The process in psychological debriefings. *J Trauma Stress* 1997;10:589–605.
9. Emergency Nurses Association. *Position statement.* Mount Prospect, IL: Emergency Nurses Association, 1998.
10. Saint Joseph Hospital. *Workplace violence policy.* Ann Arbor, MI: Saint Joseph Hospital, September 1, 1997.
11. Mitchell JT, Everly GS. *Critical incident stress debriefing.* Ellicott City, MD: Chevron Publishing, 1996.
12. Deangelis T. Firefighters PTSD at dangerous levels. *APA Monitor* 1995;26:36–37.
13. Everly GS, Lating JM. *Psychotraumatology: key papers and core concepts in post-traumatic stress.* New York: Plenum Press, 1995.
14. Freud S. *Introductory lectures on psychoanalysis.* London: Hogarth Press, 1963.
15. Aghababian RV. *Emergency medicine: the core curriculum.* Philadelphia: Lippincott-Raven, 1998.
16. David D, Kutcher GS, Jackson EI, et al. Psychotic symptoms in combat related post traumatic stress disorder. *J Clin Psychol* 1999; 60:1.
17. Ivezic S, Oruc L, Bell P. Case report: psychotic symptoms in post-traumatic stress disorder. *Journal of Military Medicine* 1999;164: 1073.
18. Kaplan HI, Sadock BJ. *Comprehensive textbook of psychiatry,* 6th ed. Vol. 1. Baltimore: Williams and Wilkins, 1995.
19. Kawana N, Ishimatsu S, Kanda K. Psycho-physiological effects of the terrorist sarin attack on the Tokyo subway system. *Mil Med* 2001;166:23–26.

7

COMPLEX HUMANITARIAN EMERGENCIES

FREDERICK M. BURKLE, JR.

In past decades, armed conflicts and wars were primarily international in scope. Armies fought each other across the borders of existing nation states. In 1945, at the conclusion of World War II and the beginning of the Cold War, the United Nations (UN) Charter and other legal frameworks such as treaties, conventions, and covenants were written to address the consequences of these interstate wars. In the post-Cold War era, war and conflict increasingly have become an internal problem for fragile nation states as they have emerged from the control of colonial and repressive regimes. These disrupted states often suffer from inequalities in social, economic, and political development that are exacerbated by long-term ethnic, religious, and minority animosities and the fierce competition for existing resources. Once disrupted states deteriorate into war, they are commonly termed *complex emergencies* (CEs) because of the myriad causative characteristics that lead them into collapse. Zwi defines CEs as "situations in which the capacity to sustain livelihood and life are threatened primarily by political factors and, in particular, by high levels of violence" (1). In the 1990s, at least 38 conflicts, including events in Northern Iraq, Somalia, Rwanda, the Congo, the former Yugoslavia, the Province of Kosovo, and East Timor, have been classified as CEs.

With the internal disruption of states comes the lack of responsible authority and security that are needed to govern. National authorities, which are no longer in effective control, compete with various warring factions, rebel groups, undisciplined gangs, and paramilitary. Common characteristics of CEs are the erosion and the eventual destruction of essential public health infrastructure, flagrant violations of human rights, and the forced migration of massive numbers of civilians, either as internally displaced populations or as refugees in a neighboring country. The legal frameworks developed during Cold War interstate conflicts do not apply well in these internal wars. The major confusion is grounded in the right of national sovereignty, a legal protection under the UN Charter that guarantees the inviolability of a nation's border. As a consequence, the interpretation of basic human rights and protections are argued by many as equally inviolable, without regard for whether a conflict is internal (i.e., civil war) or external (i.e., interstate). Advocates of a universal human rights position argue that the UN Charter's assumptions of sovereignty do not release states from a need to respect human rights. They suggest, in fact, that states that are guilty of gross violations of human rights forgo their right to sovereignty.

The disruption of society inherent in a CE can have catastrophic consequences to the health of a nation (2). Civilians are the primary victims of these conflicts, making up over 80% of those killed, with children predominating—over 3,000 children and adolescents were killed by snipers in Bosnia alone, and the abandoned or unaccompanied children in both Somalia and Rwanda numbered over 100,000. Half of the residents of refugee camps today were born there. Girls are at the greatest risk for not receiving proper food or education, and they are prone to being abused, harassed, or raped. Boys as young as the age of 6 years are conscripted out of these camps as child soldiers. The outcry from the international community usually forces some humanitarian intervention, but this response may be limited in scope and it may be defined primarily by political factors or the restrictions of existing laws. The goals of humanitarian intervention are to stabilize and limit mortality and morbidity, to bring order to chaos, and to provide options for diplomatic mediation.

For these reasons, health care providers have become major humanitarian actors in CEs by offering assistance to vulnerable groups, who otherwise are denied access to basic health care protections and other human rights. Vulnerable groups are defined as "a section of the population, specifically infants, pregnant and lactating mothers, the elderly, the homeless," and others who are particularly prone to be victims of illness and injury and who are likely to suffer most in a disaster (3). Unfortunately, CEs have proven to be more dangerous, longer lasting, and more widespread than initially was thought, thus necessitating long-term commitments to vulnerable populations throughout the extended emergency, recovery, and rehabilitation phases. These commitments are not performed without difficulty. As an example, health care providers, while they are making great advances in both understanding and response to the complex health issues brought about by CEs, have often been frustrated when they find themselves meeting the challenge to save lives only to see the situation sliding back into crisis again for reasons beyond their control (2). The provision of health care in these scenarios requires professionals who understand the broad international humanitarian system and how it functions. This includes a working knowledge of the major participants in CEs, international humanitarian law, assessments and epidemiology, malnutrition and communicable diseases, gender and reproductive issues, public health infrastructure, logistics and transportation, communication, security, negotiations and mediation, and critical psychosocial and cross-cultural issues, to name just a few.

MAJOR PARTICIPANTS

Initial humanitarian requirements call for a massive logistical response to meet the needs for water, food, shelter, and medical and public health care and for provisions for civil order and security. No one agency or organization has these resources. The major participants, all of which have a vital role to play, include the UN and the UN agencies, nongovernmental organizations (NGOs), the International Committee of the Red Cross (ICRC), and coalition military forces. Both national governments and the UN are limited in their ability to provide direct aid to people in need in another country. Under international law they must deal directly with their governmental counterparts in the country in question. Through international treaties and the UN Charter, certain UN agencies, NGOs, and the ICRC are specifically mandated under the right of intervention to assist vulnerable populations in all humanitarian situations.

The United Nations functions as a treaty with an administration. It is comprised of many institutions that have roles and responsibilities in complex emergencies—the Security Council, the General Assembly, and the UN agencies (4). The UN is limited, under the Charter provisions for sovereignty, in its ability to respond to intrastate conflict. Because the country in conflict is usually a member nation of the UN, the offices of the Secretary General provide a means for negotiations and for conveying the pressure of international diplomacy. Peacekeeping operations, which are covered in Chapter 6 of the UN Charter (4a), include the use of observers and civilian personnel to monitor an accord or agreement and the deployment of peacekeeping (PK) troops or civil police under a Security Council Resolution. Unfortunately, PK forces have enjoyed only limited success in controlling fragile peace processes before a formal agreement is signed, which has resulted in Security Council Resolutions requiring Peace Enforcement forces (covered in Chapter 7 of the UN Charter [4a]) to be deployed to areas in conflict. (e.g., Haiti, Kosovo, and East Timor). This development is significant, and it characterizes the evolution of intervention as moving purely from one of human-

itarian assistance alone to a recognition that nothing is resolved without a political solution, which may necessitate the added provision of military security and protection.

UN Coalition force duties are usually limited to providing security, although they routinely supply the international relief system with heavy lift logistics, engineering, airfield operations, public health infrastructure repair, and even emergency health and food (e.g., air drops) during times of conflict when the relief system is not yet operational. A certain degree of civil-military coordination and information sharing is required, especially under the umbrella of Peace Enforcement. This can be a problem for international organizations and NGOs who must maintain the operational neutrality and impartiality required under international law. The UN uses open and transparent lateral organizations at the operational level for the coordination of policy issues (Humanitarian Operations Centers) and of relief and security at the field level (Civil-military Coordination Centers).

UN agencies are independent of the Secretary General and the General Assembly, and they have mandates to meet humanitarian needs under existing international law. The Office of the UN High Commissioner for Refugees (UNHCR), which is represented in over 100 countries, is mandated to protect, repatriate, and resettle refugees who have fled across the border from both interstate and intrastate wars. UNHCR also has an increasing responsibility for coordinating assistance programs for the large number of internally displaced persons (17 million in 1999). The World Food Program (WFP) is the food aid arm of the UN with the mission of providing emergency aid and long-term developmental assistance. The UN Children's Fund (UNICEF) provides assistance, particularly health, nutrition, and education, to children and women and to all victims of disaster. The emergency responsibilities of these and other UN agencies have been expanded tremendously because of CEs. The initial lack of operational experience, the inability to coordinate functions, and weakening budgetary support has plagued UN agencies. Under recent UN reforms, an Office of the Coordinator of Humanitarian Affairs (OCHA) was organized to provide coordination of the UN humanitarian response. Coordination is implemented through an Emergency Relief Coordinator (ERC), the designation of a lead agency role for one of the UN agencies, and the provision of a coordinating and policy steering committee of representative UN agencies, NGOs, and the Red Cross (Fig. 7.1).

NGOs are best known for their work in developing countries. Their defining characteristics are that they are voluntary, independent, and not-for-profit. They vary in size, mission, and capability. With the onset of CEs, NGOs specializing in humanitarian relief have grown in number. A count of NGOs in a sampling of CEs reveals 28 in the refugee crisis in Northern Iraq, 78 in Somalia, 170 in Rwanda, 350 in Bosnia, and over 700 in Haiti. With the increasing emphasis on emergency relief, governments, the UN, and private donors rely

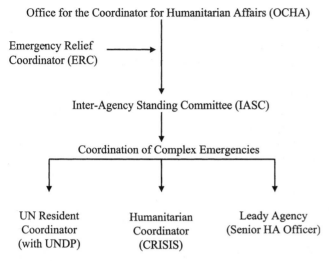

FIGURE 7.1. Organization of the Office for the Coordinator for Humanitarian Affairs (OCHA).

increasingly on NGOs to distribute the bulk of humanitarian aid on the ground. Currently, over 90% of all relief assistance coordinated by the UN are implemented through NGOs.

NGOs remain the only major component in the international relief system that directly represents the interests of the civilian victims. NGOs may specialize in water and sanitation, food, shelter, and medical care and in specific vulnerable group activities, such as reproductive services for women and protective services and therapeutic feeding centers for children. Examples of NGOs that field medical and public health teams are Medecins sans Frontieres (MSF), International Medical Corps (IMC), International Rescue Committee (IRC), Merlin, and Doctors of the World. Advocacy NGOs promote human rights protections and support efforts to uncover and record abuses (e.g., uncovering and documenting mass gravesites). Indigenous NGOs, which may be better able to represent local and traditional practices within developing countries, now number over 20,000 worldwide. These frequently are supported by and work in tandem with international NGOs from developed nations.

The *ICRC* is an all-Swiss private institution mandated to respond, under international law (Geneva Conventions), to victims of war and conflict. They are the largest and the oldest of all international humanitarian organizations, and they are involved wherever international or internal civil conflict is found. The ICRC functions, under authority mandated by the Geneva Convention, as a neutral intermediary to protect all victims. With its neutrality, impartiality, and independence (i.e., it is separate from all NGOs and other humanitarian organizations), the ICRC has a unique mandate to monitor the treatment of prisoners and to assist in finding, tracing, and protecting those missing as a result of conflict. The ICRC Medical Unit is well recognized and well respected for its capabilities in fielding hospitals during conflict and in the performance of war surgery (5,6). The

Red Cross symbol is universally recognized, and it is easy to spot in the chaos of war. Unfortunately, the ICRC and its symbol have recently become a target for attacks. Violations such as these have further characterized CEs in this decade, and they highlight the seriousness of the security issues that all relief workers face. The predeployment education of all relief workers requires security and evacuation training similar to that which has been developed by the ICRC over the years.

The Federation of Red Cross and Red Crescent (IFRC) headquarters in Geneva represents the interests of all national Red Cross and Red Crescent Societies throughout the world. IFRC coordinates relief in natural disasters and assists refugees outside areas of conflict. When a conflict stabilizes and security is established, the ICRC turns over many assistance operations to the IFRC and NGOs. With the demand for services increasing in CEs, the IFRC international staff are frequently seconded to support ICRC activities in conflict areas. During such an ICRC operation in Chechnya, six IFRC workers were singled out and assassinated.

MEDICAL AND PUBLIC HEALTH ASPECTS OF COMPLEX EMERGENCIES

Epidemiology

Burkholder and Toole (7) described CEs as having acute, late, and postemergency phases (Table 7.1), each of which is characterized by predictable patterns of health indicators and expected public health responses. If these patterns are addressed with appropriate management responses, a decline in mortality and morbidity and a shortening of the duration of each epidemiologic phase will occur. In the developing country model, the acute phase is characterized by high mortality rates for infants and those under the age of 5 years from severe malnutrition and outbreaks of communicable disease. Brennan and Burkholder (8) suggest that the acute phase in developed countries (e.g., Yugoslavia, Chechnya) appears to be characterized more by violent trauma and malnutrition and the consequences of untreated chronic diseases in the elderly.

Assessments

Effective response to CEs requires timely, accurate public health information and data. The rationale for assessments is to provide objective information for planning, prioritizing needs, implementing health programs, evaluating the relief process, and identifying health issues needing further investigation (9,10). Standard World Health Organization (WHO) (11) and Sphere (12) assessment protocols exist for natural and human-generated disasters (11). The use of such standardized assessment protocols can help to determine the magnitude of the emergency, the health and nutrition needs, the availability of local resources, and the need for external

TABLE 7.1. PHASES OF A COMPLEX EMERGENCY

Parameter	Acute emergency	Late emergency	Postemergency
Time frame	0–1 mo	1–6+ mo	>6 mo
Health profile	High CMR	Declining CMR	Stable CMR
	High CFR		"Village" profile
	Outbreaks of communicable disease		
	Malnutrition		
Priority needs	Food	Security	Expand self-sufficiency
	Water/sanitation	Fuel	
	Shelter	Improve basic needs	
Public health interventions	General ration, possible elective feeding	Train community health workers Standardize treatment protocols	Develop tuberculosis and mental health programs
	Measles immunization	Expand HIS	Expand MHC and STD programs
	HIS	Develop rational drug supply	
	Primary care clinics and outreach and ORT centers	Begin MHC and STD programs	

United Nations Office of the Coordinator of Human Affairs (OCHA) organized to coordinate large-scale humanitarian emergencies.
Abbreviations: CFR, case fatality rate; CMR, crude mortality rate; HIS, health information system; MCH, maternal and child health; ORT, oral rehydration therapy; STD, sexually transmitted disease.
From Burkholder BT, Toole MJ. Evolution of complex emergencies. *Lancet.* 1995;346:1012–1015, with permission.

resources. An understanding of basic concepts in epidemiology and assessment and an appreciation of their critical role in CEs are essential for all decision-makers.

Malnutrition

Protein-energy malnutrition (PEM) is the term used to describe clinical syndromes characterized by malnutrition and micronutrient deficiency diseases. These include the more traditional entities of marasmus (loss of fat and muscle), kwashiorkor (the presence of edema from protein loss), and the clinically frequent combination of the two (marasmic kwashiorkor). PEM recognizes that the malnourished are also prone to secondary infections, which frequently lead to severe complications and death.

To define the degrees of severity of PEM requires a means of and skill for measuring and assessing victims. Malnutrition usually manifests earliest in children because they have a greater growth rate with higher protein and caloric requirements. An arm muscle circumference of less than the fifth percentile or less than 80% of the standard usually defines PEM in children. The mid upper arm circumference (MUAC) is a stable measurement in children between the age of 1 and 5 years, and it is easily performed on the left arm midpoint occurring between the tip of the olecranon and the tip of the shoulder. MUAC can also be used to assess adults. It serves as a screening tool in the initial rapid assessment for placing victims in one of the following three categories of PEM: severe, moderately severe, and minor.

More sensitive indicators include the weight for height ratio and the Z score, which expresses a child's weight as a multiple of the standard deviation of the reference population. Measurements of these indicators are usually used to

follow victims in the late and postemergency phases, and they require more time, resources, and training of relief personnel (13).

All those that have been displaced from their food sources receive general rations that are coordinated by the WFP and implemented by NGOs. These rations completely meet requirements for caloric intake, protein, and essential vitamins. Supplementary rations provide additional calories and protein for identified vulnerable groups, such as children and pregnant and lactating women. In addition, an effort is made to ensure delivery to the elderly and unaccompanied minors, who are at risk for decreased access to food. On the basis of PEM measurements, children are placed in feeding programs depending on their need, and they are not discharged until a percentage greater than 90% of the reference standard is reached. Feeding centers for the most severely malnourished require a therapeutic environment that can provide specially formulated and frequent (six or more per day) wet feedings and the ability to monitor and treat infectious disease complications.

Most victims with PEM have anemia and a combination of micronutrient deficiencies, the most common of which are deficiencies of vitamins A, C, and B_1. Supplementation can be vital in reducing mortality and morbidity. Vitamin A supplementation has drastically reduced mortality from measles in some settings, and it is now universally recommended. Vitamin A alone will decrease the mortality rate in starving children by up to 50%, and a measles vaccine program, a priority second only to the emergency provision of food, can save the lives of those at risk from starvation. Other causes of mortality in PEM include dehydration, hypoglycemia, severe anemia, cardiac failure, and hypothermia.

Communicable Diseases

Traditionally, relief workers have worried about disease epidemics in CEs. Of importance, however, is the realization that epidemics cannot be caused by pathogens that are not present, so public health efforts should concentrate on those pathogens endemic to each setting. Infectious disease epidemics in CEs can be caused by poor sanitation, poor nutrition, the destruction of public health infrastructure, low immunization rates in the vulnerable populations, and overcrowding in refugee camps.

The incidence of infectious disease is increased in all CEs taking place in developing countries in Africa. The major diseases are acute respiratory illnesses, which often lead to pneumonia, and diarrheal diseases. Measles, malaria, meningitis, hepatitis, tuberculosis (TB), and skin infections are also common, and they may present as a severe complication of malnutrition. The conflict in Kosovo did not show an increase in the incidence of infectious disease, which, in part, was due to the early and extensive effort to control and manage the public health environment in refugee camps. The management of infectious diseases should first be directed toward primary prevention and the implementation of public health programs in water, sanitation, vector control, and health education (14,15). Infectious diseases must be confirmed by a reference laboratory (field deployable laboratories are often available). Implementing WHO standards for clinical case definitions, case finding, outbreak investigations, and surveillance must be a coordinated activity of all involved relief programs.

Other priorities include the rehabilitation of essential health services, surveillance studies, standard treatment protocols, the training of community health workers, vaccinations based on strict WHO protocols and indications, a health information system, and a health care policy consistent with national guidelines.

Critical Indicators in Support of Public Health Infrastructure

Critical indicator categories are water, food, shelter, sanitation, fuel, and health, and these represent international standards based on research and field trials (Table 7.2). They are essential for planning, logistics, assessment, and response (5,9,12). Many factors can contribute to success or

TABLE 7.2. CRITICAL INDICATOR CATEGORIES

Water (in L/person/d)
  15 L
  Minimum: 3–6 L
  With hygiene: 20 L
  Feeding centers: 25–30
  Health centers: 60
  Field hospitals: 150 (ICRC: 310)
Food
  Suggested requirements: 1,900–2,200 kcal/person/d
  Minimum: 1,900 kcal/person/d
  General feeding rations—mainstay of relief effort
  Assume supplementary or therapeutic rations will be required
    for some vulnerable groups
  Dependent upon measures indicating malnutrition and
    micronutrient deficiencies
  15,000 tons of food: feeds 1 million for 1 mo
  Grain: 85%
  Vegetable oil: 3%
  Beans/protein: 12%
Shelter
  Minimum living conditions
    3.5 m² floor area per person
  Minimum, inclusive of whole camp settlement
    30 m² per person
  Tents: family, 6 persons
    Traditional, fire resistant, low cost
    Blankets: 1/person (wool and cotton)
    Plastic sheeting: 1/household (woven and fire resistant)
    Water containers: 1/household (5 gallons)
    Cooking pots: 2/household (with lids)
    Pot stirrer: 1 per household
    Soap: 200 g/person/mo
    Matches: critical item

Sanitation
  Minimum for public: 1 latrine/50 persons
  Optimal: 1 latrine/20 persons
  15 m from water source (minimum)
  30 m from water source (preferable)
  Dependent upon type of soil
Fuel
  1 kg of wood/person/d
  5–10 kg/household/d
  Refugees may forage >10 km/d for fuel
  Found locally or supplied
  Resources: kerosene, wood or peat, charcoal, stove
Health
  Crude mortality rates (CMR): deaths per 10,000 persons/d
  Normal in developing countries: 0.3–0.6
    Range, 0.25–1.0; serious, >1.0; crisis, >2.0
  Primary objective of mission: diminish CMR
  CMR most sensitive measure of mission success
  Under age 5 (U5) mortality rate (U5MR)
    U5 age group is most vulnerable
    U5 age group is usually double that of CMR
    Normal: 0.6–2.0
    Serious: 2.0–4.0
    Crisis: >4.0
  Malnutrition indicators
    Mid upper-arm circumference
    Weight for height
    Z scores
    >20% malnourished: Alarm!
    >30% malnourished: Disaster!

Abbreviation: ICRC, International Committee of the Red Cross.

failure in meeting these guidelines. For example, in the Cambodian refugee camps on the border with Thailand, the use of emergency transportation measures (e.g., barges, refurbished trains, and trucks) was necessary to ensure critical water supplies. The initial planning called for 100 L per person per day. Due to evaporation, spillage, and theft, only 20 L per person per day arrived at the campsites. In other CEs, raids on feeding centers, the diversion of convoy food to warring factions, washed out roads, and failures to plan for hospital and clinic needs and those of essential livestock have impacted the ability of relief workers to respond to critical indicators.

Triage

The criteria in the triage process aim to improve the likelihood of recovery and to conserve scarce resources. In conventional emergency situations, triage is used to identify the sickest or the most seriously injured individual and to treat them first. In disaster medicine, with limited resources, the emphasis will normally shift toward providing the greatest good for the greatest number. The method by which this is done is the triage process, and it results in decisions whereby injured persons whose care exceeds local capacities may be excluded from all but palliative measures.

When a robust supply of resources, personnel, and opportunities for evacuation exists, the decision-making method for triage is based on the use of inclusion criteria. These criteria are the basis of basic and advanced cardiac and trauma life supports courses, and they use standardized protocols as guidelines for triage management. In these scenarios, the providers of care assume that available resources and easy access exist at every echelon of care.

Inclusion criteria–based triage is not always realistic in CEs. The epidemiologic study of casualty care in CEs conducted by Coupland (16) clearly demonstrated that personnel, equipment, medical care, and evacuation are severely compromised. Hospitals are often insecure and easily overwhelmed, and they may lack water, electricity, and the capacity to resupply. In CEs, managing triage in terms of resource-driven exclusion criteria is more realistic. Triage personnel must have a knowledge of the available resources and must make decisions accordingly. In Rwanda, for example, two expatriate surgical teams were faced with over 20,000 casualties and very few resources. To ensure that the limited resources would be directed to those with a realistic chance of survival, the triage decision was to treat only those left standing while providing little more than palliative care to the others.

Triage should provide the most realistic opportunity to survive for those with a chance for survival (17). Before the triage process begins, a mandatory step is for triage personnel and decision-makers in a CE to meet to determine what resources are available and, based on this knowledge, to determine what the criteria will be for a minimal qualifica-

tion for survival. The minimal qualification criteria identifies specific medical and surgical conditions (i.e., cardiac resuscitation) for which resources are not available; therefore, expending critical resources in their care would only compromise others. Such decisions from those who are more experienced will not be easily tolerated or fully understood by the uninitiated without education. Debriefing counseling should be offered for these persons.

Strict adherence to exclusion and minimal qualification criteria is necessary. In the Rwandan refugee camps on the Tanzanian border, dysentery and cholera were prevalent, and they caused many deaths. Oral rehydration salts, which are the mainstay of dehydration treatment for diarrhea and dehydration in developing countries, were in short supply as was personnel expertise. Initially, coordination failed, and some decision-making events allowed scarce resources to be expended on children with little chance of survival. In one instance, a severely moribund child died despite multiple resuscitation attempts, expending valuable personnel time and scarce fluid and medication resources. Later, the mother of the child also died for lack of timely resources, orphaning the three remaining children. In review, the mother's death would probably have been prevented had the triage process been sensitive to minimal qualification for survival and exclusion criteria.

Refugee camp triage is unique. Adequate equipment and field hospitals are rare before camps become established entities. Both inclusion and exclusion criteria are used, depending on the fluctuation of personnel, resources, patient access, and security indicators. In general, the triage process must be sensitive enough to seek out severe, treatable cases, especially those cases that pose a risk to an overcrowded refugee camp; and it must exclude chronic non-risk patients. Recognizing the sentinel case of measles, bloody diarrhea, and a plague-like bubo has great significance. Mobile laboratories are essential to the triage process, and they are organized to identify critical infectious diseases endemic to the region. The triage process also functions to direct the proper supply of resources, such as oral rehydration salts, specific antibiotics, and chlorine for safe water (6,16). Coupland further emphasizes that quality surgical outcomes in CEs are most dependent on good nursing care, hospital infrastructure and supply, judicious preventive care, and initial patient access.

All health resources in CEs are scarce, they are rarely expendable, and they must be protected. Abdominal wounds causing low velocity perforation without bleeding may fare well without abdominal exploration if circumstances require conservative management or operative delay. The nonoperative management of soft tissue wounds often benefits from tetanus antitoxin and antibiotics alone (16). ICRC's decision to open a surgical facility in an area of conflict is subject to nonmedical considerations. For example, the degree of security available for staff may take precedence over surgical indications. This is especially true where warring factions have not demonstrated a respect for the rules of the Geneva Conventions, which protect health care providers and facilities. Cross-cultural issues and deep-seated ethnic animosities may pressure the triage process to favor males over females or the military over civilians or to exclude totally (under threat) certain ethnic, minority, or religious groups.

Psychosocial Issues

Psychosocial issues, for victims and providers alike, have been neglected. Some common psychic trauma in victims are the loss of a loved one; physical injury, disability or disfigurement; destruction of a home or livelihood; persecution; detention; torture; imprisonment; witnessing atrocities; and sexual violence. Often multiple pathologic conditions are found in each victim, with anxiety, depression, and posttraumatic stress disorder (PTSD) predominating (18–21). Multiple community-based interventions have been started in the former Yugoslavia and Kosovo, but few psychosocial programs have been initiated in developing countries. In addition, good cross-cultural data collection and case definitions are lacking. Studies suggest, however, that PTSD is a major problem and that suicide remains an unattended public health problem, especially in raped or abused women, long-term refugees, and the elderly. Interventions for children must take into account parental stresses. Traditional practices for healing must not be ignored.

Sources of psychologic stress in relief personnel include personal loss, separation from family, culture shock, intense physical work, overwhelming responsibilities, austere conditions, and illness. Managing stress in relief workers begins with predeployment screening and education, followed by field-based debriefings and finally by support groups and reintegration counseling on their return home.

Reproductive Health and Women's Issues

Major advances have occurred in the recognition, advocacy, and management of gender-based issues in CEs (22–24). In particular, the Women's Commission for Refugees and Children in New York, working with UN agencies and NGOs, has actively advocated and produced management standards to protect females of all ages. Early assessments include attention to breastfeeding practices, requirements for traditional birth attendants, contraception programs, sexually transmitted disease case detection and management, sexual and gender violence prevention and counseling, and the early initiation of women's organizations and leadership, especially in refugee camps.

FUTURE EXPECTATIONS

The frequency of CEs will remain high for the next decade. Over 70 countries have predictive indicators for CE vulner-

ability. Small-scale conflicts average 25 to 35 a year, and they require political and economic efforts to prevent them from declining further (25). The UN reform movement has placed responsibility on the UN Development Program (UNDP) for initiating preventive development programs with an emphasis on governance projects designed to educate fledgling states in democratic growth and management. UNDP has the responsibility for promoting disaster preparedness in developing countries. Research suggests that a useful barometer of stable governance is the measurement of the resilience of a nation in their response to a major disaster.

Humanitarian assistance is rapidly moving from rural to urban settings as the Third World's poor migrate to urban slums. The projected global population increase of over 35% by the year 2020 will exacerbate some CEs, especially those which already have dense populations and those lacking a public health infrastructure. The lack of food and water security will contribute to the migration of populations.

Some regions of the world, especially Asia, suffer environmental risks in water, air pollution, and too little arable land per capita. These risks do not stop at the border of neighboring countries, and they may lead to the migration of people for environmental and ecologic insecurity reasons. Such migration may force governments to take military action (2).

Natural disasters in the 1990s have worked to catalyze CEs (e.g., drought in Somalia). Natural disasters work to keep governments honest—disasters can demonstrate the efficacy of the public health infrastructure of a nation and can expose its vulnerabilities, causing political upheaval and civil unrest if the response is not what is expected (e.g., in earthquakes in Armenia, Turkey, and Columbia).

A growing concern is the potential effect that terrorist events (including nuclear, chemical, and biologic) might have in destabilizing a government and precipitating a CE. Managing the consequences of these events is beyond the capacity of most nations. Both the potential for widespread public health consequences and the international multiagency response requirements are similar to those seen in CEs (2).

SUMMARY

Complex humanitarian emergencies are the ultimate challenge for disaster management and medicine. Health care management has shown great growth and maturity during the CEs of the 1990s. However, political factors and security risks continue to limit the capacity of the international relief community to respond. CEs are long-term events requiring both civil and military professional management. Health care professionals face great challenges in controlling communicable diseases, starvation, age-based and gender-based abuses, trauma care, and complex public health infrastructure loss.

REFERENCES

1. Zwi A, Uglade A. Political violence in the third world: a public health issue. *Health Policy Planning* 1991;6:203–217.
2. Burkle FM. Lessons learnt and future expectations of complex emergencies. *BMJ* 1999;319:422–426.
3. Gunn SWA. *Multilingual dictionary of disaster medicine and international relief.* Dordrecht, The Netherlands: Kluwer Academic Publishers, 1990:87.
4. Natsios AS. The international humanitarian response system. *Parameters* Spring 1995;68–81.
4a. United Nations. *Charter of the United Nations and Statute of the International Court of Justice.* New York: United Nations Department of Public Information, 1945.
5. Perrin P. *Handbook on war and public health.* Geneva: International Committee of the Red Cross Health Division, 1996.
6. Coupland RM. *The Red Cross wound classification.* Geneva: International Committee of the Red Cross, 1991.
7. Burkholder BT, Toole MJ. Evolution of complex emergencies. *Lancet* 1995;346:1012–1015.
8. Brennan R, Burkholder BT. Centers for Disease Control and Prevention, unpublished data, 1997.
9. Centers for Disease Control and Prevention. Famine-affected, refugee and displaced populations: recommendations for public health issues. *MMWR* 1992;41:RR-13.
10. Toole MJ, Waldman RJ. Prevention of excess mortality in refugee and displaced populations in developing countries. *JAMA* 1990;263:3296–3302.
11. World Health Organization. *Rapid health assessment protocols for emergencies.* Geneva: World Health Organization, 1999.
12. Sphere Project. *Humanitarian charter and minimum standards in disaster response,* 1st ed. Geneva: Sphere Project, 1998:2–56.
13. Médecins sans Frontieres. Nutrition guidelines. In: *Médecins sans Frontieres* Paris: Medicins Sans Frontieres, 1995.
14. Toole MJ. Mass population displacement: a global public health challenge. *Infect Dis Clin North Am* 1995;9:353–365.
15. Centers for Disease Control and Prevention. Mortality rates in displaced populations of central Somalia during 1992 famine. *MMWR* 1992;41:913–917.
16. Coupland RM. Epidemiological approach to surgical management of the casualties of war. *BMJ* 1994;308:1693–1697.
17. Burkle FM. Triage in complex emergencies. In: Burkle FM, ed. *Combined humanitarian assistance response training (CHART) course.* Hawaii: COE, 1999.
18. Zivcic I. Emotional reactions of children to war stress in Croatioa. *J Am Acad Child Adolesc Psychiatry* 1993;32:709–713.
19. Macksoud MS, Aber JL. The war experiences and psychological development of children in Lebanon. *Child Dev* 1996;67:70–88.
20. Dahl S, Mutapic A, Schei B. Traumatic events and predictive factors for post traumatic symptoms in displaced Bosnian women in a war zone. *J Trauma Stress* 1998;11:137–145.
21. Thabet AA, Vostanis P. Post-traumatic stress reactions in children of war. *J Child Psychol Psychiatry* 1999;40:385–391.
22. Women's Commission for Refugees and Children. *Report on the situation of women in UN and UNHCR administered refugee operations as observed by members of the Women's Commission for Refugees and Children.* New York: International Rescue Committe, 1989.
23. United Nations Children's Fund. *Analysis of the situation of women and children in the refugee camps of Ntega and Marangara.* New York: UNICEF, 1988.
24. Kozaric-Kovacic D, Folnegovic-Smaic V, Skrinjaric J, et al. Rape, torture and traumatization of Bosnian and Croatian women: psychological sequelae. *Am J Orthopsychiatry* 1995;65:428–433.
25. National Defense Council Foundation World Conflict List. Available at www.ndcf.org/97list.html. Accessed June 1, 1998.

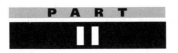

PART

II

DISASTER RESPONSE PLANNING AND COORDINATION

PRINCIPLES OF HOSPITAL DISASTER PLANNING

ERIK AUF DER HEIDE

OVERVIEW

The purpose of this chapter is to outline the basic principles of hospital disaster planning. It differs from those in other textbooks on disaster and emergency medicine, as the emphasis is not so much on the clinical aspects of preparedness but rather on the organizational, social, and political aspects because these aspects are where most of the disaster response problems occur. This chapter also focuses not just on what ought to happen but rather on what actually happens in disasters and why it happens.

Disaster planning is only as good as the assumptions on which it is based. Unfortunately, many of these assumptions have been shown to be inaccurate or false when they have been subjected to empirical assessment (1,2). A great deal of planning is based on what is logically to be expected, but what is logical is not always what happens. To avoid this problem to the extent that one can, the information found in this chapter has been culled from field research studies of hundreds of domestic disasters over the last few decades. However, anecdotal reports have also been used to illustrate the points from the research.

This chapter will address primarily domestic, peacetime disasters because these are the types of events most likely to be faced by United States hospitals. This chapter points out more problems than solutions, which might prove somewhat frustrating to the disaster medical planner. Nevertheless, one hopes that, where no definitive answers are presented, an accurate perception of the problems will bring the solutions closer. In the meantime, some of the proposed solutions must be treated like hypotheses that still require testing.

To cover completely the subject of hospital disaster planning in a single book chapter is impossible. Thus, the reader should not be surprised that some important issues have been omitted. The author tried to select the most important material for inclusion, particularly that which has not been adequately covered in other book chapters on disaster medical planning. For those who wish to pursue the topic in greater depth, a list of information sources is included at the end of this chapter. In addition, readers are referred to *Disaster response: principles of preparation and coordination*, which is now available at no charge on the Internet from http://www.coe-dmha.org/dr/flash.htm, and *Community medical disaster planning and evaluation guide*, which is available from the American College of Emergency Physicians (http://www.acep.org or by telephone at 1-800-798-1822 [press 6]).

Why Is it Necessary for Hospitals to Plan Specifically for Disasters?

Hospitals take care of emergencies every day, so why is additional planning specifically for disasters necessary? Some have argued that disasters are just like daily emergencies, only larger. Therefore, they conclude that the best disaster response is merely an expansion of the routine emergency response, supplemented by the mobilization of extra personnel, supplies, bed space, and equipment (2–5).

However, years of field research on medical disaster responses has shown this strategy is not successful because disasters are not simply large emergencies. Instead, disasters pose unique problems that require different strategies. Disasters are not only quantitatively different, but they are also qualitatively different. For example, disasters tend to disrupt normal communications systems (e.g., telephones and cellular telephones), damage transportation routes, and disable normal response facilities. As this chapter will illustrate, disaster response involves working with different people, solving different problems, and using different resources than those for routine emergencies (2,6–8).

The material in this chapter reflects solely the views of the author. It does not necessarily reflect the policies or recommendations of the Agency for Toxic Substances and Disease Registry or of the U.S. Department of Health and Human Services. Any reference to commercial products does not imply endorsement; it is provided solely as an example of what is available.

Fortunately, disasters in the United States are low-probability events. Paradoxically, this poses a problem for hospital planners, because few planners have had enough disaster experience on which to base realistic and effective plans. Furthermore, no nationally institutionalized process exists for collecting, analyzing, and disseminating the lessons learned from past disasters so that future planning can benefit from them. This chapter is an effort to fill that need, at least in part.

Finally, one should recognize that planning and response are different. Planning is an organized effort to anticipate what is likely to occur and to develop reasonable and cost-effective countermeasures. Response is the process of dealing with what actually happens, regardless of whether it was anticipated. When planning is effective, ad hoc, fly-by-the-seat-of-your-pants responses are reduced. However, the benefits of planning are relative, not absolute. Utopian planning efforts that seek to address every possible disaster contingency simply are not realistic. Even if these types of efforts were possible, the planners would never have the funding to implement them (6). Thus, the goal of this chapter is somewhat limited—to identify for planners the most common problems and tasks they will face in virtually any disaster.

Some believe that every disaster is unique, meaning that effective planning is not even possible. However, empirical disaster research studies have identified a number of problems and tasks that appear to occur with predictable regularity, regardless of the disaster. These problems and tasks are the most amenable to planning. For example, almost every major disaster requires collecting information about the disaster and sharing it with the multiple agencies and institutions that become involved in the response. Other tasks include warning and evacuation, resource sharing, widespread search and rescue, triage, patient transport that efficiently utilizes area hospital assets, dealing with the press, and overall coordination of the response. Effective planning involves identifying and planning for what is likely to happen in disasters. It also requires procedures for planned, coordinated improvisation to deal with those contingencies that have not been anticipated in the plan (6). (Details of this two-pronged approach will be discussed in more detail in this chapter.)

The Paper Plan Syndrome

Just because a hospital has completed a written plan does not mean the hospital is prepared for a disaster. Although a written plan is important, it is but one requirement for preparedness. In fact, a written plan can be an illusion of preparedness if other requirements are neglected. This illusion has been called *the paper plan syndrome* (2,6,9). To avoid the creation of impotent paper plans, the following must be true of the planning:

- Based on valid assumptions about what happens in disasters (2).
- Based on interorganizational perspective. (Often, hospitals, as well as other emergency and disaster response organizations, plan in isolation, rather than collaborating with other agencies likely to become involved in the response [e.g., ambulance services, emergency management agencies, blood banks, 911 dispatchers, law enforcement agencies, fire departments, health departments, Red Cross personnel, news media, and other hospitals].) (2,10).
- Accompanied by the provision of resources (time, funding, supplies, space, equipment, and personnel) to carry out the plans (6).
- Associated with an effective training program so that users are familiar with the plan (10).
- Acceptable to the end-users. (If the plan users are involved in the planning process, they are more likely to be familiar with the final product; to consider it practical, realistic, and legitimate; and, most importantly, to use it.) (11,12).

Failure to comply with these prerequisites may contribute to the development of disaster plans that are unworkable in practice, and it may explain why so often the disaster response differs from what was prescribed in the plan (2,4,5,13–26).

Example. Many hospital administrators concede that, although disaster plans are necessary for hospital accreditation, they are relatively unworkable in practice. As one administrator involved in a disaster stated, "I opened up our plan immediately after we were notified, and it said that wards 4A and 4B would be the shock and resuscitation areas for all victims. That's four floors up, and I said 'We're forgetting the disaster plan completely, this is the way we are going to run it,' and we ran it from that point on our own…" (15).

Example: Earthquake, Coalinga, California, 1983. "On the day of the disaster, the plan seemed wholly inadequate. Cooperation of the many jurisdictions necessary to meld a common disaster plan for a large community was extremely difficult. The paramedics drill their disaster responses, the hospitals drill their interhospital responses, and the multiple agencies drill both individually and collectively. However, on the day of the disaster, the various resources often seemed to be functioning with very independent plans." (27)

Example: The DC-10 Air Crash, Dallas-Fort Worth International Airport, 1985. "This was the first major airline disaster that was experienced in the Dallas area, and many of the components of the disaster plan failed." Because the telephone circuits were jammed and no radio communications were available to use as an alternate means of information sharing, adequate communications between the scene and area hospitals were not possible for hours. Communications were also complicated because the city, county, and airport all had different disaster plans (a problem that still exists). Because of the communications problem, early confusion existed as to whether a disaster actually had occurred. The hospital disaster response was first initiated by medical personnel, but it was aborted by the administration. The local broadcast radio stations announced the disaster before adequate medical information was available. They also wanted access to information from the hospital. However, the disaster plan had not identified an organized approach for information release (5).

Example: Radiation leak, Three-Mile Island, 1979. When a radiation leak occurred in 1979 at the Three Mile Island nuclear plant, the health care system was ill prepared to deal with a community-wide evacuation. Area hospitals found existing disaster plans inadequate, and thus they developed evacuation plans both spontaneously and in concert with local emergency management agencies. No plans existed for area-wide evacuation of hospitalized patients (28).

In a study of 29 United States disasters, the University of Delaware's Disaster Research Center found that, in most cases, the disaster plan was not followed to any great extent. One of the reasons this occurred was that key personnel did not fully understand the plan or know their role in it. Another reason was that common disaster problems were not anticipated by the plan. Triage occurred according to plan in only one-third of the cases they studied. In fewer than half of the cases, casualties were transported to the hospital according to the plan; moreover, a predesignated communications plan was followed in only 21% of the cases (2).

According to a 1979 report (29), city managers and county executives think that state and federal disaster agencies require very complicated and lengthy disaster plans. City managers said they had read their plan once and did not know where it was now and that they would not use it in a disaster anyway. In many cases, these plans are developed in isolation by a single person with minimal involvement from key emergency response organizations because the operational goal is simply to comply with federal disaster planning requirements. As a result, the procedures of different organizations do not form a coordinated management system (1).

Example: 1989 San Francisco Bay Earthquake. A study conducted in the aftermath of the 1989 San Francisco Bay area earthquake revealed that, although 46 of 49 (94%) hospital emergency department nurses and 35 of 49 (71%) emergency department physicians knew the location of the emergency department disaster plan, only 15 (31%) of the emergency nurses and 13 (27%) of the emergency physicians in hospitals impacted by the quake referred to the plan during the disaster (30).

Disaster planning is further complicated by the fact that many emergency departments are staffed with part-time emergency physicians, and these physicians frequently work at more than one hospital. As a result, physicians are sometimes unfamiliar with the staff, hospital procedures, and the disaster plan. During the 1989 earthquake in the San Francisco Bay area, one physician reported to her second shift at an urban hospital to find that she was designated to be in charge of the disaster with a plan she had never seen in a hospital where she could not even locate the cafeteria (30).

Importance of the Planning Process

A frequently overlooked but important factor in disaster planning is the planning process. Often the process of planning is more important than the written document that results from it. This is not only because those who participate in the planning process are more likely to accept the final product as legitimate and practical but also because of the personal contacts that result. A number of researchers have observed that predisaster contacts among members of emergency response organizations result in smoother operations when disaster strikes. Even informal contacts have been said to have this effect. Organizations and their personnel are more likely to interface successfully if they do not have to do so with total strangers. Furthermore, in the process of planning, the participants develop a trust in one another, and they also become more familiar with the roles of other individuals and organizations in the response. Finally, during the planning process, one learns how one's actions in a disaster might enhance or detract from the ability of others to carry out crucial activities (3,6,10,11, 31–36).

Importance of Administrative Commitment and the Provision of the Resources Necessary to Carry Out the Plan

Success in any organizational endeavor hinges on the extent to which the chief executive officer is committed to that success; disaster preparedness is no exception. To gain the attention, respect, and cooperation of organization members, disaster planning needs to be given the necessary status, authority, and support. Unfortunately, the disaster planning task is often relegated to a position of low status within the administrative hierarchy and is isolated from any existing sources of political power and from priority-setting, budgeting, and decision-making processes (1,19,37–39).

One of the reasons things so often do not go according to plan when disasters strike is the failure to provide the resources (e.g., personnel, time, money, equipment, supplies, and facilities) necessary to make the plan work. Plans might be developed without funding for equipment and supplies. Time and money might not be budgeted for the development of disaster training programs or for the overtime needed for training or drills. Persons assigned disaster-planning tasks might still be expected to carry out all of their regularly assigned duties, and they may receive little remuneration or recognition for their extra efforts. One should not be surprised that organizations that allow planning to occur in this context get what they pay for. If preparedness efforts are to result in more than paper plans, the planning process must be tied to the resources necessary to carry out the mandate (4,29,38,40–43).

OBSERVATIONS FROM THE RESEARCH LITERATURE

Complacency Toward Planning

Hospital disaster planners must face the reality that disaster planning is not always met with enthusiasm (1,6,24,44). Although the theoretical value of planning for disasters is accepted to some degree by the medical community, implementation is not typically given much priority (2). Often, getting chief executive officers and organizational members to support disaster preparedness is more difficult than developing the disaster countermeasures themselves (6).

> **Example: Hurricane Agnes.** In 1972, the Wilkes-Barre, Pennsylvania, area was flooded by the remnants of Hurricane Agnes. The floodwaters damaged the offices of 130 (43%) of the area's 300 physicians, 55 dentistry offices, and 50 pharmacies and public health structures. In addition, two hospitals and five nursing homes had to be evacuated. Medical records were destroyed, pharmacies were inundated, and all lines of communications were out of order. The loss of the area's backup disaster communications equipment, which had been stored in the basement of the civil defense building, compounded the problem. This building, located on the riverbank, was one of the first areas to be flooded. Wilkes-Barre is in a flood plain, and it had been flooded in 1784, 1786, 1842, 1846, 1850, 1865, 1893, 1901, 1902, 1936, and 1955. Despite this history, no comprehensive, coordinated plan existed to guide these health care institutions or professionals at the time of the 1972 calamity (45).

A number of reasons can be found for this lack of support for disaster preparedness activities. First, some of those involved in routine emergency responses believe that they already know what to do because they see disaster response as merely an expansion of daily emergency response.

Second, disasters are low-probability events. Americans tend to dismiss major disasters as something that is unlikely to happen, that is going to happen to someone else, or that is going to happen on someone else's watch (46). As the renowned disaster researcher Thomas Drabek of the University of Denver states, "The statistical probability is that when a disaster strikes, it will strike elsewhere—primarily because there is so much 'elsewhere'" (31). The improbability of occurrence is especially true with regard to large-scale disasters in the United States. Auf der Heide (6) reported that only six peacetime disasters in the entire history of the country have resulted in over 1,000 fatalities. These included the following.

- 1865—Steamship *Sultana* explosion, Mississippi River, near Memphis, Tennessee (1,547 deaths).
- 1871—Forest fire, Peshtigo, Wisconson (1,182 deaths).
- 1889—Flash flood, Johnstown, Pennsylvania (more than 2,200 deaths).
- 1900—Hurricane, Galveston Island, Texas (more than 5,000 deaths).
- 1904—Fire on the steamship *General Slocum* on the East River, New York (more than 1,021 deaths).
- 1928—Hurricane, Lake Okeechobee, Florida (more than 2,000 deaths).

Another disaster that should be added to this list is the 1918 flu pandemic that caused 500,000 deaths in the United States (47). Only about 10 to 15 disasters a year result in more than 40 injuries (48). The risk of death from a disaster (1 per 100 billion person-hours of exposure) pales in comparison to that for deaths due to tobacco use (50 per 100 billion person-hours) or automobile crashes (100,000 per 100 billion person-hours) (49, 50). These figures are given not to downplay the need for hospital disaster programs but rather to illustrate the difficulty in mobilizing resources for readiness-related efforts. Those areas of the country with the most extensive preparedness are those exposed to recurrent seasonal threats from floods, hurricanes, and tornadoes. Probably the greatest single incentive for disaster preparedness is the occurrence of a disaster. In fact, the statement has been made that the interest in disaster preparedness is proportional to the recency, magnitude, and proximity of the last disaster (5,6,18,25,33,35,38,43,51).

Third, hospital administrators must deal with other competing daily priorities. For many hospitals, the most pressing crisis is surviving the next fiscal quarter. Hospitals are increasingly faced with cutbacks in health insurance reimbursements, as well as with reductions or freezes in federal, state, and local funding. At the same time, hospitals must deal with increasing numbers of uninsured and underinsured patients who are sicker and who have fewer coping resources (52).

The extent of this adverse fiscal climate is illustrated by the $655 million budgetary shortfall faced by the Los Angeles County Health Department in the summer of 1995. Only a federal bailout prevented the closure of the Los Angeles County–University of California Medical Center, the nation's largest and busiest hospital and the provider of care to 28% of the major trauma victims in the county (53). In the face of these financial problems, a prospective mechanism for funding hospital disaster preparedness is nonexistent.

Fourth, assessing the risks from potential disasters and determining the benefits of disaster management efforts are difficult at best. Because disasters are unexpected and unique, some have the view that planning is either useless or that it is lacking in cost-effectiveness. Often, the benefits of preparedness are not obvious until after a disaster occurs. In times of economic constraints, programs whose benefits cannot clearly be demonstrated tend to get short shrift on the list of budgetary priorities (6,54). The problem of competing budgetary priorities is compounded by the lack of federal, state, and insurance-based funding mechanisms for health sector disaster readiness efforts. This lack of funding might partially be due to the widespread American attitude that the best government is the least government and that one of the best tools to achieve this objective is to reduce taxes (33).

The monetary issue is illustrated by the following hypothetical question: if you were a hospital administrator who received a $100,000 budgetary surplus, would you spend it on disaster preparedness that may never save a life or would you allocate it for the purchase of new imaging equipment with which you could start saving lives tomorrow and for which your institution will be fully reimbursed?

Planning Assumptions

The value of planning is in its ability to anticipate the problems that are likely to be faced in a disaster and to develop realistic, cost-effective, and practical countermeasures. It should not be surprising to find that, if likely problems are not anticipated, the plans will not be very useful. Furthermore, if planning is based on invalid assumptions, it may not succeed in guiding an effective response. Planners might, for example, assume the following:

- A shortage of supplies and medical personnel will exist.
- Hospitals will receive prompt notification after disaster occurs.
- Responding emergency medical services (EMS) units will triage the victims, provide stabilizing first aid or medical care, and then distribute casualties in such a manner that no one hospital is inordinately overloaded.
- Patients needing specialized care (e.g., hazardous materials decontamination or burn care) will be sent to hospitals that have the capacity to deal with patients' conditions.

Hospitals might reasonably assume these activities will occur because they are written in the disaster plan. How-

ever, numerous field disaster studies and after-action critiques have demonstrated that these and other planning assumptions, on which hospital disaster planning is based are often inaccurate or untrue (2).

Another common planning assumption is that disasters are similar to daily emergencies, except for the extreme shortages of response resources. In fact, disasters are often defined as emergencies that exceed the available resources to deal with them (6). Although this definition might hold true for disasters in underdeveloped countries or in military conflicts, this is uncommon in domestic peacetime disasters. Numerous events in the United States that have been called disasters have not been characterized by severe shortages of community medical resources (31,55,56).

In a study of 29 mass casualty disasters in the United States and its territories, the Disaster Research Center found that only 6% of the hospitals had supply shortages and that 2% had shortages of personnel. Many hospitals reported that they had more regular staff and medical volunteers than they could effectively use (2).

Example: 1989 San Francisco Bay Earthquake. A report by the California Association of Hospitals and Health Systems on the 1989 San Francisco Bay area earthquake, commonly referred to as the Loma Prieta earthquake, included this remark, "Hospitals did not experience an initial shortage of staff, and in some cases there was even an initial overflow of staff due to staff voluntarily returning to the hospital" (25). Of 54 hospital administrators interviewed after the earthquake, 51 (94%) reported adequate supplies during the earthquake period, and 47 administrators stated that they had adequate supplies for the week following the earthquake (30).

Example: Sioux City United Airlines Crash, 1989. In July 1989, when United Airlines Flight 232 suffered an engine failure accompanied by a loss of all hydraulic control, it crash-landed at the Sioux City Airport and cartwheeled into an adjacent cornfield. As a result of the crash, 193 survivors were transported to St. Luke's Regional Medical Center and the Marian Health Center. Of these victims, 59 were admitted to one of the two hospitals. On hearing of the crash, about 100 physicians closed their offices and responded to the hospitals. Six physicians went directly to the scene to help there. In addition, nearly 300 nurses, other specialists, and volunteers waited at the hospitals to help with the incoming casualties. In this situation, an abundance of both medical supplies and personnel was available (57–59).

Example: Oklahoma City Bombing, 1995. When a bomb exploded in front of the Murrah Federal Building in Oklahoma City in 1995, a call went out over the news media early in the disaster for everyone with medical training to report to various locations in town. The state's medical community responded in force. Neonatal nurses from Tulsa drove 2 hours to help care for the many injured children they had heard about. Every type of health care provider from physical therapists to neurosurgeons arrived to help. Local hospital emergency departments were quickly inundated with medical personnel wanting to offer assistance. St. Anthony's Hospital, closest to the scene, received the most casualties, but it had over 500 medical personnel on hand to treat them. About 100 physicians ended up treating fewer than 50 patients at any given time. At least one or two physicians and several nurses were providing care to each patient (60–63).

Because disasters are believed to be defined by the lack of resources, the emphasis of planning and response is often placed on the indiscriminate mobilization of large numbers of extra resources. Unfortunately, the establishment of procedures and mechanisms to coordinate these resources is frequently neglected (64,65). When resources are present in greater amounts than is needed, their presence can greatly complicate the already difficult problems of coordination and communication. In the more extreme cases, an excessive influx of resources has even been observed to impede physically effective response activity during the disaster (6).

Example. Nine minutes after a tornado hit, an ambulance was dispatched to the scene. The emergency medical technician on board reported back, saying "Send everything available; it's a big one." As a result, ambulances arrived from all over the state. However, the assessment was wrong, and outside ambulances were not needed at all. Three times the number of ambulances necessary responded, many of which got flat tires and blocked the roadways (2).

Example. When an airliner crashed in Kenner, Louisiana, in 1982, unsolicited ambulance and rescue units came from as far as 70 miles away. The response also included 14 helicopters, 42 doctors, and 100 nurses. About 200 police arrived, parked their vehicles, and proceeded on foot to the scene. The police created a crowd problem for rescue personnel, and the parked police cars blocked incoming fire trucks and ambulances. All this was for a mere four seriously injured survivors from the crash. Local command personnel were unaware that these response resources were coming, and, therefore, they could not cancel their response. While the response was well intentioned, the flood of emergency personnel and equipment overwhelmed site authorities, making management and control difficult (66).

Certainly, resource shortages can occur at any given time or place in a disaster. However, in the United States, more often than not, overall community medical resources are sufficient; but they must be used in different ways than during routine, daily emergencies. One of the reasons that disaster medical resources are not strained as much as one would expect is because disasters in the United States have been relatively small in comparison to those in other parts of the world. In addition, the United States is also comparatively well endowed with a medical infrastructure (6,55).

One factor enhancing available medical resources in disasters is that most hospitals operate on a 24-hour basis. In a crisis, therefore, many hospitals can rapidly double or triple their available staff by calling in off-duty personnel (4,67). In fact, most off-duty staff do not have to be formally called back to duty; they will report to their hospitals on their own without being asked (33,38,56,68–72). In addition, physicians, nurses, and other medical professionals not on the hospital staff will show up to volunteer their services (33, 57,69,73–75).

The assumption that emergency response personnel will abandon their professional responsibilities to attend to their families in disasters contributes to the belief that disasters are resource-deficiency phenomenon. However, field studies have not borne out that such professional role abandonment is common. The few who must choose family over professional emergency responsibilities are more than made up for by the large numbers of volunteers and off-duty staff who spontaneously show up and offer help (7,38,64).

Lack of Hospital Notification and Information on Casualties

Most community hospital and emergency medical disaster plans assume that timely and appropriate information will be received from the disaster site. Information on the nature and scope of the disaster will allow responders to prioritize the use of available resources and to mobilize the appropriate numbers and types of resources when and where they are needed. For the medical response, essential information includes (a) estimates of the numbers, types, and severities of illnesses or injuries and (b) the current abilities of medical facilities (e.g., hospitals) to accept and treat casualties. This information can be used to facilitate the distribution of casualties so as to spread the patient load among area hospitals so that no single facility is overwhelmed (2,14). While the majority of casualties will bring themselves to the closest or most familiar hospitals by nonambulance transport, the availability of the above information can still guide the destination of patients transported by ambulances over which local authorities may still have control. For example, if hospitals closest to the scene are being overloaded with patients transported by private vehicles, ambulances can be instructed to avoid those hospitals.

However, the evidence suggests that such information flow to hospitals usually does not occur. At least in part, this might be due to the fact that few plans actually specify who has the responsibility for such assessment or how exactly needs assessment at the scene will be carried out (2,5,14,23, 76,77). In one study of 29 United States disasters in the late 1970s, researchers found that communications from the disaster site to any hospital occurred in fewer than one-third of the cases (2). However, even when such communication does occur, it frequently does not include critical information on the numbers, types, and severities of casualties to expect (2,68). In fact, many hospitals learn about the disaster from the mass media, the first arriving casualties, or ambulances rather than from official sources (2,13,14,17, 25,30,56,63,68–70,74,78–86).

An overall needs assessment is unlikely to occur when coordination and control at the scene have not been accomplished, and for coordination and control to occur early in a disaster response is rare (more on this later). Although individual agencies might attempt to collect information, more often than not they use it to address their own agency-specific tactical needs. Both the pooling of observations among agencies to develop an overall strategic needs assessment and the transmission of assessment results to all who need this information are uncommon (2,14).

Compared to the situation in daily emergency responses, overall scene assessment is often complicated in disasters when the scene is very large, when multiple disaster sites exist, when streets are strewn with debris that inhibits access, and when emergency medical agencies have not been integrated into the response. The process is further complicated when, as so often happens, multiple agencies with overlapping jurisdictional authority from different levels of government and the private sector respond (6,87).

Lack of Interagency Radio Communications Networks

Lack of adequate information flow to hospitals might occur because existing radio equipment has been damaged or even because the harried emergency department staff has turned down the volume so as not to be bothered by its incessant noise. However, in many cases, the lack of information sharing occurs because many emergency response agencies, including hospitals, ambulance services, health departments, emergency management and disaster agencies, and dispatch centers, do not have mutually compatible radio networks or procedures to share needs assessment information. In other cases, the lack of information results because communication to hospitals by dispatchers and outside emergency response organizations depends on telephones (28,58,61,88,89).

Unfortunately, even if telephone lines are left intact by the disaster, the circuits will almost certainly be overloaded and unusable (61,69,88,89). Although emergency response organizations such as hospitals can arrange to receive priority with the telephone company when the telephone lines are jammed, little evidence shows that most hospitals take advantage of this option (or that they even know it exists). In recent years, as the use of cellular telephones has greatly increased, cellular telephone connections have become the victim of the same types of communications overload that wire-based telephones encounter in disasters (33,58,61, 90–92). Because wire-based and cellular telephones are unreliable in disasters, interorganizational information flow requires that emergency response organizations have common, mutual aid radio frequencies on which to carry out two-way communications. This lesson is learned over and over again in disaster after disaster (5,28,33,61,88,93–96).

Although mutual aid radio networks are important, disaster researchers have reported that most communication problems are people problems rather than equipment problems. For effective disaster communications to occur, the person who is responsible for collecting critical information, the person who needs this information but does not have it, and the method for getting the information to them promptly using terminology that is mutually understood must be clearly delineated. For example, in a hazardous chemical spill, the hospital needs to know the identity of the chemical, the numbers of casualties being transported, the severity of their symptoms, and their estimated time of arrival. However, firefighters and ambulance crews at the scene may never have received any training that tells them who is responsible for collecting and relaying this information. No amount of communications hardware can solve this kind of issue (6,97). The responsibilities for these communications tasks need to be set in the community-wide disaster plan and included in disaster training programs and exercises.

Responders Are Different in Disasters Than in Routine Emergencies

One common observation in disasters is that those who respond to them are often different than those who are dispatched to routine, daily emergencies. Responders in surrounding communities will hear about the incident on their police scanners or from news broadcasts. In many instances, the initial reports are greatly exaggerated and confused. Often, determining if outside help is actually needed is extremely difficult—not only because of the above-mentioned problems with telephone lines and mutual aid frequencies but also because who (if anyone) is in charge of the scene and who will know if outside help is needed may not be clear. Assuming that too much help is better than too little, emergency units will respond on an unsolicited basis from many miles away, even from other states. Local authorities might be completely unaware of what outside help is coming, much less be prepared to integrate it into the response effort (6,55).

Example: Coalinga, California Earthquake, 1983.
In 1983, an earthquake measuring 6.5 on the Richter scale struck the small town of Coalinga (population, 7,000) in Central California. Word went out via amateur radio that this was the "Big One," with requests to "send everything you've got." Thirty ambulances and five helicopters responded from as far away as San Francisco, which is 100 miles away. None had been officially requested, none were actually needed, and some left their communities without ambulance coverage during their response (27,98).

Example: Sioux City United Airlines Crash, 1989.
In the 1989 Sioux City air crash, all 14 of the county's basic life support ambulances were dispatched to the scene. About 80 on-duty and off-duty Sioux City firefighters arrived to help at the crash site (58). Approximately 250 troops at the Air National Guard Base adjacent to the airport for a scheduled drill responded to the scene (99). The state emergency operations center dispatched six Army National Guard helicopters from Boon, Iowa, near Des Moines. A statewide law enforcement agency teletype message requested that ambulances within a reasonable distance respond to the disaster (58). Thirty-five ambulances from 29 communities, along with four civilian EMS helicopters, responded from as far away as 70 miles from Iowa, Nebraska, and South Dakota. The response included 20 paramedics, 100 basic emergency medical technicians, and 40 outside fire departments (58,59,99). More ambulances responded than were actually needed. During the after-action critique, the concern that the law enforcement teletype request for ambulances was too vague and that it might have left some counties without adequate ambulance coverage during the disaster response was expressed (58).

Effects of Bystander Volunteers

To complicate matters further, most of the initial response (e.g., search and rescue) is not carried out by trained emergency personnel, but rather it is conducted by civilian bystanders who happen to be in the area. These bystanders might include family members, friends, neighbors, coworkers, and even those who are complete strangers to the victims (6,55,100,101) (Fig. 8.1).

Example: San Francisco Bay Earthquake, 1989. In 1989, an earthquake measuring 7.1 on the Richter scale struck the San Francisco Bay area. A random survey revealed that 3% of the residents of San Francisco county and about 5% of the residents of Santa Cruz county engaged in search and rescue activities. This amounted to over 31,000 persons (102).

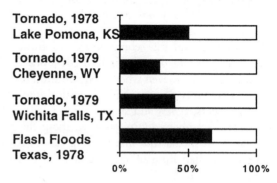

Search & Rescue by Bystander Volunteers

FIGURE 8.1. Search and rescue by bystander volunteers.

Example: Tanshan, China Earthquake, 1976. In 1976, Tanshan, China, was hit by an earthquake measuring 7.8 on the Richter scale. The earthquake killed 240,000 persons. About 200,000 to 300,000 survivors extricated themselves from the rubble and went on to rescue others. The survivors were credited with 80% of the rescue of those who were still buried (103).

For disaster victims with life-threatening injuries and illnesses, the time until arrival at the hospital is not the most important factor in survival. Rather, the time until the victims receive the appropriate definitive medical care is crucial. For example, when a disaster victim is critically injured, shortening the time from injury to arrival in the operating room is often what determines the outcome. If that victim is transported rapidly to a nearby hospital that is overloaded with trauma patients, the delay to definitive surgical treatment may be greater than if transport had been to a more distant hospital that had fewer patients competing for the available operating rooms and surgeons. Survival may also depend on transporting the patient to a hospital that has the specialists and facilities that the patient needs. Therefore, rapidly sending a patient with a serious head injury to a nearby hospital that has no neurosurgical capability is not likely to optimize survival.

To the lay public, however, the best emergency care is transport to the closest hospital as quickly as possible. If sufficient ambulances are not promptly available, these volunteers do not tend to sit idly by awaiting their arrival. Instead, they use whatever means of transportation is available to rush casualties to the closest hospital. A variant on this theme is when one hospital is particularly renowned for giving emergency care (e.g., the trauma center), in which case it may be the chosen destination (16,104). Police officers and firefighters sometimes contribute to this pattern by loading victims into various non-ambulance vehicles and sending them to these same hospitals. Thus, the majority of disaster casualties are not transported by ambulance, nor are they under the control of the EMS system (6,38,55,61,69,70,104,105). In this process, field first aid and triage stations are frequently bypassed, either because their existence or location is unknown or because first aid is perceived as a lower level of care than that which is available at hospitals (6). These patterns help to explain why hospitals have such difficulty obtaining the information necessary to guide their response. These patterns also contribute some understanding as to why so many victims arrive at hospitals without having received first aid or undergoing triage (6,100). In the late 1970s, the Disaster Research Center carried out a study of emergency medical services in 29 domestic disasters. At 75 hospitals where the initial means of casualty arrival could be determined, 54% arrived by ambulance, 16% by private vehicle, 16% by police car, 5% by helicopter, 5% by bus or taxi, and 4% on foot. Although these figures described the initial means of arrival, overall more than half of the casualties were transported by means other than ambulance (2).

Example: San Francisco Bay Earthquake, 1989. During the first night after the 1989 San Francisco earthquake (also called the Loma Prieta earthquake), only 23% of patients transported to area hospital emergency departments arrived by ambulance (106).

Example: Los Angeles Civil Disturbance, 1992. During the 1992 civil disturbance in Los Angeles, 34% of patients were transported to the hospital by ambulances, 11% were transported by police cars, and 13% were walk-ins. Koehler (107) reports that the percent of the injured who took themselves to the hospital or who were transported by friends varies by the source of data—it was 30.6% according to preliminary data from the Centers for Disease Control and Prevention and 60% to 70% according to hospital emergency department reports.

Example: Oklahoma City Bombing, 1995. After the Murrah Federal Building in Oklahoma City was destroyed by a bomb blast in 1995, 139 casualties (32%) were transported by ambulance and over 300 (68%) were transported by other means, such as buses, vans, or private vehicles (61).

Example: Tokyo Sarin Attack, 1995. When terrorists released the nerve agent sarin in the Tokyo subway system in 1995, 10% of the 640 patients arriving at nearby St. Luke's Hospital came by ambulance, 5% by fire department minivan, and 85% by private vehicle (108).

These actions by bystanders, as well as by fire and police, help explain why one (or a few) hospitals closest to the disaster site typically receive the majority of casualties while other hospitals await victims that never arrive (Table 8.1) (6,38,55,63,88,109). The Disaster Research Center found that, in 75% of the cases, a majority of casualties went to the closest hospital. In 46% of the cases, over three-quarters of the casualties went to the closest hospital. (This report did not indicate what proportion of this distribution pattern was due to decisions of bystanders versus those of fire-fighters or police officers.) A simple majority of the hospitals received one or more casualties in only about half of the disasters studied. This was despite the fact that unused hospitals had an average vacancy rate of 20% (2). This pattern appears less often in disasters that strike a large geographical area where numerous hospitals are closest to the scene.

Time Course of Casualty Arrival at Hospitals

Casualties usually start arriving at hospitals within 30 minutes of the disaster impact, and the majority arrive within 60 to 90 minutes. Early casualty flow is made up mostly of those with minor injuries, probably because they are less likely to be trapped in the rubble or because they can more easily escape or be rescued by bystanders. Because of the lack of timely casualty information from the scene, hospitals might be unaware of the fact that more serious victims are yet to arrive. When these victims do arrive, all of the emergency department beds might already be occupied (2,14,16,57,68,71,73,110,111).

Survival Versus Time Until Rescued

Although a few trapped disaster victims have been rescued alive at 5, 10, and even 14 days after impact, this occurs only in exceptional cases. In the 1980 earthquake in southern Italy, for example, 94% of the trapped people who survived were rescued during the first 24 hours. No victims were rescued alive after the third day (101). The 1990 earthquake in the Philippines yielded similar findings—88% survival was seen for those rescued on day 1, 35% on day 2, 9% on day 3, and 0% from day 4 and onward (112). In the 1976 earthquake in Tangshan, China, those rescued in the first half-hour had a 99% survival rate, followed by 81% on day 1, 34% on day 2, 38% on day 3, 19% on day 4, and 7.4% on day 5 (113). In the 1995 bombing of the Murrah Federal Building in Oklahoma City, all but three of the survivors were rescued alive within 5 hours of the explosion (61). Thus, one can expect that rescue teams responding to large-scale disasters involving trapped victims will have little impact on survival unless they arrive within 1 or 2 days (114). In other words, the local emergency response is the critical variable in the survival of trapped casualties.

TABLE 8.1. MALDISTRIBUTION OF DISASTER CASUALTIES

Disaster Location Date	Details
Tornado Flint, Michigan 1953	About 750 (80%) of victims were brought to one hospital (16).
Tornado Worcester, Massachusetts 1953	Eight hundred were injured; 90% were admitted by 3 of 15 area hospitals (16).
Tornado Waco, Texas 1953	Most of injured were taken to one downtown hospital, which was swamped before those at greater distances from the incident were filled (158).
Tornado Dallas, Texas 1957	Casualties received by each hospital: Parkland, 178; Methodist, 17; Baylor, 2; St. Paul's, 1 (109).
Aircraft carrier fire New York 1960	A nearby hospital had 35 patients and inadequate resources to care for them. Most patients could have been transported to hospitals farther away from the scene where personnel were available and provisions for treatment had been made (76).
Coliseum explosion Indianapolis, Indiana 1963	Seventy-five percent of the 374 casualties were taken to three local hospitals. Hospitals available included 7 in the city and 12 in the surrounding area for a total of over 4,600 beds (36).
Earthquake Anchorage, Alaska 1964	Twenty-two victims were taken to one of five hospitals in Anchorage; no mention of total casualties for this disaster (212).
Train crash Chicago, Illinois 1972	Of 400 injured, none were transported to Cook County Hospital, the local trauma center and a 4-minute trip by any of the 15 helicopters transporting patients from the site (140).
Train crash Chicago, Illinois 1976	Of the 381 injured, 85% were sent to 3 of 11 hospitals but none were sent to Cook County Hospital (213).
Train crash Chicago, Illinois 1977	Of the 183 injured, 48% were sent to the 2 closest of 11 hospitals; Cook County Hospital received 9% (213).
Skywalk collapse, Hyatt Hotel Kansas City, Missouri 1981	Seventeen of 26 hospitals were used; the 4 closest hospitals received 42% of the 200 victims and 55% of those admitted and did 83% of the surgery (110).
Metrorail crash Washington, D.C. 1982	Nineteen of 22 (86%) injured survivors went to one hospital (83).
Tornado Coldenham, New York 1989	Of the 26 patients transported from the scene, 19 went to St. Luke's Hospital (including the 2 deceased), 5 to Cornwall Hospital, 1 to Horton Hospital, and 1 to St. Francis Hospital (77).
Tornado Plainfield, Illinois 1990	When telephone lines were severed by the tornado, ambulance services were left with no means to contact the command post or area hospitals. In addition, many of the vehicles from surrounding towns operated on different radio frequencies and could not communicate with one another. As a result, most patients that were transported by ambulance were taken to the closest hospital. In all 221 patients were treated at this hospital; 35 of those patients were admitted and 5 were transferred (138).
Bombing Oklahoma City, Oklahoma 1995	Although there were many victims of this disaster, only one hospital—the closest geographically—became overwhelmed by the number of victims arriving. Most emergency departments triaged patients they would normally have seen on any given day to another care area to make room for "the massive wave" of critical patients that was sure to come. In reality, this massive wave never materialized, and many of the emergency departments sat idle after treating only a few victims (63).
Tornado Oklahoma City, Oklahoma 1999	Distribution of patients to the metropolitan hospitals followed the same pattern as in the 1995 Oklahoma City bombing; the two closest hospitals were overwhelmed with patients (111).

References indicated in parentheses following each item.

Adapting Plans to Deal With Typical Patterns of Disaster Behavior

Disaster planners and responders can do little to control the efforts of bystanders in disaster situations. Disaster plans are more effective if they are designed around how people tend to behave in disasters. This approach is likely to be more successful than expecting persons to conform to the plan (2). Planners and responders can influence the outcome by anticipating the likely course of bystander actions. For example, ambulances should anticipate that the closest hospitals will get the most patients and thus should avoid transporting additional patients to these if possible. Hospitals should not expect that patients will be triaged or decontaminated at the disaster site but should instead make provisions to carry out these tasks at the hospital.

Focus on Multiple Trauma Preparedness

Another common assumption in medical disaster planning is that the primary medical need will be to deal with large numbers of victims suffering from multiple trauma. Although the capacity to deal with critical traumatic injuries is important, most disaster injuries are relatively minor, and these could be managed in medical facilities other than hospitals (e.g., clinics, urgent care centers, and physicians' offices)(115–121). Many injuries, in fact, occur not during impact but during the clean-up period (93,112). The Disaster Research Center found that, on average, only 20% of the casualties were admitted—even overnight—to the hospital. Furthermore, about half of these were admitted more because they had been in the disaster than because of the seriousness of their conditions, and they were discharged the next day (2). Thus, only about 10% of disaster casualties really required even the most basic inpatient care.

Nontrauma Casualties and Loss of Access to Routine Sources of Medical Care

That, in many disasters, the majority of patients need care for conditions other than trauma is not always appreciated. This set of patients might include those who have lost access to their routine sources of custodial care, medical care, mental health care, or prescription medications (22, 45,112,115,118,122–131). For example, in Hurricane Andrew, the initial damage estimates included 1,000 physician offices, 11 private pharmacies, 7 convalescent hospitals, 90 living facilities for the aged, 2 dialysis clinics, 4 mental health facilities, 5 community clinics, 38 assisted living facilities, and 4 intermediate facilities for the developmentally disabled (132,133). Exacerbations of chronic medical conditions, such as asthma, emphysema, coronary ischemia, hypertension, and diabetes, may contribute to the situation.

Problems also occur with a lack of provisions to deal with the health needs of persons who have been evacuated to public shelters. After Hurricane Elena caused 1.25 million Florida residents to evacuate their homes, a study determined that 23% of those in shelters had some kind of medical problem. The most common were heart problems (29%), diabetes mellitus (17%), a handicap (17%), high blood pressure (5.1%), need for oxygen (2%), and other conditions (29%; this last category included pregnancy, fractures, recent discharges from hospitals, and chronic illnesses such as cystic fibrosis) (127).

Although disaster medical planning tends to focus on hospital and EMS readiness, most patients could be cared for in nonhospital settings, such as physicians' offices, clinics, and free-standing urgent care or ambulatory care centers. Unfortunately, these valuable medical assets are often not included in community disaster plans. For example, although 70% of the urgent care centers in San Francisco were open at the time the 1989 earthquake struck, only 50% stayed open. Sixty-seven percent of the urgent care centers had no disaster plan, and 70% had no backup electrical generator (134).

By assuring that routine sources of medical care survive and function after a disaster, the patient burden on hospitals might be reduced, leaving them more able to treat the critically ill and injured. After Hurricane Andrew, one Miami hospital administrator commented that most home health care agencies providing dialysis or ventilator care had not provided for backup electrical power arrangements for their patients (132). When Hurricane Iniki struck the island of Kauai, it knocked out the island's electrical power, putting 60 dialysis patients in peril (133). Reportedly, when both Hurricane Iniki and Hurricane Andrew struck, no hard-copy lists existed that showed the locations of patients on dialysis or home ventilators (133). A 1994 study of home health care agencies in San Diego found that, although 90% had a plan, only 33% had tested the plan. Forty-seven percent had made no backup arrangements for their patients, and 31% of those surveyed thought that they would not be able to meet their patients' needs in a disaster (135).

Donations

Public altruism in disasters is not limited to providing direct contributions in the form of search, rescue, and transportation. Unsolicited donations of all kinds and in every imaginable form are common (6,55,136). Citizens, merchants, and businesses from all over the country are quick to offer whatever might be of help in dealing with the aftermath of disasters. This assistance might include offers of food, laundry service, free long-distance telephone calls, chiropractic and massage services for rescuers and relief workers, clothing, money, vehicles, tools, rescue equipment, medical supplies, pharmaceutical agents, cellular telephones, heavy construction equipment (e.g., heavy cranes), the free use of company personnel, and even leather booties for rescue dogs (63,64).

Sometimes the magnitude of the response results in a situation where on-site personnel have to be diverted from other duties to process and track the excessive quantities of donated material (6,55,64). When donations include perishable items, the problem of inventory tracking is magnified (64). Pharmaceutical donations often create a problem because they are sent in amounts greater than what is needed, they include inappropriate and out-of-date medications, and they are not sorted and categorized before arrival (see Chapter 5).

Example: Armenia Earthquake, 1988. After the December 1988 earthquake in Armenia, over 5,000 tons of drugs and consumable medical supplies were donated for the relief effort, not including materials for dialysis, field hospitals, or laboratory equipment. Within a few days, these donations filled local warehouse and hospital storage capacity, and authorities had to open 32 new warehouses. By January, the new warehouses were also full, and storage had to be found in Moscow. Eighteen percent of the items were unsorted (with many different drugs all in the same box), and pharmacists wasted about two-thirds of their time merely looking for and identifying useful drugs. Eleven percent of the donated materials was of no use to the recipients, including items such as vitamins, nasal spray, and antibiotics only usable for infectious diseases not found in the region, and 8% of the drugs had passed their expiration date. Only 30% of the drugs were both easily identifiable and relevant to the emergency situation. Fifty people worked for 6 months merely to get a clear picture of the drugs donated (137).

Example: Oklahoma City Bombing, 1995. In the aftermath of the 1995 Oklahoma City bombing, medical donations came by the truckloads from across the country. "However, except for dressing and bandage materials, almost all of this equipment was wasted. One conservative estimate from a representative of the Oklahoma Hospital Association put the dollar amount of wasted medical supplies and equipment at over $1.5 million." (63).

Example: Plainfield, Illinois Tornado, 1990. In 1990, Plainfield, Illinois, was hit by a tornado. Problems occurred in discerning the official rescue workers from the well-meaning citizens who came to offer their help or to lend equipment such as dump trucks and backhoes. So many donations were received that they filled two warehouses; some donations were in danger of spoiling because the items could not be used fast enough (138).

Blood Donors

Hospitals and blood banks are often caught off-guard and are unprepared for the quantities of blood donors that show up during disasters (65,136,139) The situation is aggravated when local elected officials or mass media representatives issue mass appeals for blood donors, often without consulting the recipient organizations regarding the actual need for blood (5,56,67,136,140).

Example: Athens, Georgia Tornado, 1973. When a tornado struck Athens, Georgia, in 1973, "a request for blood donors produced a deluge of willing donors, far in excess of the number that could be handled by the hospitals. These people left their vehicles parked illegally and blocked traffic around the hospital." (65)

Example: Dallas, Texas DC-10 Crash, 1985. After a DC-10 crashed during a thunderstorm at Dallas-Fort Worth International Airport in 1985, radio stations announced the disaster before adequate medical information was available. "These stations suggested that blood would be needed. Four hundred ninety-one blood donors responded to the media's call for blood. This inundated the local hospital's blood bank, causing a problem with crowd control. Personnel had to be diverted from the emergency department to the blood bank to manage the people trying to donate blood." Some donors were actually turned away from the blood bank because personnel were unable to process them at the time (5).

Example: Oklahoma City Bombing, 1995. After the Oklahoma City bombing, "the Oklahoma Blood Institute opened satellite centers where citizens stood in line for 2 or 3 hours to donate blood. The blood centers closed in the late afternoon because the institute had received all the blood it could process." (64)

Example: Sioux City United Airlines Crash, 1989. At the time of the Sioux City air crash, the "blood supplies at the local hospitals and at the Siouxland Community Blood Bank were adequate to meet all of the demands. Though officials made no public appeal for blood donors, more than 400 persons turned out to donate blood. Offers of additional blood from blood centers in Des Moines, Omaha, and other areas much further away were declined." (58)

Hospitals as Disaster Victims

Although hospital plans often focus on disasters that may affect the community, insufficient attention is given to the possibility that the hospital itself might become a victim (141,142).

Example: San Fernando Valley Earthquake, 1971.
After the 1971 San Fernando Valley earthquake in Southern California, several hospitals sustained heavy damage or collapsed. In response to this tragedy, the 1972 Hospital Seismic Safety Act was passed. This act required the implementation of design and construction practices to ensure that hospitals could survive a major earthquake. The law applied to new construction and alterations or remodeling but not to hospitals constructed before the act was passed. The planner envisioned that the pre-Act, nonconforming buildings would be replaced by new, conforming facilities through attrition. However, a 1990 report by the California Office of Statewide Health Planning and Development (OSHPD) indicated that fewer than 17% of California's hospital beds were in hospitals that conformed to the Hospital Seismic Safety Act (less than 33% of the hospital buildings in the state) (143). A subsequent study by OSHPD in 2001 indicated that 51% of the hospital buildings were in compliance with the act and that they would not be expected to collapse in a major earthquake. However, the study could only identify 13% of the state's hospital buildings that could reasonably be expected also to resist the nonstructural damage (defined below) that would limit their ability to function after a strong motion earthquake (144).

Nonstructural damage can cause injury to hospital occupants, and it can interfere with the ability of the facility to care for patients. Nonstructural damage includes that which affects the nonload-bearing components of the building, such as the windows, ceilings, light fixtures, electrical circuits, water storage tanks, and sewer and water pipes. It also includes the contents of the hospital, such as shelves, cabinets and their contents, refrigerators, laboratory supplies and equipment, cardiac monitors, imaging equipment, computers, communications equipment, and cafeteria appliances.

Earthquakes (and other disasters) also interrupt utility services, such as electricity, sewer, water, and telephone lines, to the hospital. However, the 2001 California study could document fewer than 1% of the state's hospital buildings whose contents were adequately anchored or braced and that had sufficient backup power, water, and wastewater systems to operate for 72 hours (144).

Numerous case reports illustrate the lack of attention to basic measures to assure hospital survival and function after disasters. Generator failure is frequently mentioned (20–22, 71,75,82,142,145–147). Hospital function has also been compromised by inadequately anchored generators, unan-chored generator batteries, damage to the lines carrying natural gas to power the emergency generators, and the loss of the water supply to cool emergency generators (18,30, 148). Generators and generator-switching equipment have failed because they were located in basements subject to flooding (21,22,79,149). Failures have also resulted from inadequate electrical surge protection (21,30), dead batteries, and an inadequate fuel supply for the generators (30,148).

The ability of hospitals to function after a disaster has been compromised when inadequate emergency generator capacity exists (21,150,151) or when essential areas and equipment have not been included in backup generator circuits. Examples of the latter include x-ray developers (30), x-ray machines (33), air-conditioning needed for sensitive computer equipment (33), cafeteria refrigerators and freezers (30), bells and button lights on telephones (21), computed tomography scanners (25), two-way radios (25), computers (25), central supply areas (18), and ambulatory care units (150).

Although the need for backup water provisions is frequently mentioned as a necessity for preparedness, hospitals continue to suffer when water supplies are interrupted (18,25,75,148). Hospital functions that have been interrupted because of their dependence on water include operating room temperature and humidity systems, sterilization equipment, water-cooled refrigerators and freezers, hydrotherapy, x-ray film developers, telephone switchboard and computer mainframe cooling systems, air conditioning systems, fire sprinkler systems, medical suction, cooling systems for lasers, and emergency generators (142,150,152,153).

Other factors that have impaired hospital ability to function after disasters, particularly earthquakes, have included unanchored pharmaceutical storage shelves (25); severed oxygen lines (18); leaking natural gas lines (18); boilers with no backup fuel source (21); broken windows and glass (145,154); elevator malfunctions (33); and the lack of battery backup lighting to stairwells, elevators, operating room corridors, radiology, laboratory, outpatient units, and areas of the emergency department (142).

Summary of Field Research Findings

1. Most initial postdisaster search and rescue, field medical, or first aid care (to the extent that it occurs at all) and victim transportation is provided by civilian bystanders (e.g., family, neighbors, coworkers, and even passersby). This contributes to the following:
   - Most casualties are typically transported to the closest hospitals or to those most locally renowned for providing emergency care, while other hospitals await casualties that never arrive.
   - A minority of disaster victims actually receive effective first aid, medical care, or triage in the prehospital setting.

■ Little useful information about the disaster site or the numbers, types, or severities of casualties is communicated to area hospitals. Hospitals will often first become aware of the disaster from the news media or the first arriving casualties.

2. Casualties generally begin arriving at hospitals within 30 minutes; the majority arrive within 60 to 90 minutes. Thus, disaster responders to the scene will have little effect on emergency patient care unless they can arrive within a very short time. The first arriving casualties are usually those in the least serious condition. Because of the lack of scene-to-hospital information flow, hospitals might be unaware of the more serious casualties who subsequently arrive to find the emergency department already full of victims.

3. Few critically injured victims are rescued alive after the first day or two. Outside search and rescue teams arriving after that time will have little impact on the overall survival of trapped disaster casualties.

4. Little need exists in United States disasters to evacuate casualties to distant communities or for outside medical teams to provide critical care or surgical services; however, a locally increased demand for family practice type medical care services might exist.

5. Many disaster casualties can be treated in medical facilities other than hospitals. This can reduce the burden on hospitals so that they can care for the more serious patients.

6. When routine sources of medical care become inaccessible in disasters, the burden on hospitals can increase, lessening their ability to care for serious illnesses and injuries caused by the disaster. Therefore, nonhospital medical assets (e.g., physician offices, urgent care centers, clinics, dialysis centers, pharmacies, home health care agencies, nursing homes, and custodial care or assisted living facilities) need to be integrated into community disaster medical plans.

7. Hospitals can be casualties too. Effective planning requires the implementation of mitigation measures to ensure that hospitals can survive and function.

8. Effective disaster planning must include strategies for overcoming complacency toward disaster preparedness. Often, this is more difficult than implementing the disaster countermeasures themselves.

9. Effective planning requires the active participation of a diversity of emergency response organizations from multiple levels of government and the private sector (e.g., private physicians, hospitals, and ambulance services). However, hospitals and other emergency medical and health sector response organizations often plan in isolation and are often divorced from other community disaster planning efforts. The establishment of regional and statewide disaster planning bodies with representation from these organizations is essential for effective planning.

IMPROVING HOSPITAL PREPAREDNESS

Standards and Guidelines for Hospital Preparedness

The Joint Commission on Accreditation of Healthcare Organizations (JCAHO) promulgates standards for hospital preparedness. These standards (155) require, among other things, that hospital disaster plans include provisions for the following:

■ Carrying out a hazard vulnerability assessment;
■ Activating the plan;
■ Integrating the hospital plan with the community disaster plan;
■ Notifying external authorities that a disaster has occurred;
■ Alerting hospital personnel that the plan has been activated;
■ Identifying hospital personnel;
■ Housing and transporting staff;
■ Providing for staff family support;
■ Maintaining supply management (e.g., pharmaceutical agents, medical supplies, food, water, and linen);
■ Controlling access, crowds, and traffic;
■ Maintaining media relations;
■ Evacuating and establishing alternative sites for patient care when necessary;
■ Tracking patients and managing patient medications and medical records during evacuation;
■ Establishing and maintaining backup communications and utilities;
■ Setting up facilities to deal with and isolate patients contaminated by hazardous materials;
■ Assigning staff responsibilities during disasters;
■ Using a command structure consistent with that used by the local community in disasters;
■ Training;
■ Evaluating the plan annually.

Mitigation

The first duty of the hospital in a disaster is to avoid becoming a disaster victim. One of the best ways for the hospital not to become a disaster victim is for it not to be in locations where disasters tend to occur. Hospitals should not be constructed in areas where recurrent flooding occurs, near earthquake faults, on sandy river bottom soil that amplifies seismic shaking, near coastal areas subject to hurricane winds or storm surge, near chemical plants or storage areas, or in forested areas subject to recurrent wildland fires. When considering the construction of new hospital facilities, the local disaster office can be contacted for information on areas vulnerable to disasters that should be avoided.

The use of modern, hazard-resistant building codes for new construction or retrofitting is another important strategy to prevent hospitals (and other medical assets) from becoming disaster victims. For more information on building codes, see the web site for the Institute for Business and Home Safety (IBHS) at http://www.ibhs.org/building_codes/, the International Code Council at http://www.intlcode.org/ and http://www.intlcode.org/download/index.htm, the Building Seismic Safety Council at http://www.bssconline.org/ (the *2000 NEHRP Provisions for New Buildings and Other Structures*, FEMA 368, and FEMA 369), and the Federal Emergency Management Agency—Mitigation web site at http://www.fema.gov/mit/hseries1.htm. Attention also should be paid to the contents of the hospital building that might be vulnerable to damage in a disaster. For example, hospitals commonly locate heating systems, backup generators, and electrical switching equipment in the basement, the most vulnerable area in the event of flooding or water system leakage. More than one hospital suffered internal water damage during the 1994 Los Angeles earthquake because of disruption to the large water storage tanks on their roofs. Earthquakes commonly disrupt hospital utility, heating and cooling, and electrical backup systems. Simple and comparatively inexpensive engineering measures can avert these problems. One of the simplest and most inexpensive mitigation measures that can be taken in earthquake-vulnerable regions is to survey the hospital interior to identify those items that could fall or tip over during seismic shaking. The simple use of Velcro and adhesive straps to anchor equipment can prevent damage. Latched cabinets, wall bins, and ledges on shelves can prevent supplies, pharmaceutical agents, and equipment from falling. L-brackets can be used to anchor shelves, file cabinets, and other furniture to the wall studs to prevent the items from falling and damaging their contents or injuring staff and patients. An extensive listing of hospital mitigation measures can be found in *Community medical disaster planning and evaluation guide* by Auf der Heide (available from the American College of Emergency Physicians on the Internet at http://www.acep.org/ or by telephone at 1-800-798-1822 [press 6]).

Do Not Plan in Isolation

One lesson that is clear from the disaster research literature is that most response problems are due to the lack of interorganizational coordination and communication. However, most hospitals and other emergency response organizations plan as if they existed in isolation. Hospital planners should contact their local municipal or county disaster or emergency management office to find out if a community disaster planning committee exists. If no committee exists, they should consider starting one (1). Table 8.2 lists examples of the types of organizations that should be represented on such a committee. One alternative to establishing a community disaster planning committee is to use the Local Emergency Planning Committee (LEPC). LEPCs are

TABLE 8.2. EXAMPLES OF ORGANIZATIONS REPRESENTED ON A COMMUNITY DISASTER PLANNING COMMITTEE

Hospitals or hospital association
Medical society
Emergency physician groups
Nursing association
Health maintenance organizations (HMOs)
Local emergency medical services agency
Ambulance and rescue services
Helicopter services
Municipal or county disaster or emergency management office
Fire chiefs
Sheriff and police chiefs
Public works and highway departments
Local government chief executive officers or managers
Local military establishments
Local health department
Red Cross
Local ports and airports
Urgent care centers
Clinics
Home health care agencies
Nursing homes
Assisted living facilities
Pharmacies
Dialysis centers
Outpatient surgery centers
News media organizations
Flood control and dam officials
Local office of the United States Weather Service
Churches and social welfare agencies
Mental health facilities
Local businesses or chamber of commerce
Local utilities and communications providers
Local building inspectors and civil engineers

required under the Superfund Amendments and Reauthorization Act of 1986 Act (SARA Title III) for chemical emergency planning. More information on LEPCs can be obtained via the Internet at http://www.rtk.net/lepc/.

Such a planning committee can be an effective means of addressing a number of issues related to disaster preparedness. The committee can be the stage for developing not only regional plans for mitigation, response, and recovery but also for the establishment of a joint training program. Moreover, it provides the opportunity for the cost-sharing of training, which can reduce the financial outlay of the individual organizations. Standardization and the cost-sharing of items such as equipment for communications networks can also be addressed by the committee (156). Finally, plans, procedures, and training that have buy-in from a committee with broad community participation assures that they are more likely to be used.

Health and medical care responsibilities that should be addressed by the committee include the following:

- Warning and evacuation;
- Mitigation activities for health care facilities;

- Establishment of training programs for health care providers;
- Overall coordination of the health sector response;
- On-scene medical assessment;
- Overall coordination of site search and rescue;
- Triage;
- Hospital notification (including information on numbers, types, and severities of casualties);
- Inventory of current hospital patient loads and capacity to receive additional patients;
- Transport and distribution of casualties;
- Use of nonhospital facilities for patient care;
- Health facility recovery activities;
- Public health and environmental health activities (e.g., management of infectious disease outbreaks and chemical spills) and development of messages on disaster-related health issues for the media and the public (e.g., food safety when the power is lost, the effects of hazardous chemicals, and the prevention of chain saw injuries and carbon monoxide poisoning during cleanup and recovery).

Plan for Communications

Communication difficulties are one of the most recurrent and enduring problems identified in the analysis of disaster responses. Most commonly, when planners think of communications problems, they think of deficiencies in the hardware (two-way radio equipment, in particular). Decades of experience have shown that telephone systems are unreliable in disasters. Even if the circuits are not damaged, telephone systems are subject to communications traffic overload that rapidly makes them unusable. Despite this experience, most disaster plans still rely on telephone communications for postdisaster information exchange. Furthermore, with the rapid expansion of cellular telephone use, these systems often suffer from the same overload as land-line–based systems.

One must realize that, with the advent of modern mass communications technology, even a relatively small disaster becomes an international media event literally within minutes. Often initial media reports are greatly exaggerated, confused, and dramatic. These reports can cause a great deal of concern in those who think their loved ones are in the impacted area.

For example, consider the nationwide, if not worldwide, concern that would be generated by the following television announcement, "Flash! 747 jetliner crashes into suburban Los Angeles freeway and plows into adjacent neighborhood. Hundreds of dead and injured. Details at six."

One result of this concern would be a large number of telephone calls into the impacted area checking on the welfare of loved ones. If those telephoning are unable to make contact, attempts will be made to get information from police departments, hospitals, government offices, and the local news media. If telephone calls are unsuccessful in obtaining the needed information, many will show up and will try to get it in person (156a). Although this information-seeking behavior cannot be controlled, it can be substantially reduced by providing accurate information via the news media to describe the areas not impacted by the disaster. If, for example, the above television announcement gave details about the airline company, flight origin and destination, freeway name, suburb name, and the names of streets on which the damaged buildings were located, a much smaller number of people would be concerned about their loved ones as victims of the disaster. Also, another helpful technique would be for area hospitals to collect joint information on disaster patients and to transmit it by encrypted radio to a distant location where it can be provided (e.g., via the Red Cross) to the public through a toll-free telephone number. This will route call volume away from local telephone circuits, thus reducing the demand on them. Although some may hesitate to release patient information unselectively, information certainly can be released on what persons are not patients.

Calls are also received volunteering assistance, offering donations, and asking for disaster-relevant advice. In addition, local emergency response organizations will generate an increase in communications traffic as they try to ascertain the nature and scope of the disaster, to determine what actions to take, and to marshal resources. This volume of communication can overwhelm the information-processing capacity of local authorities. Planning needs to include provisions not just for collecting information but also for processing and prioritizing it. Therefore, having procedures and plans for augmenting those in communications processing and decision-making roles, such as dispatchers, administrators, and telephone operators, is also important.

Hospitals and other emergency response organizations can take some simple measures to reduce the possibility that they will not be able to use the telephone system. Sometimes, fax and pay phone communications are possible when telephone and cellular circuits are unusable. In addition, local telephone service providers can designate local emergency response organizations that receive priority when the circuits have reached capacity. In some parts of the country, this is called "essential service" status. Different terminology might be used in other parts of the country.

The Government Emergency Telecommunications Service (GETS) under the National Communications System (NCS) provides another mechanism for assuring telephone communications access when the phone circuits are overloaded. GETS is accessed through a universal telephone access number and an assigned personal identification number (PIN) via common telephone equipment (e.g., telephone, fax, modem, or cellular telephone). Once an organization has been authenticated as a valid user, its call receives special treatment such as enhanced routing and priority. Federal civilian or military agencies are eligible for this service. State and local governments and industries can participate if they are sponsored by an NCS member organization. (Table 8.3 lists NCS member organizations.) State and local organizations wishing to be designated as GETS users should request a sponsorship letter by contacting the Office of the Manager at the National Communications System, Programs Division (N2), 701 S. Court House Rd., Arlington, VA 22204-2198 (or via telephone at 703-607-6225; via fax at 703-607-4801; or via e-mail at GETS@NCS.gov). Next, one must establish a billing code account with the Defense Information Technology Contracting Office to pay for usage. After a billing code account is established, a billing code, a point of contact for PIN cards, and the PIN card requirements (GETS User Form) will be provided. The Office of the Manager will then issue a PIN card directly to the organization using the service.

However, for effective disaster communications, no reliable substitute exists for the use of two-way radio networks. The main challenge in establishing such networks is that the Federal Communications Commission has assigned incompatible radio frequencies to the various emergency response organizations in the United States. Frequencies are made available for radio communications on several radio bands. Each band represents a range of communications frequencies. For example, the ultra-high frequency (UHF) band is occupied by frequencies in the 450-MHz range, and the very high frequency (VHF) band has frequencies in the 150-MHz range. Although the industry is beginning to make some exceptions, radios that communicate on one band cannot, for the most part, communicate on other bands. Thus, UHF radios are incompatible with VHF radios. For various response organizations to communicate

TABLE 8.3. NATIONAL COMMUNICATIONS SYSTEM MEMBER ORGANIZATIONS

Central Intelligence Agency
Department of Commerce
Department of Defense
Department of Energy
Department of Health and Human Services
Department of the Interior
Department of Justice
Department of State
Department of Transportation
Department of Treasury
Department of Veterans Affairs
Federal Communications Commission
Federal Emergency Management Agency
Federal Reserve System
General Services Administration
Joint Staff (works under the Joint Chiefs of Staff)
National Aeronautics and Space Administration
National Security Agency
National Telecommunications and Information Administration
Nuclear Regulatory Commission
United States Information Agency
United States Postal Service

by radio, therefore, they must either have radios on the same band, or they must purchase a second set of radios, an expense that few organizations can afford (96).

One approach to dealing with the radio-band problem is the technique of cross-banding (using multiband scanning radio receivers). This equipment is relatively inexpensive, and it can receive radio transmissions on several bands, scanning them in quick succession and locking on frequencies where radio traffic is occurring. The strategy works like this—in the particular community or region in question, the various bands that emergency response organizations use are identified. In each band, one or more frequencies are identified for mutual aid emergency use. All of these frequencies are programmed into multiband scanning receivers. When an agency wants to initiate mutual aid communications with another, it broadcasts on a mutual aid frequency in the band for which its radio transceivers are designed. The agency then listens for reply traffic, using the scanning receiver, on the frequencies on which the other organization can transmit (Fig. 8.2).

Satellite communications is another promising technology, although it has not yet experienced even a moderate level of implementation. Newer communications technology allows communications among several radio bands using a device called a transpeater (for an example, contact Transcrypt Secure Technologies on the Internet at http://www.transcrypt.com/ or by telephone at 402-474-4800). Regardless of the technology approach used, two-way radios should include a setting where they remain silent until a tone alert is sent by someone wishing to communicate with the recipient. With this setting, the alerts would be less likely to be ignored or to be turned down so low that incoming messages cannot be heard.

The previous discussion not withstanding, the research on disasters suggests that most communications problems are people problems rather than equipment problems (6). Although communication equipment might be in short supply, more often than not a physical means of communication is available. Often what are thought to be communications problems are actually coordination problems—that is, a lack of mutual agreement on the following:

- What information needs to be collected;
- Who should collect it;
- Who needs it;
- How to get it to those who need it expeditiously, in a form that it useful to them, using terminology they understand.

These are the crucial aspects of communications that no amount of radio equipment is likely to solve (97). The quality of information is more important than quantity. Crucial information is that which can assure appropriate decision-making (6). Sometimes, even the rather simple use of communications can facilitate a more coordinated and effective response.

Fire Department   Highway Patrol

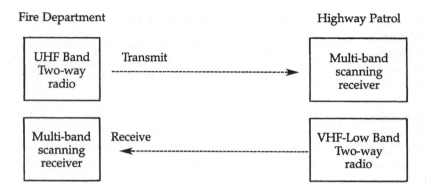

FIGURE 8.2. Two-way radio cross-banding.

Example: Waco Tornado, 1953. After a tornado struck Waco, Texas, in 1953, military personnel brought organization to the rescue efforts by incorporating civilian workers in their teams. These teams were commonly composed of 15 men under a leader and an assistant leader with walkie-talkies, which were used to contact headquarters and other nearby teams (157).

Effective communications in disasters requires that those responding have an agreed understanding of what the communications tasks are and who is responsible for them. (This implies the implementation of community-wide, or better yet, joint, regional, or statewide communications planning and training.) For effective communications to occur, responders need to agree on the following:

- Who is responsible for collecting information and who needs to receive information about the scope and extent of damage at the disaster site;
- Who will have overall responsibility for coordinating site operations;
- Who needs to receive notification of the disaster;
- What areas or facilities are still in the path of the disaster;
- What secondary threats exist (e.g., dam or levee collapse or toxic spills);
- Estimates of numbers, types, severities, and location of casualties;
- Damage to emergency response facilities (e.g., hospitals);
- Capacity of surviving facilities to handle incoming patients;
- Resources needed to combat the disaster threat or damage;
- Resources available to respond;
- Resources committed to the incident (including volunteers and donations);
- Where incoming resources (including unsolicited volunteers) should report;
- When disaster operations have been concluded.

Management of Donations and Volunteers

One of the key issues that is often overlooked in disaster plans is the lack of adequate provisions for dealing with volunteers (1). Community planning can also help to avoid some of the problems posed by excessive or unneeded donations and volunteers while maximizing the usefulness of those donations and volunteers. Members of public safety organizations need to receive training in how to organize citizen volunteers, and someone needs to be charged with the responsibility of community-wide coordination of volunteers and donations. Those charged with this responsibility need access to situation-assessment information on resource needs, a clearance process before public appeals are made by elected officials or the news media, and procedures for processing donations and volunteers. As a group, hospitals should develop common procedures for checking-in, credentialing, and providing workers' insurance and liability coverage for medical volunteers who are not on the hospital staff.

Working With the News Media

One of the predictable problems in disasters is the lack of planning for interactions with the media (1). Although interaction with the media is often perceived as an adversarial relationship, the media have definite roles and responsibilities in disasters. Planning with the media, rather than for the media, can maximize their potential contribution while lessening the disruptive aspects of their involvement (6,158). The insatiable appetite of the media for information can be a drain on emergency response organizations who are trying to carry out their responsibilities under conditions of great urgency and uncertainty. However, in disasters, the media, especially the local media, has been observed to become more altruistic in disasters and to make valuable contributions (6). Although the planning might focus on how to deal with the information demands from the media, planners often do not appreciate the frequency with which the media are sources of information for emergency response organizations.

Example: San Francisco Bay Earthquake, 1989. After an earthquake struck the San Francisco Bay area in 1989, emergency physicians, emergency nurses, and hospital administrators reported a lack of information from government and emergency medical services on the effects of the earthquake, the status of hospitals and roads, and the estimates of the number of injured. The primary source of information turned out to be the news media (30). In addition, the Oakland City Fire Department reported that a lack of clear information about the overall conditions hampered and delayed a coordinated response to the earthquake. Telephone communication with the local fire stations was knocked out, the two functioning radio communications frequencies were overloaded, the county medical radio communications were disabled, and an insufficient number of dispatch personnel were available for adequately answering the telephones and radios. Aerial reconnaissance information was requested from the Oakland Police Department, but their helicopter was down for repairs. During the first crucial hour after impact, fire department headquarters staff relied on television news coverage, including the televised pictures from the news helicopters, for information on the extent of the earthquake damage (81). Clearly, preplanned information-sharing and two-way radio communications capability between the fire department and the local news media could have been a useful asset in this disaster.

The potentially disruptive activities of the media can be reduced by having a single point of information release. Media pools are another useful technique where one or a few news journalists (e.g., one each from television, radio, and print media) are allowed into the impacted area or command posts to collect reports that will be shared with other media organizations (6). Often, the use of these procedures for information release is welcomed by the press corps (6).

News media present a valuable opportunity for efforts at preventing postimpact injuries and illnesses by publicizing precautions about heat stress, food and water safety, carbon monoxide poisoning, and the avoidance of the danger of fires from damaged electrical circuits or from using incorrect methods for reigniting gas pilot lights. The involvement of the news media before disasters can provide a source of public education and support for community disaster mitigation and planning. Finally, remembering not to neglect the media that reach domestic, non-English speaking audiences when planning for disasters is important. Auf der Heide (6, see Chapter 10 in reference) provides more information on planning with the news media.

Postimpact Hospital Safety Assessment

When mitigation measures fail, hospitals can become a safety hazard to patients and staff. Thus, a rapid postimpact hospital safety assessment might be needed to determine if the facility is safe for occupation and the continuing provision of patient care. California uses a cadre of volunteer structural engineers to provide this service after earthquakes, but such an arrangement might also be valuable after severe weather disasters such as floods, tornadoes, and hurricanes. Repeated assessments might need to be carried out when earthquakes are followed by repeated aftershocks (148).

Hospital Evacuation

Hospitals might need to be evacuated when threatened or damaged by disasters. Several tasks need to be planned for, including (a) warning of an impending disaster threat, (b) conducting a postimpact safety assessment, (c) deciding to initiate evacuation and determining destinations for evacuated patients, (d) safely moving out of damaged facilities, (e) moving patients to host facilities, (f) avoiding patient influx to other facilities that are in need of evacuation, (g) tracking patients, (h) provisioning staff to care for the evacuated patients, (i) transporting patient records and medications, and (j) determining when returning is safe and making the return arrangements (148).

Evacuation can be especially challenging when the loss of electrical and backup electrical power for lights, telephones, radios, and elevators occurs or when spillage of hazardous materials inside the facility occurs. Difficulties are also encountered when the plans do not include provisions for adhering to federal regulations on patient transfers (148). In 1986, Congress passed legislation that was intended to prevent hospitals from transferring to other hospitals patients who were unable to pay for their care. This legislation was appended to the Consolidated Omnibus Budget Reconciliation Act (COBRA) as the Emergency Medical Treatment and Active Labor Act (EMTALA). The legislation applies to hospitals that participate in Medicare, and it requires that hospitals with an emergency department provide medical evaluation and emergency medical stabilizing treatment (within the hospital's capacity) to all patients that present for care. If the patient has not been stabilized, EMTALA specifies several requirements before the patient can be transferred to another medical facility as follows (159):

- Such patients cannot be transferred unless they, or their legally acting representative, first consent.
- The transferring physician must certify that the potential medical benefits of the transfer reasonably outweigh the risks.
- The transferring hospital must provide all medical treatment within its capacity to reduce the risk of the transfer.

- The receiving hospital must have the capability of providing the care the patient needs and must agree to accept the patient.
- The sending hospital must provide the receiving hospital with all medical records and materials related to the patient's condition at the time of the transfer.
- The transferring hospital must provide for qualified medical personnel and equipment appropriate to the needs of the patient during the transfer.

Adherence to these requirements can be especially challenging when the transferring and receiving hospitals do not have two-way radio communications capability and the telephone and cellular telephone systems are damaged or rendered inoperable due to circuit overload.

Hazardous Materials Problems

Although a detailed discussion of hazardous materials disaster preparedness is beyond the scope of this chapter, making a few comments and observations is appropriate. (For more detailed information, see the Chapters 25, 26, and 33. See also "Managing Hazardous Materials Incidents" available from the Agency for Toxic Substances and Disease Registry and *Hospitals and community emergency response—what you need to know*, available from the Occupational Safety and Health Administration [OSHA]. [Contact information for these documents is listed at the end of this chapter.]) Regulations administered by OSHA and standards promulgated by the JCAHO require hospitals to be capable of providing care to those exposed to or contaminated by hazardous substances (e.g., accidental releases from chemical plants and storage facilities; accidents involving transportation of hazardous materials; hazardous materials spills within hospitals; terrorism; and hazardous materials releases resulting from natural disasters, such as tornadoes, hurricanes, floods, wildland fires, and earthquakes). Although the planners might believe that most victims will be decontaminated before reaching the hospital (160), evidence suggests that this is not a reliable assumption (161).

A great deal of controversy exists about what constitutes adequate personal protective equipment (PPE). Although some believe that surgical gowns, gloves, masks, and booties are sufficient, others believe that the minimal level of gear should include a full-faced respirator, chemically resistant suit, hood, boots, and gloves. The type of respirator is also a subject of debate—some advocate masks that use a cartridge to filter out toxic substances, and others favor air-supplied (hose or tank) respirators (160,162–164).

Several other proposals have been made for preparedness, including the following:

- Development of a plan for hazardous materials casualties;
- Training (including annual refresher training) for staff involved in the decontamination process;
- Availability of appropriate PPE for staff involved in treatment or decontamination of contaminated casualties;
- Facilities for carrying out decontamination, even under inclement weather conditions. If such facilities are located indoors, they should be in an area isolated from other patients and staff;
- Contaminated patients should have a separate entrance; an isolated, negative-pressure ventilation system; and a means for collecting contaminated water used in the decontamination process;
- Access to sources of information on the toxicity of specific chemicals that can be rapidly accessed even when the telephone system is nonfunctional;
- Antidotes for hazardous material (hazmat) substances (e.g., pralidoxime, atropine, and cyanide kits).

The theoretical benefits of these various options continue to be argued, and some may feel meeting some of these requirements may be ideal but impractical. Little in the way of empirical observations exists to clarify the issue. The regulatory situation, however, is more clear. OSHA regulations stipulate that a filter mask can be used only when the chemical and its air concentration can be identified, when the chemical has adequate warning properties (e.g., smell or mucous membrane irritation) that occur before its toxic effects, and when a cartridge is available for the specific chemical. When the chemical is unknown, the minimal level of protection required by OSHA is an air-supplied respirator (160).

Given that the conditions are limited for allowing filter masks, reliance on air-supplied respirators as the standard might be more practical. Planners should also be aware that persons expected to use respirators (whether cartridge or air-supplied) must also be fit-tested using National Institute for Occupational Safety and Health (NIOSH)-approved procedures. A listing of additional reading materials on hospital and medical preparedness for hazardous materials incidents is provided in the "Further Reading and Sources of Information" section at the end of the chapter.

LEPCs, required by SARA Title III, must designate a local hospital that has agreed to accept and treat victims of emergencies involving hazardous substances (165). Unfortunately, this can create a false sense of security for other hospitals if they believe they are relieved of responsibility because they are not the designated hospital. As has been demonstrated, most disaster casualties are transported completely outside the local EMS system, and local authorities have little control over which hospitals will receive them. Thus, regardless of what any community disaster plans might stipulate, any hospital might receive such patients and therefore must be prepared for them.

Recently, a great deal of national concern has been focused on the threat of mass casualty events resulting from terrorism. As a result, large amounts of money have been appropriated in an effort to prepare first responders to deal with this threat. Unfortunately, as was noted earlier in this chapter, this effort has failed to recognize that in most mass casualty events, including those involving hazardous chemicals and infectious disease outbreaks, *the hospital is the primary first responder*. Furthermore, a paucity of funding for hospital preparedness for these events is seen, even though numerous studies have pointed out that most hospitals are not adequately prepared for even one patient contaminated by hazardous material, much less for a multitude of such casualties (169–176). In a survey of all the nation's level 1 trauma centers, fewer than 3% of the respondents were adequately prepared for a patient exposed to hazardous materials (177). Because nonterrorist hazardous materials incidents are more common and they frequently involve a greater variety of toxic substances, these should be the focus for preparedness efforts. Likewise, building the public health infrastructure for dealing with epidemics and disease outbreaks should be the foundation for preparing for terrorism involving infectious agents (160,178).

Some have suggested that, in terrorist attacks, psychologic casualties will predominate. However, the proponents of this assertion offer no empirical evidence to support their claims (164,179). Others have expressed concern over the probability of mass hysteria or mass psychogenic illness as a result of chemical spills (161). However, often, these diagnostic conclusions are made because of patients who arrive at hospitals complaining of symptoms not accompanied by physical findings. While psychologic casualties certainly may occur as a result of disasters involving terrorism, current evidence does not support the assertion that they will predominate. While the *Diagnostic and statistical manual of mental disorders*, 4th edition, (DSM-IV) describes psychiatric problems that may occur in disasters, such as post traumatic stress disorder (PTSD), "mass hysteria" and "mass psychogenic illness" are not recognized psychiatric disorders (180).

Persons without demonstrable clinical abnormalities may have other reasons for seeking help besides psychologic disorders. Phosgene gas, for example, can produce hyperventilation and shortness of breath without hypoxia or abnormal x-ray findings in the early stages. Victims can subsequently develop a delayed but rapid onset and potentially fatal pulmonary edema (181). Many who think they may have been exposed to a hazardous substance may want to be examined as a precaution (e.g., for insurance purposes) in case they later develop a disability due to any exposures. Furthermore, one should recognize that neurotoxicants, by their physiologic effects, can create psychologic symptoms and can be misdiagnosed as psychologically induced illness. Sarin, the nerve agent used in the 1995 terrorist attack on the Tokyo subway system, can cause chronic neurobehavioral effects (182). Other examples of neurotoxic chemicals that can cause psychologic dysfunction include mercury vapor (183), carbon monoxide (183), hydrogen sulfide (184), and organic solvents (185).

Psychogenic illness is a diagnosis of exclusion (186–188). The conclusion that symptoms are psychogenic is always tenuous because it is based primarily on the absence of physical evidence rather than on the presence of a clearly defined set of precipitating psychologic conditions (189). The success in excluding other causes of illness is often related to perseverance on the part of the investigator.

Many of the papers alleging cases of "mass hysteria" have not reported enough information to rule out chemical toxicity as the cause of patient complaints (187,189–192). In some cases when delayed sampling has been done, the presence of toxic substances during the actual onset of symptoms could not be ruled out (187,193). Some articles on "mass hysteria" have still applied the label even when toxic chemicals or other causes of physical illness were present at the site (193–196).

Sometimes, because of the presumption that the incident was due to "mass hysteria," a deliberate decision is made to forgo detailed epidemiologic investigation (197) because of the belief that such an inquiry will perpetuate or exacerbate the "hysteria" (198). Some have suggested that mass psychogenic illness is common, and they have even gone so far as to state that "many more outbreaks are unreported" (199) (how one identifies an unreported case is not made clear). However, Sirois, in an extensive review on the subject, could identify only 78 purported outbreaks during a 100-year period (200).

Many of the symptoms attributed to "mass hysteria," such as nausea, headache, fatigue, dizziness, fainting, and shortness of breath (195), can also be caused by toxic chemicals and other illnesses. Other attributes that have been suggested as suspicious for a hysterical or psychogenic etiology include young age and female gender. However, because these attributes are often used, *a priori*, as diagnostic criteria for "mass hysteria," their presence in such "diagnosed" cases is not particularly surprising, nor does their incidence inspire confidence in the diagnosis.

In summary, "mass hysteria," if it exists at all, is a rare phenomenon. At best, "mass hysteria" is a diagnosis of exclusion; therefore, it is difficult to make in the acute aftermath of a mass casualty incident. In addition, a misdiagnosis could result in a medical, as well as a public relations, disaster. The best strategy when faced with large numbers of casualties with unexplained symptoms is probably to provide facilities (e.g., an auditorium) where medical supervision can be undertaken for a large number of victims by relatively few medical personnel. Facilities and provisions should be made for rapid intervention if the condition of the victims deteriorates during the observation period. In the meantime, environmental health authorities can carry out detailed investigations to determine whether a hazardous exposure has occurred.

Officials should be quite reticent to attribute symptoms to a hysterical cause. Communications with the media should identify the situation as an illness of unknown cause that is under investigation. Meanwhile, the information given to the media should state that, until a diagnosis is made or the symptoms resolve, every precaution is being taken to assure the victim's safety and well-being.

Triage

Although disaster triage is often preached as an ideal, field observations indicate that most casualties do not undergo triage in the prehospital setting. To a large extent, this is because most patients are rescued and transported to hospitals by the efforts of bystanders. Because much of the search and rescue done by formal emergency response personnel is carried out by firefighters and peace officers, their lack of training in the triage system can contribute to the problem (6). Some triage systems call for the use of tags to identify the patient's priority and other limited patient information, as well as for patient tracking (6). However, in numerous cases, these tags have not been used (59, 77,110,201), sometimes because they were not available when and where they were needed (2,71,202). In other cases, the use of tags was abandoned because of the perception that it slowed down the triage process (40,58). In some instances, tags were not used in normal emergency responses, so personnel were not familiar with them and they did not use them in disaster triage (99).

> **Example: San Francisco Earthquake, 1989.** In a survey carried out after the 1989 San Francisco Bay area earthquake, approximately 70% of emergency department physicians and nursing staff stated that they were familiar with the disaster tags to be used by their facilities. However, less than half reported that the tags were actually used the night of the disaster (30).

No standard or universal method of triage exists. In the various systems that have been described, the numbers of triage categories vary from two to five or more. Various colors, numbers, and symbols have been used to identify these categories. The subject of triage is also covered in Chapter 2. A paucity of empirical studies exists for demonstrating the efficacy of one triage system over another. However, as has been noted previously, only about 10% of disaster casualties on average require admission to the hospital even overnight. Thus, even the most crude forms of triage can identify the more than 90% of casualties that do not require emergency surgery or critical care (6). Because people do not stop having heart attacks, exacerbations of chronic lung disease, diabetes, high blood pressure, and obstetric and gynecologic problems, the triage system used must be able to prioritize these conditions, as well as disaster-related injuries.

One method of promoting the use of triage by ambulance and rescue personnel is to require them to assign a triage category to each patient transported on a day-to-day basis in nondisaster times. This category becomes a part of the prehospital patient record and the radio report to the hospital. EMS personnel and, secondarily, hospital staff therefore become oriented to the process. Thus, when disaster strikes, triage categories are not an unfamiliar procedure. How many ambulance, rescue, fire, and law enforcement personnel have received formal training in triage is unclear. To the extent that such training does not occur, one cannot expect a high level of field triage to be carried out in disasters.

Security and Staff Identification

One need that has been described repeatedly in the disaster literature is for some sort of identification gear to indicate key players in the disaster response. Arm bands, helmets, and vests are among the techniques suggested. Despite the presence of numerous recommendations as lessons learned from various disasters, the failure to make provisions for identification continues to be a problem (40,57,59,65,70, 71,81,110,128,203,204). In some cases, this failure has resulted in disaster medical personnel being unable to get through roadblocks on their way to the hospital (202,205). One possible solution to this problem is to assign a person from the hospital to report to a check-in area outside any security perimeter that blocks access to the hospital. That person would be provided with preprinted generic plastic badges to identify authorized hospital staff. A list of hospital staff and employees would also be provided to indicate who is eligible for the badges. Employees would need to present a picture identification (e.g., driver's license) so that their name could be compared with the staff listing. This could be done in collaboration with the local law enforcement agency.

The Incident Command System

In the fall of 1970, Southern California was ravaged by a series of devastating wildland fires that burned over 600,000 acres and 772 structures in 13 days and resulted in the loss of 16 lives. As the result of extensive coordination problems identified in a report on the emergency response, Congress funded a consortium of state, county, and city fire departments, which was led by the United States Forest Service, to address some of the response problems. Among the accomplishments of the consortium called Firefighting Resources of Southern California Organized Against Potential Emergencies (FIRESCOPE) was the development of the incident command system (ICS). ICS is a standardized organizational structure and set of procedures for various fire departments to use in large-scale emergencies. Subsequently, ICS users found it to be useful for other incidents, such as earthquakes and floods. The system has been widely adapted by fire departments, as well as by other emergency response organizations, such as law enforcement agencies, emergency medical services providers, and hospitals (6,206). A number of variants of the original FIRESCOPE ICS have arisen over the years. Some of these variants are simpler to use, but they lack key elements for dealing with large-scale disaster operation. While a detailed discussion of ICS is beyond the scope of this chapter, further information on FIRESCOPE ICS is available. See Auf der Heide (6, see Chapter 7 in reference), and consult the sources of information listed in "Further Reading and Sources of Information" at the end of this chapter.

Planned Improvisation

As was mentioned at the beginning of the chapter, effective planning involves the following two strategies: (a) planning for what is likely and (b) planned improvisation. Planned improvisation is particularly important where overlapping jurisdictional responsibilities are present and where problems or tasks arise for which no organization has clear-cut jurisdiction.

For example, in June 1978, a tornado suddenly appeared and capsized a showboat carrying 60 passengers and crew on Lake Pomona in Kansas. This incident took place on a federal reservoir in a state park in an unincorporated area of the county. Unfortunately, no existing state law defined who should be in charge. Even if one had existed, it would not have applied to federal authorities. The matter was only resolved after the county attorney was consulted and declared the sheriff to be in charge (207).

Planned improvisation might include mutually agreed-on preplanned responsibility and procedures for the following:

- Identifying areas stricken by the disaster and the nature and scope of damage and health effects;
- Determining what agencies have disaster responsibilities;
- Agreeing on one agency to assume the overall coordination role for the response;
- Identifying those who have responded and notifying those that still need to respond;
- Establishing a joint, multiagency command post and, if needed, an off-site joint emergency operations center;
- Creating a means of rapid information sharing among the response organizations (two-way radio networks);
- Agreeing upon a joint incident response strategy;
- Establishing check-in or "staging" areas to which incoming responders and volunteers should report;
- Identifying what resources are committed, what is needed, and what is available;
- Deciding what tasks are to be carried out by whom
- Determining priorities for the use of available resources, including those that are volunteered and donated;
- Monitoring the progress of the disaster, including any secondary threats, and the response;
- Adjusting the incident strategy as conditions change;
- Deciding when to terminate the response.

The need for improvisation in disasters should be expected so that it can be planned for. The FIRESCOPE ICS provides procedures for most of these planned improvisation activities.

Training, Drills, and Critiques

Even if a community develops a plan that addresses the recommendations provided in this chapter, the implementation of these plans is unlikely in the absence of an effective training program. Several advantages exist for establishing a joint training program. First, as has been shown, disaster responses are more effective when formal and even informal relationships have been previously established among the various responders. Joint training is one strategy for encouraging such relationships. Secondly, joint training fosters an understanding not only of what activities and responsibilities need to be carried out but also of how those activities facilitate or inhibit the abilities of others to carry out their responsibilities. Finally, a community-wide or statewide training program can reduce the costs of training and can make carrying out training at multiple times and locations economically feasible, so that the training is more available to the potential users (156).

The usefulness of disaster drills in improving the response to subsequent disasters has been mentioned in a number of reports (2,10,58,208,209). However, one could also say that having a drill without the prerequisite training is like having the final examination without having attended the course. The usefulness of drills is enhanced if they are based on valid assumptions about what happens in disasters and if they have multiagency participation. Unfortunately, disaster drills are often a means of satisfying minimal requirements (e.g., those imposed by JCAHO) rather than being processes that impart a significant amount of learning to the participants (1). Other learning techniques that can enhance institutional disaster response capacity include holding brief critiques after small emergencies involving multiple casualties, maintaining a community disaster planning body, and regularly reviewing mutual aid agreements with other involved organizations. Finally, no community preparedness program is complete without the establishment of a method of learning from disasters and disaster drills and of implementing the lessons learned to improve disaster management procedures and training.

POSTSCRIPT: THE WORLD TRADE CENTER ATTACK OF SEPTEMBER 11, 2001

The terrorist attack on the World Trade Center is the eighth peacetime disaster in United States history with more than 1,000 fatalities. As in previous disasters, telephone and cellular telephone circuits were overloaded. A newspaper arti- cle estimated that the predisaster cellular traffic of 115 mil- lion calls a day in the New York metro area reported by Ver- izon Wireless doubled during the disaster (210). Even calls using the GETS would not go through. A number of pat- terns were seen in this disaster that have been described in previous disasters. As in previous disasters, the number of offers of voluntary assistance was overwhelming. According to an article in *EMToday*, a newsletter published by the American College of Emergency Physicians, the Healthcare Association of New York State established a hotline for medical volunteers. On the first day, over 40,000 calls were received. The line was so congested that it took over 4 hours for some physicians to get through. Over 10,000 medical volunteers were put on standby with state emergency man- agement officials. By 5 PM on Wednesday, September 12, the hotline was shut down. Those who called after the shut- down received a message stating, "We have received an overwhelming response to our call for assistance. Thank you for your concern. We are are unable to accept any more calls" (211). Discussions with emergency physicians from New York City revealed that no interhospital radio com- munications network was present and that hospitals were not able to receive timely information from the scene. By the end of the second day after the attack, New York City had in excess of 3,000 surplus hospital beds available for disaster victims. Television news reports showed the exten- sive preparations being made at area hospitals, which waited for the arrival of disaster victims that never came. Blood donors came out in droves. Despite the massive amount of destruction, most surviving casualties had relatively minor injuries. As in other large building collapses, most surviving victims were rescued on the first day. At the time of this writing, 12 days after the attack, no additional live rescues have occurred since the five survivors were pulled out of the rubble on the second day.

CONCLUSION

This chapter has attempted to point out a number of prin- ciples for effective hospital disaster planning. Some of the most important points are summarized below.

1. Disaster planning is only as effective as the assump- tions upon which it is based. Unfortunately, many commonly held assumptions are inaccurate or untrue. The effectiveness of planning is enhanced when it is based on information that has been empirically verified by systematic field disaster research studies.

2. Most disasters cannot be adequately managed merely by mobilizing more supplies, equipment, and person- nel. Disasters are different from daily emergencies, and they pose problems that have no counterpart in routine emergency responses. Many of these disaster-related

problems have been identified by disaster researchers, and they can be anticipated and planned for.

3. While completing a written plan is important, it, by itself, is insufficient to assure preparedness. Plans must be practical for, acceptable by, and familiar to the users. Plans must also be interorganizational, and they must be based on valid information about what happens in disasters. Finally, resources (e.g., time, personnel, fund- ing, facilities, and equipment) must be made available to carry out the plan.

4. The process of planning is more important than the written plan because those who participate in the plan- ning process are more likely to accept the end product. The process is also important because the relationships that develop enable smoother responses.

5. Disaster planning often has to overcome apathy and complacency. Dealing with barriers to and incentives for planning is one of the most important steps to insure preparedness.

6. Cost-effective planning can be accomplished by means of a two-pronged strategy—plan for what is likely, and develop procedures for planned, coordinated improvi- sation. The ICS provides some useful procedures for coordinated improvisation.

7. A large portion of the care given to disaster casualties is carried out by volunteers. In many cases, these volun- teers are untrained and their response is unsolicited and therefore unexpected. Effective disaster planning needs to anticipate volunteers and to develop guide- lines and procedures for dealing with them.

8. Numerous studies and anecdotal reports clearly show that telephones and cellular telephones are unreliable in disasters and that the lack of interagency mutual aid radio networks frequently hampers effective response.

9. In disasters, emergency response units will often come from many miles away. For this reason, the establishment of regionwide, or even better, statewide disaster plans, is helpful in promoting a coordinated response.

10. Most disaster casualties will arrive at the hospital within 1 hour of the impact, and very few trapped casualties are rescued alive after the first day. Thus, the effectiveness of the local response is a key determinant in preventing death and disability. National rescue and medical teams that come from across the country will have little overall impact on casualty survival.

11. While hospital treatment of the critically injured is often the focus of disaster planning, most casualties tend to have minor injuries that could be treated in the non-hospital setting. Non-hospital medical assets (e.g., private physicians' offices, clinics, and urgent care cen- ters) should be integrated into disaster medical plan- ning. When patients lose access to their routine sources

of medical care in disasters, they can increase the burden on hospitals. Disaster planning should include provisions to assure the survival and function of these routine sources of care (e.g., pharmacies, dialysis clinics, home health care agencies, nursing homes, assisted living facilities, and psychiatric facilities).

12. The news media has a vital role in disasters, and failure to include the media in planning can lead to a dysfunctional response.

13. Preventing hospitals from becoming disaster victims is crucial. Hospitals should not be constructed in areas of the community at high risk for disasters (e.g., in flood plains or near earthquake faults). Construction according to up-to-date building codes will reduce the damage to hospitals that might result from a disaster. Even if the hospital survives the disaster, the lack of adequate utility backup arrangements can greatly impede patient care. To assess whether a hospital is still safe for occupation and use after a disaster, the importance of planning postimpact assessment by trained structural engineers cannot be minimized. When hospitals are disabled by a disaster, community-wide plans for patient evacuation to other medical facilities must be in place.

14. JCAHO standards and federal regulations require hospitals to prepare for patients contaminated by hazardous substances. Some have recommended designating one hospital in each community to which contaminated patients should be sent. However, most disaster casualties tend to go to the closest or most familiar hospital, and this may not be the one designated for contaminated patients. Thus, every hospital needs to prepare for these patients. Sufficient preparedness requires the development of a plan; the establishment of a training program; and the availability of personal protective equipment, decontamination facilities, and appropriate antidotes.

15. While some have claimed that most casualties in disasters due to chemical terrorism will be pyschogenic or hysterical, little evidence supports this assertion. Many who show up at hospitals, however, may be among the "worried well" or those suffering from mild exposures. Some exposures to chemicals used by terrorists (e.g., inhalation of phosgene or skin exposure to sarin) can have life-threatening effects, the onset of which may be delayed by many hours. When large numbers of casualties are seen and the cause of their symptoms cannot be immediately identified, the best strategy may be to provide a large-scale medical observation capacity until a serious exposure can be ruled out (e.g., observation in an auditorium or gymnasium where a few medical personnel can watch a large number of people with access to rapid medical care if any patient's condition deteriorates).

FURTHER READING AND SOURCES OF INFORMATION

The contact information given here provides the reader with instructions for acquiring a copy of the publication listed.

Applied Technology Council. *Procedures for postearthquake safety evaluation of buildings (ATC-20).* Redwood City, CA: Applied Technology Council, 1989. **Contact information:** 3 Twin Dolphin Drive, Suite 275; Redwood City, CA 94065.

Auf der Heide E. *Community medical disaster planning and evaluation guide.* Dallas: American College of Emergency Physicians, 1995. **Contact information:** Don Kerns, American College of Emergency Physicians; P.O. Box 619911; Dallas, TX 75261; 800-798-1822 [press 6]; or http://www.acep.org/bookstore/.

Auf der Heide E. Disaster planning, part II: disaster problems, issues, and challenges identified in the research literature. *Emerg Med Clin North Am* 1996;14:453–480.

California Office of Emergency Services. *Hospital earthquake preparedness guidelines.* Sacramento, CA: California Office of Emergency Services, 1991.

Drabek TE, Hoetmer GJ. *Emergency management: principles and practice for local government.* Washington, D.C.: International City Management Association, 1991. **Contact information:** ICMA Distribution Center; P.O. Box 2011; Annapolis Junction, MD 20701; or 1-800-745-8780.

Drabek TE. The professional emergency manager. Monograph no. 44. Boulder, CO: Natural Hazards Research and Applications Information Center at the University of Colorado, 1987. **Contact information:** Natural Hazards Research and Application Information Center, IBS #6; Campus Box 482; University of Colorado; Boulder, CO 80309; or http://www.colorado.edu/hazards/.

Drabek TE. *Emergency management: strategies for maintaining organizational integrity.* New York: Springer-Verlag, 1990.

Dynes RR. *Organized behavior in disaster.* Newark, DE: Disaster Research Center at the University of Delaware, 1974. **Contact information:** Disaster Research Center Publications; University of Delaware; Newark, DE 19716; or http://www.udel.edu/DRC/.

Federal Emergency Management Agency. *Non structural earthquake hazard mitigation for hospitals and other health care facilities.* Washington, D.C.: Federal Emergency Management Agency, SM 370/May 1989. **Contact information:** Federal Emergency Management Agency; P.O. Box 70742; Washington, DC 20023.

Kartez, JD, Kelley WJ, Lindell MK. *Adaptive planning for community emergency management: a summary for public managers.* Pullman, WA: Washington State University

Environmental Research Center, 1997. **Contact information**: Washington State University; Environmental Research Center; Pullman, WA 99164-4430.

Landesman LY. *Emergency preparedness in health care organizations*. Oak Brook Terrace, IL: Joint Commission on Accreditation of Healthcare Organizations, 1996. **Contact information:** Joint Commission on Accreditation of Healthcare Organizations; One Renaissance Blvd.; Oakbrook Terrace, IL 60181.

Lindell MK, Perry RW. *Behavioral foundations of community emergency planning*. Bristol, PA: Hemisphere Publishing, 1992. **Contact information:** Hemisphere Publishing; 1900 Frost Rd., Suite 101; Bristol, PA 19007.

Mileti DS, Sorensen JH. Determinants of organizational effectiveness in responding to low probability catastrophic events. *The Columbia Journal of World Business* 1987;22: 13–21.

Morres CA, Burkle FM Jr, Lillibridge SR. Disaster medicine. *Emerg Med Clin North Am* 1996;14:xiii–xiv.

Noji EK. *The public health consequences of disasters*. New York, NY: Oxford University Press, 1996.

Perry RW. *Comprehensive emergency management: evacuating threatened populations*. Greenwich, CT: JAI Press, 1985.

Reitherman R. How to prepare a hospital for an earthquake. *J Emerg Med* 1986;4:119–131.

San Bernardino County Medical Society. *Earthquake disaster preparedness: a guide for medical offices*. Colton, CA: San Bernardino County Medical Society, 1993. **Contact information:** San Bernardino County Medical Society; 952 S. Mt. Vernon Ave.; Colton, CA 92324.

State of California Emergency Medical Services Authority. *Hazardous material medical management protocols*, 2nd ed. Sacramento, CA: Emergency Medical Services Authority, 1991. **Contact information:** State of California, Emergency Medical Services Authority; 1930 9th St., Suite 100; Sacramento, CA 95814.

State of Carlifornia Governor's Office of Emergency Services. *Hospital earthquake preparedness guidelines*. Sacramento, CA: Governor's Office of Emergency Services, 1997. **Contact information:** State of Carlifornia, Governor's Office of Emergency Services; P.O. Box 9577; Sacramento, CA 95823.

Wenger DE, James TF, Faupel CE. *Disaster beliefs and emergency planning*. New York: Irvington Publishers, 1985.

FURTHER SOURCES OF INFORMATION ON THE INCIDENT COMMAND SYSTEM

Free Documents on the Internet

Agency for Toxic Substances and Disease Registry (ATSDR), U.S. Department of Health and Human Services. *Managing hazardous materials emergencies*. Atlanta, GA: U.S. Department of Health and Human Services,

2001. Available at: http://www.atsdr.cdc.gov/mhmi.html. To request the material in print hard copy or on CD, contact the ATSDR Information Center, Mailstop E-57, 1600 Clifton Rd, NE, Atlanta, GA 30333. 888-422-8737. E-mail: atsdric@cdc.gov.

Auf der Heide E. *Disaster response: principles of preparation and coordination*. St. Louis: CV Mosby, 1989. Available free at: http://www.coe-dmha.org/dr/flash.htm.

Federal Emergency Management Agency. *Incident Command System Self-study CD*. Washington, D.C.: Federal Emergency Management Agency. Available at: http://www.usfa.fema.gov.nfa/tr_ertss.htm.

Governor's Office of Emergency Services. *Law enforcement guide for emergency operations*. Sacramento, CA: Governer's Office of Emergency Services. Available at: http://www.oes.ca.gov/. Click on "OES Divisions, Regions and Partners" in the left frame of the page, then click on "OES Law Enforcement Branch," then scroll down to "Redbook.pdf" (next to "Law Enforcement Guide for Emergency Operations").

Incident command system forms and manuals. Available at: http://www.firescope.oes.ca.gov/. Select "ICS Documents FREE downloads."

Irwin RL. The incident command system. In: Auf der Heide E, ed. *Disaster response: principles of preparation and coordination*. St. Louis: CV Mosby, 1989:133–163. Available at: http://www.coe-dmha.org/dr/flash.htm.

National Aeronautics and Space Administration (NASA). *Incident command system slide series*. Houston, TX: National Aeronautics and Space Administration.

State of California Emergency Medical Services Authority. *Hospital emergency incident command system*. Sacramento, CA: Emergency Medical Services Authority. Available at: http://www.emsa.cahwnet.gov/dms2/dms2.asp.

U.S. Coast Guard. *Incident command system field operations guide*. U.S. Coast Guard. Available at: http://www.uscg.mil/hq/g-m/nmc/response/.

Wildland Fire Net. *Incident command system training materials*. www.wildlandfire.net/.

Print Documents on the Incident Command System

Federal Emergency Management Agency. *Exemplary practices in emergency management: the California FIRESCOPE program*, monograph series no. 1, Federal Emergency Management Agency 117, February 1987. **Contact information:** Federal Emergency Management Agency; National Emergency Training Center, Emergency Response Institute; P.O. Box 70742; Washington, D.C. 20023; or 1-800-238-3358.

Governor's Office of Emergency Services. *The standardized emergency management system* (available on computer disk). *Student manuals, instructor manuals, and slides* (in PowerPoint). San Luis Obispo, CA: Governor's Office of

Emergency Services . **Contact information**: Tracy Blake; Governor's Office of Emergency Services, California Specialized Training Institute; P.O. Box 8123; San Luis Obispo, CA 93403-8123; or 805-549-3343. (This is the California iteration of the Incident Command System. It is a statewide emergency and disaster incident management system [the "next generation" of the Incident Command System]. Although the Incident Command System only dealt with on-scene coordination, SEMS is an expanded version for use both on-scene and at local, area-wide, and state emergency operations centers.)

Incident Command System. *Basic orientation course training package.* Sacramento, CA: California Fire Service Training and Education System, 1982. **Contact information:** California Fire Service Training and Education System; 7171 Bowling Drive, Suite 500; Sacramento, CA 95823.

Incident Command System. *Hazardous materials operational system description.* ICS-HM-120-1. Riverside, CA: Incident Command System, 1990. **Contact information:** FIRESCOPE; P.O. Box 55157; Riverside, CA 92517; or 714-782-4174.

Incident Command System. *Multi-casualty operational system description.* ICS-MC-120-1. Riverside, CA: Incident Command System, 1992. **Contact information:** FIRESCOPE; P.O. Box 55157; Riverside, CA 92517; or 714-782-4174. (This is an Emergency Medical Services version of ICS.)

National Fire Protection Association 1561. *Fire Department Incident Management System.* Quincy, MA: ANSI/NFPA 1561, 1990. **Contact information:** National Fire Protection Association; 1 Batterymarch Park; P.O. Box 9191; Quincy, MA 02269-9101; or 800-735-0100.

National Interagency Incident Management System (NIIMS). *Information and guides.* Boise, ID: Boise Interagency Fire Center, 1983. **Contact information:** Boise Interagency Fire Center; 3905 Vista Ave.; Boise, ID 83705; or 208-334-9807. (NIIMS is the version of the FIRESCOPE ICS used by federal wildland fire-fighting agencies.)

Office of Emergency Services. *Region IV multi-casualty incident plan.* Stockton, CA: OES region IV multiple casualty/mutual aid planning project, 1993. **Contact information:** Clarence Teem; San Joaquin EMS Agency; P.O. Box 1020; Stockton, CA 95201; or 209-468-6818. (A regional medical mutual aid plan incorporating the Incident Command System: Multi-Casualty Operational Description—that is, the ICS component used for medical disasters.)

Oklahoma State University. *Incident command system.* Stillwater, OK: Fire Protection Publications, 1983. **Contact information**: Oklahoma State University, Stillwater, OK 74078.

For additional publications lists for FIRESCOPE ICS training materials, including those for individual positions within the ICS organizational structure, contact the Boise Interagency Fire Center, Division of Training, Bureau of Land Management at 3905 Vista Avenue, Boise, ID 83705; or at 208-334-9202. Alternatively, contact the Support Services Manager, FIRESCOPE, Operations Coordination Center at P.O. Box 55157, Riverside, CA 92517; or 714-782-4174.

Periodicals and Journals

Disaster Recovery Journal (dedicated to business continuity). **Contact information:** Richard Arnold. Telephone at 314-894-0276; fax at 314-894-7474; e-mail at drj@drj.com; or visit on the web at http://www.drj.com/. Free.

Disaster Research Newsletter. Boulder, CO: University of Colorado. **Contact information:** Telephone at 303-492-6819; e-mail at hazctr@spot.colorado.edu; or visit on the web at http://www.colorado.edu/hazards/. Free.

International Journal of Mass Emergencies and Disasters. Los Angeles: University of Southern California. **Contact information:** Telephone at 213-740-6842; e-mail at ijmed@usc.edu; or visit on the web at http://www.usc.edu/schools/sppd/ijmed/.

The Natural Hazards Observer. Boulder, CO: The Natural Hazards Research and Applications Information Center. **Contact information:** Mail requests to The Natural Hazards Research and Applications Information Center, IBS #6; Campus Box 482; University of Colorado; Boulder, CO 80309; telephone at 303-492-6819; e-mail at hazctr@spot.colorado.edu; or visit on the web at http://www.Colorado.edu/hazards/. Free.

Disasters: preparedness and mitigation in the Americas. Washington, D.C.: Pan American Health Organization (PAHO). A newsletter. **Contact information:** Telephone at 202-974-3527; fax at 202-775-4578; e-mail at disaster@paho.org; or visit on the web at http://165.158.1.110/english/ped/pedtm3en.htm.

DISASTER BIBLIOGRAPHIES

1997 Information sources. *Natural Hazards Observer,* special edition, June 1997. **Contact information:** Direct mail to Natural Hazards Research and Applications Information Center, IBS #6; Campus Box 482; University of Colorado; Boulder, CO 80309; telephone at 303-492-6819; e-mail at hazctr@spot.colorado.edu; or visit on the web at http://www.Colorado.edu/hazards.

Bibliodes: a selected bibliography series. This is a series of specialized bibliographies that extract information by the individual topic area from DESASTRES, the master database of the Regional Disaster Documentation Center. Washington, D.C.: Pan American Health Organization (PAHO). **Contact information:** Telephone at 202-974-3527; fax at 202-775-4578; e-mail at disaster@paho.org; or visit on the web at http://165.158.1.110/english/ped/ped-bibdi.htm.

California Seismic Safety Commission publications. Sacramento, CA: California Seismic Safety Commission. **Contact information:** Telephone at 916-322-4917; or visit on the web at http://www.seismic.ca.gov/.

Disaster humanitarian assistance. Publications and training materials. Washington, D.C.: Pan American Health Organization (PAHO). **Contact information:** Telephone at 202-974-3527; fax at 202-775-4578; e-mail at disaster@paho.org; or visit on the web at http://165.158.1.110/english/ped/pedhome.htm.

Disaster medicine bibliography. **Contact information:** Visit on the web at http://www.mother.com/~hxgarzon/biblio.htm. (This bibliography has a focus on material relevant to urban search and rescue teams.)

Disaster research center publications. Newark, DE: University of Delaware. **Contact information:** Telephone at 302-831-6618; fax at 302-831-2091; e-mail at susan.castelli@mvs.udel.edu; or visit on the web at http://www.udel.edu/DRC/publications.html.

Internet Sources Of Disaster Information

Many of the following are sources of research information. Many have extensive links to other disaster information sources.

Agency for Toxic Substances and Disease Registry. **Available at:** http://www.atsdr.cdc.gov/.

Building Seismic Safety Council. **Available at:** http://www.bssconline.org/. (See *Building code information: the 2000 NEHRP provisions for new buildings and other structures*, FEMA 368, and FEMA 369.)

California Seismic Safety Commission. **Available at:** http://www.seismic.ca.gov/.

California Office of Statewide Health Planning and Development. **Available at:** http://www.oshpd.ca.gov/index.htm. (This site has information on hospital compliance with seismic resistant building practices.)

Centers for Disease Control and Prevention. **Available at:** http://www.cdc.gov/.

Centers for Disease Control and Prevention. *Prevention guidelines.* **Available at:** http://www.phppo.cdc.gov/CDCrecommends/AdvSearchV.asp. (This site includes a number of documents dealing with disasters.)

Disaster Central. **Available at:** http://www.disaster-central.com/.

Disaster Management Higher Education Project, Emergency Management Institute, Federal Emergency Management Agency. **Available at:** http://www.fema.gov/emi/edu/higher.htm. (Several academic texts on disaster management are available for free downloading. Several of the texts are excellent sources of information from the disaster

research literature and are a good basis for evidence-based disaster planning.)

Disaster Net. **Available at:** http://www.disaster.net/disaster/disaster.html.

Emergency Management Gold! 2000. **Available at:** http://www.disasters.org/emgold/index.htm.

EPIX (Emergency Preparedness Information Exchange). **Available at:** http://hoshi.cic.sfu.ca/epix/.

Federal Emergency Management Agency (FEMA). **Available at:** http://www.fema.gov/.

Federal Emergency Management Agency (FEMA). Global Emergency Management System. **Available at:** http://www.fema.gov/gems/. (Links to information on preparedness, listed by topic.)

Federal Emergency Management Agency. Mitigation. **Available at:** http://www.fema.gov/mit/.

International Code Council. **Available at:** http://www.intlcode.org and http://www.intlcode.org/download/index.htm. (Information on building codes.)

Occupational Safety and Health Administration. *Hospitals and community emergency response—what you need to know.* OSHA 3152. **Available at:** http://www.osha-slc.gov/Publications/OSHA3152/osha3152.html. (A pamphlet about preparedness for chemically contaminated patients.)

Institute for Business and Home Safety. **Available at:** http://www.ibhs.org/ibhs2/. (Several free documents on how to build and retrofit buildings to withstand natural disasters.)

Pan American Health Organization (PAHO). **Available at:** http://165.158.1.110/english/ped/pedhome.htm.

University of Colorado. Natural Hazards Center. **Available at:** http://www.Colorado.edu/hazards/.

University of Delaware, Disaster Research Center. **Available at:** http://www.udel.edu/DRC/.

World Health Organization (WHO) Handbook for Emergency Related Field Operations. **Available at:** http://www.who.int/disasters/tg.cfm?doctypeID=25.

World Health Organization (WHO) Health Library for Disasters. Available at: http://www.helid.desastres.net/. (Downloadable full-text documents.)

REFERENCES

1. International City Management Association. Emergency planning: an adaptive approach. *Baseline Data Report* 1988;20: 1–14.
2. Quarantelli EL. *Delivery of emergency medical care in disasters: assumptions and realities.* New York: Irvington Publishers, 1983.
3. Tierney KJ. *A primer for preparedness for acute chemical emergencies.* Book and monograph series no. 14. Columbus, OH: Disaster Research Center, Ohio State University, 1980.
4. Dynes RR, Quarantelli EL, Kreps GA. *A perspective on disaster planning,* 3rd ed. Columbus, OH: Disaster Research Center, Ohio State University, 1981.
5. Klein JS, Weigelt JA. Disaster management: lessons learned. *Contemp Probl Trauma Surg* 1991;71:257–266.

6. Auf der Heide E. *Disaster response: principles of preparation and coordination.* St. Louis, MO: CV Mosby, 1989.

7. Barton A. Communities in disaster: a sociological analysis of collective stress situations. Garden City, NY: Doubleday, 1969.

8. Gibson G. Disaster and emergency medical care: methods, theories and a research agenda. *Mass Emerg* 1977;2:195–203.

9. Barton AH. *Social organization under stress: a sociological review of disaster studies.* Disaster study no. 17, publication no. 1032. Washington, D.C.: Disaster Research Group, National Academy of Sciences—National Research Council, 1963.

10. Adams CR. *Search and rescue efforts following the Wichita Falls tornado.* Technical report no. 4, SAR research project, Department of Sociology. Denver: University of Denver, 1981.

11. Gordon D. High-rise fire rescue: lessons from Las Vegas. *Emerg Med Serv* 1986;15:20–30.

12. Gratz DB. *Fire department management: scope and method.* Beverly Hills, CA: Glencoe Press, 1972.

13. Neff JL. Responsibility for the delivery of emergency medical services in a mass casualty situation: the problem of overlapping jurisdictions. *Mass Emerg* 1977;2:179–188.

14. Golec JA, Gurney PJ. The problem of needs assessment in the delivery of EMS. *Mass Emerg* 1977;2:169–177.

15. Worth MF, Stroup J. Some observations of the effect of EMS law on disaster related delivery systems. *Mass Emerg* 1977;2: 159–168.

16. Rosow I. *Authority in emergencies: four tornado communities in 1953.* Columbus: Disaster Research Center, Ohio State University, 1977.

17. Henry S. Mississauga hospital: largest evacuation in Canada's history. *Can Med Assoc J* 1980;122:582–586.

18. Arnold C, Durkin M. *Hospitals and the San Fernando earthquake of 1971: the operational experience.* San Mateo, CA: Building Systems Development, Inc., 1983

19. Tierney KJ. Report on the Coalinga earthquake of May 2, 1983. Publication no. SSC 85-01. Sacramento: Seismic Safety Commission, State of California, 1985.

20. Chavez CW, Binder B. A hospital as victim and responder: The Sepulveda VA medical center and the Northridge earthquake. *J Emerg Med* 1996;14:445–454.

21. Friedman E. Updating disaster plans: a tale of three hospitals. *Hosp JAHA* 1978;52:95–102.

22. Blanshan SA. A time model: hospital organizational response to disaster. In: Quarantelli EL, ed. *Disasters: theory and research.* Beverly Hills, CA: Sage Publications, 1978:173–198.

23. Form WH, et al. *Final report on the Flint-Beecher tornado.* Detroit, MI: Social Research Service, Continuing Education Service, Michigan State College, 1954.

24. Angell L. Watsonville hospital: the day of the quake. *Business and Industry Council for Emergency Planning and Preparedness News* 1990:10–14.

25. California Association of Hospitals and Health Systems. *Hospital earthquake preparedness: issues for action. A report on the Loma Prieta earthquake issued October 17, 1990.* Sacramento: California Association of Hospitals and Health Systems, 1990.

26. Vogt BM. *Evacuation of institutionalized and specialized populations, ORNL/SUB-7685/1 & T23.* Oak Ridge, TN: Oak Ridge National Laboratory, 1990.

27. Kallsen G. Collapse of Coalinga. *J Emerg Med Serv* 1983;8: 24–29.

28. Maxwell C. Hospital organizational response to the nuclear accident at Three Mile Island: implications for future-oriented disaster planning. In: Cowley RA, ed. *Mass casualties: a lessons learned approach.* Proceedings of the First International Assembly on Emergency Medical Services, Baltimore, June 13–17, 1982. DOT HS 806 302. Washington, D.C.: U.S. Department of Transportation, National Highway Traffic Safety Administration, 1982.

29. Seismic Safety Commission. *Public official attitudes toward disaster preparedness in California.* Publication no. SSC 79-05. Sacramento, CA: Seismic Safety Commission, 1979.

30. Martchenke J, Pointer JE. Hospital disaster operations during the 1989 Loma Prieta earthquake. *Prehospital Disaster Med* 1994;9:146–153.

31. Drabek TE. *Emergency management: principles and practice for local government.* Washington, D.C.: International City Management Association, 1991.

32. Grollmes EE. *Air disaster response planning: lessons for the future.* Emmitsburg, MD: National Emergency Training Center, Federal Emergency Management Agency, 1985.

33. Seismic Safety Commission. *Planning for the next one: transcripts of hearings on the Loma Prieta earthquake of October 17, 1989.* SSC 91-02. Sacramento, CA: State of California, Seismic Safety Commission, 1991.

34. Federal Emergency Management Agency. *Emergency planning.* Student manual, SM-61. Washington, D.C.: Federal Emergency Management Agency, 1983.

35. Adams CR, Drabek TE, Kiliganek TS, et al. *The organization of search and rescue efforts following the Wichita Falls, Texas tornado.* Presented at the Annual Meeting of the American Sociological Association, New York, August, 1980. Denver: University of Denver, 1980.

36. Bush S. *Disaster planning and multiagency coordination.* Littleton, CO: City of Littleton, 1981.

37. Stevenson L, Hayman M. *Local government disaster protection: final technical report.* Washington, D.C.: International City Management Association, 1981.

38. Drabek TE. *Human system responses to disaster: an inventory of sociological findings.* New York: Springer-Verlag, 1986.

39. Washington State University. *Adaptive planning for community emergency management.* Pullman, WA: Washington State University, 1987.

40. Kilijanek TS. *There she blows: the search and rescue response to the Mount St. Helens volcano.* Technical report no. 11, SAR research project. Denver: Department of Sociology, University of Denver, 1981.

41. May PJ. FEMA's role in emergency management: examining recent experience. *Publ Admin Rev* 1985;45:40–48.

42. Mushkatel AH, Weschler LF. Emergency management and the intergovernmental system. *Publ Admin Rev* 1985;45:49–56.

43. Cigler B. *Emergency management and public administration.* Report #86-12. Chapel Hill: University of North Carolina at Chapel Hill, 1986.

44. Burke YB, Carlucci FC, Dempsey CL, et al. *Coping with catastrophe: building an emergency management system to meet people's needs in natural and manmade disasters.* Washington, D.C.: National Academy of Public Administration, 1993.

45. Smith RA, Traum CC, Poole LH. The provision of primary care during a period of natural disaster or large scale emergency. *Mass Emerg* 1977;2:19–23.

46. Levy LJ, Toulmin LM. *Improving disaster planning and response efforts: lessons from Hurricanes Andrew and Iniki.* McLean, VA: Booz, Allen & Hamilton, 1993.

47. Centers for Disease Control and Prevention. *Preparing for the next influenza pandemic.* Atlanta, GA: Centers for Disease Control and Prevention, 1999.

48. Wright JE. The prevalence and effectiveness of centralized medical responses to mass casualty disasters. *Mass Emerg* 1977;2: 189–194.

49. Foster HD. *Disaster planning: the preservation of life and property.* New York: Springer-Verlag, 1980.

50. Starr C. Social benefit versus technological risk: what is our society willing to pay for safety? *Science* 1969;165:1232–1238.

51. Drabek TE. Managing the emergency response. *Publ Admin Rev* 1985;45:85–92.

52. Institute of Medicine. *America's health care safety net: intact but endangered*. Washington, D.C.: National Academy Press, 2000.

53. Cornwell EE 3rd, Berne TV, Belzberg H, et al. Health care crisis from a trauma center perspective: the LA story. *JAMA* 1996; 276:940–944.

54. Wolensky RP, Wolensky KC. American local government and the disaster management problem. *Local Government Studies* 1991;17:15–32.

55. Auf der Heide E. Disaster planning, part II: disaster problems, issues, and challenges identified in the research literature. *Emerg Med Clin North Am* 1996;14:453–480.

56. Drabek TE. *Disaster in aisle 13: a case study of the coliseum explosion at the Indiana state fairgrounds, October 31,1963*. Columbus, OH: College of Administrative Science, Ohio State University, Columbus, 1968.

57. Sopher L, Petersen R, Talbott M. The crash of flight 232L: an emergency care perspective. *J Emerg Nurs* 1990;16:61A–66A.

58. Kerns DE, Anderson PB. EMS response to a major aircraft incident: Sioux City, Iowa. *Prehospital Disaster Med* 1990;5:159–166.

59. Nordberg M. United flight 232: the story behind the rescue. *Emerg Med Serv* 1989;18:15,22–31.

60. Hearn W. Disaster plan in action: Oklahoma medical teams respond well to terrifying time. *Am Med News* 1995:3,24.

61. Maningas PA, Bobison M, Mallonee S. The EMS response to the Oklahoma City bombing. *Prehospital Disaster Med* 1997;12: 80–85.

62. Quayle C. Lessons learned from the Oklahoma City bombing. *Am Hosp Assoc News* 1995;31:7.

63. Landesman LY. *Emergency preparedness in health care organizations*. Oak Brook Terrace, IL: Joint Commission on Accreditation of Healthcare Organizations, 1996.

64. Oklahoma City Mayor and City Council. *Murrah rescue and recovery operation*. Final Report to the Mayor and City Council. Oklahoma City, OK: Oklahoma City Mayor and City Council, 1996.

65. Fechtel EJ. How St. Mary's hospital, Athens, Ga. handled a recent tornado disaster. *Hosp Progr* 1973;54:38–40.

66. Morris GP. The Kenner airliner disaster: a 727 falls into a New Orleans suburb. *J Emerg Med Serv* 1982;7:58–65.

67. Dynes RR. *Organized behavior in disaster*. Columbus, OH: Disaster Research Center, 1974.

68. Stallings RA. Differential response of hospital personnel to a disaster. *Mass Emerg* 1975;1:47–54.

69. Kennedy WC. *Some preliminary observations on a hospital response to the Jackson, Mississippi tornado of March 3, 1966*. Research report 17. Columbus: Disaster Research Center, Ohio State University, 1967.

70. Morris BAP, Armstrong TM. Medical response to a natural disaster: the Barrie tornado. *Can Med Assoc J* 1986;134:767–769.

71. Beelman FC. Disaster planning: report of tornado casualties in Topeka. *J Kansas Med Soc* 1967;68:153–161.

72. Johnson JE. Tornado as teacher: lessons learned in caring for tornado victims lead to revision of one hospital's disaster plan. *Hosp JAHA* 1970;44:40–42,104.

73. Amundson SB, Burkle AM. Golden minutes: the Oklahoma City Bombing—two ED nurses' stories. *J Emerg Nurs* 1995;21: 401–407.

74. Quarantelli EL. The community general hospital: its immediate problems in disasters. *Am Behav Sci* 1970;13:380–391.

75. Anonymous. Hurricane Andrew puts Florida's hospitals to the test and leaves hundreds of nurses homeless. *Am J Nurs* 1992;October:96–100.

76. Shaftan GW. Disaster and medical care. *J Trauma* 1962;2: 111–116.

77. Davie K. It always happens "somewhere else": Coldenham 1989. *Emerg Med Serv* 1990;19:31–40.

78. Taylor V. *Hospital emergency facilities in disaster: an analysis of organizational adaptation to stress*. Columbus: Disaster Research Center, Ohio State University, 1974.

79. Alberta Public Safety Services. *Tornado, a report: Edmonton and Strathcona county, July 31st, 1987*. Edmonton, Ontario, Canada: Alberta Public Safety Services, 1991.

80. Adams R. DC disaster crisis: a fatal plane crash and deadly subway derailment challenge regional emergency forces. *Firehouse* 1982;March:50–54.

81. Oakland Fire Department. *Oakland fire department earthquake report*. Oakland, CA: City of Oakland Fire Department, 1990.

82. Haynes BE, Freeman C, Rubin JL, et al. Medical response to catastrophic events: California's planning and the Loma Prieta earthquake. *Ann Emerg Med* 1992;21:368–374.

83. Edelstein S. Metro subway accident. In: Cowley RA, ed. *Mass casualties: a lessons learned approach*. In: Proceedings from the First International Assembly on Emergency Medical Services, Baltimore, June 13-17, 1982. DOT HS 806 302. Washington, D.C.: United States Department of Transportation, National Highway Traffic Safety Administration, 1982:157–162.

84. Goodwin DV. D.C. crash problems magnified by snow, traffic snarl & EMS snafu. *Emerg Depart News* 1982;4:1,14.

85. Palafox J, Pointer JE, Martchenke J, et al. The 1989 Loma Prieta earthquake: issues in medical control. *Prehospital Disaster Med* 1993:291–297.

86. Gray C, Knabe H. The night the skywalks fell: 111 dead, 188 injured in Kansas City hotel collapse. *Firehouse* 1981;6:66–70, 132–133.

87. Federal Emergency Management Agency. *FEMA's disaster management program: a performance audit after hurricane andrew*. Washington, D.C.: Office of the Inspector General, Federal Emergency Management Agency, 1993.

88. Curry JL. A disaster that could happen anywhere—the Palm Bay massacre. *J Emerg Nurs* 1990;16:42A–48A.

89. Klein JS, Weigelt JA. Disaster management lessons learned. *Surg Clin North Am* 1991;71:257.

90. Alson R, Alexander D, Leonard RB, Stringer LW. Analysis of medical treatment at a field hospital following hurricane Andrew, 1992. *Ann Emerg Med* 1993;22:1721–1728.

91. Oklahoma Department of Civil Emergency Management. *After action report: Alfred P. Murrah federal building bombing, 19 April, 1995*. Oklahoma City, OK: State of Oklahoma, Department of Central Services, Central Printing Division, 1995.

92. Williams MS. Remarks presented by Michael S. Williams, Chief HRS Office of Emergency Medical Services to the Governor's Disaster Planning and Response Committee, 1992.

93. Tierney KJ. *Emergency preparedness and response: lessons from the Loma Prieta earthquake*. Newark, DE: Disaster Research Center, University of Delaware, 1993.

94. Reshaur LM, Luongo RP. Lessons in business continuity planning: one hospital's response to a disaster. *Disaster Recovery J* 2000;Spring:12–13.

95. McCann J. Disaster drills pay off in VT Amtrak wreck: minor problems include need to triage x-ray. *Emerg Depart News* 1984; 6:9,20.

96. Joint Committee on Fire Police Emergency and Disaster Services. *California's emergency communications crises*. Sacramento, CA: California State Senate and Assembly, 1983.

97. Cuny FC. *Disasters and development*. New York: Oxford University Press, 1983.

98. Seismic Safety Commission. *Preliminary reports submitted to the seismic safety commission on the May 2, 1983 Coalinga earth-

quake. Publication no. SSC 83-08. Sacramento, CA: Seismic Safety Commission, 1983.

99. Sundberg C. In the fiery aftermath of the crash of flight 232, Sioux City EMS proved that it has the right stuff. *Emergency* 1990;August:30–33.

100. Noji EK, Armenian HK, Oganessian A. Issues of rescue and medical care following the 1988 Armenian earthquake. *Int J Epidemiol* 1993;22:1070–1076.

101. De Bruycker M, Donato G, Isidoro A, et al. The 1980 earthquake in southern Italy: rescue of trapped victims and mortality. *Bull WHO* 1983;61:1021–1025.

102. O'Brian P, Mileti DS. Citizen participation in emergency response following the Loma Prieta earthquake. *Int J Mass Emerg Disasters* 1992;10:71–89.

103. Yong C, Tsoi K, Felbi C, et al. *The great Tangshan earthquake of 1976: an anatomy of disaster*. New York: Pergamon Press, 1988.

104. Raker JW, Friedsam HJ. Disaster-scale medical care problems: a study of medical problems experienced in the Dallas tornado. *JAMA* 1960;173:1239–1244.

105. Munninger K, Ravenholt O. Lessons from Las Vegas: the MGM hotel fire. *J Emerg Med Serv* 1981;6:37–40.

106. Tierney KJ. *Emergency medical care aspects of the Loma Prieta earthquake*. Newark, DE: Disaster Research Center, University of Delaware, 1992.

107. Koehler G, Isbell D, Freeman C, et al. *Medical care for the injured: the emergency medical response to the April, 1992, Los Angeles civil disturbance*. EMSA #393-01. Sacramento, CA: State of California, Health and Welfare Agency, Emergency Medical Services Authority, 1993:28.

108. Okumura T, Takasu N, Ishimatsu S, et al. Report on 640 victims of the Tokyo subway sarin attack. *Ann Emerg Med* 1996; 28:129–135.

109. Fogelman MJ. The Dallas tornado disaster. *Am J Surg* 1958; 95:501–506.

110. Kansas City Health Department. *Hyatt disaster medical assessment*. Kansas City, MO: Health Department, 1981.

111. Hogan DE, Askins DC, Osburn AE. The May 3, 1999, tornado in Oklahoma City. *Ann Emerg Med* 1999;34:225–226.

112. Noji EK. *The public health consequences of disasters*. New York: Oxford University Press, 1997.

113. Sheng ZY. Medical support in the Tangshan earthquake: a review of the management of mass casualties and certain major injuries. *J Trauma* 1987;27:1130–1135.

114. Kirsch TD. External emergency medical disaster response: does a need exist? *Ann Emerg Med* 1996;28:220–222.

115. Centers for Disease Control and Prevention. Hurricanes and hospital emergency-room visits—Mississippi, Rhode Island, Connecticut. *MMWR* 1986;34:765–770.

116. Romo RC. The Mexico City earthquake—an international disaster. An overview. *J World Assoc Emerg Disaster Med* 1986;1–4:4–8.

117. Durkin ME, Thiel CC Jr, Schneider JE, et al. Injuries and emergency medical response in the Loma Prieta earthquake. *Bull Seismol Soc Am* 1991;81:2143–2166.

118. Pointer JE, Michaelis J, Saunders C, et al. The 1989 Loma Prieta earthquake: impact on hospital patient care. *Ann Emerg Med* 1992;21:1228–1233.

119. Mallonee S, Shariat S, Stennies G, et al. Physical injuries and fatalities resulting from the Oklahoma City bombing. *JAMA* 1996;276:382–387.

120. Goltz JD. *The "921" Chi-Chi, Taiwan earthquake of September 21, 1999: societal impacts and emergency response*. Pasadena, CA: Seismological Laboratory, California Institute of Technology, 1999.

121. Lechat MF. Disasters and public health. *Bull WHO* 1979;57: 11–17.

122. Scott S, Constantine LM. When natural disaster strikes: with careful planning, pharmacists can continue to provide essential services to survivors in the aftermath of a disaster. *Am Pharm* 1990;NS30:27–31.

123. Centers for Disease Control and Prevention. Morbidity and mortality associated with hurricane Floyd—North Carolina, September–October 1999. *MMWR* 2000;49:369–372.

124. Leor J, Poole WK, Kloner RA. Sudden cardiac death triggered by an earthquake. *N Engl J Med* 1996;334:413–419.

125. Anonymous. Northridge, California Earthquake: Implications for the central U.S. *Central United States Earthquake Consort J* 1994;2:1–7.

126. Centers for Disease Control and Prevention. Surveillance for injuries and illnesses and rapid health-needs assessment following hurricanes Marilyn and Opal, September–October 1995. *MMWR* 1996;45:81–85.

127. Gulitz E, Carrington L. Notes from the field. Planning for disasters: sheltering persons with special health needs. *Am J Publ Health* 1990;80:879–880.

128. Blumhagen DW. Evacuation of patients during a fire at a general hospital. *Ann Emerg Med* 1987;16:209–214.

129. Roman R, Wamsley B, Clyburn E. Northridge, California earthquake: implications for the central U.S. *Central United States Earthquake Consort J* 1994;2:1–7.

130. Centers for Disease Control and Prevention. Community needs assessment and morbidity surveillance following an earthquake—Turkey, August 1999. *MMWR* 1999;48:1147–1150.

131. Centers for Disease Control and Prevention. Rapid health needs assessment following hurricane Andrew—Florida and Louisiana, 1992. *MMWR* 1992;41:687–688.

132. Sabatino F. Hurricane Andrew: south Florida hospitals shared resources and energy to cope with the storm's devastation. *Hosp JAHA* 1992;December 20:26–30.

133. Friedman E. Coping with calamity: how well does health care disaster planning work? *JAMA* 1994;272:1875–1879.

134. Martchenke J. Abstract for the EMS Earthquake Project Study. San Francisco: Department of Health, San Francisco City and County, 1994.

135. Phreaner D, Jacoby I, Dreier S, McCoy N. Disaster preparedness of home health care agencies in San Diego county. *J Emerg Med* 1994;12:811–818.

136. Fritz CE, Mathewson JH. *Convergence behavior in disasters: a problem in social control*. Disaster study no. 9, publication no. 476. Washington, D.C.: Committee on Disaster Studies, National Academy of Sciences—National Research Council, 1956.

137. Autier P, Ferir MC, Hairapetien A, et al. Viewpoint: drug supply in the aftermath of the 1988 Armenian earthquake. *Lancet* 1990;335:1388–1390.

138. Nordberg M. Rapid rescue: the Illinois tornado. *Emerg Med Serv* 1991;20:25–29.

139. Cihlar C. Hospitals respond efficiently to Chicago's worst train wreck. *Hosp JAHA* 1972;46:17–17b.

140. Dynes RR. Interorganizational relations in communities under stress. In: Quarantelli EL, ed. *Disasters: theory and research*. Beverly Hills, CA: Sage Publications, 1978:49–64.

141. Breo DL. Tragedy's aftermath: town pulls together. *Am Med News* 1986;May 1:1.

142. Aghababian RV, Lewis CP, Gans L, Curley FJ. Disasters within hospitals. *Ann Emerg Med* 1994;23:771–777.

143. Office of Statewide Health Planning and Development. *A recommended program to seismically strengthen pre-hospital act hospital facilities: a response to milestone 4, initiative 1.2, "California at risk", December 1990*. Sacramento: Building Safety Board, Office of Statewide Health Planning and Development, Division of Facilities Development and Financing, 1990.

144. Office of Statewide Health Planning and Development. *Sum-*

mary of hospital seismic performance ratings: as submitted to California's office of statewide health planning and development by California's general acute care hospitals in accordance with the Alquist Hospital Facility Seismic Safety Act. Sacramento: Building Safety Board, Office of Statewide Health Planning and Development, Division of Facilities Development and Financing, 2001.

145. Wolfson J, Walker G. *Hospital disaster preparedness: lessons from hurricane Andrew.* Tampa, FL: The Florida Public Health Information Center, College of Public Health, The University of South Florida, 1993.

146. Reitherman R. How to prepare a hospital for an earthquake. *J Emerg Med* 1986;4:119–131.

147. Staver S. Hospitals, MDs battle blackout. *Am Med News* 1977:1,10.

148. Olson RA, Schultz CH, Koenig KL, Auf der Heide E. *Critical decisions: evacuating hospitals after the 1994 Northridge earthquake.* National Science Foundation Grant Number CMS-9416277. Sacramento, CA: Robert Olson Associates, Inc., 1998.

149. O'Brian PE. The hospital isn't closed—we've just relocated: a New Brunswick disaster plan. *Can Med Assoc J* 1979;120:1132–1138.

150. Cushing TS, Whittington KE, Boyd HD. *Hurricane Andrew afteraction report.* Indianapolis: Department of Veterans Affairs, Veterans Health Administration, Emergency Medical Preparedness Office, 1993.

151. Anonymous. Two hospitals treat majority of casualties as Midwest tornadoes kill 70, injure 1300. *Hosp JAHA* 1968;42:128.

152. Peters MS. Hospitals respond to water loss during the Midwest floods of 1993: preparedness and improvisation. *J Emerg Med* 1996;14:345–350.

153. Fisher HL. Emergency evacuation of the Denver Veteran's Administration medical center. *Mil Med* 1986;151:154–161.

154. Freeman C, Van Ness C, Morales JE. *Hurricane Andrew: lessons for California.* Sacramento, CA: State of California, Emergency Medical Services Authority, 1993.

155. Joint Commission on Accreditation of Healthcare Organizations. *Emergency management standard.* Oak Brook Terrace, IL: Joint Commission on Accreditation of Healthcare Organizations, 2001.

156. Mileti DS, Sorensen JH. Determinants of organizational effectiveness in responding to low probability catastrophic events. *Columbia J World Bus* 1987;22:13–21.

156a. Fritz CE, Mathewson JH. *Convergence behavior in disasters: a problem in social control.* Disaster study no. 9. Publication no. 476. Washington, D.C.: Committee on Disaster Studies, National Academy of Science, National Research Council, 1956.

157. Moore HE. *Tornados over Texas: a study of Waco and San Angelo in disaster.* Austin: University of Texas Press, 1958.

158. Arnett N. The Las Vegas jinx. *Emerg Prod News* 1981;May:76–90.

159. Diekema DS. Unwinding the COBRA: new perspectives on EMTALA. *Pediatr Emerg Care* 1995;11:243–248.

160. National Institute for Occupational Safety and Health. *NIOSH-DOD-OSHA sponsored chemical and biological respiratory protection workshop,* Lakeview Resort and Conference Center, Morgantown, WV, March 10-12, 1999. Cincinnati, OH: National Institute for Occupational Safety & Health, 2000.

161. Sorensen JH, Vogt BM. *Interim report on lessons learned from decontamination experiences.* Oak Ridge, TN: Oak Ridge National Laboratory, 2000.

162. Levitin HW, Siegelson HJ. Hazardous materials: disaster medical planning and response. *Emerg Med Clin North Am* 1996;14:327–348.

163. Olson KR. Hazmat-o-phobia: why aren't hospitals ready for chemical accidents? *West J Med* 1998;168:32–33.

164. Burgess JL, Kirk M, Borron SW, Cisek J. Emergency depart-

ment hazardous materials protocol for contaminated patients. *Ann Emerg Med* 1999;34:205–212.

165. Occupational Safety and Health Administration. *Hospitals and community emergency response — what you need to know.* OSHA 3152 1997. Washington, D.C.: United States Department of Labor, Occupational Safety and Health Administration, 1997.

166. Occupational Safety and Health Administration. *OSHA regulations (standards—29 CFR). General requirements—1910.132 personal protective equipment.* Washington, D.C.: United States Department of Labor, Occupational Safety and Health Administration, 1975. Amended in 1994.

167. Occupational Safety and Health Administration. *OSHA regulations (standards—29 CFR). General requirements—1910.134. App A fit testing procedures (mandatory).* Washington, D.C.: United States Department of Labor, Occupational Safety and Health Administration, 1998.

168. Occupational Safety and Health Administration. *OSHA regulations (standards—29 CFR 1910.120). Hazardous waste operations and emergency response, 1990.* Washington, D.C.: United States Department of Labor, Occupational Safety and Health Administration, 1990.

169. Cone DC, Davidson SJ. Hazardous materials preparedness in the emergency department. *Prehospital Emerg Care* 1997;1:85–90.

170. Burgess JL, Blackmon GM, Brodkin CA, Robertson WO. Hospital preparedness for hazardous materials incidents and treatment of contaminated patients. *West J Med* 1997;167:387–391.

171. Kuhn JM. *A study of factors associated with emergency department preparedness for employee safety during the treatment of hazardous material patients: implications for hospital emergency planning.* Honolulu: University of Hawaii, 1997.

172. Parker D, Dart R, McNally J. Critical deficiencies in the treatment of toxicologic emergencies: antidote stocking in Arizona hospitals [abstract]. *Vet Hum Toxicol* 1990;32:376.

173. Chyka PA, Conner HG. Availability of antidotes in rural and urban hospitals in Tennessee. *Am J Hosp Pharm* 1994;51:1346–1348.

174. Woolf AD, Chrisanthus K. On-site availability of selected antidotes: results of a survey of Massachusetts hospitals. *Am J Emerg Med* 1997;15:62–66.

175. Dart RC, Stark Y, Fulton B, et al. Insufficient stocking of poisoning antidotes in hospital pharmacies. *JAMA* 1996;276:1508–1510.

176. Teresi WM, King WD. Survey of the stocking of poison antidotes in Alabama. *South Med J* 1999;92:1151–1156.

177. Ghilarducci DP, Pirrallo RG, Hegmann KT. Hazardous material readiness of United States level 1 trauma centers. *J Occup Environ Med* 2000;42:683–692.

178. Committee on R&D Needs for Improving Civilian Medical Response to Chemical and Biological Terrorism Incidents. *Chemical and biological terrorism: research and development to improve civilian medical response.* Washington, D.C.: National Academy Press, 1999.

179. United States Army Soldier and Biological Chemical Command. *Domestic preparedness: hospital provider course.* Aberdeen Proving Ground, MD: United States Army Soldier and Biological Chemical Command, 1998.

180. American Psychiatric Association. *Diagnostic and statistical manual of mental disorders,* 4th ed. Washington, D.C.: American Psychiatric Association, 1994.

181. Sidell FR, Takafuji E, Franz DR. *Medical aspects of chemical and biological warfare.* Washington, D.C.: Office of the Surgeon General, Borden Institute, Walter Reed Army Medical Center, 1997. Textbook of Military Medicine series.

182. Yokoyama K, Araki S, Murata K, et al. Chronic neurobehavioral effects of Tokyo subway sarin poisoning in relation to posttraumatic stress disorder. *Arch Environ Health* 1998;53:249–256.

183. Hartman DE. Missed diagnoses and misdiagnoses of environmental toxicant exposure. The psychiatry of toxic exposure and multiple chemical sensitivity. *Psychiatr Clin North Am* 1998; 21:659–670.

184. Agency for Toxic Substances and Disease Registry. *Toxicological profile for hydrogen sulfide.* Atlanta, GA: Agency for Toxic Substances and Disease Registry, 1999.

185. Xiao JQ, Levin SM. The diagnosis and management of solvent-related disorders. *Am J Indus Med* 2000;37:44–61.

186. Colligan M. Mass psychogenic illness: some clarification and perspectives. *J Occup Med* 1981;23:635–638.

187. Faust H, Brilliant L. Is the diagnosis of "mass hysteria" an excuse for incomplete investigation of low-level environmental contamination? *J Occup Med* 1981;23:22–26.

188. Boxer P. Occupational mass psychogenic illness: history, prevention and management. *J Occup Med* 1985;27:867–872.

189. Colligan M, Urtes MA, Wisseman C, et al. An investigation of apparent mass psychogenic illness in an electronics plant. *J Behav Med* 1979;2:297–309.

190. Chew P. How to handle hysterical factory workers. *Occup Health Saf* 1978;47:50–53.

191. Ruiz M, Lopez J. Mass hysteria in a secondary school [letter]. *Int J Epidemiol* 1988;17:475–476.

192. Small GW, Propper MW, Randolph ET, Eth S. Mass hysteria among student performers: social relationship as a symptom factor. *Am J Psychiatry* 1991;148:1200–1205.

193. Bell A, Jones A. Fumigation with dichlorethyl ether and chlordane: hysterical sequelae. *Med J Aust* 1958;45:258–263.

194. Araki S, Honma T. Mass psychogenic illness in school children in relation to Tokyo photochemical smog. *Arch Environ Health* 1986;4:159–162.

195. Baker P, Selvey D. Malathion-induced epidemic hysteria in an elementary school. *Vet Hum Toxicol* 1992;34:156–160.

196. Levine RJ. Epidemic faintness and syncope in a school marching band. *JAMA* 1977;238:2373–2376.

197. Moffat M. Epidemic hysteria in a Montreal train station. *Pediatrics* 1982;70:308–310.

198. Nitzkin JL. Epidemic transient situational disturbance in an elementary school. *J Florida Med Assoc* 1976;63:357–359.

199. Wessley S. Responding to mass psychogenic illness. *N Engl J Med* 2000;342:129–130.

200. Sirois F. Epidemic hysteria. *Acta Psychiatr Skand Suppl* 1974; 252:5–45.

201. Vukmir RB, Paris PM. The Three Rivers rigatta accident: an EMS perspective. *Am J Emerg Med* 1991;9:64–71.

202. Orr SM. The Hyatt Regency skywalk collapse: an EMS-based disaster response. *Ann Emerg Med* 1983;12:601–605.

203. Glass RI, Craven RB, Bregman DJ, et al. Injuries from the Wichita Falls tornado: implications for prevention. *Science* 1980;207:734–738.

204. Orr SM, Robinson WA. The Hyatt disaster: two physicians' perspectives. *J Emerg Nurs* 1982;8:6–11.

205. Mangum WP, Kosberg JI, McDonald P. Hurricane Elena and Pinellas County, Florida: some lessons learned from the largest evacuation of nursing home patients in history. *Gerontol* 1989; 29:388–392.

206. Federal Emergency Management Agency. *Exemplary practices in emergency management: the California FIRESCOPE program.* Monograph series no. 1. Washington, D.C.: Federal Emergency Management Agency, 1987.

207. Kilijanek TS. *The night of the whippoorwill: the search and rescue response to a boating disaster.* Technical report no. 2, SAR research project. Denver, CO: Department of Sociology, University of Denver, 1980.

208. United States General Accounting Office. *Disaster assistance: federal, state, and local responses to natural disasters need improvement.* GAO/RCED-91-43. Washington, D.C.: United States General Accounting Office, 1991.

209. Dynes RR, Quarantelli EL. *Organizational communications and decision making in crises.* Columbus, OH: Disaster Research Center, Ohio State University, 1977.

210. Emerson B. Cellphones come through when emergencies strike. *The Atlanta Journal-Constitution* 2001:G7.

211. Uraneck K. Emergency physicians offer help—but find few takers. *EMT Today* September 21, 2001.

212. Yutzy D. *Community priorities in the Anchorage, Alaska earthquake, 1964.* Columbus: Disaster Research Center, Ohio State University, 1969.

213. Mesnick PS. Value of disaster critiques as demonstrated by the management of two "L" crashes in the city of Chicago. In: Frey R, Safar P, eds. *Types and events of disasters: organization in various disaster situations.* New York: Springer-Verlag, 1980:133–139.

EMERGENCY MEDICAL SERVICES IN DISASTER

MICHAEL F. MURPHY

"I've got patients "coming out of the woodwork—literally."
—Paula Clay, Oklahoma City Tornado, May 3, 1999.

OVERVIEW

The Role of the First Responder

Emergency medical services (EMS), fire departments, and police departments of the local jurisdictions are invariably the first responders to arrive at the scene of a disaster. The level of preparedness, planning, and coordination among these agencies and the actions taken in the first few minutes will dictate their level of success in mitigating the medical consequences of a disaster. The level of preparedness often varies from jurisdiction to jurisdiction and from agency to agency. The type of EMS organization, its size and geographical location, and its leadership affect how much emphasis is placed on disaster preparation. The roles played by first responders may vary depending on the situation. Traditionally, emergency medical services have been responsible for the triage, treatment, and transport of victims. Fire departments have provided incident command, fire suppression, rescue, and manpower assistance. Police departments have provided security, perimeter control, and access and egress management.

Recent disasters have shown that these "traditional" roles are actually less clear, with first responders and bystander citizens performing functions that are not according to plan (1). Paramedics have performed rescue alongside police officers. Firefighters have set up treatment areas and have rendered patient care. Police officers and citizens have transported injured victims to local hospitals for treatment. Although traditional roles for first responders are generally understood, a more flexible response process may be required.

Service Type and Preparedness Level

The preparedness level for prehospital management of medical casualties will differ depending on certain variables. The type of service, its size and leadership, the political and economic environment in which it operates, and its geographic location all affect the level of readiness to respond to a disaster. Large, well-funded organizations in a disaster-prone location usually prepare and exercise more readily than smaller organizations in relatively stable environments. The leadership of an organization responding to the political and economic environment often dictates the level of preparedness. A local jurisdiction that is genuinely concerned about the safety of its citizens with a leadership who is aware of the need to prepare will result in exercises and procedures that rival the best services. Conversely, complacency, lack of concern or awareness, low economic priority, and a lack of leadership will result in a large organization that is totally unprepared.

The Prehospital Mission

The mission assigned to prehospital providers varies within each jurisdiction. The most consistent theme is the need to identify, extricate, triage, and transport victims from a scene to a definitive care facility. The reality of prehospital activities, however, often differs from the plan (see Chapter 8). How the patient is triaged often differs from what has been written in protocols. Patients are often transported by means other than ambulances. The receiving facilities are often separate from the prehospital system. Notification and patient disposition outcomes are frequently different from the expectations of those receiving facilities. The nature and amount of prehospital medical care that is provided frequently differs from the expectations of receiving facilities. Most of the time, care in the field is limited to dressing and C-spine protection. Few disasters have established treatment areas where anything beyond basic care is provided (2,3).

Current Perspectives: The Classic Model

The evolution of civilian response systems has resulted in a standard for mass casualty management that has been adopted in various forms across the country (4,5). This standard system includes the concept of triage, triage classifications, triage tags, choke points, and treatment areas. Transport officers load patients onto ambulances or buses to go to a designated definitive care facility. The transport units are directed to go to hospitals farther from the scene to decrease the overloading of geographically closer hospitals. Buses are directed to transport the less injured still farther away from heavily impacted hospitals. The EMS system, either in the form of a transport officer or the communications center, is supposed to notify hospitals of incoming patients.

While effective on paper and occasionally in real life, this system has inherent weaknesses. It assumes a static and cooperative patient population that will wait until it is either picked up or until it is directed to the choke point. It is applicable to a one-sided or a one-dimensional scene, and it does not adequately address patients flowing out in a 360-degree pattern. Attempts at scene control may limit flexibility and may result in frustration. The standard plan does not adequately address the self-referring patient population. In addition, EMS units, for a variety of reasons, tend to go to the closest hospital rather than to transport to locations on the perimeter.

Rethinking the Classic Model

Recent experiences in managing medical disasters suggest that the classic system needs to be revisited. Experience has shown that up to 80% of the patients involved in an incident will seek medical help on their own and that they will not interact with either the EMS system or the incident command structure (1,6). Victims and bystanders will also be involved in the rescue effort, whether or not they are asked. Volunteer medical personnel often arrive to the disaster site with good intentions, but they then actually become a management problem (6,7). Patients often refuse treatment, feeling that medical resources should go to "help someone who really needs it." The media can be either an asset or a problem depending on prior planning and the flow of accurate information. EMS units will initially transport to the closest hospital, which inevitably is heavily laden with patients who have received minimal treatment. Outlying hospitals may call in extra staff members when they are not needed and then question why they incurred the expense without receiving an appropriate number of patients. Many patients triaged at hospitals subsequently have to be transferred to other facilities due to the lack of specialty services. The current concern about weapons of mass destruction has forced planners to look at methods for decontaminating large numbers of patients before treating or transporting them (8,9).

By examining the past and learning from it, planners and response personnel can recognize the strengths and weakness of the current systems. They can then take steps to emphasize procedures that work, change procedures that do not, and add new procedures to fill the voids that are found. Clearly, some behaviors will consistently occur during disasters. Modification of the standard approach to the EMS disaster response should take these behaviors into account to improve its effectiveness.

EMERGENCY MEDICAL SERVICE DISASTER TYPES AND DEFINITIONS

Definitions

Various EMS organizations often have different criteria for defining a disaster. In addition, the definition of a disaster from the EMS point of view is different from that of emergency medicine, public health, or the research disciplines. Because EMS organizations respond to disasters, they tend to look at disasters from a response-related point of view. A car crash with six victims is absorbed into a large metropolitan EMS without notice, while the same crash may result in the activation of the disaster plan of a rural EMS. Some definitions related to EMS disaster response are as follows:

- *Disaster:* any event that overwhelms the EMS *resources available at that time* in a jurisdiction.
- *Multiple Patient Incident (MPI):* any event that causes more than one individual to become ill or injured.
- *Mass Casualty Incident (MCI):* any event that causes a large number or individuals to become ill or injured.
- *Medical Disaster:* any event that causes a large number of individuals to become ill or injured and that overwhelms the *resources* of the health care delivery system *available at that time.*

A key concept is that medical disasters are defined by the amount of available medical resources in relation to the needs of individuals requiring care at a specific place and time. The overall medical capability of a large community's health care system rarely will be totally overwhelmed by the number of patients produced by a disaster in the United States. However, disasters do result in a maldistribution of victims and medical resources, thus causing local treatment sites to be overwhelmed (10).

An event can be a disaster without necessarily becoming a medical disaster. An earthquake may cause the disruption of the public works, police, and fire departments without creating enough patients to overwhelm the health care delivery system. The Kansas City Skywalk collapse, the Oklahoma City bombing, and the events of September 11 all created patient counts that overwhelmed the local EMS system. However, the hospital infrastructure was quite capable of handling the increased patient load (11,12). Conversely, a medical disaster may occur without the infrastructure of a city being adversely affected. A flu pandemic may tax the healthcare delivery system to the breaking point long before employee absence due to illness adversely affects the city infrastructure.

Medical disasters may not always be a sudden, unanticipated event. The ice storm in upstate New York in 1998 did not immediately overwhelm the medical infrastructure. After several days, however, the number of visits to the emergency department doubled due to injuries from debris clearing and heater-induced carbon monoxide exposure. Fragile patients that had been receiveing care at home were sheltered in nursing homes. Elderly patients in shelters began to deteriorate from poor diet and hydration. Normal discharge options were compromised, and the hospitals became overwhelmed. In another example, tropical storm Allison also compromised the medical community in Houston, Texas, in 2001. The storm created massive flooding, and several large hospitals lost total power from flooded electrical switches in their basements. One hospital had to be evacuated, and several others had to transfer scores of patients out of their facilities. At the same time, patient volume increased, and normal discharge patterns were disrupted. Tropical storm Allison in Houston is an example of a health care system that became overwhelmed not by the number of patients requiring resources but by a significant disruption in the facilities providing those resources.

Disaster and Mass Casualty Types

Open

An open disaster occurs over a large geographic area and presents many patient management issues. These events are usually natural in origin, and they can include earthquakes, hurricanes, and tornados. Because the incident covers a large area, the control of patient flow and their disposition becomes more difficult. The disaster may be ongoing for several days, and it may require EMS managers to consider seriously resource allocation and mutual-aid assistance. The incident management system (IMS) is essential for effective management and mitigation. The incident must be broken down into workable response units that may be dictated by the numerous simultaneous events occurring at different locations. The incident and medical commanders need to avoid focusing on particular areas and must strive to visualize the total picture.

Closed

A closed disaster occurs within a small or confined area. These disasters tend to be technologic, and they occur with little or no warning, usually in urban areas. They include building collapses, chemical explosions, and transportation accidents. The resources deployed for the management of these incidents are more concentrated. Management may be difficult because the patient load is primarily located in a small area, and it overwhelms the first responder units. Overcrowding of response units and traffic gridlock often are problems with these events. Hospitals located in prox-

imity to the incident tend receive a sudden surge of patients, often without warning (the geographic effect). The infrastructure of a city usually remains intact, and resources are available to respond to the incident. At times, the number of resources available can present a management problem; this has been called the second disaster (2).

Finite

A finite disaster has a beginning and a defined end point that is measurable. A hurricane will eventually leave the affected area. A tornado strike will be over within a few minutes. In "normal" aircraft crashes, no further aircraft will follow the aircraft that just crashed. The fact that the causative agent is now gone makes planning and management of the incident easier. A finite number of injuries will have occurred, and further injuries will be minimal. Local health care institutions will receive the vast majority of the patients within 2 hours of the incident. Following the initial patient influx, patient flow will slow to a trickle. The damage and injuries from a finite disaster may be extensive, but the causative process has stopped; efforts may be concentrated on rescue and recovery.

Ongoing

An ongoing disaster may have a sudden start, but the forces or factors that have overwhelmed the available resources may continue to do so for an extended time. The initial events may also be rather insidious and difficult to recognize until the situation gets bad enough to warrant attention. By then, responders may find that they are behind, and they may have to expend resources to catch up. Examples of ongoing disasters include a pandemic of an infectious respiratory virus, floods, sustained armed conflicts, and complex humanitarian emergencies. Initial efforts must be focused on limiting or eliminating causative factors as quickly as possible, and they may require resource allocation to that end. Planning is extremely difficult because no clear end is in sight and the situation may keep deteriorating. This planning for mitigation will require long-range vision. Resource requirements will exceed those for a finite event due to the need for commitment to the elimination of the causative factors. Affected patient populations will continue to grow, and they may overwhelm a system that is quite capable of handling a single finite event. Resources may become scarce enough to require decisions on allocation that may prove difficult to make. Intensive care unit beds and ventilators may become scarce, thus requiring hospital committees to set qualification criteria for patients who are critically ill and in need of ventilatory support. Communities become dependent on outside aid as local resources become saturated or depleted.

Terrorism

The addition of terrorism to the disaster equation raises several unique issues responders must navigate while handling a disaster. A terrorist's goal is to create mass casualties, to strike fear into the general population, and to make the responding agencies appear powerless to stop them. Additionally, a terrorism incident may involve a weapon of mass destruction (e.g., a nuclear, chemical, or biologic agent). All terrorism events are crime scenes, and care must be taken to preserve evidence while triaging and treating patients (11). Chemical or biologic agents may still be on patients, and mass decontamination may be required before most treatment and transport can begin. The presence of secondary devices will always be a possibility (11,13). Psychologic stress will create additional casualties who will add to the already burdensome number of patients. Biologic attacks may require the health care system to engage in mass prophylaxis and immunization. Medical resources may become so scarce or so controlled that the population seeking medical attention will threaten the medical providers. The basic tenets of disaster response for EMS are sound even during a terrorist event. However, additional training and resources are needed to meet the unique challenges associated with potential terrorist actions (13).

PREHOSPITAL MASS CASUALTY PLANNING AND TRAINING

Principles Behind Planning and Training

Thorough planning coupled with realistic and effective training has proved to be one of the strongest factors in the successful response to a disaster. Without these, personnel do the best they can in a disjointed helter-skelter manner. All the patients will eventually be transported and treated despite the level of training, but the response will not result in the best care for the victims. Planning and training should focus around several basic principles as follows:

- When personnel are stressed and overwhelmed, they will fall back on prior training and experience. Equipment and protocols will be used only if they are commonly used during day-to-day operations. In other words, "you play as you practice."
- Most patients will arrive at local hospitals within 2 hours of the event, either with or without EMS assistance.
- If medics are not trained in incident command and mass casualty management, they will not think of setting up the early structures vital to the successful organization of an incident.
- An influx of outlying transport units and a spontaneous civilian medical response will occur.
- A paper plan that sits on a shelf without being exercised is worthless.

The military learned long ago that, for personnel to function effectively in combat, they had to be trained to a very high level so that actions would become second nature in times of stress. Fortunately, combat action does not occur

with regularity. Training, therefore, becomes necessary to bridge the time gap and to keep personnel sharp. The same concept holds true for disaster management. Mass casualty incidents or disasters are rare events that are stressful, and they require a high degree of competence to manage them successfully. EMS organizations, as well as the health care community as a whole, need to plan and to train to react to such events.

The planning process should incorporate disaster management skills and operational procedures into everyday operations as much as possible (daily doctrine). Although the unique nature of a disaster will not allow this to be done completely, every effort should be made. One EMS commander used a legal pad when handling incidents on a day-to-day basis. When faced with a mass casualty incident, despite the management forms that were available, he resorted to what was familiar to him—a yellow legal pad. Paramedics not familiar with triage tags will be less likely to use them in a mass casualty incident. One EMS system organized "triage Tuesday," a day when all EMS units used disaster triage tags on routine runs to increase EMS and hospital familiarity with their use (see Chapter 2).

The real challenge of handling a disaster is time. Experience has shown that patients will get to hospitals within 2 hours of an incident unless they are trapped or geographically isolated (11). Any plans that call for an elaborate system that takes hours to establish will not effectively serve the needs of the vast majority of patients.

Almost every mass casualty incident stimulates a spontaneous and unrequested response of other EMS agencies. The Oklahoma City bombing resulted in an overwhelming volunteer medical response (1,6). When unmanaged, these spontaneous responders can actually prove to be an impediment to the operation. Plans need to include provisions for managing these extra resources so that they become an asset instead of a liability.

Training Methods

Training programs should focus on getting the most benefit out of the resources committed to any exercise (see Chapter 37). Each tabletop or field drill should have a clear objective of what is to be tested and taught. Too often, exercises are performed to meet a requirement set by a jurisdiction, and a minimal number of personnel are used. The tertiary players (e.g., hospital staff and support personnel) that are so vital in a real event are rarely mobilized. Occasionally, a wild and unlikely scenario will be presented (e.g., incident commander has a heart attack after the tornado strikes the earthquake damage area), and the limited resources are overwhelmed. Players then go through the motions or throw their hands up in the air in frustration. Exercises should practice the plan, not just the chaos associated with the disaster. If a full-scale exercise is planned, then it should be just that—full-scale. All the involved agencies and hospitals should be included. Enough "real" victims should be moulaged and coached to provide actual stress to the paramedics in the field and the receiving hospitals. Several hours should be planned for the drill. The scenario should be simple and forthright without technical glitches to confuse the players further.

If agencies are not willing to commit resources to a full-scale practical exercise, then a "tabletop" should be used. A "tabletop" requires far less commitment of personnel and resources, yet it can still give the players a sense of the challenges presented by the scenario (14).

A predesignated time and location for a debriefing should be arranged after the exercise, and *all* the agencies involved should be invited. The objectives of the drill and the results should be discussed with input from all parties concerned. Operational solutions to the encountered difficulties should be discussed. Once the debriefing is completed, the planners and players should return to their respective agencies and should *implement* the operational changes discussed. Too often, the drill ends and everyone meets for a 5-minute pep talk on how well it went. Then everyone returns home, and nothing is changed.

TOOLS OF THE TRADE

EMS agencies carry a variety of items to assist in organizing and processing the patients encountered during a disaster. These tools can be quite helpful, but they work only if the user is familiar and comfortable with them. Such equipment needs to be immediately accessible, or the responders will carry on without it, thus rendering lost whatever benefit it may have offered.

Triage tags. The one item carried by most, if not all, EMS agencies. These tags are designed to designate the patient's condition and to allow those providing treatment and transport to record what has been done. They should be unique for each community's needs, and they should be practiced with often.

Triage ribbons. Sections or rolls of colored surveyor's tape that can be tied around a patient's ankle to designate the triage category of the patient. They are inexpensive and easy to use. They do have the downside of not having specific treatment information recorded on them, but they can be effective for the initial triage sorting at the scene and rescue level.

Triage tarps and flags. Colored tarps or flags designed to identify specific areas in the treatment or triage areas. A colored tarp provides a clear location to direct patients and/or rescuers. Colored coded flags serve the same purpose. The tarps tend to be more visible in a cleared area while the flags offer the benefit of being visible above the heads of people working in the area. Most commercially available tarps and flags are designed for use in grass or dirt. Urban systems need to make sure they have a mechanism to set them up *and secure them* on asphalt or concrete.

Triage signs. A more formal way of accomplishing the objective of identifying designated areas of triage and treatment areas. They need to be of appropriate size, visibility, and stability. The inclusion of appropriate languages should be considered.

Traffic cones. Cones are carried by some agencies to create desired traffic paths and borders for operational areas. They are costly and bulky, but they can be of great assistance in controlling the flow of personnel and patients.

Scene tape. These rolls of tape are similar to police crime scene tape. They allow one or two individuals to define the area of operation quickly and to provide some security for the boundaries. They should be set up in a double row to deter individuals from lifting them over their heads and walking through them. Scene tape use depends on having something to tie it to, but medics can use vehicles or stakes carried for that purpose. With scene tape in place, onlookers and well-intended helpers can be controlled to some degree.

Lighting. Many disasters occur during the night. Proper lighting of an area is essential. Most EMS agencies rely on other agencies to provide lighting. Waiting on this lighting from another agency may delay effective operations in the treatment and triage areas. Ambulances can be parked so their scene lights will cover the area, but this involves tying up transport resources and exposing the area to diesel fumes.

Prompt cards and organizational sheets. These preprinted sheets delineate the responsibilities for the first arriving units and subsequent command positions. They can be effective in organizing the thoughts of medics overwhelmed by the scene. Responding personnel must have immediate access to the cards, and they must be familiar with their use. The cards should be printed on weather-resistant materials.

Radios. Some agencies have dedicated radios for use whenever a large incident puts a strain on normal communications. These radios can be inexpensive ones with a short broadcast range. They are designed to give personnel operating in a particular area the ability to communicate with others operating in the same area. They should be maintained properly, and their use should be practiced with regularity.

Mass casualty kits. These preestablished tubs, boxes, or kits are designed for use during a disaster response. Located inside are many of the tools listed above, along with basic medical supplies. These kits are created for a crew, and they enable it to establish a triage and treatment site where it is located. Additionally, these supplies can be moved to a location away from the unit. Such kits, if they are located on each unit, ensure that the unit can operate independently for a short time. These are particularly useful in incidents where a large geographic area is involved. The one caution associated with such kits is the possibility that *every* unit responding to a disaster will set up an operation wherever they arrive. This may diminish the transport capability of the system.

Mass casualty response unit. A vehicle stocked with extra supplies, such as bandaging material and backboards, that is designed to respond to the treatment area may deliver its load of supplies and return for more. These vehicles are valuable in getting a large amount of needed supplies to an operational area. The downside of the units is the fact that they require a vehicle dedicated for use that can be guaranteed to respond. In addition, the vehicles and stocks require maintenance over time.

Protective equipment. Hard hats, gloves, and eye protection for EMS crews are needed for operating in a disaster area. With the advent of potential terrorist attacks, this protective equipment may include respiratory protection, as well as chemically resistant suits, gloves, and boots. Sufficient amounts of this equipment should be on each unit.

Bullhorn and/or public address system. First responders will commonly be confronted by a large group of patients and bystanders. These individuals are often confused, shocked, and looking for direction. A bullhorn will allow directions to be given to a large group of people quickly. Careful consideration should be given to any statements made to the group. Standardized statements for first responders should be developed so that scene crowds are rapidly organized according to a designated plan.

COMMUNICATIONS

The one constant factor in disaster response is the breakdown in communications (10,15). Several reasons exist for this; they include the following: the lack of radio channels, the incredible radio traffic volume, unclear communication chains, differing radios and frequencies, and the interruption or loss of communication capability from the event itself. In a disaster, EMS agencies have five primary communication functions as follows:

1. Communication with system units not responding to the incident and providing service to unaffected areas.
2. Communication with units responding to the incident.
3. Communication with mutual aid response units.
4. Communication with other agencies through the IMS.
5. Communication with hospitals and other health care facilities about patient disposition and condition.

The prospect of getting all this done at the same time under stressful circumstances can prove daunting. Most EMS systems in large metropolitan areas have access to multiple radio frequencies. Smaller systems may only have one or two frequencies. Some systems operate with one frequency for dispatch, and they make hospital notifications via cellular telephone. Cellular systems are often disrupted or overwhelmed during a disaster making this mode of communication highly vulnerable to failure (see Chapter 8).

The most common approach, when frequencies are available, is to put units responding to a disaster on a separate channel from those responding to other calls. Each frequency should have its own dispatcher dedicated to controlling the traffic. Medical command may channel all the incident traffic through the command position and may then relay it to the communications dispatcher, or the dispatcher may be the funnel through which all communications flow. This process must be established through the planning process before the incident occurs.

Communication with mutual aid units is difficult because most EMS systems do not have a "mutual aid" frequency that is routinely used. If one exists, it can be used to direct units to staging areas. Mutual aid units are dependent on radio traffic with their own communications centers, which, in turn, relay the information gathered by telephone. Eventually, these units are out of radio range, out of information, and out of the direct control of medical command. Mutual aid units should be directed to a specified staging area where they receive explicit instructions. If assigned to transport, they should report back to a specified staging location following transport. Some units responding from outside may "shop around" for the most damage. Additionally, units will show up spontaneously without being asked. Mutual aid units must be identified and controlled. Planners should identify ways of regulating and communicating with such units during a disaster.

Medical command needs to be a conduit of information for the IMS. The incident commander will need to know about resource needs and victim disposition. In return, medical command must be updated on the operational progress and situational changes, and it must be able to gain instant access to decision makers from all the various agencies involved in the incident. This is usually done face to face in the command post, and this has been proven over the course of many disasters to be a reliable and effective way of communicating.

The responsibility of notifying hospitals about incoming patients traditionally falls on medical command. This consistently is a difficult task, particularly when multiple sites are involved. Usually the transport officer notifies the communication center when a unit leaves the transport area en route to a hospital and apprises them of which units are going where and the number and condition of the patients. The communications center then notifies the hospital and receives feedback on the capacity and capability of the hospital. This, in turn, is relayed back to the transport officer. Large incidents, where the number and spread of patients is extensive, usually place an overwhelming load on the communications center. Most communication centers have a fixed number of positions. One position will be controlling the incident radio traffic; another will be controlling the calls to unaffected areas, while another may be controlling mutual aid units. Meanwhile, the center is literally flooded with incoming requests for information and assistance.

Multiple transport officers may be calling in from several sites. The communication center may not be able to allocate the people or time to make hospital notifications. Units may be directed to encode the destination hospital on their own. This may be difficult due to the normal encoded radio channels being used for the incident, as well as the sheer volume of radio traffic. Another option is to use an unaffected hospital as a "resource" hospital to relay patient and scene information to receiving hospitals. This takes the burden off the communications center while still providing reliability and control.

PREHOSPITAL MASS CASUALTY OPERATIONS

Planning

The most effective way to respond successfully to a mass casualty incident starts with planning and education. Once an agency has developed a plan for how to respond to such an incident, frequent, quality training must take place with *all personnel* that will be asked to respond. This training should involve *all agencies* that may interact on a large incident. The first responding agencies need to be familiar not only with their own operational areas but also with the those of the other agencies. They must be comfortable (and they should be on a first-name basis) with the personnel who will occupy the command positions in the traditional fire, police, and EMS systems, as well as with those for the other nontraditional responders (e.g., public works, utilities, and Red Cross). When one is immersed in a crisis situation, this is not the time to try to establish a working relationship with someone that he or she is meeting for the first time.

Some disasters occur with a limited amount of advanced warning. Responders may have 15 to 30 minutes before a tornado strikes a city. A hurricane may allow several days of advanced planning time. Large mass gatherings can be planned in advance for weeks or months. Even with advanced warning, one can only plan so far. No one is exactly sure where a tornado is going to strike and for how long. The exact landfall of a hurricane remains uncertain until shortly before it hits. Knowing exactly *what* will go wrong at a mass gathering is impossible. First response agencies should take advantage of every available minute of time to prepare in advance.

Operations

Medical command has the responsibility for identifying the injured and coordinating resources so that those injured can be stabilized, treated, and transported to a definitive care facility. The success of this mission will depend on the level of training, equipment, and planning by the EMS agencies involved. Traditionally, this operation has been broken down into the following functional areas: (a) command, (b) staging, (c) triage, (d) treatment, (e) transport, and (f) logistics (5,16). Each of these functional areas has specific responsibilities. Failure to perform well in one area will prove a detriment to the others as well.

Command

Medical command refers to the position within the operations section of the IMS that is responsible for all aspects of the care and transportation of victims of a disaster. The medical commander will direct the activities of all first responders, paramedics, and other health personnel assigned to patient care activities. He or she interacts with the incident commander, who oversees all operations of the disaster. This position is extremely busy and stressful for the first several hours of an incident. The medical commander will require help, and he or she should assign at least one individual to be an assistant to help keep track of the flurry of details flowing in. The medical commander needs to set up the structure of the medical response, and he or she should assign individuals to fill the various functional areas specific to patient care and transport. These individuals report to the medical commander, and a two-way conduit of information must be established to ensure that both the provider needs and the operational needs of the incident are fulfilled. The medical commander acts as the gatekeeper for this flow of information. This position is normally filled by a paramedic on the first arriving advanced life support unit on the scene; this person may, in turn, hand the position to the first arriving field supervisor. If numerous incident sites are found, each site may have a person designated as medical command for that location. He or she reports to the overall medical commander. The biggest challenge facing the medical commander is making the initial decisions that set up the medical response structure in a short time to gain whatever control is possible of a chaotic scene.

Staging

The staging officer is responsible for keeping track of arriving and returning transport resources and sending them to the appropriate requested location. Staging areas need to be identified early in a disaster. Both local and mutual aid resources should be assigned to the identified areas, and they should report to the designated staging officer. This action will allow control of the resources and will avoid too many units being sent to one scene. Medical command will request resources from the staging officer and will provide direction regarding their destination. The staging officer keeps medical command updated as to the number and type of resources available. The staging officer can also give instructions and directions to hospital locations to the

TRADITIONAL ORGANIZATIONAL SET-UP FOR MASS
MANAGEMENT

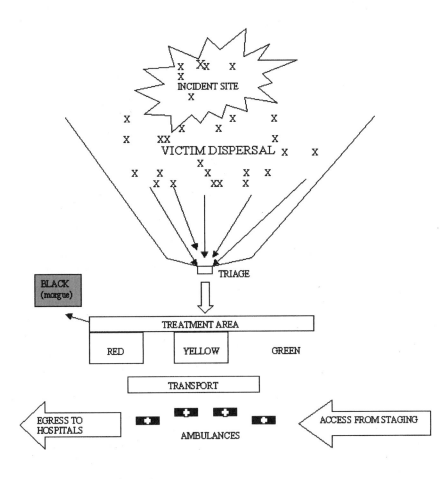

FIGURE 9.1. Traditional mass casualty management scheme.

mutual aid units. Without a clearly defined and controlled staging area, mutual aid units may respond directly to the scene(s) in which case they may not be under the control of the IMS. Medical resources from hospitals and other areas can also be sent to the staging area to be deployed as needed. The traditional method of mass casualty management is depicted in Fig. 9.1.

Triage

This position is probably the most difficult to perform, and the ablest individual should be assigned to it. One of the first requirements during a disaster is the sorting of patients by their respective medical need. This sorting will determine which patients receive treatment and transport and in what order. Although every system promotes the concept of triage, few are fully prepared or are capable of rapidly sorting a large group of patients using the system in their plans. The triage that goes on during everyday activities is quite different from the triage needed during a disaster, as Chapter 2 discusses.

Treatment

When the number of triaged patients exceeds the number of available transports, a holding area should be established and treatment of the patients should be initiated. This treatment area should be under the supervision of a clinically experienced paramedic, nurse, or physician. The treatment officer is responsible for ensuring that all patients in the area receive good quality basic care, as well as appropriate advanced care if resources allow. The level and amount of care will be dictated by the time spent in the area, the number and capability of the providers, the equipment available, and the nature of injuries present. Most patients will receive only basic C-spine immobilization, airway control, bandaging, and splinting. More advanced treatment is usually done in the transport unit, at the casualty collection point, or in the health care facility. Logistics plays a major role in making sure that adequate materials and supplies are available within the treatment area. Volunteer medical help can be used in this area if they are properly supervised. The emphasis should be on ensuring that basic care is provided and that advanced procedures are performed only when all of the basics have been covered.

Transport

The transport officer is responsible for allocating patients to units arriving to transport, tracking their movements, and notifying hospitals of their pending arrival. If access and egress to the disaster site are under control and effective staging has been established, allocating patients to units usually proceeds easily. The primary decision is often that of how many patients to assign each vehicle. That decision must be based on the available transport resources and the number of patients. Placing two immediate patients in one unit should be avoided, if possible, unless that unit has enough manpower to care for their needs. However, the number of units available and the number of critically injured patients may dictate transporting two at a time. Other resources for transportation should be considered as well. Busses and vans can carry the walking wounded to a distant hospital. Depending on the resources available, patients may be transported via private vehicle, but medical personnel should accompany the patient while en route whenever possible. Consideration should be given to keeping families and loved ones together.

The hospital destination will depend on the scene location, the number of triage and transport areas involved in the incident, the response structure established, and the capability of the destination hospitals. The scene may involve a compromised hospital, or the roads to a treatment facility may be impassable for a time. The structure of the response may include the establishment of casualty collection points or field hospitals, which will offer more options for the transport officer. Lastly, hospitals may be compromised or overwhelmed, and thus they may not be able to take patients.

Tracking patient movement usually does not occur in the early chaos surrounding a disaster. Initial responding units often load patients and transport them before any tracking structure has been established. Some commercial triage tags have tear-off corners for the transport officer to use to track patients, but these are difficult to keep hold of during the initial confusion. Some newer triage tags have a barcode sticker system designed to assist in tracking patients. Other services use preprinted transport charts and assign one individual the responsibility of keeping the charts up to date.

Hospital notification can be accomplished in a number of ways. The most common practice is the use of radios at the scene to notify each hospital when a transport leaves or the relay of notification through the communications center. Other systems depend upon cellular telephone notification. Several problems with these methods exist. Establishing radio contact with a hospital takes time, and several hospitals may have different frequencies. An EMS system may be limited in the number of available radio frequencies. Cellular telephones will usually be inoperable for a period of time following the disaster. The EMS communications center will be flooded with calls, and they may not be able to make notifications. Using a resource hospital may be an effective way of distributing transport information. The transport officer establishes communication with an unaffected hospital by whatever means is available. That hospital receives the information and in turn relays it to the appropriate hospital. This system is dependent on the cooperation of the hospital and on the establishment of reliable communication links between the hospitals. These should be clearly established *before* any incident if a resource hospital is to be used.

Logistics

An important support function for the medical command is the logistics officer. He or she is responsible for ensuring that the equipment and materials needed by triage, treatment, and transport are available. The logistics officer must think for both the long term and the short term and must make plans for anticipated, as well as actual, needs.

Supplies are one of the most important commodities during a disaster response. One must resist the temptation to send large quantities of supplies to a disaster site without proper coordination. In the Oklahoma City bombing disaster, an estimated $3 million of medical supplies were wasted because hospitals sent supplies to the disaster site (1). Hospitals should refrain from sending supplies to the disaster site unless they are specifically requested by the incident or medical commander.

A push-pull concept should be developed by EMS logistics for supply during a disaster response. The pull concept requires field units to order supplies as needed during a disaster response. This system of resupply has the disadvantage of being slow and of requiring intact communications for requesting supplies. The push concept has the advantage of making available only the supplies that are planned for in advance. The push concept places preplanned supplies at specific locations at the disaster scene. These supply packets may be brought forward to the triage or casualty collection points, or they may be distributed at predetermined locations throughout the city. In other words, push puts supplies forward for easier pull.

OTHER ASPECTS OF DISASTER RESPONSE
Spontaneous Response of Medical Personnel

EMS providers responding to the Murrah Building Incident in Oklahoma City encountered an interesting phenomenon. The incident occurred downtown, close to several medical centers. A large number of health care providers showed up early during the incident and continued to respond for several days afterward. While this assistance was welcome during the initial minutes of the response, it quickly became a management problem that occupied a large segment of the medical command's time and attention. EMS systems in urban areas need to anticipate the potential problems of such a large volunteer medical response, and they should plan accordingly.

Patient Self-Referral

In some mass casualty incidents, up to 80% of the injured patients will seek medical care themselves; they thus will not be encountered by the EMS responders. Many think that the ambulances are needed for more serious patients, some are just independent, and others do not want to wait for help to arrive. They tend to go to the closest facility, and this can place a significant burden on the emergency departments. Thus, the majority of the injured in a disaster situation do not get processed and directed by the responding EMS units. This occurs through no fault of the system or its performance—it is just a matter of numbers and human behavior. The percentage will vary according to the type of disaster. A plane crash at the end of a runway will have few, if any, self-referring patients. An incident located in an urban area or spread over a large geographic area will have a large percentage of patients transporting themselves in either their own vehicles or in some willing civilian's vehicle.

To control better the patient flow from the field to the receiving health care facilities, planners must anticipate the self-referring patient population. While controlling all of patients is impossible, some methods do help direct these patients to outlying facilities. The media can play a major role in advising these patients to seek assistance, if their injuries are minor, at hospitals farther from the incident. Officers and National Guardsman manning perimeter blockades can direct patients to outlying hospitals when the vehicles pass through the perimeter. The key is for medical command to decide where those patients need to go and to relay that information to the media and the perimeter checkpoints. A significant number of patients with minor injuries will comply.

Ambulance Transport Destinations

Within the hospital community, by either a formal written agreement or a tacit understanding, the ambulances will transport to hospitals farther away from an incident exists. This is true because of the understanding that the closest hospitals will receive a flood of self-referring patients due to the geographic effect. In reality, ambulances tend to transport to the closest destinations, particularly in the first minutes of an incident. Ambulances will add to the geographic effect by transporting victims to the closest facility for seven primary reasons as follows:

1. The crews know that more patients exists than ambulances, and they want to get back to the scene as soon as possible. The transport resources are stretched, and longer transports mean units out of service for longer periods of time.
2. Once a unit transports to a distant hospital and goes back in service, it may not be sent back to the incident, but instead it may be directed to provide system coverage.
3. Paramedics are trained to take a seriously injured patient to the closest appropriate facility. The patients transported by ambulances usually have more serious injuries, and they often are in critical condition. The paramedic does not think the patient can survive a longer transport.
4. Ambulance crews transport to one hospital, and they see that the hospital is geared up and ready to receive patients. The crew then returns and transports as many patients as possible to that one facility.
5. Roads may be impassable due to debris, downed lines, or land changes. Once a route has been established to the hospital, the crew will take the sure way instead of getting stuck trying to reach an outlying hospital.
6. Directing a mutual aid transport unit to a closer facility may be easier then risking the unit getting lost trying to make it to an outlying hospital
7. Hospitals do not want to go on a divert or reroute status during a disaster for a multitude of reasons. As long as the hospital states that it can take more patients, then the transport officer is likely to send more, even if that hospital is genuinely overwhelmed.

The impact of EMS on the geographic effect may be diminished by an evaluation of the seven reasons and subsequently taking measures to decrease their validity where this is possible.

Casualty Collection Points

One method to assist in distributing the patient flow is to establish casualty collection points relatively close to the impacted areas. These areas may be staffed by medical personnel, and they offer immediate care and intervention to victims of the disaster. Units will have a short transport time when bringing patients from the field to the casualty collection points, and they can then return for more patients. A more disciplined distribution of patients can be accomplished from the casualty collection point. The spontaneous medical staff response can be referred to these points to offer assistance and to stage for situations where they may be needed. Medical teams needed out in the field can be coordinated from these points. The critical interventions performed may allow a safer and longer transport to a definitive care facility. Self-referring patients may be sent to the casualty collection points, where they can be treated and released without requiring an emergency department visit. During a weapons of mass destruction event or an industrial disaster with contaminated patients, the casualty collection point may act as a buffer to prevent contaminated

CASUALTY COLLECTION POINTS

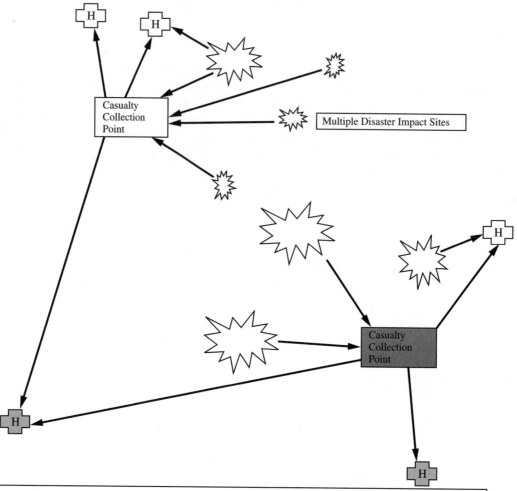

In disasters that cover a large area and involve multiple impact sites (i.e. earthquake, tornado, hurricane, terrorist attack), it may be advantageous to establish patient treatment/collection areas closer to the scenes and. initially, to transport or refer patients there. This organization offers several advantages: 1) Critical interventions can be done sooner. 2) Self-responding medical personnel can be sent there and relieve scene confusion. 3) If needed, scene medical response teams can be formulated, controlled and dispatched. 4) Patient disposition to definitive care can be efficiently coordinated. 5) Patients needing decontamination can be controlled and decontaminated prior to arriving at a hospital. 6) The CCP will be far less susceptible to a secondary device attack in a terrorist event.

FIGURE 9.2. Casualty collection points.

patients from reaching the hospitals. The location of a casualty collection point is often spontaneous, and thus it may offer some protection from a terrorist-planned secondary explosive device.

Using a casualty collection point means that the patients will be transported twice before they reach a hospital and that more transport units will eventually be required. The casualty collection point will need to be identified and staffed early to be effective. The site should be equipped from a predesignated cache of equipment and not by donations from various hospitals that may not release the equipment for use. The equipment and staff need to be transported to the site of the

casualty collection point, which places a further drain on the logistics sector of the command. Casualty collection points may be difficult to organize, support, and manage if they are not provided for early and if they are not practiced as part the overall disaster plan. Casualty collection point organization is depicted in Fig. 9.2.

MEDICAL EMERGENCY RESPONSE CENTER

One of the problems facing the medical community when it is confronted with a mass casualty incident is the separa-

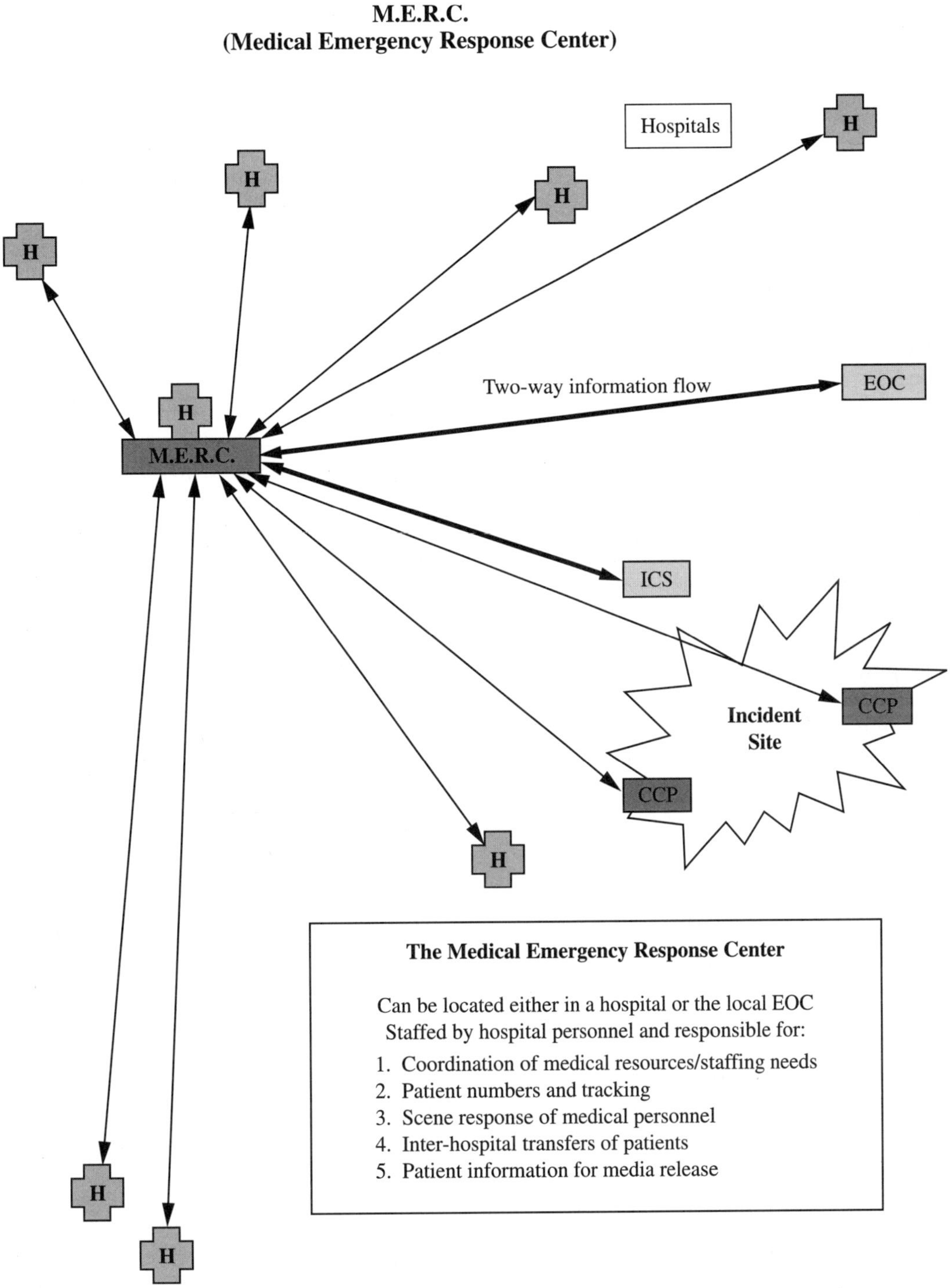

M.E.R.C.
(Medical Emergency Response Center)

FIGURE 9.3. The medical emergency response center.

tion of the hospitals and the response elements at the scene. The bridge between these two entities is often the EMS system, of whom much is expected during a disaster. Hospitals want to know what is going on at the scene, how many more patients may arrive, and how seriously they are injured. The EMS system can provide some of this intelli-

gence, but usually it is busy briefing the IMS. The hospitals never seem to get enough information.

Most hospitals do not traditionally communicate among themselves during a disaster. Hospitals have grown more competitive in recent years, and they are often reluctant to share bed counts, resources, and staff availability. When a disaster occurs, the hospitals have a great need to communicate among themselves, yet, frequently, no mechanism exists for accomplishing that. During the Oklahoma City bombing, hospitals did not communicate with each other. During tropical storm Allison in Houston, hospitals communicated with other hospitals within their own system, but they did not initially coordinate with the hospital across the street. New York's hospital communications collapsed with the destruction of EOC in the World Trade Center.

The medical emergency response center (MERC) concept provides a clearinghouse for information to the medical community through which information from the scene may be distributed to all the hospitals. Hospitals may keep a running update on the amount of beds and resources available. Staff from unaffected hospitals may be precredentialed and sent to assist an overtaxed facility. Other allied facilities can be incorporated into the patient disposition flow. The MERC may accommodate a two-way flow of information between the field and the health care community. This is crucial in the event of a biologic attack or a naturally occurring pandemic. Each community can decide exactly how to establish its own resource center. The important issue is to have one established before a disaster occurs.

Several communities have already responded to the need for interhospital communications. The Washington, D.C. Hospital Association has a mutual aid and communication memorandum of understanding with all the hospitals within the organization. Oklahoma City, Tulsa, and northern Virginia have established MERCs or clearinghouse hospitals. Other cities, such as Dallas/Ft. Worth and Phoenix, are actively organizing ways for the local hospitals to communicate.

The MERC can be located in either the city's emergency operations center, or it can be situated within a particular hospital. The hospital community needs to exercise the MERC on a frequent basis until clear operation roles and responsibilities can be established. Having this communication and decision-making network in place and functioning will allow hospitals to mitigate the medical consequences of a disaster better. The functional diagram of a MERC is depicted in Fig. 9.3.

AFTER THE INCIDENT

The EMS system's major role in a disaster response will begin to tail off after several hours once the patients have all arrived at a definitive care facility. The units still dedicated to the incident will go from a primary response and transport mode into a back-up or standby mode while awaiting any additional trickle of patients, and they will provide EMS support for ongoing rescue and recovery operations. The medical commander still has many details to address at this point. Mutual aid units need to be released back to

their own service areas. Those service areas need to be notified that the resources are being sent back. The medical system needs to be informed that the patient care aspect has slowed down so that they can release some of their resources that are standing by. Crews need to be debriefed, and the critical incident stress management counselors need to be available. Plans need to be made for the next 10 hours and the next several days. Equipment needs to be retrieved, and patient care forms must be filled out to the best degree possible. A formal operational debriefing should be scheduled for some time in the near future. Except for the units dedicated to the incident standby mode, all other units should be placed back in service and attempts should be made to bring the system back to a predisaster state.

The EMS system's responsibility does not end when units go into a standby mode. A segment of the population may have been displaced by the disaster. A large shelter-dependent population may exist. The EMS commander must make sure that the special needs of this population have been addressed.

SPECIAL NEEDS POPULATION

The EMS system must be aware of the needs of the population base under 5 years and over 55 years of age. These two age groups have special needs when faced with a disaster (17,18). The elderly in particular often have a difficult time adjusting to life after being displaced to a shelter. They may do well initially, but the lack of diet, hydration, and security may lead to medical problems. Numerous elderly patients lead a tenuous existence at home that is dependent on electricity, oxygen, and home health and meal visits. If the area is disrupted by a hurricane, earthquake, or ice storm, these resources may not be available to the house. The elderly patient may have to be evacuated to a shelter where care is provided. Most shelters do not plan to provide medical care. The EMS system should identify these high-risk individuals within the community whenever possible, and it should make sure their medical and personal care needs are being met.

SUMMARY

Emergency medical services are a key part of the response to a disaster, but they do not function in a vacuum. EMS operations are generally organized via the IMS, and they must be integrated into the overall community disaster response. An understanding of the organizational structure and function of the parts of the IMS is crucial to a good disaster response by the EMS. Reasonable education and training of EMS personnel for disaster response will improve the quality of the response. New challenges in the types and frequency of disasters in recent years make the preparation and performance of the EMS systems more critical because of the lives entrusted to them.

REFERENCES

1. Hogan DE. *The Oklahoma City terrorist blast: a case study in disaster. Environment of care.* Oak Brook Terrace, IL: Joint Commission on Hospital Accreditation Publications, 1997:3–17.
2. Quarentelli EL. *Delivery of emergency medical services in disasters: assumptions and realities.* New York: Irvington, 1983.
3. Tierney KJ, Taylor VA. EMS delivery in mass emergencies: preliminary research findings. *Mass Emerg* 1977;2:151.
4. Leonard RB. Planning EMS disaster response. In: Roush WR, ed. *Principles of EMS systems*, 2nd ed. Dallas: American College of Emergency Physicians 1994:203–226.
5. Irwin RL. The incident command system (ICS). In: Auf Der Heide E, ed. *Disaster response: principles of preparation and coordination.* St. Louis: Mosby, 1989:133–163.
6. Nordberg M. The big one. *Emerg Med Serv* 1995;24:58–66, 84–86.
7. Maningas PA, Robison M, Mallonee S. The EMS response to the Oklahoma City bombing. *Prehospital Disaster Med* 1997;12:80–85.
8. Richards CF, Burstein JL, Waeckerle JF, et al. Emergency physicians and biological terrorism. *Ann Emerg Med* 1999;34:183–190.
9. Brennan RJ, Waeckerle JF, Sharp TW, et al. Chemical warfare agents: emergency medical and emergency public health issues. *Ann Emerg Med* 1999;34:191–204.
10. Waeckerle JF. Disaster planning and response. *N Engl J Med* 1991;324:815.
11. Hogan DE, Waeckerle JF, Dire DJ, et al. Emergency department impact of the Oklahoma City terrorist bombing. *Ann Emerg Med* 1999;34:160–167.
12. Waeckerle JF. The skywalk collapse: a personal response. *Ann Emerg Med* 1983;12:651.
13. Eckstein M. The medical response to modern terrorism: why the "rules of engagement" have changed. *Ann Emerg Med* 1999;34:219–221.
14. Hogan DE, Kallas L. Education in disaster medicine. In: Aghababian R. *Emergency medicine: the core curriculum.* Philadelphia: Lippincott-Raven, 1998:1381–1385.
15. Garshnek V, Burkle FM Jr. Telecommunications systems in support of disaster medicine: applications of basic information pathways. *Ann Emerg Med* 1999;34:213–218.
16. Christen HT, Maniscalco PM. *The EMS incident management system: EMS operations for mass casualty and high impact incidents.* Jersey City, NJ: Prentice Hall, 1998:1–15.
17. McIntire MS, Sadeghi E. The pediatrician and mental health in a community wide disaster: lessons from the aftermath of a tornado. *Clin Pediatr* 1977;16:702–705.
18. Bolin R, Klenow DJ. Older people in disaster: comparison of black and white victims. *Int J Aging Hum Dev* 1988;26:29–43.

MUNICIPAL AND EMERGENCY HEALTH CARE PLANNING IN DISASTERS

ADEN HOGAN, JR.

Most municipal disaster planning agencies are familiar with emergency medical services (EMS) and its function within the local disaster response plan. These planners may not, however, be aware that the medical response to a disaster spans a wide array of other emergency health care providers who should be represented in the disaster response planning process. Emergency health care (EHC) providers incorporate a spectrum of EMS, emergency medicine, trauma, and public health responders providing immediate assessment and care to victims of a disaster. For the EHC community to be successful in a disaster response, they must be able to interface effectively with the local governmental jurisdiction and its emergency operations plan (EOP). Key to this interface is an understanding of how local government operates both during an emergency and in their day-to-day activities. This understanding can greatly improve the speed and quality of the EHC disaster response. Having medical input at the local level is also important in the initial disaster planning, as it leads to a better integration of EMS and other EHC elements into the community's emergency response to disasters (1).

Involvement in planning may seem difficult at first because local governments often appear too bureaucratic to EHC providers. However, both the local government and the EHC community exist to preserve the health, safety, and welfare of the citizens. Therefore, close coordination and cooperation between local government and the EHC community is not just a convenience, *it is a necessity*. At stake are the lives of the people in the community who will be affected by the disaster.

This chapter is intended to provide the EHC professional with a basic understanding of how local government is structured and how it operates. The intent is to prepare EHC personnel for working with these municipal agencies to enhance their emergency response.

STRUCTURE, ORGANIZATION, AND OPERATIONS OF LOCAL GOVERNMENT

Several types of governmental structures exist in the United States today, fulfilling a variety of community governmental functions. Obviously, the federal government and the 50 state governments have the largest geographic scope and range of services. However, local governments, such as cities, towns, villages, boroughs, counties, and townships, are closest physically to the citizens. Therefore, as might be expected, these units of government provide most of the basic services people expect to use on a daily basis. Some of the more common services might include trash collection services, police and fire protection, street maintenance, parks, recreation, or water treatment. Complicating a clear-cut definition of local government for EHC is the proliferation of special districts throughout the United States. These districts provide a myriad of services, including schools, infrastructure, water, sanitation, parks, recreation, and irrigation.

Special districts have their own governing board, which is made up of people elected from the district's service area. These boards are quite often separate and autonomous from the city and county within which their district lies. Some areas in the United States may have more than 90 separate taxing entities overlying a single location. Meaningful, effective EHC coordination for a disaster response with this many agencies and their various officials is nearly impossible. Fortunately, however, the county and municipal (city) levels are those with which EHC providers will most likely need to interface for disaster planning and response.

Unlike the federal and state governments, which are governed by executive, legislative, and judicial branches, most cities and counties simply have elected officials and appointed officials. Elected officials, such as city council members, county commissioners, sheriffs, and others serve at the pleasure of the voters of each jurisdiction. Appointed officials, such as city managers, county administrators, and executive directors of special districts, serve at the discretion of the entity's elected officials. The next level of key officials will generally be operational department directors, such as the police chief, fire chief, finance director, and emergency manager. Local government agencies are often much less bureaucratic than the state or federal agencies; one is more likely to work directly with the senior officials at the municipal or county level than at the state or federal level.

In local government, elected officials are responsible for setting the organization's policies and mission. They normally do not play a major operational role in disaster response. The responsibility of city and county managers, police chiefs, fire chiefs, public works directors, and other operational managers is to carry out the elected officials' policy directives in the form of operations and programs. The degree of participation by elected officials in an emergency response will vary depending on the structural form used by that entity.

City Governmental Structures

The most common form of local government used in cities is the council–manager form, which is shown in Fig. 10.1. In this form, a city manager or administrator is hired to serve as the entity's chief administrative officer, and this official is responsible for the day-to-day operation of orga-nization. The manager conducts operations through department heads, such as the police chief, public works director, fire chief, and others. The manager also works with the elected officials on policy analysis, research, and setting goals and objectives. In the council–manager form, EMS and other emergency health care providers will likely deal with the manager or one of his or her department directors during disaster planning and emergency response.

Other common forms of municipal government are the strong mayor form (Fig. 10.2), in which the elected mayor is both the chief executive officer and the chief administrative officer, and the commissioner form (Fig. 10.3), in which individual elected officials assume administrative authority over specific areas, such as public safety, utilities, and streets. In these two forms of local government, direct involvement by the mayor or other elected officials in the disaster response is much more likely.

The form of local government is determined by either the state statutes or the incorporation charter of the municipality. Size has no bearing on the form of government used. Cities such as Chicago, New York City, Cincinnati, and Denver use the strong mayor form, while other large communities such as San Diego, Oakland, Dallas, and Oklahoma City use the council–manager form. Although the council–manager is the prevalent form, a mix of methods are found in both large and small communities. Understanding the form of government in use is the first step in understanding how best to interface emergency health care into the community's emergency operations planning.

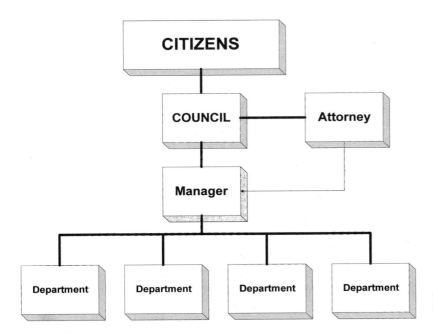

FIGURE 10.1. The council–manager municipal government format.

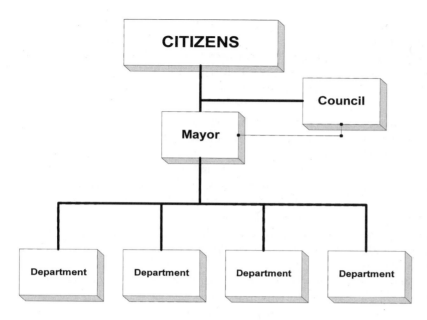

FIGURE 10.2. The strong mayor municipal government format.

County Government

County government is somewhat different from municipal government in that its elected officials have more day-to-day involvement in operations. Normally, from three to five elected commissioners serve as county government's main policymakers. In this structure, the board of county commissioners has both significant policy-making and administrative powers. In the past 15 to 20 years, some counties have also hired professional managers. These managers often have less direct power over operations than their counter-

parts in municipal government due to the high level of involvement of elected county officials. County governments further differ from the vast majority of cities in that some department heads such as the county clerk, sheriff, and coroner may also be elected officials. The county sheriff will most likely be the incident commander for any county disaster and should be one of the primary contacts. One must keep in mind the fact that the sheriff is an elected, not appointed, official. Understanding the true power structure in county government may be challenging, and it can be difficult to accomplish.

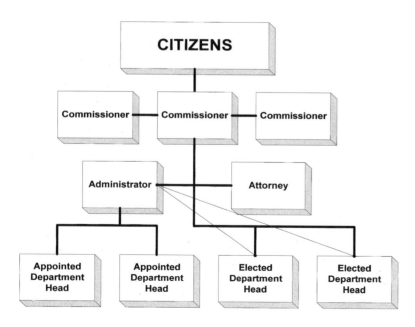

FIGURE 10.3. The commissioner format of municipal government.

THE IMPORTANCE OF EMERGENCY HEALTH CARE INTERACTION IN GOVERNMENT

Regardless of the local government's structure, EHC providers will have to work cooperatively through the entity's lead operational managers to plan and coordinate activities both before and during a disaster response. In emergency situations, the local jurisdiction's fire chief, police chief, or sheriff most commonly will assume the lead role as incident commander. This person will be responsible for coordinating activities for emergency response, rescue, and recovery. Many smaller communities do not have a high level of expertise in the EMS or other EHC functions. The ultimate success of any disaster medical response will largely be determined by how involved EHC providers have been in the local community's emergency planning process. The earlier EMS and other EHC providers become key players in local emergency planning, the greater the likelihood is that the medical response will be timely, coordinated, and well managed. If ten rules for success in disaster management were given, the first eight would relate to planning. This is, quite simply, the foundation of a quality emergency response. Contrary to the old saying, "Nothing happens without a plan," something *does* happen without a plan, and it will likely be what one *does not* want to occur. Early involvement in the local emergency planning process and frequent testing of the plan through exercises, drills, and tabletop evaluations are critical components to successful performance during the actual disaster response (see Chapter 37) (2).

EMERGENCY HEALTH CARE AND LOCAL EMERGENCY RESPONSE

In the past, local governments have used almost as many methods of managing an emergency response as they have structural forms of government. Cities with strong mayor forms have responded somewhat differently than do those with council manager forms. County governments may also react slightly differently than municipal governments in the way they choose to manage an emergency situation. Most local governments do not have the resources to respond to a large-scale emergency or a mass-casualty disaster on their own, and they will require assistance from other agencies. The size of the entity and a lack of funds for maintaining people and equipment that will only be used in a large-scale event contribute to this problem. Most local governments use intergovernmental agreements (IGAs) with neighboring entities to help insure that adequate people and equipment are available in emergency situations (1). The IGA documents things such as liability, reporting protocols, risk assumption, and other sorts of operational and financial details necessary to facilitate resource sharing.

In recent years, the nation has seen the myriad of disasters that can befall a community. The terrorist bombings of the World Trade Center in New York City and the A.P. Murrah Federal Building in Oklahoma City; the shootings at Columbine High School in Jefferson County, Colorado; the floods in North and South Dakota; the hurricanes in Florida; the earthquakes and fires in California; and many other civil, natural, and technologic disasters are comprised in this litany. All these events, as well as the terrorist attack on September 11, 2001, have demonstrated the need for close intergovernmental and interagency cooperation in mounting an effective emergency response at the local level. IGAs are good tools for the local jurisdiction and EMS because they help assure that needed assets that could never be maintained by the entity on its own are available during an emergency response. Depending on local situations, EMS and other EHC elements may want to be tied to a local community through an IGA or similar agreement. These agreements can be very simple and straightforward. The key to a good IGA is having it in place before it is needed.

THE INCIDENT COMMAND SYSTEM FROM A MUNICIPAL PLANNING VIEWPOINT

As has been noted, each community may use a slightly different approach to emergency planning and response. EHC coordination can sometimes be complicated by these differences. Recently, however, more and more local governments are using the incident command system (ICS) to organize and manage their emergency response. ICS is designed to help to organize and allocate people, to activate services, and to provide resources during an emergency response. ICS provides an organizational structure that can be used in virtually any emergency response. It provides the framework for quickly responding to the dynamics of an emergency or major disaster, and it allows the emergency response to be managed effectively. ICS was once largely limited to use by the fire service and the military. Only in the past 10 years or so have law enforcement and emergency management agencies started using ICS.

ICS was founded in the field at the scene of the emergency. Its use has evolved slowly over the past three decades due, in part, to the system's complex nature. The difficulty was creating a mirror image of the field ICS in the municipal emergency operations center (EOC). Recently, new emergency management concepts have brought ICS into the EOC to coordinate the emergency response better. One must still remember that ICS is not a simple system. It is designed to manage chaos, and, as such, it is a difficult technique to master. This simply means that a greater emphasis needs to be placed on education and training for using the ICS. Today, more and more police, fire, public works departments; emergency managers; and other key emergency planners and responders are working together to incorporate ICS as their management tool of choice.

ICS is promoted by national organizations, such as the Federal Emergency Management Agency (FEMA), the National Fire Academy, and National Wildfire Coordinating Group, as a compatible system for emergency incident management. ICS training is available through a variety of agencies. Check with the local county emergency manager or fire chief for training resources.

Using the Incident Command System

The key to ICS as an effective emergency management tool is its flexibility. It can be modified to fit each jurisdiction's specific needs without losing its compatibility with other entities that may be involved in emergency response. It is also effective regardless of the size of the incident. The Oklahoma City Fire Department, for example, routinely uses ICS in nearly every response. In most cases, the event is very small, and the system is never expanded beyond the initial responding fire unit. However, ICS easily expands to match the ever-changing scope of an emergency. It is also just as easily collapsed as the incident winds down. By using ICS on a daily basis, emergency response agencies become familiar with its application. Once everyone is comfortable with using ICS, applying it in its larger scope to deal with a major emergency becomes simple.

No disaster or emergency is ever the same. Therefore, logically, no one management approach can adequately deal with every situation. The real functionality of ICS comes from its flexible nature. The ICS structure can be scaled up or down to match the nature of the emergency. Tasks and responsibilities can be added or created to deal with problems arising out of the disaster. This ability to grow the necessary command, control, operational, and support functions as needed is the true strength of ICS.

ICS can significantly enhance the timeliness and quality of an emergency response. Therefore, an understanding of its theory and application and, most importantly, how the EHC function fits into the ICS process is critical for the EMS community.

A typical ICS structure might look something like the one shown in Fig. 10.4. As this illustrates, adding or activating the various ICS components as necessary is easy for coping with the unique problems associated with each disaster or emergency.

Incident Command Structure

ICS has five major management activities—command, operations, planning, logistics, and finance. These functions, at some level, are present at every incident. Any event, regardless of size, can use ICS to manage the situation better. The first step is establishing an incident commander at the scene. The incident commander has the ultimate responsibility for the execution of each of the five activities. On a small incident, the incident commander may perform all of these functions. Key in this arrangement is the ability of the incident commander to make assignments or decisions before they are needed. Incident command has the overall responsibility for the management of incident activity. Even if the other functions are not filled, an incident commander will always be designated.

Command

The command staff works for the incident commander. Routinely, the command staff will consist of a public information officer, a safety manager, an emergency management coordinator, and a liaison officer. Each of these peo-

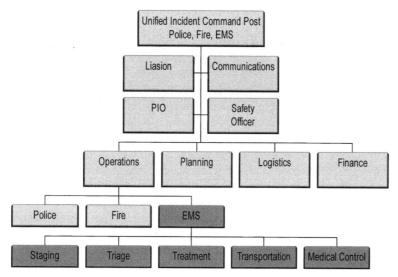

FIGURE 10.4. Generic structure for incident command

ple may have a number of subordinates within the ICS structure depending on the size of the event. Each of these command staff leaders are charged with handling problems and decisions within their area of responsibility, thus relieving the incident commander from the need to deal with these matters.

Operations

The operations section is responsible for activities in the field at the scene of the disaster. These activities usually include emergency first aid, triage, rescue, emergency medical services, fire fighting, debris removal, and shelter for the victims. These functions, or branches as they are called in ICS, are placed under the direction of the operations section chief, and they may be broken down further into divisions or groups depending on the situation and response needs. Only the operations section has direct contact with the general public in a response mode. All the other functions of ICS are in support of the operations section.

Planning

The planning section is responsible for the continued evaluation of the incident situation. They will collect information, prepare situation reports for the incident commander, display situational information, maintain resource status reports, develop an incident action plan, and prepare documentation of the incident. The planning section normally includes functions such as a situation unit (to collect and process information on the current incident situation and develop reports and summaries), a resources unit (to handle all check-in activity and to account for personnel and equipment resources), a documentation unit (to maintain all incident-related records and documentation), a damage assessment unit (to collect information regarding the extent and value of damages suffered to structures), a special needs population unit (to prepare plans to protect people with special needs), a technical specialists and/or volunteers unit (to access people with knowledge specific to the incident in support of the emergency workers), and a demobilization unit (to plan for a safe, orderly, and cost-effective deescalation of personnel and resources). The damage assessment unit and the special needs population unit are usually only used in the emergency operations center (EOC). The planning section has the responsibility to get ahead of the incident by anticipating the problems, issues, and needs of the other ICS sections. It also plays a critical role in keeping the incident commander apprised of the incident's current status.

Logistics

The logistics section provides services and support for all the needs of the event. Logistics has the following seven main activities: a communications unit (to develop the communications plan and to maintain the incident communication system), an information systems unit (to establish and to preserve telephone, computer, and network access for emergency workers), a medical unit (to develop a medical plan and to provide first-aid for incident personnel), a food unit (to supply the emergency workers with food and drinking water), a supply unit (to order personnel, equipment, and supplies for the emergency workers), a donated goods unit (to manage inventory and to distribute clothing and other donated goods), and a facilities unit (to set up and maintain whatever facilities may be required for the emergency workers and to provide for facility security). The donated goods unit and medical unit are usually only used in the EOC.

Finance

The finance section is responsible for tracking incident-related costs and administering the procurement of any necessary resources to be used in responding to the incident. This section has four key functions as follows: a time unit (to record all personnel time used on the incident), a procurement unit (to administer the contract and rental paperwork associated with the equipment and supplies), a compensation or claims unit (to document and investigate injury and damage claims), and a cost unit (to collect cost information and to recommend any cost-saving techniques). All of these functions are usually used only in the EOC. The incident commander has the responsibility to develop and assign the positions and units within this section to manage the incident properly.

THE EMERGENCY OPERATIONS CENTER

ICS is a *management activity*, and it should not be confused with the EOC. The EOC is the *location* from which the key members of the ICS structure manage overall operations. During a large-scale disaster, the responding entity may also have a forward command center near the disaster area, as well as a logistics center, an EMS or triage area, and other such key support functions. The EOC may have additional functions, assignments, and so on, but it exists to support ICS and the emergency workers. The EOC is the place from which the disaster response is coordinated.

As with disaster management structures, a variety of forms can be used for EOCs. They are sometimes located near the law enforcement dispatch center or a major public facility. However, with the use of computers, cellular telephones, video conferencing, and other technology, the EOC can be located nearly anywhere. During the response to the Oklahoma City bombing, for example, the city's Myriad Convention Center served as the EOC, leaving the city's main dispatch center available for routine, day-to-day operations. A critical component to the EHC response is to have a representative capable of making operational decisions and of allocating resources as a member of the EOC.

THE LOCAL EMERGENCY OPERATIONS PLAN

The overall success of a local government's response to an emergency will be largely dependent on the quality of the people who will carry it out. Most cities and counties have an emergency operations plan (EOP). Unfortunately, many of them are long out of date, and thus they will be of little use during the disaster response. Many local jurisdictions also probably have not practiced their EOP or drilled with the outside agencies with which they will have to interact during an actual emergency response.

Most EOPs that have not been revised in 5 or 6 years contain significant amounts of boilerplate information that was required by FEMA in order to receive federal emergency management funds. While this information may be good as training material, much of it proves to be of little use during an actual disaster response. Even those communities who have tried to keep their EOP updated will find that the contact and resource lists are inaccurate, that equipment that has not been frequently tested will fail, and that communications will be a problem in the actual disaster response.

In the past few years, the philosophy about what should be contained in an EOP has started to change. Today, the idea of smaller is better is beginning to take hold as the preferred approach to developing a workable EOP. Beginning with the lessons learned in the Oklahoma City bombing response and continuing through the Columbine High School event, emergency responders are finding that simple action plans are preferable to the big book approach common to most EOPs in the past. Another new technique is the inclusion of action checklists in the EOP rather than the pages of verbiage seen in the past. This approach allows people to be quickly tasked, and it provides a much clearer and more concise description of their duties and responsibilities. The entire emergency response gears up more quickly when the participants have less to read; thus they can focus on actions.

The simpler and more concise the EOP is, the more useful a tool it becomes during the event response. EMS should obtain a copy of the EOP for the community they serve to determine how their role has been defined by local government. This is the first step in getting involved in the local emergency planning process.

LOCAL DISASTER AND EMERGENCY PLANNING

The importance of EMS involvement in the local emergency planning process cannot be overemphasized. Planners must realize that the active involvement of EHC elements in developing and updating these plans is imperative.

Planning is the foundation component of a workable disaster plan and emergency response. Unfortunately, it is one of the first activities to be cut during when local governments have fiscal constraints. Without a strong local emergency planning function to forecast possibilities, to identify potential problems, to anticipate alternatives, and to develop responses, the EOP is relatively impotent as a useful tool for directing the disaster response, and the community's quality of response can suffer.

Do local governments sufficiently plan for their disaster responses? The answer is, unfortunately, not as well as they should. This is usually a function of not enough time, people, or money, rather than of a lack of interest on the part of local officials. Those communities with less than ideal preparations will usually elevate their daily operational functions to a higher, emergency level to deal with the unexpected disaster event. Those communities with good emergency planning will still find that things go wrong or that things that were not anticipated complicate their emergency response. These findings only accentuate the importance of EHC involvement as early as possible in whatever planning processes might exist. This will help assure adequate coordination and control during an emergency. While some communities across the United States are putting a stronger emphasis on disaster planning, it has not become a routine activity in a majority of cities and counties.

When citizen surveys are conducted to determine the activities deemed most important by the taxpayers of a community, services such as water, sewer, trash removal, parks, recreation, and animal control all rank above disaster planning (if it is mentioned at all!). Most local officials are consumed by the day-to-day activities of keeping their entity running. They are hard-pressed to respond to the citizens' immediate needs. Activities such as planning, disaster exercises, and coordinating sessions seem a luxury in their hectic worlds. The simple fact is that for most local governments today, no disaster is conceivable until a disaster occurs. The failure to address disaster planning locally as a normal function of the public safety process significantly complicates the EMS interface.

ACCESSING THE LOCAL EMERGENCY PLANNING PROCESS

The ease of accessing a local jurisdiction's emergency planning process will vary depending on the make-up, philosophy, and politics germane to that organization. In the event of an emergency or disaster, they are very likely to want or to need the involvement of the EHC community. With this in mind, a look at the issues surrounding EMS participation in local EOPs is appropriate.

EMS is generally accepted into emergency planning in most municipalities. EMS, however, represents only one part of the overall emergency health care response that is needed during a disaster. If other EHC providers are not currently involved in planning efforts, some municipal planners may have difficulty in understanding the need for the involvement of emergency physicians, emergency nurses, and public health professionals. Their involvement in interfacing other elements of the emergency health care response with the overall disaster response and EMS is critical.

Using the access to the planning process already available through the EMS medical director is a good way to start. In addition, presenting a unified and organized front for the EHC community through mutual aid committees, hospital associations, trauma committees, or medical societies is a good first step. National organizations, such as the American College of Emergency Physicians, can provide guidance in organizing the overall emergency health care response for a community.

The key to EHC participation in the local government's emergency planning process is knowing who to contact. To that end, this chapter has offered some insight on how local government works and on how it is structured to assist the reader in that objective. One advantage is knowing where to try to access the local government structure. The theory of POSDCORB developed by Luther Gulick and Lyndall Urwick in the 1930s is a good tool (3). POSDCORB is an acronynm standing for **P**lanning, **O**rganizing, **S**taffing, **D**irecting, **CO**ordinating, **R**eporting, and **B**udgeting. While the theory was long on organizational structure and

a bit short on the human relations element, it does provide seven areas through which to find access to the local government's emergency planning process. For example, involvement in the planning function would be best. But, if for some reason this is not possible, try involvement through staff relationships or in the budgeting process. More than one door always exists through which one can access the entity.

Make sure whatever approach is used, it brings something to the table. This can be expertise, resources, assistance, or even a process. But, sometimes the local government entity needs to think that they get an even exchange for what they give up by letting an outsider into their planning process.

Do not forget to connect with the private sector. Hospitals, chambers of commerce, citizen groups, airports, and state or federal offices in the community all offer potential relationships through which one can become more involved in local emergency planning issues.

EHC involvement in the local government's emergency operations plan is not only good management; it is also imperative to a successful emergency response. Not only should the people the EHC serves expect this; they should, in fact, demand it. FIND A WAY TO GET INVOLVED! This is fundamental to the goal of saving lives in an emergency response.

REFERENCES

1. Godschalk DR. *Natural hazard mitigation: recasting disaster planning policy and planning.* Washington, D.C.: Island Press, 1999.
2. Erickson PA. *Emergency response planning: for corporate and municipal managers.* San Diego: Academic Press, 1999.
3. Lindbolm C. The science of muddling through. *Public Admin Rev* 1959;19:79–88.

URBAN SEARCH AND RESCUE

CARL S. GOODMAN
DAVID E. HOGAN

INTRODUCTION

Urban search and rescue (USAR) is the process of locating, extricating, and providing for the immediate medical treatment of victims trapped in collapsed structures. The goal is to recover live victims in a manner that maximizes their chances of recovery to their previous states of health (1). Confined space medicine (CSM) is the emerging body of knowledge concerned with the treatment and rescue of victims trapped in a collapsed structure. Examples of confined spaces include mines; caves; tunnels; collapsed buildings, elevated roadways, and farm silos; manholes; sewers; utility tunnels; and crawl spaces (1).

Several unique pathophysiologic entities have been described in the literature when injury occurs in a confined space. In addition, special techniques are needed to evaluate and treat the entombed individual before extrication. In response to the increased need, USAR and CSM are evolving specialties.

History

Much of the epidemiology related to USAR and CSM has been obtained from descriptive studies following major earthquakes (2–6). The clinical entity of crush injury and crush syndrome were first reported by the Germans in World War I. In 1941, following the Blitz in London, Bywaters (7,8) first fully described the entity.

The scope of USAR is quite varied, and the lessons learned from confined space rescue are essential to the operational success of the mission. In the late 1980s and early 1990s, several domestic events were investigated and reported by the United States Fire Administration (9–14). These events demonstrated the need for an organized and coordinated approach to USAR and confined space rescues. Local cave-in and collapse response teams were developed in California; New York City; Fairfax, Virginia; and Montgomery County, Maryland (15). In addition, a volunteer group of emergency physicians and paramedics trained and equipped in rescue and CSM, called the special medical response team (SMRT), was formed in southwestern Pennsylvania. While the team was originally developed to respond to entrapments in coal mining, industrial, and farming accidents, it has also responded to confined space incidents involving building collapse, mine explosion and fires, cave-in accidents, and well-drilling mishaps (16).

The first well-known national effort to develop a multidisciplinary task force to respond to and to assist local resources with the location and extrication of entrapped individuals was pioneered by the Office of United States Foreign Disaster Assistance (OFDA) (15). The capability of these teams was demonstrated in Mexico City, Philippines, and Soviet Armenia. The OFDA, as a part of the Agency of International Development, is prohibited from developing USAR teams domestically, so, as a result, domestic development became the responsibility of the United States military.

In 1988, public law 93-288 (the Robert T. Stafford Disaster Relief and Emergency Assistance Act) gave the federal government authority to respond to disasters; to provide assistance to save lives; and to protect public health, safety, and property. Hurricane Hugo and the Loma Prieta earthquake focused the attention of the nation on deficiencies in USAR capabilities. As a result, the Federal Emergency Management Agency (FEMA) received a federal mandate to develop a national USAR system as emergency support function (ESF) no. 9 of the federal disaster response plan (FRP). At the inception of the FRP's development, the Department of Defense had the logistical capabilities to support heavy urban search and rescue operations but not the technology, skills, and experience. They did, however, have the personnel for light search and rescue and the ability to support civilian heavy rescue teams. Through the coordinating efforts of FEMA, civilian and military teams work together to maximize USAR operations.

Operational Considerations

ESF no. 9 functions within the scope of the FRP, and it will interface with health and medical services (ESF no. 8). The locus of interface during the operation is outside the collapsed structure. The USAR (ESF no. 9) medical and rescue personnel hand the patient off at the casualty collection point or at the transportation sector to ESF no. 8 personnel (Fig. 11.1).

Currently, 28 equipped and trained USAR task teams exist (*personal communication*, William Gluckman, 2002). The USAR team is made up of a 56-member task force (TF), consisting of the following four functional TF elements (17): the search team, the rescue team, the medical team, and the technical team. Each team is composed of at

least two persons. This structure allows the TF to operate 24 hours a day, working in 12-hour shifts, with sufficient time for rest.

The TF leader is the central point of coordination. The leader must be able to integrate the activities of each of the four functional elements. The TF leader's role is to blend the team into the incident command structure of the local authorities and the Department of Defense for implementation of their tactical assignment. The search team's primary function is to locate victims using canines, special techniques, and tactics with the assistance of fiberoptic cameras and sensitive acoustic listening devices. The purpose of the rescue team is the evaluation of the collapsed structure, stabilization of the structure, and extrication of victims. The technical team is responsible for hazardous materials assess-

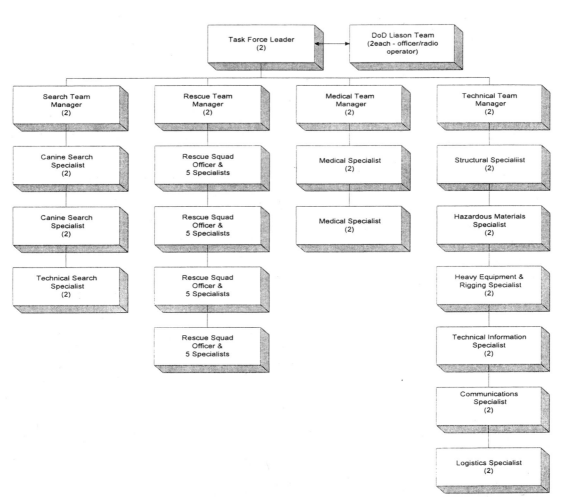

FEMA US&R Task Force Organization

FIGURE 11.1. Federal Emergency Management Agency (FEMA) and Urban Search and Rescue (US&R [generally USAR]) task force organization (From Federal Emergency Management Agency. *Urban search and rescue response system: field operations guide.* Washington, D.C.: Federal Emergency Management Agency, September, 1993:III-1, with permission).

TABLE 11.1. EQUIPMENT CACHE

Rescue equipment	Communications equipment	Technical equipment
Electric generators	Portable radios	Atmospheric monitoring equipment
Pneumatic air compressors	Charging units	Structural specialist items
Power tools	Telecommunications items	Technical information specialist items
Hand tools	Repeaters	Technical search specialist items
Electrical equipment	Batteries	Logistics equipment
Lighting	Power source	Water and fluids
Maintenance items	Satellite phone	Food
Rope and rigging equipment	Cellular phones	Shelter
Safety equipment		Sanitation items
Search equipment		Personal safety gear
Search cameras		Administrative support items
Seismic and acoustic listening devices		Personal gear
Thermal imaging devices		

From Federal Emergency Management Agency. *Technical rescue program development manual.*
United States Fire Administration, August 1995, with permission.

ment, structural stabilization advice, communications, local system liaison, and logistics management.

The medical team provides sophisticated and possibly prolonged emergency medical care during the mission. Unlike traditional United States disaster field care, the USAR team is designed to deliver more sophisticated care to fewer patients (1). The team must be medically self-sufficient, and it should not rely on the local medical system. The health care of the team members is the first priority. The physician is not only responsible for acute injuries occurring during the mission, but he or she should also be prepared to deal with common complaints, such as upper respiratory infections, gastroenteritis, and even sunburn. Once the care of the task force is ensured, attention can be turned to entrapped victims, search team canines, and the surrounding community. The team should not serve as a free-standing medical resource at the disaster site (18). It will hand off patients to local EMS agencies or other disaster medical assistance teams.

Development considerations include that the team have the capacity to be rapidly deployable and fully self-sufficient for food, water, shelter, and sanitation. It should be self-

TABLE 11.2. MEDICAL SUPPLIES

Pharmacologic agents	Airway equipment	Miscellaneous
Antibiotics	Endotracheal tubes: adult and pediatrics	Assorted bandages and dressings
Intravenous and intramuscular	Laryngoscope: straight and curved	Assorted tape
Oral medication	End tidal carbon dioxide colormetric	Stokes basket
Ocular medication	monitor	Canine supplies
Topical medication	Stylet	Personal protective equipment
Steroids	Spare bulbs and batteries	Helmet
Cardiac drugs	Fiberoptic flexible scope	Personal locating device
Respiratory drugs	Flexible guide wire	Goggles
Analgesia	No. 11 blade and handle	Sturdy shoes or boots
Sedatives, anesthetics, and paralytics	Umbilical tape	Safety glasses
Comfort medication	Bag valve mask: adult and pediatrics	Nomex jumpsuit
Antacids	Portable ventilator	Work gloves
Hemorrhoidal preparations	Oxygen	Tyvex coveralls
Insect repellent	Assorted oxygen masks	Latex gloves
Sunblock	Nasal cannula	Dust mask
Immunizations	Eye care	
Tetanus toxoid	Saline solution	
Assessment/monitoring	Flourosceine	
Stethoscope	Metal shield	
Blood pressure cuff manual and automated	Immobilization devices	
pulse oximeter	Kendrick extrication device	
End-tidal carbon dioxide monitor	Long spine board or full body	
Thermometer: oral, rectal, tympanic	vacuum splint	
Otoscope	Assorted board splints	
Ophthalmascope		

From Federal Emergency Management Agency. *Technical rescue program development manual.*
United States Fire Administration, August 1995, with permission.

sufficient for 72 hours and able to operate for up to 10 days (16,17). The team brings its own equipment. In addition to rescue equipment, lighting, heating, and generators are cached (Table 11.1). Medical equipment includes basic and advanced life support supplies, an expanded pharmacology stock, personal protective equipment, patient monitoring devices, and supplies for treating the canine team members (Table 11.2).

Scientific Background

A study of the health effects of earthquakes in the mid 1990s revealed that building collapse was the principle source of casualties (19). Most injuries and death that occur in a collapsed structure are the result of energy transmitted to the body that exceeds the body's threshold to withstand the transfer (20). Frequently cited causes of death include multiple injury (21), dust asphyxiation, and head trauma (20,21). Furthermore, the risk of death is significantly higher in individuals trapped beneath the rubble (2,3,21), and the death rate is higher for individuals located on higher floors before structural collapse (3,21).

The literature is replete with the concept of the Golden Day. The chance of extricating a victim alive drops dramatically after 24 hours following the structural collapse. In Soviet Armenia, of the patients rescued alive, 89% were extricated during the first 24 hours (2). Similarly, in the Tangshan earthquake, 81% of those extricated in the first 24 hours were alive, while only 7.4% beneath the rubble were found alive at 5 days after the event (23). Analysis of the data from the Guatemalan earthquake suggests that most of the deaths took place almost immediately (4). After the bombing of the Murrah Federal Building in Oklahoma City, the mean extrication time was 20 minutes, and only three persons were found alive after 3 hours (24). Most victims trapped in a collapsed building have been shown to die within the first minutes to hours following injury. As a result, USAR teams providing assistance are often performing body recovery (14,19). However, many anecdotal reports are found of victims who have survived after being entombed for up to 6 days and longer (2,19,23). Thus, efforts should not be delayed or abandoned after 24 hours.

When rescuers are reaching an entrapped patient who is alive, routine prehospital procedures do not apply. The scoop and run philosophy is not possible with the trapped or pinned individual (16). The most significant medical advance in reducing the morbidity and mortality of pinned individuals is the prevention of renal failure due to crush injury.

Advances in incident management, particularly the incident command system, further support the scientific basis for USAR (15). Technical developments in the detection of hazardous materials and in protective gear allow rescue workers to mitigate their risk when working in a confined space. Search equipment, such as fiberoptic cameras, thermal imaging, and ultrasensitive listening devices, have advanced the ability to locate trapped persons. Rescue capa-

bilities for shoring, cutting, and lifting have allowed rescue personnel a better chance of extricating the individual without creating further injury.

Confined Space Medicine

A confined space has limited access and egress and unfavorable environmental conditions, and it is not designed for continuous occupancy. Persons trapped beneath rubble may be in a confined space, and knowledge of the associated dangers is essential to the safety of both the patient and the emergency care worker. Confined spaces are subject to temperature extremes, and this can present an added problem for the trapped patient and the rescuers.

Atmospheric conditions may be dangerous. Hazardous atmospheres include oxygen-deficient, flammable, and toxic conditions (25). An environment that contains less than 19.5% available oxygen requires the use of supplemental oxygen. Oxygen may be delivered via a self-contained breathing apparatus or an airline respirator. An airline has a remote source, and it is delivered by a hose to a mask worn by the operator. Oxygen cannot be simply pumped into the confined space because this may lower the threshold of flammability in the air. Even in the absence of an oxygen-enriched atmosphere, flammable gas and dust may be present. In addition to delivering sufficient oxygen to the rescuer and patient, proper ventilation is essential. The use of sparking or electric tools is extremely dangerous without taking this necessary precaution.

Before entering a confined space, the atmosphere should be properly tested. Carbon monoxide may result from nearby fires and portable generators. Carbon dioxide may accumulate from the expired respiratory products of the patient and rescuers, and methane may be present from broken gas lines. Consideration also needs to be given to the presence of hazardous materials stored in the collapsed structure. If the environment is found to have unfavorable conditions, ventilation and oxygen supplementation is essential. Other safety measures include isolating and shutting off gas lines and electrical service and the removal of hazardous material.

In addition to the atmospheric concerns, the risk of secondary collapse must be taken seriously. Proper stabilization will mitigate further risk to rescuers. Although the collapse hazard cannot be completely eliminated, measures may be taken to lessen the chance of a second catastrophe. Numerous reports are found of coworkers and rescuers who enter confined spaces before establishing safe environmental conditions only to become casualties themselves (25).

Search and Rescue Operations

Rescue of victims from a collapsed structure is never a rushed operation. The safety of the rescuer is of paramount importance. Becoming a victim creates more of a problem than it solves. Many victims are extricated by laypersons soon after the collapse of a structure using the simple hand removal of debris. However, living individuals may be trapped, thus requiring specially trained personnel to locate and extricate these people. Appropriate personal protective equipment is essential. Respiratory protection should be selected depending on the nature of the atmospheric hazards. At a minimum, a dust mask will be required; and, in extreme situations, a self-contained breathing apparatus or a supplied air respirator may be needed. Barrier protection, such as Tyvek coveralls and latex gloves, should be worn, even under leather work gloves, if the risk of fluid contamination exists. A helmet is essential for protecting the rescuer from falling debris. Safety glasses or goggles should be put on when the potential for eye injury exists. Hearing protection may be needed when operating heavy rescue tools. Appropriate footwear is essential to provide adequate footing on uneven rubble and to protect against injury from heavy debris. A safety lifeline should be used when appropriate, and a personal locating device should be carried. A safety officer is essential for oversight of the operation; he or she is part of the incident command system. An important initial consideration is the decision of rescue versus recovery.

The Fire Department of New York has developed a five-step collapse rescue plan (10) as follows: (a) the site is surveyed; (b) victims on the surface are rescued; (c) voids are explored; (d) selected debris is removed; and (e) then general debris is removed. The type of collapse and void spaces are identified as lean-to, V-type, pancake curtain-fall, or cantilever collapse. Most structural collapses result in a combination of collapse and void space types (1). Surviving victims will be in the voids that have been formed. When the rubble pile is deemed acceptable for entry by trained rescue teams, shoring is undertaken to support the structure and to prevent secondary collapse. Victim location occurs with the assistance of the canine team and of specialized acoustic, video, and infrared devices.

When a victim is located, the patient can be remotely assessed and triaged. The process of extrication can begin with simple bucket brigade hand removal of debris and power tools. Trenching and tunneling occurs until the patient can be reached by medical personnel and is further assessed; treatment is initiated, and the patient is ultimately removed from the rubble. After all known victims are accounted for or the assessment is made that the persons remaining are not salvageable, general debris removal occurs. Heavy equipment may be required, and caution must be used because a victim may be unexpectedly found alive.

MEDICAL CONSIDERATIONS

An understanding of the unique environment and knowledge of CSM will enhance the survival of and reduce morbidity in the extricated patient. Assessment and treatment needs to begin as soon as possible to maximize survival potential. Assessment may not initially involve any physical contact with the patient, and it may take place remotely, either by voice contact alone or by visualizing the patient using devices such as fiberoptic cameras. When the patient is finally reached, a minimal portion of their body may be accessible until rubble can be fully removed. Assessment for respiratory impairment, hypovolemia, crush injury, skeletal injury, burns, and thermoregulatory problems in the rubble is very important. Once the airway, breathing and circulation have been attended to, attention can be focused on immobilization of the spine and fractures. However, priorities may need to be adjusted according to accessibility. Analgesia should be used liberally to assist in the extrication process.

Anticipation of Prolonged Field Management

Although most victims extricated alive are rescued within 24 hours, rescuers must be prepared for prolonged extrication and patient management. Emergency physicians should expect the patient to be hypothermic and dehydrated at best secondary to no food or water intake. In addition, victims may develop an ileus and vomit, they may sustain blood loss, and they may experience third space fluid accumulation. To minimize the risk of vomiting, patients should not take anything by mouth, and intravenous hydration is preferred. Bodily functions, such as urination and bowel movements, may have occurred, and these may complicate procedures requiring a clean environment. Infectious disease issues need to be addressed. The elderly, as might be expected, are prone to developing pressure sores and ulceration, thus providing a source of sepsis. Victims may develop rhabdomyolysis from crush injury or immobilization.

Environmental concerns pose a problem not only to the patients but to the rescuers as well. Patients are subject to potential environmental temperature extremes (1). Medical causes of hypothermia likely to be encountered are trauma and hypoglycemia. Other causes may contribute, such as being improperly dressed for outdoor exposure because the victim was inside the building when it collapsed, which can be further complicated because the victim may be lying on a cold slab of concrete or in a pool of water from a ruptured water line. Temperature should be monitored, and intravenous fluids should be warmed, if possible. Oxygen tanks should be kept warm.

Heat-related medical problems may be more common in the rescuer. The spectrum of illnesses expected ranges from minor heat exhaustion to severe life-threatening heat stroke. The rescuer is prone to heat injury secondary to personal protective clothing limiting heat escape. Rescuers, in addition, are hypermetabolic secondary to the strenuous activity in which they are engaged, and they may not be consuming adequate amounts of fluids and electrolytes. Team members need to be encouraged to remove their heavy outer protective clothing and helmets when they are outside the danger zone and to drink plenty of fluids.

Confined Space Medicine Pharmacology

The pharmacy cache of the medical team includes medications not traditionally used by paramedics. The expanded pharmacy includes analgesia, sedatives, paralytics, antibiotics, and common over-the-counter remedies. One should not overlook the fact that trapped patients may have underlying medical conditions; thus, maintenance medications, such as insulin or cardiac drugs, may need to be administered.

The use of analgesia is essential when dealing with the trapped patient who likely is in considerable pain that will only be made worse by the extrication process. The removal of debris and the movement of the patient without appropriate analgesia may hinder the extrication efforts. Narcotic analgesia, such as morphine, may be required for routine procedures or for extremes, such as an in-field amputation. Nitrous oxide has a quick onset of action and elimination, and it does not have the risk of respiratory depression. When thoracic or intraabdominal injury is suspected, the use of nitrous oxide is contraindicated. The use of nitrous oxide in a confined space mandates adequate ventilation to prevent intoxicating the rescuers. Simple remedies, such as acetaminophen and ibuprofen, should also be on hand for team members' minor complaints.

Respiratory problems need to be managed more aggressively in the trapped patient. In addition to bronchodilators, mucolytics may be necessary, as well as steroids. Management of the airway becomes more difficult as has been previously mentioned, and the cache should include short-acting and intermediate-acting paralytic agents, such as succinylcholine, rocuronium, and vecuronium; sedatives, such as midazolam and thiopental; and the dissociative anesthetic, ketamine. Caution should be exercised when using succinylcholine because of the potential risk of increasing intracranial and intraocular pressure, as well as of worsening hyperkalemia (26).

Infectious Disease Issues

Disasters have the potential to increase the risk of infectious disease emergencies (27). The predisaster health infrastructure is paramount in mitigating this risk; however, disruption of host defense and the breakdown of infection control measures may lead to an increased risk even in the isolated trapped victim. The patient may be contaminated with airborne and waterborne infectious agents, in addition to those from their own vomit and feces. Those with chronic diseases (thus already predisposed to infection) are at additional risk (27).

Trapped patients with open wounds are subject to wound infection and sepsis if they are not treated promptly.

Battlefield experience has demonstrated that the early administration of antibiotics is of utmost importance (28). Antibiotics administered more than 6 hours after injury will prevent local wound infection (28). The incidence of sepsis may be reduced if antibiotics are administered later. A broad-spectrum antibiotic that is safe, easy to administer, and stable in various environments and that has a long half life is well suited for initial antibiotic coverage. A first-generation cephalosporin is a good choice for wound infection, but it can become a problem because of a dosing requirement of every 6 to 8 hours. Ceftriaxone, a third-generation cephalosporin, although it is not as good for gram-positive organisms, has better gram-negative coverage for intraabdominal and pulmonary organisms. It also has the advantage of being administered in one intramuscular dose with adequate blood levels for 24 hours.

Pulmonary disease is also a concern. Patients trapped in a moist environment may be subject to infection by *Legionella*. Rare clinical entities, such as acute pulmonary coccidiomycosis, following the Northridge earthquake were believed to be due to high dust and spore levels (27).

Teams responding to international requests for assistance need to be prepared to deal with pathogens indigenous to the locality. The safety of the team depends on the use of appropriate surveillance and prophylaxis by the medical team. Vaccines need to be up to date, and medicine must be on hand to treat local pathogens. The prompt recognition of foreign diseases is essential to prevent their introduction into the United States (27).

Blast Injury

Buildings collapse as a result of many different factors. Seismic activity has been a known cause of structural collapse. The structural support of aging buildings may fail. Recently, terrorism has become a greater concern. Prior to the collapse of the World Trade Center Towers, building collapse from terrorist activity had occurred at the Murrah Federal Building in Oklahoma, the Marine Corps barracks in Beirut, the Khobar Towers in Saudia Arabia, and the Musgrave Park Hospital in Belfast (21,29,30).

As a result of this rise in the incidence of the use of explosive devices to collapse buildings, the clinical entity of blast injury must be considered when evaluating the patient trapped in collapsed rubble. Blast injury occurs as blast waves impact susceptible organs. Air-filled structures, such as the lungs, gastrointestinal tract, and tympanic membrane, are most frequently injured (31). Secondary injury occurs when blast fragments and debris strike the victim. Injury may result from shrapnel, glass, and any other debris that has become airborne. Injury occurring due to the collapse of the structure can be considered a secondary injury. Tertiary injury occurs when the victim is thrown against a solid object. Head injury, thoracic injury, lacerations, contusions, fractures, and burns are frequently encountered when the structure's collapse is secondary to an explosive device (30). The presence of fire can result in carbon monoxide poisoning, which should be considered in the trapped unconscious victim without signs of head injury or hypoglycemia. Assessment of tympanic membranes for rupture may indicate exposure to a significant blast load (29). However, the absence of tympanic membrane rupture does not rule out blast injury.

A metaanalysis reported by Hodgetts (29) indicated that the incidence of blast lung was 0.6% in 2,394 immediate survivors. Persons situated close to the explosive device suffer a higher frequency of primary blast injury. Death in this setting is most likely to be caused by air embolism (30). Although adult respiratory distress syndrome (ARDS) and other pulmonary blast complications are uncommon, they may develop in the victim. Intestinal perforation, pneumoperitoneum, and splenic rupture may also be found (32). Serious ocular injury from flying debris is a frequent occurrence (21).

Blast injuries that occur in confined spaces differ from those seen in open-air bombings (32). A comparison of four terrorist events in Israel demonstrated increased mortality and morbidity when the victim was in a confined space. Blast injury to the pulmonary system and burns were also more extensive and more frequent. Individuals situated closer to the explosion in a confined space are likely to have more severe injuries.

Airway Management

Effective management of the trapped individual's airway may be difficult. Obstacles include patient access difficulties, suboptimal positioning, dirty conditions, poor lighting, and prolonged extrication. Proficiency in alternative techniques to standard oral tracheal intubation is essential when working in this austere environment.

Often, the patient's head may not be accessible. If the head is visible, debris may prevent oral intubation from the usual position. Alternatives to standard direct laryngoscopy endotracheal intubation include nasal tracheal intubation, digital technique, retrograde Seldinger technique, cricothyroidotomy, transtracheal jet insufflation, and the Tomahawk approach. The Tomahawk approach is performed by straddling the patient over their torso, holding the laryngoscope in the right hand like a tomahawk or ice pick, and introducing the tube with the left hand (33) (Fig. 11.2). Once the patient is intubated, a portable ventilator device is preferred because of the potential need for prolonged extrication and the lack of space for a second rescuer to bag. Pulse oximetry and end tidal carbon dioxide monitoring are essential when the medical team does not have direct visibility of the patient.

Pulmonary Concerns

The patient trapped in a collapsed building may suffer from numerous respiratory problems, including airway obstruc-

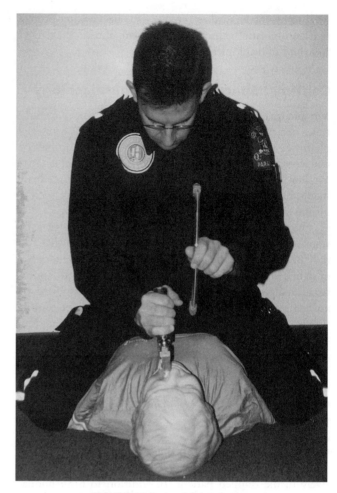

FIGURE 11.2. Icepick intubation

tion, particulate contamination, restriction of ventilation, inhalation injury, and blast lung (1). The airway may be obstructed by vomitus or broken teeth. In addition, building collapse generates the unique clinical entity of particulate respiratory compromise. Ventilation may be limited by rubble, limiting chest wall expansion. Significant crush injury to the chest will be fatal (1). Inhalation injury may be secondary to thermal burns when gas mains rupture or electrical fires are started. Oxygen-carrying capacity may be limited as a result of carbon monoxide, methane, and other toxins, such as phosgene. The end result may be a patient requiring respiratory support in a less than optimal situation for endotracheal intubation. Additional procedures, such as chest decompression, chest tube insertion, and surgical airway, may be required. Measures, such as monitoring oxygen saturation and end tidal carbon dioxide, using positive end expiratory pressure, and performing gastric suction, will assist in monitoring the patient and optimizing oxygenation.

When a building collapses, the respiratory system may be severely compromised from the dust cloud that results (20). The effects of dust on airways are related to the physical and chemical properties of the dust, as well as the particulate size (34). Particles in the respirable range are those less than 10 μm (34). Building collapse results in suspended particles within the respirable range. Building materials include masonry (concrete, block, brick), sheet rock, plaster, paint, tiles, drop ceiling, and insulation. Constituents of these materials contain calcium, silica, asbsestos, wood, and other mineral fibers. These particles have the capacity to induce acute and chronic pulmonary toxicity, primarily by their fibrogenic effects and by injury to the lung cellular defense mechanism (34–36).

Death by dust asphyxiation may be the sole cause of death in some (37). Postmortem examinations of earthquake victims in Soviet Armenia revealed large amounts of dust in the nasal cavities, throat, and respiratory passages, suggesting that airway obstruction and asphyxiation were the cause of death (2). Data from the Kobe, Japan earthquake revealed that choking and suffocation was a major cause of death (19). Inhalation of dust contaminated with *Pseudomonas pseudomallei* has been reported in a victim following a fireworks factory explosion, resulting in adult respiratory distress (ARDS) (38). Other causes of ARDS in the trapped patients include sepsis, thermoregulatory disorders, volume depletion, and multisystem organ failure from overwhelming trauma.

Volume Concerns and Vascular Access

The entombed patient is subject to volume problems as a result of numerous factors, including hemorrhage, dehydration, and third spacing. Hemorrhage from trauma may be delayed until extrication when the compressing rubble is removed from a trapped extremity. Many victims trapped in Kobe died as a result of dehydration before they were rescued (19). Crush injury, which will be discussed later, contributes to fluid shifts. Early fluid administration is essential to prevent delayed complications when the individual is freed.

Vascular access needs to be initiated as soon as possible (16). Two large-bore (14G) peripheral intravenous sites should be established. Invasive procedures, such as central lines and venous cutdown, are subject to a high degree of complications, including contamination and dirt emboli. However, if peripheral access is difficult, these procedures may be necessary. Bladder catheterization may be needed to monitor urine output (1). Intraosseous lines should be considered, particularly in children. Fluid administration by evacuating all air from the intravenous set and using a pressure infuser ensures flow in tight spaces where gravity flow is not possible (15).

Crush Injury and Crush Syndrome

The most dangerous time for the victim is during the extrication phase of the rescue when the compressive forces are suddenly released from the pinned extremity (20). The patient may look deceptively well, only to deteriorate shortly after being freed (16). The crush syndrome is referred to as the smiling death because the victim will be smiling when you free him or her yet will be dead a few minutes later (20). In the Tangshan, China earthquake, 20% of victims suffered crush syndrome (37). In Armenia, crush injury was the third most common injury and the leading cause of death in patients reaching medical care (39). Significant impact on morbidity and mortality reduction is seen when crush injury and crush syndrome are treated properly.

Crush injury results from the pressure applied to a limb, which causes skeletal muscle damage. Muscle death occurs immediately following mechanical disruption. The death of muscle tissue by ischemia is delayed by several hours (40). Crush injury only occurs to the limbs, most commonly the lower extremities (8). It may occur in as little as 1 hour (16). Crush syndrome is the systemic manifestation of crush injury, and, if it is not treated expediently, it will lead to electrolyte problems, acid-base shifts, and acute renal failure (7,8,40).

The two major entities that need to be dealt with are the local crush injury to the tissue and the subsequent systemic complications when the pressure forces are released. The severity of crush syndrome is proportional to the amount of injured muscle (8). Crush syndrome essentially is traumatic rhabdomyolysis. When the muscle is injured, the contents of the myocytes are released into the plasma; therefore, an influx of myoglobin, potassium, and phosphorus into the circulation is observed (40,41). The deceptive feature of the syndrome is that it does not develop until the limb is free from entrapment. The syndrome is further complicated by hypovolemia from edema, third spacing, and lactic acidosis from muscle ischemia (7,41). Rhabdomyolysis may occur in the absence of ischemia (7). Third spacing of fluid into the tissue of the injured extremity may be significant enough to cause shock. No limb edema occurs initially, but, once it develops, it is quite striking (8). Additional injury is created by oxygen free radicals, the intracellular influx of calcium, and polymorphonuclear leukocyte activation through toxic products and during reperfusion (41).

After release from entrapment, sudden death may result from cardiac arrhythmias—either asystole or ventricular fibrillation—and acute renal failure (ARF) (7,8,41). Severe hypocalcemia and hyperphosphatemia may contribute to cardiac instability (16). The intracellular level of calcium increases, while the serum level falls. A mitochondrial increase in calcium impairs cellular respiration and adenosine triphosphate production (41). This intracellular increase in calcium increases the activation of phospholipase A_2, which results in the activation of leukotrienes, prostaglandins, and lysophospholipase, causing cellular injury (41). Calcium administration is not recommended, unless the calcium is needed to resolve ventricular ectopy (7,16). Calcium administration will correct hypocalcemia

TABLE 11.3. TREATMENT PROTOCOL TO PREVENT ACUTE RENAL FAILURE IN CRUSH SYNDROME

1. Combat hypovolemia with crystalloids.
2. Infuse hourly 500 mL of crystalloid and 22.4 meq of bicarbonate.
3. If diuresis is <300 mL/hr, give mannitol 1 g/kg per dose.
4. If blood pH is >7.45, give 250 mg of acetozolamide.
5. Monitor vital signs hourly, plus urine pH and volume.
6. Monitorr osmolarity and electrolytes in blood and blood gases every 6 h.

From Michaelson M. Crush injury and crush syndrome. *World J Surg* 1992;16:899–903, with permission.

only transiently, and the calcium will be deposited in the injured muscle (7). Calcium deposited in the muscle is referred to as metastatic calcification; it will worsen rhabdomyolysis.

Direct renal toxicity is not fully understood, but it is thought to be due to the decomposition products of myoglobin, such as ferriheme, and the direct obstruction caused by myoglobin and uric acid crystals (41). The iron component of myoglobin is also believed to play a role in kidney damage (7,41). Hypovolemia potentiates the problem, so prevention is the mainstay of treatment.

Treatment of the patient and steps to prevent crush syndrome begin as soon as the patient is reached. Intravenous access is essential, with the anticipation of infusing large amounts of fluid (6–10 L) in the immediate postrelease period (16). Urinary pH of greater than 6.5 has been demonstrated to protect the kidneys by increasing myoglobin solubility and by enhancing its excretion (Table 11.3) (7,8,40). Diuresis is also protective (8).

Crush injury results in local tissue destruction (7,8,40). Mechanical disruption causes instant cell death, whereas ischemia leads to the death of muscle within 6 hours at a normal body temperature (40). The cell begins to swell as a result of the intracellular accumulation of solutes—sodium chloride and calcium pull water in osmotically. An efflux of substances from the damaged muscle cell, including potassium, purines, phosphate, lactic acid, myoglobin, thromboplastin, creatine kinase, and creatinine, occurs (7) (Table 11.4). Because the muscle groups are encased in a watertight fibrous sheath, additional pressure and cell damage are caused as the intracompartmental water content rises (7). This causes a cycle of edema, leading to an increase in compartment pressure. Compartment syndrome develops and leads to additional ischemia and muscle damage.

The initial presentation of the crushed extremity may be misleading. The victim may have no pain, the development of edema may be delayed, and pulses may be present. If pulses are absent, injury such as vascular disruption should be sought (7,8). Limb swelling does not occur immediately, but, when it does, it may be significant enough to cause hypovolemic shock (7,8). Sensory findings in the crushed extremity may mimic spinal cord injury, resulting in the complete loss of motor and sensory function (40). Preservation of anal sphincter tone and the lack of saddle anesthesia argue against a complete spinal cord injury.

Controversy has arisen regarding the indications and benefits of fasciotomy. Better and Stein (7) recommend fasciotomy when the intracompartmental pressure exceeds 40 mm Hg (or the diastolic pressure minus 30 mm Hg) and remains at that level for more than 8 hours. Michaelson (8) and Reis (40) do not specify a particular pressure. They state that fasciotomy in crush injury is only indicated in open injury in an attempt to avoid infection and/or when the intracompartmental pressure is high enough to compromise the vascular supply to the distal extremity. Both authors agree that, if fasciotomy is to be performed, radical debridement of the dead muscle must take place. One note of caution is that traditional methods of identifying viable tissue do not apply (8,40). Dead muscle from crush injury may

TABLE 11.4. FLOW OF SOLUTES AND WATER ACROSS SKELETAL MUSCLE CELL MEMBRANES IN RHABDOMYOLYISIS

Flow	Consequence
Influx from extracellular compartment into muscle cell	
Water, sodium chloride, and calcium	Hypovolemia and hemodynamic shock, prerenal and later acute renal failure; hypocalcemia, hyperkalemia; increased cytosolic calcium, activation of cytotoxic proteases
Efflux from damaged muscle cell	
Potassium	Hyperkalemia and cardiotoxicity
Purines from disintegrating cell nuclei	Hyperuricemia, nephrotoxicity
Phosphate	Hyperphosphotemia
	Worsening of hypocalcemia and metastatic calcification
Lactic and other organic acids	Metabolic acidosis
Myoglobin	Nephrotoxicity
Thromboplastin	Disseminated intravascular coagulation
Creatine kinase	Extreme elevation of serum level
Creatinine	Increased serum creatinine to urea ratio

Modified from Better MD, Stein JH. Early management of shock and prophylaxis of acute renal failure in traumatic rhabdomyolyisis. *N Engl J Med* 1990;322:825–829.

bleed profusely. Viability should be determined by the response to electrical or mechanical stimulation (40). Fasciotomy, if indicated, should never be performed in the field.

Field Amputation

The need for a prehospital amputation is a rare occurrence (42). The indication for field amputation is the inability to extricate the patient by any other means or when the need for rapid extrication is paramount, such as in cases of impending secondary collapse, hazardous materials, or fire (1). Ideally, the decision should be made by two physicians who agree, in conjunction with the rescue team, that amputation is the only option that exists.

Performing an amputation is a difficult procedure, and it results in significant long-term morbidity (1). The procedure may take place with inadequate analgesia and anesthesia. Hemorrhage is difficult to control, and the risk of infection and subsequent sepsis is obvious in this austere environment.

Psychoemotional Considerations

By itself, responding to a disaster is a significantly stressful event. A response involving a collapsed structure with entrapped live persons or, even worse, dead victims is a tremendous burden, and it has the potential to place a significant psychologic burden on performance. Extreme empathy is required when making contact with the trapped patient. Prolonged relationships often develop as, for hours, the rescuer may be the patient's only contact to the outside world.

Many medical response obstacles and risks are present for USAR personnel. Problems encountered include the loss of local infrastructure, the medical system chaos, delays in treatment, nonselective victim processing, unusual medical problems, and a race against time. The rescuers themselves incur considerable risks, such as secondary collapse, hazardous materials exposure, austere living conditions, long work hours, intense physical labor, and psychoemotional stress. Part of the responsibility of the medical team is to ensure that team members are properly hydrated and fed and that they have obtained sufficient rest. Signs of stress need to be recognized and dealt with effectively so that the overall mission and safety of others are not compromised. Part of the overall plan of the medical team must include appropriate critical incident stress debriefing and defusing.

SUMMARY

USAR is an important part of disaster response, and CSM supports the overall mission. CSM is the unique body of knowledge concerned with the medical needs of the trapped individual. The emergency physician should be familiar with problems encountered in the victim trapped in a confined space and in those who, in addition, have sustained a crush injury. Scientific advances in the treatment of these victims has reduced morbidity and mortality. The overall success of the mission depends on all aspects of the disaster response. Furthermore, one must remember that the extraordinary efforts of the USAR team will go unrecognized unless the emergency department is prepared to receive the extricated casualty.

ACKNOWLEDGMENTS

We acknowledge Joseph Barbera, M.D., for his foresight in recognizing the "Medical Response to Urban Search and Rescue; Andy Jagoda, M.D., for his guidance through the writing of this chapter; and Dario Gonzalez, who provided early assistance on this project. Any discussion of urban search and rescue would not be complete without giving our deepest sympathy to the entire urban search and rescue community for their efforts at the World Trade Center collapse and their eternal bond with the late Raymond Downey, who made the ultimate sacrifice on September 11, 2001.

FURTHER READING

Barbera JA, Lozano M. Urban search and rescue medical teams: FEMA task force system. *Prehospital Disaster Med* 1993;8:349–355.

Campbell DA, Walker MA. Hypothermia and the crush syndrome. *J R Coll Surg Edinb* 1992;37:257–256.

Centers for Disease Control and Prevention. Heatstroke—United States, 1980. *MMWR* 1981;30:277–279.

Federal Emergency Management Agency. *Confined space rescue on SS Gem State*. Washington, D.C.: United States Fire Administration, 1990.

Federal Emergency Management Agency. Emergency support function no. 9—urban search and rescue. *The Federal Response Plan* P.L. 93-288, April, 1992.

Federal Emergency Management Agency. *Federal response plan, notice of change*. FEMA publication no. 229. Washington, D.C.: Federal Emergency Management Agency, 1994.

Grande CM, Baskett PJF, Donchin Y, et al. Trauma anesthesia for disasters: anything, anytime, anywhere. *Crit Care Clin* 1991;7:339–361.

Koenig KL, Schultz CH. The crush injury cadaver lab: a new method of training physicians to perform fasciotomies and amputations on survivor of a catastrophic earthquake [abstract]. *Ann Emerg Med* 1992;21:613.

National Institute for Urban Search and Rescue. Available at: http://www.NIUSR.org. Accessed March, 2002.

O'Donnell TF Jr. Acute heat stroke: epidemiologic, biochemical, renal and coagulation studies. *JAMA* 1975;234:824–828.

Restall J, Knight RJ. Analgesia and anesthesia in the field. In: Baskett PJF, Weller RM, eds. *Medicine for disasters.* Bristol: Wrights, 1988.

Urban Search and Rescue Response System. Aviailable at: http://www.fema.gov/usr/index.htm. Accessed March 2002.

REFERENCES

1. Federal Emergency Management Agency. *FEMA USAR response system task force medical team training manual.* Washington, D.C.: Federal Emergency Management Agency, November, 1993.
2. Noji EK, Kelen GD, Oganessian A, et al. The 1988 earthquake in Soviet Armenia: a case study. *Ann Emerg Med* 1990;19:891–897.
3. De Bruycker M, Greco D, Lechat MF. The 1980 earthquake in southern Italy: morbidity and mortality. *Int J Epidemiol* 1985;14:113–117.
4. de Ville de Goyet C, Jeannee E. Epidemiological data on morbidity and mortality following the Guatemal earthquake. *IRCS Med Sci Soc Med* 1976;4:212.
5. Kunkle RF. Emergency medical care in the underground environment. *J Wilderness Assoc Emerg Disaster Med* 1986;10:54–55.
6. Kunkle RF. Medical care of entrapped patients in confined spaces. *International workshop on earthquake injury: epidemiology for mitigation and response.* Baltimore: John Hopkins Proceedings, July 10–12, 1989.
7. Better OS, Stein JH. Early management of shock and prophylaxis of acute renal failure in traumatic rhabdomyolyisis. *N Engl J Med* 1990;322:825–829.
8. Michaelson M. Crush injury and crush syndrome. *World J Surg* 1992;16:899–903.
9. Federal Emergency Management Agency. *Urban search and rescue in the Crested Butte, Colorado, state bank following an explosion collapse.* FA-120. Washington, D.C.: United States Fire Administration, 1992.
10. Federal Emergency Management Agency. *Urban search and rescue in New York City following a commercial building collapse.* FA-121. Washington, D.C.: United States Fire Administration, 1992.
11. Federal Emergency Management Agency. *Urban search and rescue in Brownsville, Texas, following a commercial building collapse.* FA-123. Washington, D.C.: United States Fire Administration, 1992.
12. Federal Emergency Management Agency. *Urban search and rescue in the Santa Cruz area following the Loma Prieta earthquake.* FA-124. Washington, D.C.: United States Fire Administration, 1992.
13. Federal Emergency Management Agency. *Urban search and rescue in San Bernardino, California, following a major train derailment in a residential neighborhood.* FA-125. Washington, D.C.: United States Fire Administration, 1992.
14. Eberhart-Philips JE, Saunders TM, Robinson AL, et al. Profile of mortality from the 1989 Loma Prieta earthquake using coroner and medical examiner reports. *Disasters* 1994;18:160–170.
15. Barbera JA, Macintyre A. Urban search and rescue. *Emerg Med Clin North Am* 1996;14:399–412.
16. Barbera JA, Cadoux CG. Search, rescue and evacuation. *Crit Care Clin* 1991;7:321–337.
17. Federal Emergency Management Agency. *Technical rescue program development manual.* Washington, D.C.: United States Fire Administration, 1995.
18. Federal Emergency Management Agency. Urban search and rescue response system. In: *Field operations guide.* Washington, D.C.: Federal Emergency Management Agency, 1993.
19. Alexander D. The health effects of earthquakes in the mid 1990s. *Disasters* 1996;20:231–247.
20. Moede JD. Medical aspects of urban heavy rescue. *Prehospital Disaster Med* 1991;6:341–348.
21. Mallonee S, Shariat S, Stennies G, et al. Physical injuries and fatalities resulting from the Oklahoma City bombing. *JAMA* 1996;276:382–387.
22. Sanchez-Carillo CI. Morbidity following Mexico City's 1985 earthquakes: clinical and epidemiological findings from hospitals and emergency units. *Public Health Reports* 1989;104:482–488.
23. Zhi-Yong S. Medical support in the Tansghan earthquake: a review of the management of mass casualties and certain major injuries. *J Trauma* 1987;27:1130–1135.
24. Hogan DE, Wackerle J, Dire DJ, et al. The emergency department impact of the Oklahoma City terrorist bombing. *Ann Emerg Med* 1999;34:160–167.
25. National Institute for Occupational Safety and Health. *A guide to safety in confined spaces.* Department of Health and Human Services publication 87-113. Washington, D.C.: United States Government Printing Office, 1987.
26. Rosen P, Barkin RM, Braen GR, et al., eds. *Emergency medicine concepts and clinical practice,* 3rd ed. St. Louis, MO: Mosby, 1992:2147.
27. Howard, MJ, Brillman, JC, Burkle FM. Infectious disease emergencies in disasters. *Emerg Med Clin North Am* 1996;14:413–428.
28. Hell K. Characteristics of the ideal antibiotic for prevention of wound sepsis among military forces in the field. *Rev Infect Dis* 1991;13:S164–S169.
29. Hodgetts TJ. Lessons from the Musgrave Park hospital bombing. *Injury* 1993;24:119–121.
30. Fryberg ER, Tepas JJ III, Alexander RH. The 1983 Beirut airport terrorist bombing injury patterns and implications for disaster management. *Am Surg* 1989;55:134–141.
31. Gans L, Kennedy T. Management of unique clinical entities in disaster medicine. *Emerg Med Clin North Am* 1996;14:301–326.
32. Leibovici D, Gofrit ON, Stein M, et al. Blast injuries: bus versus open-air bombings—a comparative study of injuries in survivors of open-air versus confined-space explosions. *J Trauma* 1996;41:1030–1035.
33. Koetter KP, Hilker T, Genzwuerker HV, et al. A randomized comparison of rescuer positions for intubation on the ground. *Prehospital Emerg Care* 1997;1:96–99.
34. Baxter PJ, Ing R, Falk H, et al. Mount St. Helens eruptions: the acute respiratory effects of volcanic ash in a North American community. *Arch Environ Health* 1983;38:138–143.
35. Baxter PJ, Ing R, Falk H, et al. Mount St. Helens eruptions, May 18 to June 12, 1980. An overview of the acute health impact. *JAMA* 1981;246:2585–2589.
36. Martin TR, Wehner AP, Butler J. Pulmonary toxicity of Mt. St. Helens volcanic ash. A review of experimental studies. *Am Rev Resp Dis* 1983;128:158–162.
37. Yong C, Tsoi K, Felbi C, et al., eds. *The Great Tansghan earthquake, 1976: an anatomy of a disaster.* New York: Pergamon Press, 1988.
38. Wang CY, Yap BH, Delilkan AE. Meliodosis pneumonia and blast injury. *Chest* 1993;103:1897–1899.
39. Klain M, Ricci E, Safar P, et al. Disaster reaminatology potentials: a structured interview study in Armenia. *Prehospital Disaster Med* 1989;4:135–152.
40. Resi ND, Michaelson M. Crush injury to the lower limb: treatment of local injury. *J Bone Joint Surg Am* 1986;68:414–418.
41. Odeh M. The role of reperfusion-induced injury in the pathogenesis of the crush syndrome. *N Engl J Med* 1991;324:1417–1422.
42. Kampen KE, Krohmer JR, Jones JS, et al. In-field extremity amputation: prevalence and protocols in emergency medical services. *Prehospital Disaster Med* 1996;11:36–60.

THE UNITED STATES FEDERAL RESPONSE PLAN

REUBEN G. PINKSON, JR.

FOREWORD

I am conducting, late in September 2001, the final manuscript review for this chapter on the federal response plan (FRP), which I wrote some time earlier. Like many others, I am sad and angered, and my mind and heart are elsewhere. The United States has just experienced the largest terrorism attack of this era. Recovery operations continue in New York City where the Twin Towers once stood and at the Pentagon in Washington, D.C. A crash site located in Pennsylvania marks where more lives were lost. The loss of lives to these attacks still seems unimaginable, and the ongoing performance of the local and supplemented responders and rescue workers is simply and purely heroic and inspiring.

This catastrophe was global in nature, and thus the world is uniting for justice and the eradication of terrorism as it exists today. At this moment, the national mobilization is ongoing, coalitions are forming, and the world is coming to the aid and support of the United States. The country itself seems to be patriotically uniting in its determination to address this wrong, and potentially, it will soon enact a global remedy in order to remove this disruptive threat. However, the country must also accept that a significant change in the grand American ways is likely. No doubt, however, it will adapt, heal, and rise again to the standards of freedom and justice for all.

How this experience may require functional modifications to the highly valued FRP is still unknown. I doubt that any significant core changes will occur. However, the FRP, like the United States, has always adapted to any new challenges in the past, and it will do so again. Nevertheless, the reader should note that the information offered in this chapter precedes the attack on the World Trade Center.

OVERVIEW

The United States government has a fundamental obligation to provide for the security of the nation and to protect its people; values; and social, economic, and political structures. Inherent in that obligation is the requirement to have an emergency mobilization preparedness program that will provide an effective capability to provide defense and to meet the essential civilian needs during national security emergencies and major domestic emergencies (1). The head of each federal department and agency must be prepared to respond adequately to all national and domestic emergencies. These and many more responsibilities are generally captured in one primary contingency document entitled the "Federal Response Plan."

Since 1965, over 1,200 presidential disaster declarations have been made. The FRP describes the mechanism and structure by which the federal government mobilizes resources and conducts activities to address the consequences of any major disaster. Major disasters include any incident or event that overwhelms the capabilities of state and local governments. The decisions to mobilize federal resources are generally made by the President of the United States. The federal assistance, available under the Robert T. Stafford Disaster Relief and Emergency Assistance Act, as well as under individual agency authorities, seeks to save lives; to protect public health, safety, and property; to alleviate damage and hardship; and to reduce future vulnerability (2). The President makes disaster-stricken areas eligible for federal assistance by declaring an emergency or major disaster. The process normally begins when a state governor asks the president for federal help. The Federal Emergency Management Agency (FEMA) evaluates the request and makes an immediate recommendation to the president. On his approval, the requested federal agencies move immediately to assess needs and to meet the state's request for help. Today, 27 federal departments and agencies, including the American Red Cross, support the FRP. Under the previously mentioned Stafford Act and Executive Orders 12148 (3) and 12656 (4), FEMA has been delegated the primary responsibility for coordinating federal emergency preparedness, planning, management, and disaster assistance functions. Thus, FEMA has the lead in developing and maintaining the FRP.

THE ORGANIZATION OF THE FEDERAL RESPONSE PLAN

The FRP is divided into a number of primary sections, including (a) basic plan elements, (b) the emergency support function annexes, (c) recovery function annexes, (d) support annexes, and (e) appendices. The FRP organization is demonstrated in Fig 12.1.

EMERGENCY SUPPORT FUNCTIONS

Each section under the FRP is organized further into specific functional areas. The most important for health care providers are the emergency support functions (ESFs). Each ESF has been created to cover a specific task or set of tasks during a disaster response. Each ESF is headed by a primary agency and is supported by several support agencies. The ESFs, their primary agencies, and area of responsibility under the FRP consist of those listed below.

ESF 1: Transportation
Primary Agency: Department of Transportation (DOT).
Responsibility: provide civilian and military transportation support.
ESF 2: Communications
Primary Agency: National Communications System (NCS).

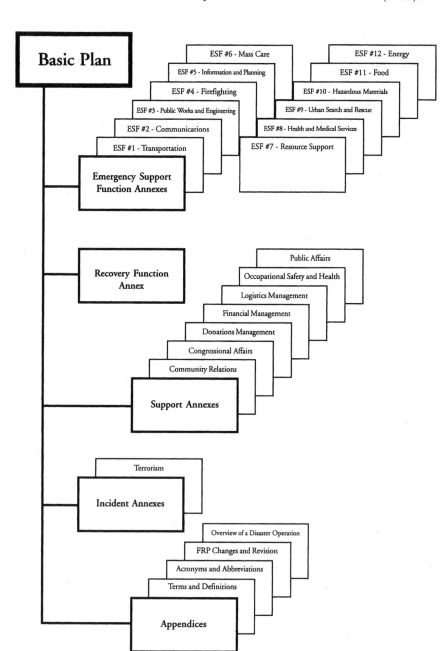

FIGURE 12.1. Organization of the federal response plan. This denotes components of the basic plan, annexes, and appendixes. (From Federal Emergency Management Agency. *Federal response plan.* 9230.1-PL. Washington, D.C.: Federal Emergency Management Agency, 1999, with permission.)

Responsibility: provide telecommunications support.

ESF 3: Public works and engineering

Primary Agency: United States Army Corps of Engineering (COE), Department of Defense (DOD).

Responsibility: restore essential public services and facilities.

ESF 4: Firefighting

Primary Agency: United States Forest Service (USFS), Department of Agriculture (USDA).

Responsibility: detect and suppress wildland, rural, and urban fires.

ESF 5: Information and planning

Primary Agency: Federal Emergency Management Agency (FEMA).

Responsibility: collect, analyze, and disseminate critical information to facilitate the overall federal response and recovery operations.

ESF 6: Mass care

Primary Agency: American Red Cross (ARC).

Responsibility: manage and coordinate food, shelter, and first aid for victims; provide bulk distribution of relief supplies; implement a system to assist family reunification.

ESF 7: Resource support

Primary Agency: General Services Administration (GSA).

Responsibility: provide equipment, materials, supplies, and personnel to federal entities during response operations.

ESF 8: Health and medical services

Primary Agency: United States Public Health Services (USPHS), Department of Health and Human Services (DHHS).

Responsibility: provide assistance for public health and medical care needs.

ESF 9: Urban search and rescue

Primary Agency: Federal Emergency Management Agency (FEMA).

Responsibility: locate, extricate, and provide initial medical treatment to victims trapped in collapsed structures.

ESF 10: Hazardous materials

Primary Agency: Environmental Protection Agency (EPA).

Responsibility: support federal response to actual or potential releases of oil or hazardous materials.

ESF 11: Food

Primary Agency: Food and Nutrition Service (FNS), Department of Agriculture (USDA).

Responsibility: identify food needs; ensure that food gets to areas affected by the disaster.

ESF 12: Energy

Primary Agency: Department of Energy (DOE).

Responsibility: restore power systems and fuel supplies.

Fig. 12.2 provides a summarizing matrix of all ESFs, including both primary and support agencies.

PLANNING ASSUMPTIONS

For a disaster plan to work, it must be based on a set of valid assumptions. The FRP is based on the following five primary assumptions:

1. The FRP assumes that a major disaster or emergency will cause numerous fatalities and injuries, property loss, and the disruption of normal life-support systems and that it will have an impact on the regional economic, physical, and social infrastructures.
2. The extent of casualties and damage will reflect factors such as the time of occurrence, the severity of impact, the weather conditions, the population density, building construction, and the possible triggering of secondary events, such as fires and floods.
3. The large number of casualties, heavy damage to basic infrastructures, and the disruption to basic public services will overwhelm the capabilities of the state and local governments to meet the needs of the situation. The president will therefore declare a major disaster or emergency.
4. Federal agencies will need to respond on short notice in order to provide timely and effective assistance.
5. The degree of federal involvement will be related to the severity and magnitude of the event, as well as to the state and local needs for external support. The most devastating disaster may require the full range of federal response and recovery assistance. Some disasters may require only federal recovery assistance. Regardless, the federal government has proven exceedingly responsive to the needs of United States citizens.

Fig. 12.3 provides a summary of Presidential Disaster Declarations from January 1965 to December 31, 1998, separated by FEMA regions and by disaster types.

CONCEPT OF OPERATIONS

Local and state responders can effectively handle most disasters and emergencies. They are at the leading edge of the response. The federal government is generally called on to provide supplemental assistance when the consequences of the disaster or incident exceed the local and state capabilities. The FRP can mobilize an array of resources, including emergency teams, support personnel, specialized equipment, operating facilities, and assistance programs, and it has access to private sector resources. It uses a multiagency operational structure that is based on the principles of the incident command system (ICS). Consistent with these principles, the FRP can be partially or fully implemented in the anticipation of a significant event or in response to an actual event. This flexibility allows the effective operational merging of response and recovery resources. The plan, however, makes no provisions for the direct federal support of law enforcement functions in a disaster or emergency. That becomes a state func-

Agency \ ESF #	1 Transportation	2 Communications	3 Public Works and Engineering	4 Firefighting	5 Information and Planning	6 Mass Care	7 Resource Support	8 Health and Medical Services	9 Urban Search and Rescue	10 Hazardous Materials	11 Food	12 Energy
USDA	S	S	S	P	S	S	S	S	S	S	P	S
DOC		S	S	S	S		S			S		
DOD	S	S	P	S	S	S	S	S	S	S	S	S
DOEd					S							
DOE					S		S	S		S		P
HHS			S		S	S		P	S	S	S	
HUD					S							
DOI		S	S	S	S					S		S
DOJ					S			S	S	S		
DOL			S				S		S	S		
DOS	S									S		S
DOT	P				S		S	S		S		S
TREAS	S				S		S					
VA			S			S	S	S				
AID								S	S			
ARC					S	P		S			S	
EPA			S	S	S			S		P	S	
FCC		S										
FEMA	S	S		S	P	S	S	S	P		S	
GSA	S	S			S	S	P	S			S	
NASA					S		S		S			
NCS		P			S		S	S				S
NRC					S					S		S
OPM							S					
SBA					S							
TVA	S		S									S
USPS	S					S		S				

P = Primary Agency: Responsible for Coordination of the ESF

S = Support Agency: Responsible for Supporting the Primary Agency

FIGURE 12.2. Emergency support functions (ESF) designation matrix. This denotes 12 emergency support functions (ESFs) and the primary and support agencies. (From Federal Emergency Management Agency. *Federal response plan.* 9230.1-PL. Washington, D.C.: Federal Emergency Management Agency, 1999, with permission.)

tion. However, other mechanisms outside the FRP allow a governor to request this type of assistance from the attorney general of the United States. The FRP does describe policies and structures for coordinating FRP operations with the Department of Justice (DOJ) response to threats or acts of terrorism within the United States.

In addition, a myriad of teams and facilities is involved in making the plan happen once it has been activated. These are complex, yet functional, and highly effective. The disaster field office (DFO) becomes the primary field location in each affected state for the coordination of the federal response and recovery operations. It will operate under a schedule or 24 hours per day when necessary to sustain federal operations. The federal coordinating officer (FCO) and the state coordinating officer (SCO) generally collocate at the DFO, with the relevant federal agency regional representatives and state and local liaison officers. A special team called the emergency response team (ERT) supports the FCO. It ensures that federal resources are made available to meet the states' requirements, as communicated by the SCO. The majority of the medical-specific functions of the FRP are contributed by ESF 6 and ESF 8.

ESF 6 coordinates federal assistance in support of state and local efforts to meet the mass care needs of victims of a

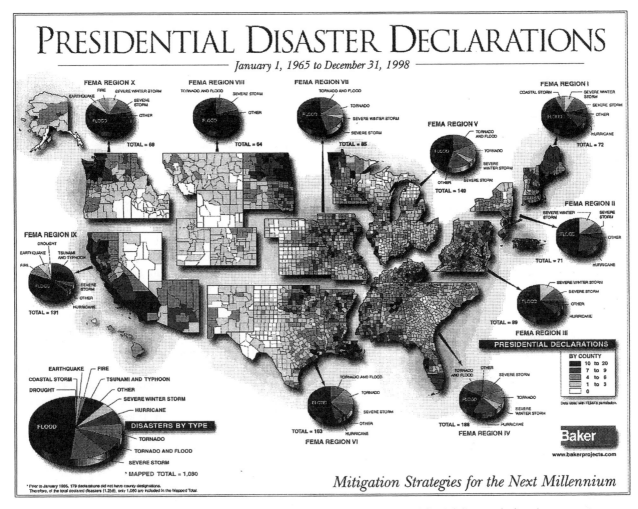

FIGURE 12.3. Presidential disaster declarations. This represents presidential disaster declarations by Federal Emergency Management Agency (FEMA) regions, from January 1, 1965 to December 31, 1998. (From FEMA Chart. Available at: http://www.bakerprojects.com/fema/mapmain.htm. Accessed February 13, 2002, with permission.)

disaster. This federal assistance will support the delivery of mass care services for shelter and feeding. It also provides emergency first aid to disaster victims and the establishment of systems to allow the bulk distribution of emergency relief supplies. In addition, ESF 6 collects information for operating a disaster welfare information (DWI) system in order to report victim status and to assist in family reunification. Initial response activities focus on meeting the urgent needs of disaster victims on a mass care basis. Initial recovery efforts may commence as response activities are taking place. As recovery operations are introduced, close coordination is required between those federal agencies responsible for recovery operations and the voluntary organizations providing recovery assistance, including the ARC. Emergency first aid will be provided to disaster victims and workers at mass care facilities and at designated sites within the disaster area. The ARC also contributes superb counseling services to victims and responders alike. These services will be supplemental to the emergency health and medical services that have

been established to meet the needs of disaster victims. The organization of ESF 6 is depicted in Table 12.1.

ESF 8, or health and medical services, provides coordinated support to supplement state and local resources in response to public health and medical care needs following

TABLE 12.1. EMERGENCY SUPPORT FUNCTION 6 (MASS CARE)

Eight support agencies aid the Mass Care Annex (ESF-6), which is led by the American Red Cross.
    Department of Agriculture (USDA)
    Department of Health & Human Services (DHHS)
    Department of Veterans Affairs (VA)
    General Services Administration (GSA)
    Department of Defense (DOD)
    United States Postal Service (USPS)
    Federal Emergency Management Agency (FEMA)
    Department of Housing & Urban Development (HUD)

TABLE 12.2. EMERGENCY SUPPORT FUNCTION 8 (HEALTH AND MEDICAL SERVICES)

The Health and Medical Services Annex (ESF-8), led by the Department of Health and Human Services (DHHS), is ably supported by 13 support agencies.
> Department of Agriculture (USDA)
> Department of Energy (DOE)
> Department of Transportation (DOT)
> Agency for International Development (AID)
> Environmental Protection Agency (EPA)
> General Services Administration (GSA)
> United States Postal Service (USPS)
> Department of Defense (DOD)
> Department of Justice (DOJ)
> Department of Veterans Affairs (VA)
> American Red Cross (ARC)
> Federal Emergency Management Agency (FEMA)
> National Communications System (NCS)

a major disaster or emergency or during a developing medical situation. Resources are furnished when state and local capabilities are overwhelmed and public health and/or medical assistance is requested from the federal government to meet the medical needs of victims of a major disaster, emergency, or terrorist attack. The organization of ESF 8 is depicted in Table 12.2.

MEDICAL FUNCTIONAL AREAS OF FEDERAL SUPPORT

Federal medical support can be categorized into the following 15 functional areas:

- Assessment of health and medical needs;
- Health surveillance;
- Medical care personnel;
- Health and medical equipment and supplies;
- Patient evacuation;
- In-hospital care;
- Food, drug, and medical device safety;
- Worker health and safety;
- Radiologic, chemical, and biologic hazards consultation;
- Mental health care;
- Public health information;
- Vector control;
- Potable water and wastewater and solid waste disposal;
- Victim identification and mortuary services;
- Veterinary services.

Also included are the overall public health response; the triage, treatment, and transportation of victims of the disaster; and the evacuation of patients outside the disaster area, as needed, into a network of DOD, Department of Veterans Affairs (VA), and preenrolled nonfederal hospitals located in the major metropolitan areas of the United States. The National Disaster Medical System (NDMS), a nationwide medical mutual aid network connecting the federal and nonfederal sectors, provides many medical options, including medical response, patient evacuation, and definitive medical care.

MEDICAL AREAS OF CONCERN

Depending on the magnitude of the disaster, resources within the affected area could be inadequate for clearing casualties from the scene or treating them in local hospitals. Medical resupply, medical bed availability, movement and evacuation of patients, and definitive medical care requirements are important areas of interest. A terrorist release of weapons of mass destruction; damage to chemical and industrial plants, sewer lines, and water distribution systems; toxic environments; exposure to hazardous chemicals and biologic and radiologic substances; and contaminated water supplies, crops, livestock, and food products are all potential areas of medical concern. If the event results in a large number of deaths and injuries, the state and local mental health system may be overwhelmed. An urgent need for mental health crisis counseling for victims, families, and responders alike may develop. The office of the medical examiner may need supplementation and assistance to be able to expand to meet the forensic and mortuary loads.

The basic medical infrastructure of the community may be disrupted. In addition, a widespread disruption of sanitation services and facilities, as well as the loss of electrical power, may occur. Massing of people in shelters increases the potential for disease and injury, thus requiring the operation of epidemiologic surveillance programs. Primary medical treatment facilities may be damaged or inoperable. Assessments and emergency restorations to necessary operational levels are required to stabilize the medical support system.

MEDICAL RESPONSE ACTIONS

Federal health and medical assistance is generally categorized into the major functions of prevention, medical services, mental health services, and environmental health. Upon receiving notification of a disaster, the lead administrator of ESF 8 (the Assistant Secretary of Health) will request DHHS and its support agencies to initiate actions for identifying and reporting the potential need for federal health and medical support to the affected disaster area. A brief synopsis of which DHHS agency leads the efforts and what primary actions are generally executed in each of the 15 functional areas follows.

Assessment of Health and Medical Need

Lead DHHS Agency: Office of Public Health and Science, Office of Emergency Preparedness, National Disaster Medical System (OPHS/OEP/NDMS).

Action: mobilize and deploy an assessment team to the disaster area to assist in determining specific health and medical needs and priorities.

Health Surveillance

Lead DHHS Agency: Centers for Disease Control and Prevention (CDC).

Action: assists in establishing surveillance systems to monitor the general population and special high-risk population segments, to carry out field studies and investigations, and to monitor injury and disease patterns and potential disease outbreaks; provides technical assistance and consultation on disease and injury prevention and precautions.

Medical Care Personnel

Lead DHHS Agency: OPHS/OEP/NDMS.

Action: provide disaster medical assistance teams (DMATs) and individual public health and medical personnel to assist in providing care for ill or injured victims at the location of a disaster or an emergency. The DMATs are capable of providing triage, medical or surgical stabilization, and continued monitoring and care of patients until they can be evacuated to locations where they can receive definitive medical care. Specialty DMATs can also be deployed to address mass burn injuries, pediatric care requirements, chemical injury or contamination, and so forth. Additionally, active and reserve component field medical units for casualty clearing and staging and other missions are available to multiply these special capabilities effectively. Individual clinical health and medical care specialists may be provided to assist state and local personnel. The VA is one of the primary sources that can expeditiously deliver these staffing complements. Additionally, the VA can provide medical emergency radiological response teams (MERRTs) and emergency medical response teams (EMRTs). The VA is also capable of mobilizing other health professionals who are not necessarily part of a formal team, depending on ESF 8 requirements.

Health and Medical Equipment and Supplies

Lead DHHS Agency: OPHS/OEP/NDMS.

Action: provide health and medical equipment and supplies, including pharmaceutical agents, biologic products, and blood and blood products. These are generally provided in support of DMAT operations and for restocking health and medical care facilities in an area affected by a major incident or emergency. In this area, the VA again has a valued network of medical centers throughout the nation that has proven to be operationally capable in the delivery of these emergency medical resources.

Patient Evacuation

Lead DHHS Agency: OPHS/OEP/NDMS.

Action: provide for the movement of seriously ill or injured patients from the area affected by a major disaster or emergency to a location where definitive medical care is available. NDMS patient movement will be accomplished using fixed-wing aeromedical evacuation resources from the DOD. However, other suitable transportation options may be applied as the situation may warrant. Special patient regulation systems are available to track the movement and transfer of casualties effectively.

In-Hospital Care

Lead DHHS Agency: OPHS/OEP/NDMS.

Action: provide definitive medical care to victims who become seriously ill or injured as result of a major disaster or emergency. For this purpose, the NDMS has established and maintains a nationwide network of voluntary precommitted, nonfederal, acute care hospital beds in the largest metropolitan areas in the United States. Fig. 12.4 provides a summary of these capabilities throughout the United States. Both the DOD and the VA provide federal coordinating centers (FCC) to oversee the management and training of this unique bed expansion system.

Food, Drug, and Medical Device Safety

Lead DHHS Agency: Food and Drug Administration (FDA).

Action: ensure the safety and efficacy of regulated foods, drugs, biologic products, and medical devices following a major disaster or emergency. Arrange for the seizure, removal, and destruction of contaminated or unsafe products.

Worker Health Safety

Lead DHHS Agency: CDC.

Action: assist in monitoring health and well-being of emergency workers; perform field investigations and studies addressing worker health and safety issues; provide technical assistance and consultation on worker health and safety measures and precautions.

Radiologic, Chemical, and Biologic Hazards Consultation

Lead DHHS Agency: CDC.

Action: assist in assessing health and medical effects of radiologic, chemical, and biologic exposures on the general population and on high-risk population groups; conduct field investigations, including the collection and analysis of relevant samples; advise on protective actions related to direct human and animal exposure and on indi-

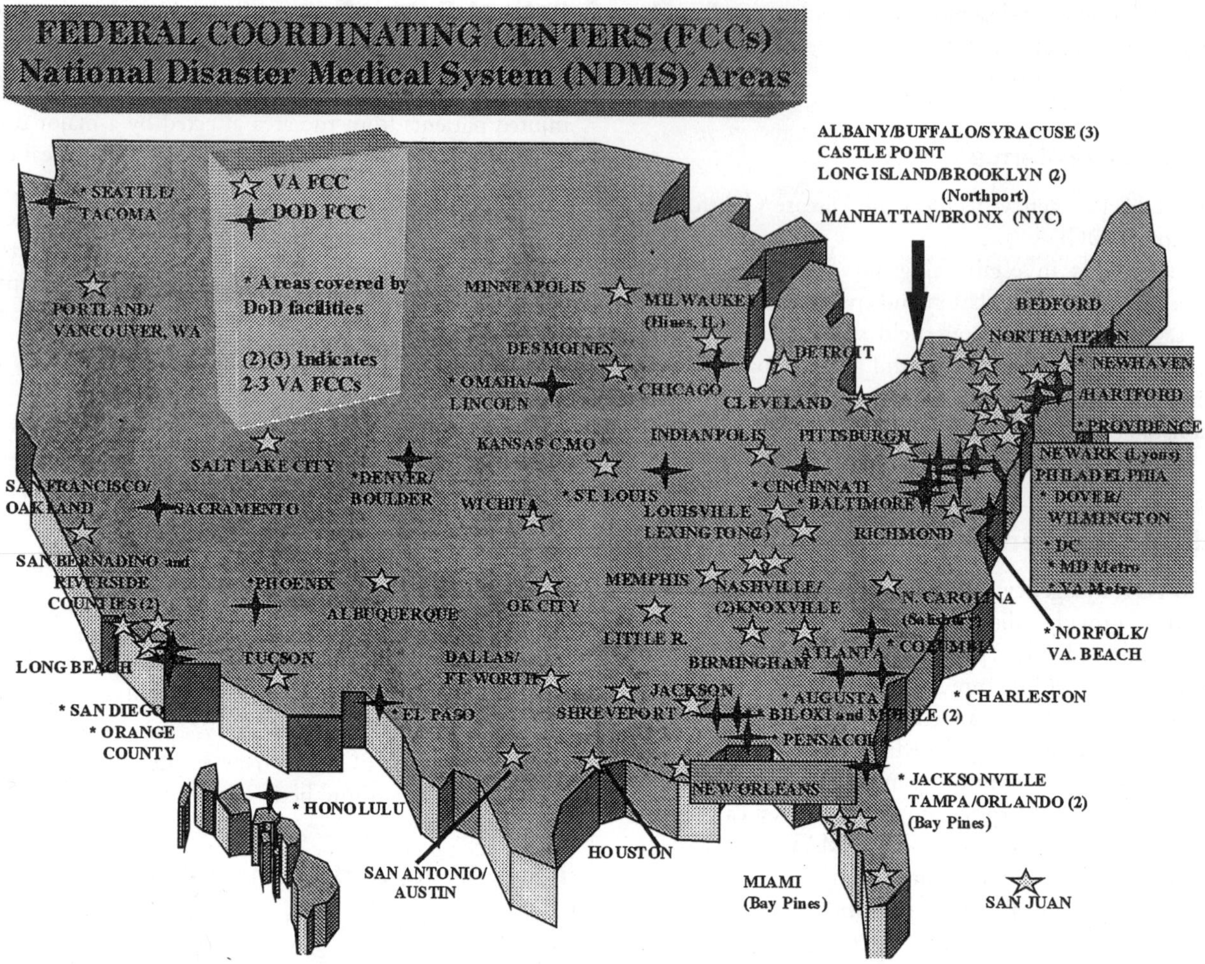

FIGURE. 12.4. National Disaster Medical System (NDMS) areas. The figure designates both Veterans Affairs (VA) and Department of Defense (DOD) federal coordinating centers (FCCs). (From the Emergency Management Strategic Healthcare Group (EMSHG). Department of Veterans Affairs, March 1999, with permission.)

rect exposure through radiologically, chemically and biologically contaminated food, drugs, water supply, and other media; and provide technical assistance and consultation on medical treatment and decontamination of casualties.

Mental Health Care

Lead DHHS Agency: Substance Abuse and Mental Health Services Administration (SAMHSA).

Action: assist in assessing mental health needs; provide disaster mental health training materials for disaster workers; and provide a liaison with assessment and training and program development activities undertaken by federal, state, and local mental health officials.

Public Health Information

Lead DHHS Agency: CDC.

Action: assist by providing public health and disease and injury prevention information that can be transmitted to members of the general public who are located in or near areas affected by a major disaster or emergency.

Vector Control

Lead DHHS Agency: CDC.

Action: assist in assessing the threat of vector-borne diseases following a major disaster or emergency; conduct field investigations, including the collection and laboratory analysis of relevant samples; provide vector control equipment and supplies; provide technical assistance and consultation on protective actions regarding vector-borne diseases; and provide technical assistance and consultation on medical treatment of victims of vector-borne diseases.

Potable Water and Wastewater and Solid Waste Disposal

Lead DHHS Agency: Indian Health Service.

Action: assist in assessing potable water and wastewater and solid waste disposal issues; conduct field investigations, including collection and laboratory analysis of relevant samples; provide water purification and wastewater and solid waste disposal equipment and supplies; and provide technical assistance and consultation on potable water and wastewater and solid waste disposal issues.

Victim Identification and Mortuary Services

Lead DHHS Agency: OPHS/OEP/NDMS.

Action: assist in providing victim identification and mortuary services, including NDMS disaster mortuary teams (DMORTs); the provision of temporary morgue facilities; victim identification by fingerprint, forensic dental, and/or forensic pathology and anthropology methods; and processing, preparation, and disposition of the remains.

Veterinary Services

Lead DHHS Agency: OPHS/OEP/NDMS.

Action: assist in delivering health care to injured or abandoned animals and in performing veterinary preventive medicine activities following a major disaster or emergency. This also includes conducting field investigations and providing technical assistance and consultation as required.

MEDICAL SUPPORT TEAM

Before the deployment of federal medical resources, the national ESF 8 will also alert, organize, and deploy a management support team (MST) to the disaster area to liaison with and provide support to the fielded ESF 8 resources. The MST will be as self-contained as possible, and it will provide operations, administration, logistics, planning, and communication support to the medical team. It is generally staffed by experienced emergency preparedness specialists from the United States Public Health Services Office of Emergency Preparedness (OEP) and the DVA Emergency Management Strategic Healthcare Group (EMSHG).

PATIENT REGULATION

Through the Global Patient Movement Requirement Center (GPMRC), national NDMS hospital bed reports can be made available. Reports are sent locally to the assigned VA or DOD FCC, who then consolidates the acute bed data and forwards it electronically to the GPMRC for review

and consideration. Additionally, the GPMRC will arrange medical transportation resources and will manage patient regulation if patient or casualty evacuations are required.

DOMESTIC TERRORISM

Before closing this FRP chapter, this exceedingly important area warrants some discussion. Terrorism threats within the continental United States continue to expand. The potential use of weapons of mass destruction (WMD) by both domestic and international terrorists is now a threatening possibility. This terrorism challenge has generated the development of numerous mandated emergency management initiatives that are now being applied throughout metropolitan areas within the United States. The federal government, noting the need to improve the emergency preparedness postures of local metropolitan areas significantly in order to address WMD terrorism incidents, has made Herculean efforts to develop, train, and equip local responders with functional and proven capabilities for responding effectively to these potential challenges.

The requirements are not simple to develop, and they mandate the utmost commitment from local responders and the supplementing private and public sector health care facilities. These Domestic Preparedness Programs (DPP) and Metropolitan Medical Response Systems (MMRS) initiatives cannot be left to chance. The stakes are too big to simply ignore. Incidents like the 1993 bombing of the Twin Towers in New York City by international terrorists and the 1995 bombing of the Oklahoma City Alfred P. Murrah Federal Building by domestic terrorists sparked these mandated preparedness efforts. No longer were citizens at potential risk only when abroad. The challenge has now become domestic as well.

Presidential Decision Directive 39 (PDD 39), *U.S. Policy on Counterterrorism*, establishes policy for reducing the nation's vulnerability to terrorism, for deterring and responding to terrorism, and for strengthening the capabilities to detect, prevent, defeat, and manage the consequences of terrorist use of WMD. The directive states that the United States will have the ability to respond rapidly and decisively to terrorism directed against Americans wherever it occurs, to arrest or defeat the perpetrators using all appropriate instruments against the sponsoring organization and governments, and to provide recovery relief to victims as permitted by law (5). Responding to terrorism involves instruments that provide crisis management (led by the DOJ). This includes measures to identify, acquire, and plan the use of resources needed to anticipate, prevent, and/or resolve a threat or act of terrorism. It is a law enforcement response. Consequence management, which is led by FEMA efforts, refers to measures to protect public health and safety, to restore essential government services, and to provide emergency relief to governments, businesses, and individuals affected by the consequences of terrorism. These are carefully described in the FRP's Terrorism Incident Annex.

The DHHS is a signatory agency to the annex, and it has a functional plan that includes threat assessment, consultation, agent identification, epidemiologic investigations, hazard detection and reduction, decontamination, public health support, medical support, and pharmaceutical support operations. At the time of this writing, local metropolitan areas have continued to develop and validate their programs. Health care facilities also need to energize their preparedness efforts and pace to ensure that they can effectively institute their critical link in this chain of preparedness initiatives.

SUMMARY

Today, both natural and manmade disasters continue to grow in magnitude and frequency. These mass casualty–producing events will continue to task medical systems, sometimes beyond their capabilities. The unpredictability of these events, when coupled with proximity variables, will continue to overload the most capable medical facilities. Past and recent events indicate that approximately 60% to 65%

of the injured will self-refer to the closest medical facilities. When these odds are applied to a WMD event or incident, special medical preparedness and capabilities take on a greater importance. To say that the valued medical community must become a part of the solution before an incident or disaster strikes is sufficient. These special medical capabilities must already be in place, and they must be validated routinely. This must be true because the federal medical supplementation may not be an immediate possibility for enhancing the capabilities of first responders. Local medical preparedness remains key if the goal is to save lives, limbs, and eyesight and to avoid unnecessary suffering.

REFERENCES

1. National security decision directive 47. *Emergency mobilization preparedness.* July 22, 1982 (unclassified).
2. Federal Emergency Management Agency. *Federal response plan.* 9230.1-PL. Washington, D.C.: Federal Emergency Management Agency, 1999.
3. Executive order 12148. *Federal emergency management.* July 20, 1979.
4. Executive order 12656. *Assignment of emergency management responsibilities.* November 18, 1988.
5. Presidential decision directive 39. *U.S. policy on counterterrorism,* June 21, 1995.

NATIONAL DISASTER MEDICAL SYSTEM: DISASTER MEDICAL ASSISTANCE TEAMS

ARTHUR G. WALLACE, JR.

Civilian and federal medical planners who were concerned about the ability to respond to the needs of victims of a major disaster developed an initial concept paper in August 1981. It envisioned a single national system that could provide backup support to the Department of Defense (DOD) and that could organize resources to care for civilian victims of major domestic disasters. In December of the same year, the President established the Emergency Mobilization Preparedness Board (EMPB) and twelve Principal Working Groups (PWGs), including the Principle Working Group on Health (PWGH). The board and groups were directed to develop improved policies and programs for national preparedness. Chaired by Edward N. Brandt, the Assistant Secretary for Health in the Department of Health and Human Services, the PWGH designed the system that is in place today—the National Disaster Medical System (NDMS) (1).

Development and continuance of the NDMS was directed to the following four federal agencies: the Department of Health and Human Services (DHHS), the DOD, the Federal Emergency Management Agency (FEMA), and the Department of Veterans Affairs (VA), with DHHS serving as the administrative lead agency. The lead policy official for the DHHS health and medical response is the Assistant Secretary of Health (ASH). The Director of the Office of Emergency Preparedness (OEP) is the action agent, and he or she is responsible for coordinating the implementation of the delivery of health and medical services with partner DHHS agencies. The NDMS is an interagency program that provides a nationwide medical mutual aid system.

NATIONAL DISASTER MEDICAL SYSTEM ORGANIZATION AND PURPOSE

The NDMS has the following three primary functional elements: medical response, patient evacuation, and hospitalization.

Medical response. NDMS responds to a disaster area with Disaster Medical Assistance Teams (DMATs), specialty teams, management support teams (MSTs), medical supplies, and equipment.

Patient evacuation. Arrangements are coordinated for patients who cannot be cared for locally to be evacuated to designated locations throughout the United States.

Hospitalization. NDMS has created a network of hospitals spanning the major metropolitan areas of the country. All hospitals in this network have agreed to accept patients in the event of a national emergency.

The NDMS is designed to care for as many as 100,000 victims of any incident that exceeds the capability of the state, regional, or federal health care system. Some of the events that may require its activation are earthquakes, floods, hurricanes, industrial disasters, a refugee influx, and military casualities from overseas.

NATIONAL DISASTER MEDICAL SYSTEM ACTIVATION

Activation of NDMS may be accomplished by a presidential declaration. This authority is granted by the Robert T. Stafford Disaster Relief and Emergency Assistance Act, commonly referred to as the Stafford Act. When a presidential declaration has not occurred, DHHS, under the Public Health Service Act as amended, may still activate the NDMS (2). In the event of a military contingency, the Assistant Secretary of Defense (Health Affairs) has the authority to activate the NDMS. Individual states may activate health and medical teams that are participating in the NDMS under several emergency conditions. States may choose to activate a health and medical team within their state to augment local resources responding to an emergency event. In addition, states may request health and medical teams from another state when either their own resources are overwhelmed

TABLE 13.1. COMPONENTS OF THE FEDERAL RESPONSE PLAN: EMERGENCY SUPPORT FUNCTIONS

ESF 1	Transportation
ESF 2	Communications
ESF 3	Public works and engineering
ESF 4	Firefighting
ESF 5	Information and planning
ESF 6	Mass care
ESF 7	Resource support
ESF 8	Health and medical services
ESF 9	Urban search and rescue
ESF 10	Hazardous materials
ESF 11	Food
ESF 12	Energy

Abbreviation: ESF, Emergency support function.

and/or they do not have the particular type of resource available in a nearby jurisdiction.

Under the provisions of the Stafford Act, which is often referred to as the Federal Response Plan, the federal government may, when requested, provide assistance to state and local agencies by coordinating relief efforts in those specific areas of need. Within the Stafford Act, specialized response provisions known as emergency support functions (ESFs) exist, delegating the responsibility for these functions to various federal agencies. Twelve ESFs cover various response needs, such as transportation, mass care, communication, and firefighting (Table 13.1).

The DHHS Public Health Service (PHS) is the primary agency for ESF 8, health and medical services. The purpose of ESF 8 is to assist in coordinating a response to supplement state and local agencies in identifying and mitigating public health and medical care needs following a significant natural disaster or manmade event. The scope of ESF 8 includes health assessment and surveillance, medical supplies, victim evacuation, hazards (chemical, biologic, and radiologic), mental health, vector control, victim identification, and mortuary services provided by disaster mortuary operational response teams (DMORTs) and medical care personnel provided by DMATs.

DISASTER MEDICAL ASSISTANCE TEAM

A disaster medical assistance team is a volunteer group of medical and nonmedical individuals, usually from the same state or region of a state, that have formed a response team under the guidance of the PHS. Hospitals, public safety agencies, or local governments sponsor most DMAT teams. The sponsor agrees to recruit, train, and maintain the team. The credentialing of the medical licenses and assisting with maintenance and storage of equipment is part of the sponsorship. Providing a point of contact for NDMS and DMAT administrative issues and releasing the team to PHS for federal disaster service when requested are also expected.

DMATs are often used in local or state disasters to assist with health and medical concerns.

Prospective members apply by completing a federal employment application; the purpose of this is to enable NDMS to place the team members into temporary federal employee status in the event that the federal declaration of a disaster occurs. The process of federalizing team members eliminates a number of issues. Health care personnel are allowed to practice in areas other than where they have licensure; liability issues are covered by the Federal Tort Claims Act; and Federal Workers Compensation Insurance coverage is enabled. In addition, team members are compensated by federal wage guidelines according to their government equivalent pay grade. Transportation to and from a disaster area can also be arranged and provided by the federal government. The temporary federal status is issued only for the duration of the team deployment. Local and state activation of DMATs may or may not be covered by this process, depending on the arrangements with various agencies.

Team Composition

Team composition is quite varied. Typically, the medical personnel include physicians, nurses, nurse practitioners, physician's associates, pharmacists, pharmacy technicians, nurse's aides, mental health specialists, dentists, environmental and laboratory specialists, and emergency medical technicians. Technical or nonmedical members may consist of engineers; radio operators; administrative specialists; and logistic, security, mechanics, and computer specialists. The technical and logistics support group is as important as the medical group. Without these support personnel, the team cannot function. This is also true for each individual on the team—because deployed team sizes are relatively small compared to the assignment, everyone and his or her individual function is vital to the success of the mission. Prospective nonmedical members frequently ask what they might have to offer. Usually, someone who qualifies and who has the energy and desire to be involved will be welcome.

Physical fitness is a requirement because fieldwork usually requires above-average endurance and physical conditioning. Occasionally, extended periods will involve extraordinarily heavy work with long periods of standing, walking, climbing, twisting, bending, and moderate lifting at the pace set by the specific situation. The highest demands of physical activity occur with loading and unloading the equipment, setting up the operations, and taking down the site. In between those times, light-to-moderate physical activity is typically the norm.

Most teams follow the incident command system (ICS) or some local variation thereof in their organizational development. Each team has a unit commander who has the overall responsibility. Delegation of specific duties and responsibilities are given to other members, usually based on their activity level and their experience or by membership election. During activation, an incident commander (IC) is identified. The IC will have the overall responsibility for the deployed team during that particular mission. This position may be filled by the unit commander or another team member. Under the IC are the medical, operations, logistics, communications, and administrative sections, with each section having its own assigned leader.

A typical team size for a deployment may vary according to the mission assignment. Strike teams, a concept developed during the Atlanta 1996 Summer Olympic Games, are five- to six-member squads usually made up of medical personnel that have the capability to move quickly into an affected area to provide limited medical treatment and assessment (3). A full team deployment is expected to be 33 to 35 personnel and is made up of medical, technical, and support personnel. The full team is usually the configuration that is used for a large event like a hurricane or an earthquake.

An example of a team composition for a field response assignment is outlined in Table 13.2; this, of course, can vary according to the situation. The final team composition is guided by the specific health needs of the mission. The entire roster of a team is built on this configuration and has the goal of being at least three deep for every deployed posi-tion so that adequate personnel are available for mobilization when some members may not be able to be present due to the demands of their family, employment, or other situations. The complete roster for some teams ranges from 20 members (level three teams) to 250 members. Individual members selected for deployment are left to the team command; often, a point system is used so that those who participate in training and team functions are usually given first consideration.

Disaster Medical Assistance Team Readiness Levels

The National Disaster Medical System has developed a standardized DMAT evaluation process, using the organizational development, team staffing, training, and the availability of team supplies and equipment. Using this format, the various teams in different stages of development are assigned a readiness level (Table 13.3). Level One status, the

TABLE 13.2. DISASTER MEDICAL ASSISTANCE TEAM COMPOSITION EXAMPLE FOR A FIELD RESPONSE ASSIGNMENT

34 Deploying personnel:
  7 Nonmedical positions
    2 DMAT leaders (may be medical personnel but do not
      count toward fulfilling medical billet) (required)
    1 Safety officer (required)
    1 Administrative or finance chief (required)
    1 Administrative assistant (encouraged)
    1 Logistics chief (required)
    1 Communications officer (required)
  26 Medical positions
    3 Medical officers (required)
    1 Pharmacist (required)
    1 Pharmacy assistant (or second pharmacist) (required)
    2 Supervisory nurse specialists (required)
    6 Staff nurses (required)
    4 Advanced practice nurses or physician assistants
      (encouraged)
    4 Paramedics (encouraged)
    5 Positions determined by DMAT
    1 Home base (nondeployed) support position

Note: Teams should fill the positions with personnel who are qualified to perform the duties of that position; they do not need to be carried in the system in that position; for example, a person may fill in for the day-to-day team leader if they could not deploy or an emergency medical technician could function as the communication officer if he or she was cross-trained. All positions requiring licensing or certification must be filled by personnel holding the appropriate licensing or certification.
Abbreviation: DMAT, Disaster medical assistance team.
From the Department of Health and Human Services, Office of Emergency Preparedness. *Team handbook.* Rockville, MD: United States Public Health Service, 2001, with permission.

TABLE 13.3. UNITED STATES PUBLIC HEALTH SERVICE DISASTER MEDICAL ASSISTANCE TEAMS AND SPECIALTY TEAMS

Level-one teams (including team designation)

Alabama (AL-1)	Arkansas (AR-1)	California (CA-1)
California (CA-2)	California (CA-4)	California (CA-9)
Colorado (CO-2)	Florida (FL-1)	Florida (FL-2)
Florida (FL-5)	Georgia (GA-3)	Hawaii (HI-1)
Indiana (IN-2)	Kentucky (KY-1)	Massachusetts
Michigan (MI-1)	North Carolina (NC-1)	(MA-1)
New Mexico	Ohio (OH-1)	Massachusetts
(NM-1)	Texas (TX-1)	(MA-2)
Rhode Island		Oklahoma (OK-1)
(RI-1)		Washington
Public Health		(WA-1)
Service (PHS-1)		

Level-two teams

California (CA-6)	Florida (FL-3)	New York (NY-4)
New Jersey (NJ-1)	New York (NY-2)	Ohio (OH-5)
Ohio (OH-6)	Pennsylvania (PA-1)	

Level-three teams

Alaska (AK-1)	Alabama (AL-2)	Florida (FL-6)
Georgia (GA-4)	Illinois (IL-1)	Indiana (IN-4)
Missouri (MO-1)	Oregon (OR-1)	South Carolina
Texas (TX-3)	Texas (TX-4)	(SC-1)

Speciality teams

California (CA-3)	California (CA-7)	Georgia (GA-1)
Illinois (IL-2)	Maryland (MD-1)	Pennsylvania
		(PA-2)

Veterinary medical assistance teams (VMATs) 1–4
TST, PST, IST, BST, Massachusetts

This designation represents very fluid classifications. These are the levels at the time of publication; however, they do often change.
Abbreviations: BST, burn special team; DMAT, disaster medical assistance team; IST, international special team; PST, pediatric special team; TST, trauma special team.
From *Personal communication.* Department of Health and Human Services, Office of Emergency Preparedness, Division of Emergency Readiness and Operations, National Disaster Medical System Branch. Rockville, MD, with permission.

highest readiness level, is given to teams that satisfy the requirements of the NDMS process for such a level. Level Two teams may only require staffing, training, or equipment adjustments to advance to Level One. Level Three teams are usually in an early stage of development; they might not have sufficient personnel or equipment to field a full team, but their personnel are used in federal responses, often to fill positions on other deployed teams. Specialty teams that focus on burn, pediatric, mental health, crush injury, and mortuary services also exist.

Disaster Medical Assistance Team Equipment

Because the DMAT's assignments are to disaster areas that have a disrupted infrastructure, each Level One team is expected to be self-sufficient for a 72-hour period. Therefore, the arriving team does not rely on the local resources because they may be quite limited or unavailable. The team must bring its own shelter, power, communications, food, and water to sustain itself for 3 days without outside assistance.

TABLE 13.4. DISASTER MEDICAL ASSISTANCE TEAM PERSONAL EQUIPMENT INVENTORY*

Uniforms
Long underwear (polypropylene)
Heavy jacket (cold-weather type)
Gloves (polypropylene)
Underclothes
Light jacket
Heavy sweater
Rain gear (Gortex-type)
Weather extreme clothing and equipment
Personal safety clothing and equipment
Photo identification and passport
Towel and washcloth
Personal grooming and hygiene kit
Two sets of eyeglasses
Sunglasses
Flashlight
Watch
Hearing protection earplugs (ANSI S.3.9-1974)
Boots (steel toe and shank, water resistant)
Personal funds and credit cards
Bottled water (32–64 oz)
Two-week supply of personal prescription medications, sunscreen, insect repellent, and applicable over-the-counter medications
If subject to working in hazardous area, add the following:
   Hard hat
   Helmet light
   Heavy work gloves (leather)
   Eye protection (ANSI 287.1)

Abbreviations: ANSI, American National Standards Institute; DMAT, Disaster medical assistance team.
*Suggested minimum equipment from the Department of Health and Human Services, Office of Emergency Preparedness. *Team handbook.* Rockville, MD: United States Public Health Service, 2001, with permission.

Shelter for the medical operations, medical equipment, supplies, and pharmaceutical agents also need to be brought with the expectation of treating up to 250 victims per 24-hour period. The field setup is quite similar to a small emergency department with adjacent outpatient clinic capabilities. To perform a field setup, a large amount of equipment must be brought with the team. The *BASIC LOAD*, as it is referred to by NDMS, can occupy at least six military pallets on a cargo aircraft. Included in the load are large commercial tents or military general purpose medium canvas tents, generators and associated power distribution systems, lighting, water purification equipment, water, fuel, and a food supply; the last usually consists of federal meals–ready-to-eat (MREs). Also included are latrines; field showers and sinks; and safety, communications, and computer equipment. The medical equipment includes monitor-defibrillators, ventilators, portable electrocardiography machines, pulse oximeters, small point-of-service laboratory capabilities, minor surgical kits, wound and orthopedic stations, intravenous setups, minor care stations, observation unit supplies, a large cache of medical disposable equipment, and the associated housekeeping equipment. Each team is responsible for the storage and maintenance of these supplies. The packaging, labeling, loading, and unloading of this equipment is the responsibility of each team. Each deploying member must carry his or her own personal gear, with weight limitations of 66 pounds for warm weather and 88 pounds for cold weather conditions. A minimum suggested equipment list is outlined in Table 13.4.

TRAINING

Training plays one of the most important roles in DMAT development. For a collective group that generally does not work together on a daily basis to go into a field situation, to live and work together in close quarters, and to perform quality medical service, ongoing training must occur. In addition to knowing their job function and the teamwork approach, hands-on experience with the basic load supply and the equipment cache provides familiarity with the setup and also allows monitoring of those items that are in need of repair or maintenance.

Training consists of classroom programs, developed by each individual team, and field training with either a partial or a full setup of the operations. NDMS, at its annual conference, offers workshops and training courses for members. At the 1999 conference, a proposed NDMS training program for DMATs was presented. The program was a composite plan created from the plans that individual teams were using for their local training (Table 13.5). When resources permit, the NDMS offers regional field training exercises in which local teams are invited to participate. During these exercises, classroom work and fieldwork are often combined. The training is usually a 3-day to 4-day event encompassing a weekend. The field exercise usually

TABLE 13.5. PROPOSED NATIONAL DISASTER MEDICAL SYSTEM DISASTER MEDICAL ASSISTANCE TEAM TRAINING PROGRAM

Module I (part A): Orientation to federal disaster medical response programs; history of various federal departments that pertain to federal disaster response programs.

Module I (part B): Orientation to the DMAT structure, function, organization, operation, and team standards; federal personnel guidelines; physical fitness standards; and criteria for DMAT levels 1, 2, and 3. Team table of organization and equipment.

Module II: Team field skills; command and control; field stations; aircraft safety; litter obstacle course; rapid shelter deployment; cache lists; equipment and supply storage and management; call down roster; alert, deployment, and demobilization procedures; aircraft cargo guidelines; equipment maintenance; and medical compound configuration. Includes various DMAT configurations for specific missions.

Module III: Personal deployment preparation and field living skills. Didactic portion of necessary skills to prepare DMAT members to live under austere conditions using the standard personal and team equipment.

Module IV: Disaster medical and traumatic emergencies. Team members learn how to make tough decisions about triage categorization, treatment priorities, transportation requirements, and patient-reporting activities.

Module V: Integration of field medical and nonmedical skills. Certain selected support applications will be reviewed with DMAT members for both their own safety and the safety and treatment of the patients.

Module VI: Comprehensive deployment exercise, including logistics and safety operations. DMAT members are provided hands on experience with the team's specialized equipment and supplies. An overnight deployment, irrespective of weather conditions, to simulate austere disaster experiences. Recreated with the design to stress the DMAT member's readiness.

Abbreviation: DMAT, Disaster medical assistance team.
From the Department of Health and Human Services, Office of Emergency Preparedness. *Team handbook.* Rockville, MD: United States Public Health Service, 2001, with permission.

uses mock victims from a disaster scenario. Evaluators follow the victims through the system from the initial contact with rescuers through evacuation to the higher echelon treatment areas. In some areas of the country, the opportunity for exercising with military assets, such as Reserve or National Guard units, is available; these military assets provide quality training involving victim loading and unloading on helicopters and large cargo aircraft.

Individual teams have different amounts of training. The recommended frequency of training sessions varies from two to four times a year. Some approaches to the field exercises have the teams identify a mass gathering event, such as an air show or outside concert. Arrangements are then made with the sponsors of these events to provide medical care to the attendees. The real-time medical encounters add more realism to the training and provide a public display of a local community asset.

Although medical care is the primary focus of training, the logistic and administrative support functions must par-

ticipate equally to develop their skills. With the DMAT operating as a stand-alone unit using internal power and resources, the logistics group deals with issues and problem solving during these real-time drills.

The administrative personnel must remain current on the latest enrollment and updates that are required for team members. The logistics section trains in disaster supply operations, military and civilian air cargo regulations, and certification. Communications operations and procedures are reviewed and practiced during exercises.

During a field training exercise, all members, both medical and nonmedical, have a part in setting up the operations; to establish a free-standing medical unit in a short amount of time takes everyone working together.

Exercises that involve actual patient or victim care may qualify as federally approved training and may allow federal liability and worker compensation to be in effect for that event. Federal exercise status may allow team members to fly on military units for the duration of the event. Federal exercise status is subject to written approval from the NDMS.

FIELD MEDICAL CARE

Activities and Limitations

This section, which is not to be interpreted as guidelines, is based on the author's observation and personal experience, the opinions of others, general common sense, and historical data from previous responses to disasters.

The United States is fortunate not to have suffered a major mass casualty incident similar to those that have occurred in other countries. Medical care is usually available within a reasonable distance for most densely populated locales in this country. Local or regional systems, although they may be temporarily inundated with victims, will likely be capable of delivering emergency medical care. Responding DMATs are not typically onsite soon enough after the impact phase of the disaster to deal with the acutely injured victims. Although the activation of a team from within the affected area may increase the probability of caring for the life-threatening, traumatized victims, this is still an unlikely occurrence. One local DMAT had a 44-member team on site within 6 hours of the 1995 Murrah Federal building bombing in Oklahoma City, but it played a minimal role because the local responders and hospital system had treated all but a few of the survivors within 3 hours of the event (4). Even in larger geographical area disasters, such as the 1999 Oklahoma City tornado, the local system treated most of the acutely affected population within 12 hours (5). Medical team members in the affected areas may be called to duty by their respective agencies in response to the event, thus making them unavailable for the local team. Because of the recognition that this may occur, NDMS activates teams to respond that are outside of the impacted area. This minimizes the compromise of local area assets.

During the postimpact phase, trauma issues usually are a result of recovery and cleanup operations or of delayed medical attention due to inaccessibility. More commonly, long-term health matters, daily urgent medical needs, mental health and stress, environmental and infectious disease concerns, public health issues, and special needs populations will make up the majority of health and medical services provided. Primary medical care will need to be addressed as early as 24 to 48 hours after the impact phase. Knowledge of the background health issues of the affected population is an invaluable tool.

Field medicine should be practiced with the same approach as conventional hospital medicine with an understanding of the limitations involved. Following the usual and customary practices, while realizing that specialty consultants or services may not be immediately available, is appropriate. Radiology and laboratory services may be limited, or they may not be immediately available. Invasive monitoring of patients usually is not possible. The transfer of patients for specialty or intensive care may be delayed, thus requiring those patients to remain onsite. Disposable medical equipment may be in short supply, or it may not be available. Adaptability is the operative word in these situations.

Field Triage

The one truism of field triage is that most victims of disasters will self-refer. They will get to a treatment facility by any means possible without waiting for emergency transport. Knowing this, two caveats prevail. First, two waves of victims are seen; the first wave are those who are ambulatory and who probably have minor injuries, and the second wave will most likely be the more critically injured who are brought by rescue squads. Second, the closest reachable medical facilities will receive the highest number of victims (5). These two facts complicate the efforts of emergency planners to distribute casualties evenly.

Both civilian and military triage categories have been formulated, each with intended agendas of who should receive treatment priority (see Chapter 2). A number of articles and references have been written regarding triage systems and casualty distribution plans (6,6a). With the assumption that a DMAT is assisting in the postimpact phase of a disaster, triage should follow the typical procedure for most emergency departments. Victims are prioritized first by those with immediate threat to life (e.g., airway, hemorrhage, and cardiovascular and neurologic insults). Those without life-threatening or limb-threatening complaints are then triaged to general medical, orthopedic, or wound care. Those who perform triage on a daily basis, such as emergency medical technicians or emergency department nurses, would be the individuals most likely to carry out field triage. A major mass casualty incident may require use of the expectant category (i.e., those victims with extreme conditions who are likely to die without intense intervention). If resources are limited, these victims would be provided with comfort care as much as possible. Currently, this is not an issue in the United States.

Acute Medical Care

Following the customary and usual practices for the emergent medical and trauma patient is appropriate if one keeps in mind the fact that resources and specialty services may be limited. Prolonged resuscitation efforts may prove futile, and they may divert resources and personnel from other victims. In particular, when considering the use of paralytic agents for airway management, one must remember that mechanical ventilator support may be limited. Team members who provide bag ventilation are temporarily removed from the functioning team. Following the stabilization of an acute condition, the patient may not be able to be immediately transferred, thus requiring monitoring and ongoing care at the site.

Aeromedical Evacuation

In the normal daily usage of air evacuation systems, emergency medical services personnel are accustomed to the rotor wing (helicopter) aircraft that carries a large array of monitoring and treatment devices, as well as advanced level paramedics, flight nurses and physicians. These aeromedical units typically transport only one or two patients at a time. If military rotor wing assets are used, one should keep in mind that the purpose of these craft is to move a larger number of patients. The capacity on some military helicopters may be up to seven combined ambulatory or litter patients. However, these airframes are usually sparsely provisioned with basic level EMTs and minimal medical equipment. If patient requirements are greater than the capabilities of the attendants, then a qualified health care provider may be needed to monitor the patients in flight. This health care provider may be provided by the DMAT, which raises the problem of covering for that team member while he or she gone. Additionally, the logistics of returning the team member to the DMAT following the flight must be worked out in advance. Problems that cannot be addressed may develop in unstable victims. Moreover, loading and unloading these aircraft can be a hazardous adventure as it is often performed while the rotors are turning. Proper training in these procedures for the DMAT team members by qualified flight crews is highly recommended. Fixed wing military aircraft are another asset that may be used, and the same concerns apply to patient selection, crew and equipment, and safety concerns regarding the loading and unloading of patients.

The physiologic changes that occur in flight due to decreased oxygen concentrations, the decreasing and increasing atmospheric pressure and its effects on the gas-containing structures of the body, the gravitational forces associated with takeoff and landing, and the changes of attitude of fixed wing aircraft must all be considered when using this mode of patient transport (7).

Wounds

As in all of medicine, different authors have varying opinions on wound management. Some believe that all wounds treated in disaster situations should be treated by delayed primary closure (i.e., left open, cleansed, and rechecked with closure occurring at a later date when infection has been either treated or ruled out). Others use knowledge of when the wound occurred to guide clinical treatment (see Chapter 17 for alternative views). For instance, if the injury occurred during the impact phase of a disaster, especially in a high wind event (e.g., tornado), it could be contaminated with an unsuspected bacterial species (e.g., *Clostridia perfringens*) and delayed primary closure may be indicated (8,9). Postimpact phase injuries occurring during clean up, if they are seen early and have minimal contamination, may be handled as a routine emergency wound.

Infectious Diseases

If a pathogen for an infectious disease was not present in the affected area before the event and is not introduced after the disaster, then that disease should not occur (see Chapter 4)(10). Communicable diseases (e.g., measles, respiratory infections) present in the community, however, may show an increased incidence, especially if mass care in close living conditions is necessary. Contaminated water supply and food spoilage may increase the cases of enteric infections. Standing water and garbage may act as a source for vector-transmitted infections. These medical issues usually become evident in the postimpact phase of a disaster. Understanding the health concerns and endemic diseases of the region before and during deployment is essential (10).

DEPLOYMENT

DMAT deployments have been increasing since the inception of the system. The first large-scale mobilization of NDMS occurred in response to Hurricane Andrew in 1992. This occurred just as the NDMS annual meeting was beginning in Oklahoma City (11). On the first day of the conference, many of the team leaders were quickly assembled and were briefed on the impending activation and then left for their home bases to begin the preparation of their teams for deployment. Most of the NDMS officials were present for the conference, and a makeshift emergency operations center (EOC) was established at the hotel hosting the conference.

The areas of DMAT use have also expanded. What was originally a plan to provide medical teams to respond to a major earthquake has now grown to include missions involving medical care in a number of circumstances. Responses have included natural disasters such as flooding, tornadoes, wildfires, ice storms, hurricanes, and earthquakes. Public health responses have included medical care

for refugees; one recent deployment was a 10-week mission providing medical services to the Kosovo population at Fort Dix, New Jersey. An airline crash in Guam in late 1998 deployed components of a DMAT to support the mortuary response team or DMORT. Teams have also been placed as a standby asset in high profile mass gatherings, such as the 1996 Atlanta Summer Olympic Games, high-level government summits, and other similar activities. DMATs are currently capable of deploying to any of the states or United States territories. In addition, international deployment capabilities have been reviewed.

Deployment Phases

Three stages of readiness exist when a federal deployment is anticipated. An advisory stage consists of the time when a team is notified that a situation has occurred or will occur that may require a team mobilization. Following this, an alert may be issued to the team, meaning that imminent deployment is expected. Activation is the final stage when the team receives travel orders and a mission assignment. All of these stages can occur simultaneously, or they may be prolonged over a period of days or longer. At any point, a team can be placed on "stand down," and all deployment activity stops. A team on alert status is expected to be at a point of departure (POD) and ready for deployment within four to eight hours. Throughout the year, the Level One teams rotate being on first call for the various areas of the country on a monthly basis.

When an advisory is received, most teams do a preliminary call up of personnel to see who is available. Packaging of equipment and supplies usually takes place during this stage. Alert status brings the likelihood of mobilizing, and a final team roster is produced and forwarded to NDMS along with the inventory of what is being transported with the team. Earlier in this progression of events, the OEP has established a 24-hour EOC at the NDMS headquarters in Rockville, Maryland. The OEP is the coordinating governmental agency for the DMATs on a daily basis and during a declared emergency.

Deployment Missions

Activation will mobilize a team, if not to the mission destination, at least to the local airport awaiting final assignment. A number of missions are possible. The DMAT could function as a casualty collection point with operations set up within or close to the affected area to receive and treat victims and to determine who needs to continue through the system for evacuation out of the area. Another assignment could be the regional evacuation point where it is collocated with a military air-medical staging facility; here, victims are prepared for airlift. Multiple DMATs can be brought together to provide a higher level of medical capability in the form of an NDMS clearing staging unit. Three DMATs are assembled to form a clearing staging unit.

Recent deployments have placed three teams plus a management support team (MST) in a staging position close to an impacted area. The MST is the command and control component in the field directing the responding teams on mission needs. The "MST plus three" concept is called a "push package." These packages can be placed in strategic locations before a slow impact disaster. This strategy was used in the responses to Hurricanes Brett and Floyd in late 1999 (12).

Team Health and Safety

Team leaders must watch for and recognize stress, both environmental and mental, and must monitor for illness and injury among the members. Any team member who becomes ill or injured becomes a priority patient. Prevention and safety play a key role in keeping the deployed team healthy. Safety officers with each team must ensure that the members are using hearing protection and gloves, as well as other personal protective equipment when indicated. A high amount of physical exertion is required to get the operations going, and this often occurs in adverse environmental conditions. Attention to fluid balances, rest breaks, and a paced approach may avoid injury and illness early in the mission. As the mission proceeds, lack of sleep, missed meals, long shifts, and exposure to contagious agents may result in some members acquiring respiratory infections. Different food and water sources may lead to gastrointestinal disorders. Musculoskeletal and dermatologic disorders may occur from heavy work, repetitive activity, and exposure to moisture and heat. A team medical cache that is used only for members should always be available, and medical attention to members should be provided on a priority basis. Toward the end of a mission, excitement has turned to exhaustion and the gung-ho attitude has come and gone. The take down and repackaging at the completion of a mission are physical and laborious. Thus, surveillance for illness and injury is an ongoing and continuous duty.

At the completion of a mission, the equipment and supplies need to be cleaned, restocked, and made ready to return the team to a readiness level. A review of the deployment is conducted, and after-action reports are generated. These assist with identifying and correcting problems that have been encountered.

SUMMARY

The NDMS is a federally coordinated system that augments the nation's emergency medical response capability. The overall purpose of the NDMS is to establish a single, integrated national medical response capability to assist state and local authorities in dealing with the medical and health effects of major peacetime disasters or armed conflicts. The DMAT is a mission-oriented volunteer organization of health professionals and support staff. It is a key asset of NDMS that can augment or replace local medical infrastructure following a disaster.

AFTERWORD: SEPTEMBER 11, 2001

Tuesday morning on September 11, the city of New York suffered an unbelievable and devastating attack when hijacked airliners struck the World Trade Center buildings. Within an hour, the Pentagon was also attacked in a similar fashion. Another airliner, apparently diverted from its intended target by onboard passengers, crashed into a field near Pittsburgh, Pennsylvania.

The loss of life was expected to be enormous, and the number of injured was anticipated to number into the thousands. The city of New York activated its OEM; the New York City Health Department and area hospitals activated their disaster plans. The New York police, fire, and emergency medical services responded to the site, establishing numerous triage and treatment areas. In addition, an overwhelming turnout of volunteer medical and nonmedical personnel responded to the World Trade Center (WTC) site.

During the hours following the initial impact while rescue, triage, and treatment operations were ongoing, the buildings of the WTC collapsed on many of the rescuers and remaining victims.

In response to the terrorist attacks, DHHS Secretary Tommy Thompson requested that the NDMS be prepared to provide assistance. In anticipation of an extensive and long-term mission and still ignorant of what other areas of the country might be requesting assistance, the NDMS placed all DMATs on advisory status. This was the first nationwide activation of the system.

FEMA immediately activated urban search and rescue teams. These self-contained teams, using search canines and sophisticated equipment, specialize in the rescue and recovery of entrapped victims. DMORTs were also activated to provide family assistance and to assist with the identification of remains. The commissioned corps readiness force was placed on advisory status. Veterinary medical assistance teams were activated to respond and care for the animals on site that were involved with the rescue and recovery efforts. The national pharmaceutical stockpile, containing pharmaceutical agents and wound and emergency treatment equipment, was delivered to New York City. The Centers for Disease Control and Prevention placed an epidemiologist in New York City to conduct medical surveillance.

The few months following the September 11 attack found the PHS conducting many varied operational missions in numerous locations throughout the country. A summation of DMAT operations is presented in Table 13.6.

On the day of the attack, NDMS mobilized the Georgia-3, North Carolina-1, and PHS-1 DMATs and the national medical response team–east (NMRT-E) to stage in the Washington, D.C. area. The NMRT is an NDMS-sponsored team specializing in victim evaluation and the decontamination of chemical-biologic-nuclear threats. At the same time, Massachusetts-1, Massachusetts-2, New Jersey-1, New York-2, and Rhode Island-1 DMATs were staged just outside New York City, while the MST from the PHS OEP

TABLE 13.6. NATIONAL DISASTER MEDICAL SYSTEM AND THE WORLD TRADE CENTER DISASTER, SEPTEMBER 2001

First-in teams: New Jersey-1, New York-2, Rhode Island-1, Massachusetts 1 and 2
Mid September: Florida-1, CCRF, PHS-1, California-2
Late September: Michigan-1, Florida-2, Alaska-1
Early October: New Mexico-1, Georgia-3, Arkansas-1
Late October: Alabama-1, California-6, Oklahoma-1
Early November: California-9, Texas-1, Washington-1
Mid November: Ohio-1, Oregon-2, Pennsyvania-1
Late November: California-4
Teams supporting all operations: Nearly every DMAT within the NDMS provided resources in support of the response to the September 11 terrorist attacks.

Abbreviations: CCRF, Commissioned Corps Readiness Force; DMAT, disaster medical assistance team; NDMS, National Disaster Medical System; PHS, Public Health Service.
From the United States Public Health Service, National Disaster Medical System, Office of Emergency Preparedness. *WTC-NYC*, 2001, with permission.

developed an operational plan. As the request for assistance came from New York City, the staged DMATs moved into the WTC site, setting up triage and treatment operations, initially just outside of the perimeter and then advancing closer to the site as debris was removed. Because the Pentagon site was being handled by the military, the responding DMATs stood down.

The rotation of DMATs to the WTC site went on for the following 10 weeks using various sizes and configurations of teams. Initially, the size of the incoming DMATs was 44 members per team, with an emphasis on medical personnel. When the number of operational sites was reduced, the team size went to 16.

In the first few days of the mission, five treatment sites were established. They were College Command, AMEX (west treatment), Liberty (Plaza), Church St., and Liberty Command, identified by the street on which they were located or the building occupied. The Liberty and Church sites were freestanding tents with power and heat supply. The AMEX and College sites were within buildings. The Church St. site changed often from tent to inside a building and then back to a tent. Each site was equipped similar to a small emergency department with advanced cardiac life support and advanced trauma life support capabilities with physician, nurse, physician's assistant, and EMT coverage on a 24-hour basis. Each team had their logistics and administrative support group on site as well. In early October, the original five treatment sites were reduced to three, with the forward element command moving from College to the Liberty location, all on the perimeter of the WTC site.

The medical treatment was focused on providing care for the many rescue personnel on site—at times, estimated to be 5,000 or more at one time—who were working in an extremely hazardous environment. In doing this, the DMATs relieved the local EMS and hospital emergency departments from a sustained influx of rescuers as patients, while remaining ready to assist with any victims that might have been found. Those treated included construction workers, New York City firefighters, New York City police, Red Cross workers, visitors to the site, and others. The local EMS had units located close to each treatment area to assist with transports out.

Illness and injury types seen by the DMATs included abrasions, blisters, burns, chest pains, contusions, dehydration, fractures, headache, lacerations, lung irritation, stress, eye injury, strains, and sprains. As part of the surveillance plan, data were sent every few hours to the New York City Health Department from the DMAT sites, as well as from hospital emergency departments; this data included certain symptoms and complaints of patients working at the site in order to identify any trends of health problems. More than 9,000 persons received care at the DMAT sites; Fig. 13.1 shows treatment on scene compared to those getting treatment at local emergency departments during the first full week of operations.

In addition to the onsite triage and treatment centers, the NDMS system provided over 50 burn specialty nurses on a rotating basis to the Cornell Presbyterian Hospital

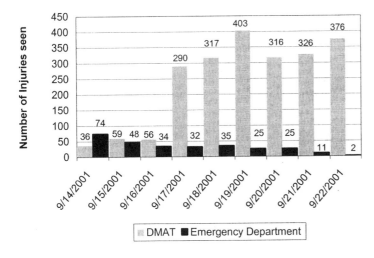

FIGURE 13.1. World Trade Center disaster. Patients seen by disaster medical assistance team (DMAT) versus hospital emergency departments. From United States Public Health Service, Office of Emergency Preparedness, Management Support Team. *WTC-NYC*. Rockville, MD: United States Public Health Service, 2001, with permission.

Burn Center. These personnel assets filled a critical need for the victims of the September 11 attacks.

The data demonstrate that proper use of these teams reduced the resource utilization and patient volume on the local EMS and hospital emergency departments, which were already stressed from dealing with the impact phase of a disaster.

REFERENCES

1. *National disaster medical system: concept of operations.* Concept paper. January 1991.
2. *Public Health Service Act,* 42 USC 243 (c)(1); 42 USC 243 (c)(2); 42 USC 319, 1985.
3. Sharp TW, Brennan RJ, Keim M. Medical preparedness for a terrorist incident involving chemical or biological agents during the 1996 Atlanta Olympic Games. *Ann Emerg Med* 1998;32:214–223.
4. Hogan DE, Waeckerle JF, Dire DJ, et al. Emergency department impact of the Oklahoma City terrorist bombing. *Ann Emerg Med* 1999;34:160–170.
5. Hogan DE, Askins DC, Osburn AE. The May 3, 1999 tornado in Oklahoma City [Editorial]. *Ann Emerg Med* 1999;34:225–226.
6. Benson M, Koenig KL, Schultz CH. Disaster triage: START, then SAVE. A new method of dynamic triage for victims of a catastrophic earthquake. *Prehospital Disaster Med* 1996;11:117–124.
6a. Auf der Heide E. Triage. In: *Disaster response: principles of preparation and coordination.* St. Louis, MO: CV Mosby, 1989:165–194.
7. United States Army Health Services Command. *Aero medical evacuation.* 28-2038-4. Washington, D.C.: United States Army Health Services Command, 1980.
8. Ivy J. Infections encountered in tornado and automobile accident victims. *J Indiana State Med Assoc* 1968;61:1657.
9. Raker JW, Wallace AFC, Rayner JF. *Emergency medical care in disaster. A summary of recorded experience.* Publication no. 457. Washington, D.C.: National Academy of Sciences, National Research Council, 1956.
10. United States Department of Health and Human Services, United States Public Health Services, Centers for Disease Control and Prevention. *The public health consequences of disasters 1989.* Atlanta, GA: Centers for Disease Control and Prevention monograph, 1989.
11. Alson R, Alexander D, Leonard RB, et al. Analysis of medical treatment at a field hospital following hurricane Andrew, 1992. *Ann Emerg Med* 1993;22:172.
12. Department of Health and Human Services, United States Public Health Service, Office of Emergency Preparedness, Emergency Operations Center, Rockville, Maryland. *Hurricane Floyd. Situation reports nos. 1–13.* Rockville, MD: Department of Health and Human Services, September 1999.

COMMUNICATION AND INFORMATION TECHNOLOGY TOOLS FOR DISASTER RESPONSE AND MEDICAL ASSISTANCE

VICTORIA GARSHNEK
FREDERICK M. BURKLE, JR.

THE DISASTER COMMUNICATIONS CHALLENGE

Disasters are extreme events. Whether natural events or manmade crises, they cause significant disruption and put lives and property at risk. Thus, they require an immediate response and a coordinated application of resources, facilities, and efforts beyond those regularly available to handle routine needs. Of all the problems experienced during disaster events, one of the most serious centers on *communication*, specifically, the lack of appropriate means to collect, process, and transmit important information efficiently in the midst of a disaster. If accurate and timely information can be made available, needless morbidity and mortality might be prevented. Thus, the establishment (or reestablishment) of efficient and reliable communications systems is one of the most important challenges that is faced.

Within the potential disaster area, the communications infrastructures often function perfectly well in the *normal* preevent environment or provide adequate capability to address everyday, minor emergencies when information needs are not complicated and only one or several agencies are involved in a localized occurrence. However, a disaster can be responsible for creating an *abnormal* communications environment in which the emergency responders must function. In this environment, the reliability and timeliness of information are now more important than ever and are also more difficult to obtain. In addition, the frequent use of single chain notification paths, which, if broken, can result in the disruption of critical information flow, may further complicate matters. Multiple path communications and redundancy have now become essential technology considerations. What is important is that critical information gets through.

Over the past two decades, a variety of telecommunications technologies have been used for humanitarian assistance and disaster medical response (1–4). Lessons that have been learned have provided important insight into the challenges and scope of utility for disaster and humanitarian applications. For example, emergency communications systems should have the ability to be quickly prepared and installed in areas where terrestrial communications lines or systems are either unreliable, damaged, or nonexistent and speed and efficiency are important for establishing contact with the outside world. This contact could be as simple as a voice lifeline, or it could be as advanced as an Internet link or broadcast quality video/audio transmission. Ideally, systems should be compact, reliably powered, easy to use, easy to repair, lightweight, rugged, and highly mobile or transportable. Disaster communications systems may not need to be special or sophisticated to deliver the required benefit. The major challenge is to match the right communications and contingency systems with a given disaster plan or scenario. Another important challenge is the ability to assess and manipulate acquired abstract information and to communicate essential results where and when they are needed.

While the recognition exists that the communications capabilities taken for granted every day can be lost in a matter of minutes during a disaster, a more effective use of existing technologies, as well as the implementation of new technologies, are important steps toward improving disaster response to save lives. This chapter explores existing and new telecommunication and information technologies and their advantages, disadvantages, and utility to disaster management and disaster medicine needs.

BASIC COMMUNICATION INFORMATION PATHWAYS

The telecommunications infrastructure provides the technology to move information electronically between geographically dispersed locations. In simple terms, it provides the conducting pathway to move electronic information. The pathway that is used is determined in large part by the available infrastructure and required capability. The pathway can take the form of any of the following:

- Land lines (single or twisted pairs of metallic wires, coaxial tubes, or fiberoptic cable);
- Air waves (radio, microwave, or television broadcast);
- Satellite link.

Tables 14.1, 14.2, and 14.3 provide descriptions of the basic telecommunication infrastructures and related information (capabilities, types of data or information transferred, advantages, disadvantages, and potential damage from disasters that can render the system useless) (5,6).

The bandwidth or bit rate of the transmission medium (terms that are used to refer to the amount of information that may be sent per unit of time) is a limiting factor on the type of telecommunication system that may be used. For example, narrow bandwidth systems, such as plain old telephone systems (POTS), are relatively inexpensive to oper-

ate, but they lack the capacity to transmit high quality full-motion video (5). Broad bandwidth networks, including fiberoptic cable and many satellite systems, are capable of carrying sufficient data to permit the use of interactive, high quality, full-motion video.

Land lines provide the links between nodes in telecommunications networks and offer point-to-point transmission along a wire or fiberoptic cable medium. Metallic twisted pairs are the most common transmission media for telephone networks. Subscriber loops consist almost exclusively of twisted pairs contained in cables. Coaxial tubes provide a higher bandwidth than twisted pairs and thus allow many channels to be carried on the same tube through multiplexing (6).

Fiberoptic communications links transmit light waves through glass fibers and offer an advantage over wire because of their high bandwidth and protection against electrical interference. With optical fibers, electrical signals

TABLE 14.1. TELECOMMUNICATION INFRASTRUCTURE: LAND LINES (GROUND OR SURFACE)

System type	Telephone (POTS)	Switched 56/64	ISDN	Fractional T-1	T-1	T-3
Frequency bands (or bandwidth)	4.8 bps or 3.3 Kbps	56/64 Kbps	$n \times 64$ Kbps or 1.544 Mbps	56 Kbps– 1.544 Mbps	1.544 Mbps	45 Mbps
Line type	Copper telephone lines	Copper or fiberoptic cable	Copper or fiberoptic cable	Copper or fiberoptic cable	Fiberoptic cable	Fiberoptic cable (28 T-1 lines)
Information transmitted	Voice, fax, data; still image video combined with real-time voice; store and forward e-mail; limited interactive motion video. Dial-up capability.	Telephone plus low-resolution, interactive motion video. Dial-up capability as needed.	Switched plus higher resolution, interactive motion video. Dial-up capability as needed.	ISDN except for dial-up. Dedicated line only.	Same as fractional T-1. Dedicated line only.	T-1 plus higher resolution, full motion interactive video. Dedicated line only.
Fixed or mobile	F (limited cordless. mobility. Additional mobility if combined with satellite van).	F (some mobility if combined with satellite van).	Same as switched.	Same as switched.	Same as switched.	Same as switched.
Advantages	Relatively inexpensive; familiar technology.	Larger bandwidth than POTS and cheaper than ISDN. as needed (cost-effective).	Bandwidth on demand; switched dial-up service	Dynamic bandwidth utilization (burst traffic to higher bandwidth)	Fully dedicated bandwidth between points. transmission time.	Fully dedicated bandwidth, more bandwidth, faster
Disadvantages	Limited capability and transmission speed. Dependent on existing (functioning) terrestrial system.	Not available in all areas. Dependent on existing (functioning) terrestrial system.	Not available in all areas; more expensive than previous. Dependent on existing (functioning) terrestrial system. Difficult to install on short notice.	Not available in all areas. Expensive (dedicated line, bandwidth related to line charges). Dependent on functioning terrestrial system. Difficult to install on short notice.	Same as fractional T-1.	Same as fractional T-1.
Affected by disaster?	Telephone lines may be overloaded; lines and electrical control center can be damaged in natural disaster.	Lines and electrical control center can be damaged in natural disaster.	Same as switched.	Same as switched.	Same as switched.	Same as switched.

Abbreviations: bps, bits per second; F, fixed; ISDN, integrated services digital network; Kbps, kilo bits per second; M, mobile; Mbps, mega bits per second; POTS, plain old telephone system.

TABLE 14.2. TELECOMMUNICATION INFRASTRUCTURE: AIRWAVES

System type	Radio AM/FM	Amateur shortwave radio	Radio pager (ground-based)	Broadcast television	Cellular telephone (ground-based)	Microwave
Frequency bands (or bandwidth)	1–100 MHz	Wide range (commonly 144–148 MHz)	160 MHz	Channels in range of 50–500 MHz (excluding aeronautical nav/com freq.)	829–849 MHz	1–40 GHz
Terminal type	Radio tower	Tower	Tower	Tower/dish	Cell tower	Tower/dish
Information transmitted	Voice/audio	Digital data, voice/audio, slow scan TV, radio-teletype, computer data exchange.	Data display and storage, numeric and text messages (some voice/e-mail).	Video, audio	Voice/audio, data, fax, voicemail, e-mail, internet.	Point-to-point communications of video, audio, telephone, fax, and data.
Fixed/mobile	F or M	F or M	M	F or M	M	F
Advantages	Independent of local telephone and electrical infrastructures (use battery power or backup generators), on-site voice communications.	Can augment normal communications in times of disaster. Long distance possible (up to hundreds or thousands of km). Amateur groups organized for emergency assistance.	Simultaneous paging possible; repeated transmission with single call; constant 24 hr/d contact; small, compact, and operates for weeks on small battery	Wide broadcast of emergency information possible.	Two-way simultaneous conversations possible; voice command dialing possible on some systems. Wide range mobility.	Cost-effective and reliable (if well engineered). Good for temporary or emergency restoration of facilities.
Disadvantages	Incompatibility with other agencies using other frequency bands. Interference due to nonavailable or crowded frequencies. Half-duplex (i.e., one person speaks at a time).	Special license, equipment, and skills necessary. Half-duplex communication. Relies on volunteers. Interference due to nonavailable or crowded frequencies.	Partial reliance on ground-based systems; only one-way alerting systems (may become two-way in future). Limited data transfer. If radio signal is blocked, sender may not know.	Expensive; not intended for directional transmission.	Expensive with extensive use; media interference; no exclusive frequency during emergencies; obstacle interference; eavesdropping possible; limited transmission speed.	Line-of-site limitations; limited range (repeaters needed). Transmission sensitive to weather (rain, fog, snow, hail) and distortion from object reflection.
Affected by disaster?	Towers, stations, and repeaters can be damaged in severe natural disaster.	Can maintain operation under a variety of natural disaster circumstances and, at times, has been the sole communication link.	Radio base stations (or their power supply) can be damaged in severe natural disaster. If phone system damaged, cannot send page.	Towers, dishes, and stations can be damaged in severe natural disaster.	Base stations, cells, and links can be damaged in severe natural disaster.	Stations, electronics, and power supply can be damaged in disaster. Failure possible in bad atmospheric conditions.

Abbreviations: F, fixed; freq., frequency; GHz, gigahertz; M, mobile; MHz, megahertz; nav/com, navigation/communication; TV, television.

are converted into light waves that are transmitted along the optical fiber and then converted back into electrical signals at the other end. The optical fibers, or lightguides, are bundled into a cable. Cables with 48 to 144 fibers are used in long-distance telephone networks, and cables with about 12 fibers are found in local networks. Where fiber is feasible, it clearly offers excellent service. The disadvantages related to disaster management are that it cannot attach to anything that moves, it cannot economically reach remote locations, and it cannot broadcast a signal simultaneously to all parts of a continent. To meet these needs, radio and satellite media are used (6).

Radio links differ from land lines in that radio signals propagate through free space and commonly use higher frequencies than line signals. They are mostly used for broad-

casting and for point-to-point communications. The entire frequency range from approximately 10 KHz to several gigahertz is available. Several different forms of radio links are used in communications networks. Microwave radio links (links using frequencies greater than 1 GHz) are used in terrestrial short-haul and long-haul links, as well as in satellite links. Cellular radio and other forms of mobile radio communications use frequencies between 30 MHz and 1 GHz. The exact frequency band alloted depends on the geographical location and the regulatory frequency allocation.

Mobile communications links, such as ship-to-shore and airplane-to-ground, operate in the high-frequency (HF) radio band. Radios provide a means of communication that is essentially independent of the local telephone and electric

TABLE 14.3. TELECOMMUNICATION INFRASTRUCTURE: SATELLITE LINK

System type	Fixed satellite service	Direct broadcast satellites	Mobile satellite (GEO)	Big LEO	Little LEO	Broad/band GEO	Broad/band LEO
Frequency bands (or bandwidth)	C and Ku C = 3.700–4.2 GHz (downlink); 5.925–6.425 GHz (uplink)	Ku Ku = 11.7–12.7 GHz (downlink); 14–17.8 GHz (uplink)	L and S L = 1.530–2.700 GHz; S = 2.700–3.500 GHz	L and S	P and below P = 0.230–1.000 GHz	Ka and Ku Ka = 18–31 GHz	Ka and Ku
Terminal type	Dish 0.5 m and larger. Fixed Earth station.	Dish 0.3–0.6 m. Fixed Earth station.	Laptop computer with antenna-mount (but mobile).	Terminals are cellular telephones and pagers; fixed telephone booth.	Terminal size of playing card; omni-directional.	20 cm, fixed.	Dual 20 cm tracking antennas (fixed).
Information transmitted	Video delivery; VSAT; news gathering; radio, telephone, TV (cable and broadcast); data networks.	Direct-to-home video; audio and computer data.	Voice and low speed data to mobile terminals.	Voice, messaging, fax, data; PC integrated for limited multimedia e-mail.	Position location; tracking; messaging.	Internet access; voice, video, data.	High-speed image transfer; data; video. Multimedia e-mail, interactive video.
Fixed/mobile	F	F	M	F or M	M	F	F
Advantages	Practical alternative to ground-based networks for fixed areas.	Transmitted information received directly from satellites on small fixed dish.	Requires few satellites to cover globe; well-known technology.	Very low latency (sub 0.03-sec roundtrip).	Same as Big LEO.	Broadband; bandwidth on demand.	Very low latency (sub 0.03-sec round trip). Broadband; bandwidth on demand.
Disadvantages	High latency (0.24-sec round trip—not ideal for interactive use).	More expensive than cable; decodes one channel at a time (without second converter); lack of local channels; digital artifacts; outages possible in thunderstorm.	High latency (0.24 sec—not ideal for real-time); limited orbital slots above each country; no polar coverage.	Requires many satellites (dozens to hundreds) to cover globe. Narrow band, relatively low data transfer rate.	Requires many satellites (dozens to hundreds) to cover globe; limited services.	High latency (0.24 sec—not ideal for real-time); limited number of orbital slots above each country; no polar coverage.	Requires many satellites (dozens to hundreds) to cover globe.
Affected by disaster?	Fixed earth station may become disabled in severe natural disaster.	Fixed earth station may become disabled in severe natural disaster.	Little possibility of damage (mobile terminal).	Same as direct broadcast satellite.	Same as direct broadcast satellite.	Fixed terminal may become damaged in disaster.	External terminal may become damaged in disaster.

Abbreviations: F, fixed; GEO, geosynchronous Earth orbit; LEO, low Earth orbit; M, mobile; PC, personal computer; TV, television; VSAT, very small aperture terminal.

infrastructures. Consequently, damage to these infrastructures as a result of disaster has minimal effect on radio communications. However, damage to radio towers, base stations, and repeaters can disable the communication (5–7).

Satellites serve places that fiber and copper wire cannot reach. Also, satellites are a broadcast medium while fiber is point to point. Satellites offer a method of long-distance communication when other means, such as land line or cellular telephone service, are destroyed by disaster or, as in many developing countries, are nonexistent or inadequate (6,8,9).

At least the following three elements are necessary to establish effective satellite communications from one site to the outside world: a satellite terminal to transmit and receive communications at the originating site, satellites and satellite services to relay the communications between the site and distant locations, and satellite gateways at distant locations to receive and transmit communications and to provide an interface with telephone or other communications networks.

The greatest advantage that satellites offer to disaster communications is their independence from the local communications infrastructure that may be nonexistent, damaged, or destroyed in a disaster. However, these advantages come at a great cost. Previously, satellite terminals have cost thousands to tens of thousands of dollars, with additional costs for satellite services and maintenance (8,10). Consequently, governments, large aid organizations, and the media have had primary access to satellite resources. Some communities and even some developing countries have not been able to afford their own emergency equipment and, therefore, have relied on outside agencies for assistance. Fortunately, lower costs are found with the more portable satellite terminals evolving into the 21st century (9,11).

In the past, even the smallest satellite terminals lacked the truly personal use that portable cellular products had achieved. Two approaches addressing the portability issue have emerged with regard to satellite systems. One approach continues along the line of geostationary satellite development. In previous years, all commercial communication satellites were geostationary (a satellite is placed in a geosynchronous Earth orbit [GEO] 22,300 miles [42,164 km] directly over the earth's equator; it appears to be stationary in the sky, turning synchronously with the earth) (9,12). Due to the long transmission distances between the Earth and geostationary satellites, gateway facilities had to be relatively powerful, thus requiring fixed facilities with large antennas. The solution for portability is to design larger, more powerful satellites that in turn require smaller (handheld) earthbound terminals (9,13). The other approach requires the use of an array of multiple nongeostationary satellites in low Earth orbit (LEO) (9). Because LEO satellites are much closer to Earth than geostationary satellites, the power requirements are reduced and handheld terminals about the size and weight of

portable cellular telephones are adequate for communicating via satellite (14,15). In the context of disaster communication, portable communication via satellite could offer immediate, reliable, and personalized communications for disaster responders, regardless of the severity and magnitude of the surrounding damage.

LEO satellites that provide "bandwidth on demand" are also an important asset for the 21st century, making high-speed data communications at up to 1.2 billion bits per second, broadband Internet access, and real-time videoconferencing available anywhere on the globe (this is the satellite equivalent of fiberoptics) (16). This is a fixed (stationary or permanently mounted) system, rather than a mobile (handheld or portable) system (the system is referred to as an Earth station; it contains radio equipment, an antenna, and satellite communication control circuitry that is used to provide access from terrestrial circuits to satellite capacity).

The advent of LEO communications satellites is a significant event, and it potentially can knit the world together with basic communications (although it is not intended to replace terrestrial circuits). On the most basic level, individuals will acquire the capability to have one cellular telephone that will operate anywhere in the world. In the midst of a disaster, even if the surroundings are totally leveled, a pocket cellular telephone user subscribing to a global LEO service can make an immediate call for help to any telephone on the planet. The major impact on disaster management is that the lack of communications no longer need to be the *paralyzing* agent in a disaster scenario.

What types of disaster medicine capabilities would be possible with satellite systems discussed here? With a LEO satellite mobile phone type system, voice, position, data, and fax can be transmitted. When connected to a personal computer (PC) (or a smaller laptop or pocket computer), spreadsheets and e-mail, as well as slow image or graphic, transfer can occur. For telemedicine use, these mobile telephones with computer interfaces can be used in the field to assist on-site workers with triage or medical advice through voice link with physicians at medical facilities and can provide a slow, but reliable, data or image transfer to medical facilities if necessary. Although limited in bandwidth, the tradeoff here would be compact mobile convenience with immediate voice communication at the cost of slow image and data transfer. For first responders in a disaster, a reliable phone voice-link may be all that is needed to communicate an initial assessment and to order appropriate medical supplies and support to the site (17). The mobile nature of these telephones and their independence from the damaged ground infrastructures make taking them directly into the field without prior preparation or setup ideal.

The "bandwidth on demand" type systems, which are rather fixed, may play an important role at a later point in the disaster flow of events by enabling a web-based, multimedia e-mail telemedicine consultation that is independent of the ground infrastructure damage. Hospitals can be equipped with the appropriate terminals and antennae well in advance as part of their emergency response system, while relief medical personnel can establish a wireless system near the disaster site where the casualties would reside. Uninterrupted medical communications could then be provided.

INFORMATION TECHNOLOGY AND DISASTER MANAGEMENT

The management, analysis, and communication of information are a challenge during a disaster. What is urgently needed are systems that reduce the information burden of disaster management and that allow the rapid entry and retrieval of notes, rapid ordering and reporting of findings, and easy and timely access to current literature, databases, and help-aids (decision support systems). The 21st century is a critical developmental period for disaster management interests in information technology. The administrative, resource management, and science and research arms of disaster management will all be affected by the growing prominence of artificial intelligence, modeling, virtual reality, the Internet, the world wide web, and computer miniaturization.

Artificial Intelligence and Decision Support Systems

For disaster applications, a useful decision support device must be easy to use and must usefully *enhance* the judgment of the user. A device that simply models the decision making behavior of the user is likely to be of limited use. Artificial intelligence (AI) provides practical and medically applicable intellectual processing capabilities. In disaster medical situations where time is especially valuable, AI systems could be the critical decision time saver that makes a significant difference in the medical outcome of casualties.

Artificial Neural Networks

An important goal of AI research is to develop computers that can learn from experience. As part of working toward this goal, a set of techniques, which offer the potential to alter the way in which knowledge is discovered and represented, have been developed in the field of machine learning. One method of particular interest is the artificial neural network (ANN).

ANNs have been described extensively (18–22). Neural nets are an approach to data analysis that is unrelated to statistical methods. An ANN uses a mathematical pattern recognition paradigm to learn the complex interactions among input variables and outputs as it trains on a known set of data. It then uses these learned patterns to estimate the expected output when presented with new inputs. The

neural net thus develops common sense and judgment for evaluating new cases based on a historical database of prior learning and experience (23,24).

For example, instead of applying multiple rules or a fixed algorithm for differential diagnosis or similar problem solving, an ANN repetitively evaluates input data (e.g., lesion descriptions, patient age, family history) paired with output data (e.g., biopsy results) of training cases to discover patterns that permit the consistent classification of test cases. Many previously difficult tasks, such as image discrimination and interpretation, pattern recognition, signal interpretation and waveform analysis (e.g., electrocardiography or electroencephalography), outcome prediction, the identification of pathologic specimens, clinical pharmacology, and the analysis of multiple streams of data in real time, have been successfully performed using ANNs; these are well referenced and documented (25). ANNs bypass the difficult and time-consuming knowledge acquisition process by learning complex associations directly from examples and experience (26). This results in a neural net decision-support tool that can adapt to perform the same task under varying conditions.

While the interpretive advantage of nets has numerous applications, the ANN is limited by its inability to explain its conclusions. The reasoning by which a neural network renders a conclusion is hidden within the distributed weights and is unintelligible as an explanation. ANNs are thus limited to interpreting patterns where no explanation or justification is necessary. Because the need to justify conclusions is recognized as an important part of the process of decision support (e.g., in clinical diagnosis), this limits the application of neural networks in certain tasks.

Neural networks can apply their estimation and classification methodologies to disaster and emergency medical decision support. For example, on the prehospital scene, first-aid disaster workers must, often in a matter of seconds with sparse information at hand, make critical decisions concerning the urgency of an injured patient's condition and the type of trauma care required. This decisional process, known as triage, is an integral component of emergency-care medicine. Avoiding undertriage is a matter of saving lives; avoiding overtriage is a matter of preventing precious emergency care resources from being overtaxed and misallocated (see Chapter 2). An ANN-based decision support tool taken into an emergency or disaster area (via compact computer) may potentially play a valuable role in producing faster triage decisions based on complex, multifaceted information.

In the disaster arena, neural networks will most likely be seen as components of larger systems that make use of expert-given rules or statistical inference techniques as required—during the acute disaster phase, they may provide decision support to individuals to help them perform at a higher level; and, at the predisaster phase, they may assist in the training of staff and may help in disaster scenario planning (e.g., "what if" situations). Developments in machine learning will allow disaster medicine and management professionals to do more than just sit on a mountain of collected information; they can then use this information to extract new knowledge.

Expert Systems

An expert system is a program that captures elements of human expertise, usually in the form of situation recognition rules, and that performs tasks that rely on specialist knowledge. Also referred to as knowledge-based systems, these computer programs analyze data in a way that, if performed by a human, would be considered intelligent. An expert system consists of a knowledge base that contains the rules necessary for the completion of its task, a working memory in which the data and conclusions can be stored, and an inference engine that matches rules to data to derive its conclusions (27).

Ideally, for medical applications, external aids (electronic tools) to improve medical decision making should be able to retrieve and link general medical knowledge and patient-specific data to identify all relevant medical options and the pros and cons of each based on the patient's unique characteristics (28).

Expert systems differ qualitatively from ANNs and are characterized by the following:

- Symbolic logic rather than just numerical calculations;
- An explicit knowledge base understandable to an expert in that area of expertise;
- Ability to explain its conclusions with concepts that are meaningful to the user.

Generally, expert systems are used in two different ways as follows: (a) for decision support (to remind an experienced decision maker of options or issues to consider that he or she once knew but may have forgotten; this is the most common use in medicine) and (b) for decision making (to allow a person to make a decision that is beyond his or her level of training and experience). Table 14.4 describes the different types of tasks enabled by expert systems (29) and their application to disaster management and disaster

TABLE 14.4. APPLICATION OF EXPERT SYSTEMS TO DISASTER MANAGEMENT

Expert system task or type	Description	Application to disaster management/medicine	Applicable disaster phase
Generating alerts and reminders	An expert system attached to a monitor can warn of changes in the external environment, injured patient, etc. It might scan data and send reminders or warnings through an electronic communications system, audio device, etc.	Environmental: multiple sites are monitored; can send alerts based on predetermined criteria for notification of a pending disaster (e.g., earthquake, tsunami) or detection of hazardous substances. Medical: patient physiologic monitoring of multiple parameters can alert of critical physiologic status.	Predisaster, acute disaster
Decision assistance	When a situation is complex or the person making decision is inexperienced, an expert system can help generate likely decisions based on given data.	Identification of unknown hazardous biologic or chemical substance; medical diagnostic or therapeutic support for the disaster victim.	Acute disaster
Planning and critiquing	Systems can look for inconsistencies, errors, and omissions in an existing plan of action, or they can be used to formulate a plan based on a specific scenario and accepted planning guidelines.	Logistics or medical supplies determined based on current consumption data and projected trends.	Predisaster, acute disaster, postdisaster
Agents for information retrieval	Software agents can search for and retrieve information (e.g., on the Internet) that is considered relevant to a particular problem. The agent contains knowledge about its user's preferences and needs; it may also possess knowledge for assessing the importance and utility of what it finds.	Retrieval of key medical information from established networks and databases (chemical/biologic contamination procedures, health consequences of disaster aftermath, etc.).	Predisaster, acute disaster, postdisaster
Image recognition and interpretation	Many images now can be automatically interpreted. In medicine, for example, this is of value in mass-screenings, where the system can flag potentially abnormal images for detailed human attention.	Mass x-ray screening of disaster casualties (e.g., specific trauma); flagging of abnormal dermatologic consequences of chemical/biologic agent.	Acute disaster, post disaster

medicine, as well as the disaster phase where the expert system type would be most useful.

A major disadvantage of expert systems is the process of manual knowledge acquisition from human experts, which can be a drawn-out affair. To counter this problem, much work has gone into developing techniques to automate the acquisition of knowledge in the form of rules or decision trees from databases (30).

Model-Based Systems

One of the important contributions of AI research has been a growing understanding of the ways in which knowledge can be represented and manipulated. Rule-based representation of knowledge is only appropriate for narrowly defined problems (e.g., diagnosing chest pain). Model-based systems (sometimes called second-generation expert systems) are designed to use the existing models in the hope that they will be able to cover a broader set of problems than that possible with rules. These models may exist as mathematical descriptions of relationships, as compartmental system models, or as statistical models. Model-based systems are perceived as being better at explanation than the shallower rule-based systems and at dealing with novel or complex problems. They are also more computationally expensive to run as it takes longer to reason a problem out from first principles than it does simply to recognize it from previous experience or input. The future will see systems that combine both, having on the one hand the facility to invoke comprehensive models should they be needed and also being able to rely on efficient rules whenever they are applicable (27).

Knowledge-based gaming modeling and analysis decision support systems can be useful as an educational or drill tool before a disaster strikes or during a disaster when multiple courses of action are being considered and the consequences must be weighed. Such tools can significantly improve the visualization, development, and assessment of alternative maneuver courses of action under the direct control of a commander and staff. Critical events could be inserted into a disaster scenario, which could then be restarted to go through an action/reaction/counteraction sequence.

Clearly, a need exists for providing decision support in areas that are difficult for humans, namely, tracking multidimensional information, visualizing abstract situational features, managing uncertainty, detecting conflicts and constraint violations, and action/reaction gaming and outcome assessment. For those in command or leadership roles to have the ability to view a complicated situation from multiple perspectives and to use this insight wisely is important.

Virtual Reality

Virtual reality (VR) is an array of computer technologies that is employed to immerse a user in a synthetic world by creating a sensory-based environment that interactively responds to and is controlled by the user's behavior. The more efficient and natural the flow of data—the sights, sounds, and sensations that mimic actual experience—the more persuasive the sense of reality is (31,32).

Virtual environments can be used effectively for training in disaster medicine and management procedures. In relation to a battlefield or disaster situation, a virtual system can provide the environment to perfect skills and rehearse procedures before entering a hostile or chaotic environment (33). A significant need exists for high-fidelity VR training tools to help develop skills for managing complex situations that must be addressed at a more abstract level. Human immersion concepts and virtual environment technology (real world display) can be applied to the development of complex mission management rehearsals for predisaster use. Such a system would allow a trainee to view, navigate, and interact with an abstract virtual world and would impart a higher level of conceptual understanding.

The Internet and World Wide Web

The Internet has emerged as an unexpected global phenomenon offering unprecedented facilities for the creation, storage, and communication of information. Worldwide networking via the Internet promises to revolutionize the way information is shared and consumed, and it can enhance communications and knowledge among and within the many areas of a given field. The rapid increase in Internet use has been significantly facilitated by diminishing technical barriers (e.g., widespread access to the Internet, increased computer literacy by end-users, and the availability of inexpensive but powerful computer hardware and software).

One of the limitations of Internet services had been that they were text-based, thus limiting the type of information that could be sent electronically across the network. However, with the advent of the world wide web (WWW), a multimedia service available through the Internet, users now can exchange not just text, but also sound, images, and video, and can access information by navigating rapidly across the global Internet.

Disaster Management Networks

Many nations have established their own disaster-related networks that are accessible through the WWW (34). An all-encompassing global source that identifies and links all nations and that makes possible the worldwide sharing of critical information and expertise would be ideal; as of the time of this writing, such information networks have emerged and are evolving (35–37).

The inclusion of medical assistance in global information systems could provide timely medical information resources in areas where medical help is scarce or in disaster situations where rapid access to medical information may be needed. Within these web-based information systems, medical assistance could take the following forms:

- Access to an online medical library;
- Access to medical consultation or advice (interactive, store-and-forward [SAF]);
- Access to medical facility and logistics information;
- Real-time interactive telementoring assistance to field personnel;
- On-line diagnostic and therapeutic decision support systems (knowledge-based systems, neural networks);
- Automated multilingual medical query capability.

Web-Based Telemedicine

The WWW has attracted considerable attention as an efficient platform for conducting telemedicine consultations, medical education, and access to medical knowledge. Developing a clinical application system based on Internet technology and using web-based commercial software is already becoming a natural choice for enhancing the practice of medicine (38–44). An overall goal is to develop a system that integrates existing systems within a single platform (workstation), that is protocol-driven with SAF or real-time teleconsulting capability, and that can operate independently on convenient multiple hardware platforms (e.g., desktop PC, laptop, or pocket-sized computer). This system would be able to access medical information from numerous sites and would have the capability to transfer and share information to remote outlying areas and throughout the world. The Internet, WWW browser technology, and online information sources are available, powerful, and cost efficient, and they are becoming the drivers to make web-based multimedia telemedicine possible. Future medical possibilities are considerable; these could include battlefield and disaster field applications.

Computer Miniaturization

Personal Digital Assistants (Pocket Telemedicine)

Computer miniaturization has downsized the familiar desktop PC to portable laptop units that provide computing power away from the desktop. Today, miniaturization has become even more dramatic, leading to the concept of a pocket-sized personal digital assistant (PDA), which has even more transparent and highly personalized interfaces, some of which are pen-based, touch-based, or even voice-driven. Interest in tailoring these devices for specialized niche areas is growing so that their unique advantages might be exploited. Health care, including emergency and disaster medicine, is one such field.

PDA devices have some key quality characteristics—information management; portability; and, to varying degrees, e-mail, fax, and graphics capability, connectivity, digital photography, and voice recording. Telephone line, ethernet, radio frequency, and diffuse infrared transmission schemes have all been used for sending and receiving information.

The ability of an individual to use a single small communicator to transmit a variety of information virtually anywhere in the world would be ideal for the disaster field worker. When equipped with WWW browser capability, a digital camera, a telephone, and a computer "all-in-one package," pocket telemedicine could be conducted immediately on site and in real time when necessary. A world in which all health care providers and disaster relief workers carry PDA devices to send, receive, and selectively retrieve electronic information can easily be envisioned. These data would be readily accessible from any place and at any time. Although personal communications services (PCS) are currently available to support PDA wireless communications, satellite links to LEO-type satellite systems may provide the most reliable PCS in times of disaster. Thus, in the midst of chaos, the field worker would have a compact powerhouse in hand linked to the world.

Wearable Computing (Personal Imaging)

The miniaturization of components has also enabled the development of personal computer systems that are wearable and nearly invisible so that individuals can move about and interact freely while supported by their personal information domain. Such systems allow hands-free operation, enhanced mobility, access to information, and shared visual experiences. The idea is not new. In 1968, Sutherland described a head-mounted display with half-silvered mirrors that let the wearer see a virtual world superimposed on reality (45,46). However, his work, as well as subsequent work by others (47), entailed the serious limitation of having to be tethered to a workstation that was powered from an electrical outlet. Since then, experiments have been conducted attaching a computer, radio equipment, and other devices to the body in a tetherless system that lets an individual roam an area and receive e-mail and that provides other capabilities commonly available on a desktop multimedia computer.

Early prototypes for wearable, tetherless computer-mediated reality used video sent to a remote supercomputing facility over a high-quality microwave communications link. The computing facility would send back the processed image over an ultra-high frequency communications link. New versions incorporate a modern commercial display product (head-mounted display) along with commercially available cellular communications. The overall goal is eventually to make this type of system nearly undetectable. An important feature of this wearable device is that it is equipped with a wireless Internet connection and camera input, making the transmission of a sequence of images to a WWW page possible and allowing the wearer to browse the page later. Other individuals, watching remotely, are able to see what the wearer sees and to interact via messages (48).

Two people equipped with wearable multimedia computers can stay in touch, sending data, voice, and video to each other. Each person can see exactly what the other person sees overlaid on a portion of his or her own screen. A community of individuals wearing such computers can also be networked. Individuals could occasionally receive an image from someone sending an important signal. For example, someone anticipating danger might trigger a distress signal to others nearby over the Internet.

Although past prototypes have been cumbersome and even present prototypes remain somewhat obtrusive, miniaturization efforts continue to progress, incorporating greater levels of functionality into smaller spaces; they may eventually disappear into clothing and eyeglasses (48,49).

Entirely new modes of human-computer interaction can be expected to arise in the future with significant applications to disaster management and medicine efforts. Wearable computing can incorporate the advantages of a PDA, but in an even more compact form that is truly hands-free, thus allowing the worker to communicate or work while moving objects, helping disaster victims, performing medical procedures, sharing visual perspectives with coworkers, and so on. This would be the ultimate wireless communications support system for the disaster responder.

CONCLUSION

In these extraordinary times of technologic advances, the ability to break distance, intellect, time, and power limitations by fashioning technologic tools to amplify and extend the reach of communication exists as never before. With this comes the ability and responsibility to assist one another in times of hardship and disaster (either locally or remotely) and to improve health and safety outcomes significantly. Technology will no doubt overcome many of the limiting factors present in disaster response today, with communications being one of them. The field of disaster medicine should acknowledge that it is in its best interest to use existing technologies to their fullest advantage while also keeping an open mind in order to understand and appropriately embrace new technologies as they become available.

REFERENCES

1. Wood M. Disaster communications. Daytona Beach, FL: Association of Public Safety Communications Officials, 1997. Available at: http://ourworld.compuserve.com/homepage/mark_a_wood/disbook.htm. Accessed April 2002.
2. Garshnek V, Burkle FM. Applications of telemedicine and telecommunications to disaster medicine: historical and future perspectives. *J Am Med Inform Assoc* 1999;6:26–37.
3. Garshnek V, Burkle FM. Telecommunications systems in support of disaster medicine: applications of basic information pathways. *Ann Emerg Med* 1999;34:213–218.
4. Garshnek V. Applications of space communications technology to critical human needs: rescue, disaster relief, and remote medical assistance. *Space Commun* 1991;8:311–317.
5. Green JH. *The Irwin handbook of telecommunications*, 3rd ed. Burr Ridge, IL: Irwin, 1997.
6. Lindberg BC. *Troubleshooting communications facilities*. New York: John Wiley and Sons, 1990.
7. Wood M. *Disaster communications. Part 1-global*, 1st ed., June 1996. Available at: http://www.reliefweb.int/library/dc1/dcc1.html. Accessed December 1997.
8. Helm N. *Satellite communications for disaster relief* (paper no. 89-533). Presented at the 40th Congress of the International Astronautical Federation, Malagna, Spain, October 7–13, 1989.
9. Lodge JH. Mobile satellite communications systems: toward global personal communications. *IEEE Commun Mag* 1991;29:24–30.
10. Wood P. Mobile satellite services for travelers. *IEEE Commun Mag* 1991;29:32–35.
11. Yoho DR. Wireless communications technology applied to disaster response. *Aviat Space Environ Med* 1994;65:839–845.
12. Newton H. *Newton's telecom dictionary*, 10th ed. New York: Flatiron Publishing, 1996.
13. Whalen DJ. Communications satellites: making the global village possible. Available at: http://www.hq.nasa.gov/office/pao/History/satcomhistory.html. Accessed November 1997.
14. Grubb JL. The traveler's dream come true. *IEEE Commun Mag* 1991;29:48–51.
15. Klass PJ. Low earth orbit communications satellites compete for investors and US approval. *Aviat Week Space Technol* 1992;136:60–61.
16. Montgomery J. The orbiting internet—fiber in the sky. *Byte* 1997;22:58–72.
17. Garshnek V, Shinchi K, Burkle FM. Disaster assessment and satellite communication: on the threshold of a new era. *Space Policy* 1998;14:223–227.
18. Boone JM, Gross GW, Greco-Hunt V. Neural networks in radiologic diagnosis. I. Introduction and illustration. *Invest Radiol* 1990;25:1012–1016.
19. Wasserman PD. *Neural computing: theory and practice*. New York: Van Nostrand Reinhold, 1990.
20. Kattan MW, Beck R. Artificial neural networks for medical classification decisions. *Arch Pathol Lab Med* 1995;119:672–677.
21. Cross SS, Harrison RF, Kennedy RL. Introduction to neural networks. *Lancet* 1995;346:1075–1079.
22. Downs J, Harrison RF, Kennedy RL, et al. Application of the fuzzy ARTMAP neural network model to medical pattern classification tasks. *Artif Intell Med* 1996;8:403–428.
23. Shufflebarger CM. What is a neural network? *Ann Emerg Med* 1992;21:1461–1463.
24. Baker JA, Kornguth PJ, Lo JY, et al. Artificial neural network: improving the quality of breast biopsy recommendations. *Radiology* 1996;198:131–135.
25. Baxt WG. Application of artificial neural networks to clinical medicine. *Lancet* 1995;346:1135–1138.
26. Hayes-Roth F, Waterman DA, Lenat DB. *Building expert systems*. London: Addison-Wesley, 1983.
27. Coiera E. Automated signal interpretation. In: Hutton P, Prys-

Rogerts C, eds. *Monitoring in anaesthesia and intensive care.* London: WB Saunders, 1994:32–42.

28. Weed LL, Weed L. Reengineering medicine. *Fed Bull* 1994; 149–182.
29. Coiera E. Artificial intelligence in medicine. In Coiera E, ed. *Guide to medical informatics, the internet and telemedicine.* New York: Oxford University Press, 1997. Available at: http://www.Coiera. com/aimd.html. Accessed March 2002.
30. Quinlan JR. Induction of decision trees. *Machine Learning* 1986; 1:81–106.
31. Pimentel K. *Virtual reality through the new looking glass,* 2nd ed. New York: McGraw-Hill, 1995.
32. Mission accomplished. *NASA Tech Briefs* 1993;17:16.
33. Stansfield S. Medisim: casualty care on the virtual battlefield. *Mil Med Technol* 1997;Fall 97/Winter 98:23.
34. Disaster-related networks in each nation. Available at: http:// apollo.m.ehime-u.ac.jp/GHDNet/Connection/national. html. Accessed November 1997.
35. Ochi G, Shirakawa Y, Tanaka M, et al. An introduction to the Global Health Disaster Network (GHDNet). *Japanese Journal of Disaster Medicine* 1997;2:18–22.
36. ReliefWeb—project description. Available at: http://www. reliefweb.int/library/descript.html. Accessed February 1998.
37. Sovereign MG. Humanitarian assistance and disaster relief in the next century—workshop report. Washington, D.C.: National Defense University, Ft. McNair, October 28–30, 1997.

38. Lareng L. Telemedicine in Europe. *Eur J Intern Med* 2002;13:1–3.
39. Wooton R. Telemedicine. *BMJ* 2001;323:557–560.
40. Bahshur RL. Where we are in telemedicine/telehealth, and where we go from here. *Telemed J E Health* 2001;7:273–277.
41. Wooton R. Telemedicine: a cautious welcome. *BMJ* 1996;313: 1375–1377.
42. Edworthy SM. Telemedicine in developing countries. *BMJ* 2001;323:524–525.
43. Henri CJ, Rubin RK, Cox RD, et al. Design and implementation of world wide web-based tools for image management in computed tomography, magnetic resonance imaging, and ultrasonography. *J Digit Imaging* 1997;10:77–79.
44. Rasberry C, Garshnek V. A web-based physician's telemedicine system for a new age. *Int J Technol Manage* 1999;1:233–238.
45. Earnshaw RA, Gigante MA, Jones H. *Virtual reality systems.* San Diego: Academic Press, 1993.
46. Sutherland I. A head-mounted three dimensional display. In: *Proceedings of the fall joint computer conference.* Los Alamitos: IEEE, 1968:757–764.
47. Feiner S, MacIntyre B, Seligmann D. Knowledge-based augmented reality. *Commun ACM* 1993;36:53–62.
48. Mann S. Wearable computing: a first step toward personal imaging. *Computer* 1997;30:25–32.
49. Satava RM, Jones SB. Military applications of telemedicine and advanced medical technologies. *Army Med Depart J* 1997; Nov/Dec:16–21.

15

MANAGING DISASTERS IN AUSTERE ENVIRONMENTS

NATHAN J. ELDER
P. GREGG GREENOUGH

Disaster response may require medical care in isolated and austere areas. This can occur both in the developed world (usually smaller, isolated incidents) and in the developing world. This chapter presents principles of response in both environments.

DEVELOPED WORLD

Wilderness and Remote Areas Without Easy Medical Access

Each year in the United States, the number of visitors to remote backcountry and wilderness areas continues to grow. Increasing numbers of people are escaping overpopulated urban centers. Interest in adventure travel and extreme sports is at an all-time high, and these groups are venturing into remote regions with limited or no medical care available. The small towns that surround these remote regions are less likely to have the resources to handle the multiple victims of the natural disasters that are likely to occur in such areas.

Disaster management in wilderness regions and remote areas without easy medical access offers unique management challenges. In these areas, smaller incidents qualify as disasters because any accident involving even a few victims can quickly overwhelm the capability of available medical care. Just locating the disaster may be a challenge. Most small towns have at least a rudimentary proactive disaster plan in place, which is usually controlled by an incident command system that includes many state and local agencies. The local search and rescue (SAR) team, if one is available, is usually part of this system, and it is likely to be the most helpful; it uses standard SAR techniques, such as map and compass and grid searches, to locate victims in remote areas. Military, police, and news helicopters may be available to assist in the search, but access to this resource varies from region to region. Once victims are located, access or fire roads requiring only a short hike may simplify access to

them; however, access may be complicated by severe terrain that requires specialized skills, such as rappelling or technical climbing, to reach the victims.

On arrival at the disaster location, the scene must be assessed for safety to prevent additional injury to the victims from the rescue effort and to prevent injury to the rescue team. If hazardous environments persist (e.g., fire, unstable terrain, bad weather), deviation from the ideal rescue protocol by distancing the patient and team from the hazards before complete stabilization of the patient's injuries may be necessary to reduce the risk of additional injury to the patient or the rescue team. The triage of multiple patients is geared toward prolonged extrication and transport times (prolonged time to definitive care), so care is directed to those most likely to survive and not necessarily to those who are the sickest at the time of the rescue team's arrival.

Knowledge of the local disaster plan and resources available is critical to the successful management of remote disasters. This includes the capabilities of the SAR team, the local fire department resources, the emergency medical service (EMS) transport capability and level of training, and the local hospital capability and their referral patterns to tertiary care trauma centers.

Evaluation of Victims in Places Without Resources

Evaluation of patients injured in austere environments begins, as in a tertiary care trauma center, with the standard primary (ABCDE) survey as follows:

A: airway with attention to maintaining cervical spine immobilization if appropriate;
B: breathing;
C: circulation, with control of external bleeding;
D: disability or neurologic status. Evaluate level of consciousness using the AVPU method (alert, response to vocal stimuli, response only to painful stimuli, or unresponsive to all stimuli) or the Glasgow coma scale (GCS);

E: exposure (undress patient) and environment (control temperature of patient).

If any abnormality is detected in a particular step, one should stop at that step and address the problem before moving on to the next step. Resuscitation with available supplies, such as oxygen, intravenous lines, dressings and splints, and ventilation equipment, should be initiated during this primary survey phase (1).

Following this initial brief evaluation, the patients should be routinely triaged for further care and transport. Patients who would ordinarily be triaged for immediate transport in an urban setting may need further stabilization before transport from a more remote setting because transport times to definitive care will likely be prolonged. When multiple casualties are evaluated, triage should recognize prolonged transport times as a factor for basic stabilization before transport, and the treatment of critically ill patients may take up too much, proportionally, of the rescue team's efforts. The principle of choosing the most salvageable also applies when limited numbers of transport mechanisms are available, such as one helicopter or a limited number of ground transport units.

After the primary survey has been completed and resuscitation has begun, a full secondary survey, including a brief history, should be obtained. The following AMPLE mnemonic can be helpful with obtaining a brief history (1):

A: allergies;
M: medications;
P: past medical illness or pregnancy;
L: last meal;
E: events or environment related to injury.

The physical examination during the secondary survey should include the following:

- *Head.* Evaluate for contusions, lacerations, fractures, visual acuity, pupillary size, penetrating injury, and maxillofacial instability.
- *Cervical spine and neck.* Evaluate for cervical spine tenderness, subcutaneous emphysema, tracheal deviation, and blunt injury to carotid arteries.
- *Chest.* Include visualization, palpation, and auscultation. Small penetrating injuries may be detected only by thorough visualization of both the anterior and posterior chest walls. Large flail segments and tension pneumothorax may be detected and may require immediate stabilization. Detection of these injuries is especially important before transportation by aircraft.
- *Abdomen.* Knowing the mechanism of injury and the associated injuries can keep the index of suspicion for abdominal injury high. Frequent reexamination is necessary.
- *Musculoskeletal.* Reduce fractures or areas suspicious for fractures if distal neurovascular compromise is present; then splint into a position of comfort.

- *Neurologic.* Complete a comprehensive motor and sensory evaluation of the patient, including the level of consciousness and pupillary size.

In remote locations, clinically clearing lucid patients with a significant mechanism for cervical spine (c-spine) injury might be necessary, if the patient is otherwise ambulatory and is without focal neurologic deficits. The criteria for c-spine clearance in the wilderness setting are similar to those in the urban setting and are as follows:

1. The patient is alert and oriented to person, place and time and is not under the influence of drugs, alcohol, or other mind-altering substances.
2. The patient has no continued distracting pain; the treatment of the patient's other injuries must have reduced pain.
3. No neurologic signs or symptoms, based on reassessments for up to 2 hours, are observed.
4. The patient has no pain with flexion, extension, and rotation of the neck.

If the c-spine is unable to be cleared clinically, full spinal immobilization is necessary with a c-collar and full backboard. However, transportation of fully immobilized patients from remote areas usually places the patient and rescuers at risk of injury secondary to prolonged weather exposure and the rough terrain.

Stabilization

For disasters occurring in a remote area, access roads may allow ambulances with the usual prehospital medical supplies close access to the scene of the disaster. If access is limited, one may need to improvise creative alternatives to standard stabilization equipment. These improvised devices rarely provide the same degree of protection, and they generally are not as useful as a specifically designed commercial product. However, with a little creative thinking and the use of materials at hand, one can stabilize a disaster victim in a remote area long enough to reach definitive care. The possibilities are limited only by the imagination. The following listing is by no means complete; it has been gathered from the useful suggestions discussed in the wilderness improvisation chapter of Auerbach's *Wilderness medicine* text and from other resources, including the Stonehearth open learning opportunity (SOLO) wilderness medicine training courses in New Hampshire and the National Ski Patrol Outdoor Emergency Care course (2–4).

Airway Management

Airway compromise in obtunded or unconscious victims most commonly is caused by the relaxation of the pharyngeal muscles, allowing the tongue to fall into the posterior pharynx and to obstruct the airway. Maintaining an open airway using the jaw thrust or chin lift method will prevent a rescuer from being able to continue with the primary or secondary survey. If no oral airway is available, improvisation of an oral airway or nasal trumpet will allow one to continue the evaluation. Any relatively small diameter tubing could be used to improvise a nasal trumpet, including tubing from a water filter, hydration bladder tubing, the inflation hose for a kayak flotation bladder, or a Foley catheter if one is kept in the medical kit. If tubing is not readily available, a safety pin or two could be used to pin the distal tip of the tongue to the lower lip or clothing to keep the relaxed tongue mass more anterior and the airway patent.

Cricothyrotomy is indicated if nasal or oral airway attempts are unsuccessful, the patient cannot maintain an open airway, and additional personnel to maintain a patent airway manually are not available. A small incision is made through the skin over the cricothyroid membrane. Once the cricoid cartilage is stabilized, the barrel of a rigid cylindrical device is passed through the cricothyroid membrane inferiorly to create a patent airway. Improvised tools include a small barrel syringe, small flashlight casings, pen casings, large bore needles, or any other small-to-medium size rigid tubes that could prevent the collapse of tissues over the newly formed airway. The improvised airway needs to be stabilized to prevent the displacement and occlusion of the trachea.

Cervical Collars

An improvised cervical collar should only be used with a backboard or other full spinal immobilization. The device should be rigid or semirigid and the appropriate size for the patient; it should not choke the patient, and it should allow for opening of the mouth if emesis occurs. SAM splints, closed-cell foam sleeping pads, padded hip belts from backpacks, and tightly rolled clothing can all be used to form a cervical collar.

Backboards

Short backboards may need to be used to extract a disaster victim rapidly from an area with continued hazards. After a cervical collar is created, a short backboard can be formed by inverting an internal or external frame backpack and using the hip belt to support the head with the belt fastened around the patient's forehead for stabilization. The body then needs to be lashed to the frame. If an avalanche shovel is available, the handle can be placed down the back of the pack, with the bed of the shovel as the head support. The shoulder straps and waist belt can then be used to attach the patient to the frame of the pack. Large snowshoes can also be improvised into a short backboard with the use of webbing or rope to secure the patient to the snowshoe. Short backboards are only temporary devices to remove the victim

from areas of continued hazard. Once the victim is extracted to an area with less risk, a long backboard should be created. Using a full-length climbing rope, several sleeping pads, and a rigid stiffening device (ski poles, branches, snowshoes, backpacks, canoe paddles, or other rigid objects), a rope litter can be created. External frame backpacks can be lashed together to form a functional litter or backboard, with rigid objects again being used to reinforce the frames. A kayak with the deck and seat removed can make an excellent backboard, as can a canoe, which requires even less modification.

Femoral Traction

Victims with suspected femur fractures should be treated with a traction splint, which counteracts muscle spasm, reduces further damage from sharp bone ends, and minimizes blood loss into the thigh. Patients with femur fractures can easily lose over 1 L of blood into the thigh, precipitating shock. In remote areas, intravenous fluid replacement may not be an option. Therefore, early splinting may help prevent subsequent shock. Many portable commercial traction devices can be purchased, including the Thomas half-ring, Hare, KTA, and Sager splints, which are relatively easy to apply. If these are not available, an improvised splint is necessary. Improvised traction splints can take some time and effort to create, but prior practice (even on uninjured group members) will allow smoother application. Improvised traction splints need the following four main elements to be effective: an ankle hitch, a rigid support that is longer than the lower extremity, the traction mechanism, a proximal anchor, and materials to secure the device to the patient. Padding should be used to ensure the patient's comfort.

Extremity Splints

Fractures, dislocations, and sprains can sometimes be difficult to differentiate in the field, so splints may be used to reduce pain, swelling, and bleeding and to prevent additional injury from sharp fracture fragments. Proper splinting immobilizes the joint above and below the injured site. Documentation of distal neurovascular status is important both before and after the application of any splint; the splint should be readjusted with any sign of decreasing function. With a little practice and creativity, closed-cell foam, self-inflating mattresses, clothing, and other natural materials can become comfortable and functional splints.

Communications, Accessing Care

Communication during or after a disaster is vital to the success of the relief effort. The medical personnel on scene must be able to communicate with the incident commander, who will coordinate the assistance from the local fire department, state police, the local SAR team, outside specialized SAR teams, EMS, and helicopter or fixed wing transport. Most communication is done by two-way radio with frequencies that have been established by protocol before an incident. Cellular and digital telephones are being used more frequently, but, in some remote areas, such service is not available. Public and military satellite telephone services could be an option if services were arranged before the incident. Amateur radio operators have formed groups of volunteers that will provide communication support for disaster operations. The Radio Amateur Civil Emergency Service (RACES) is coordinated through the Federal Emergency Management Agency (FEMA), and the Amateur Radio Emergency Service (ARES) is coordinated through the American Radio Relay League (5). The Salvation Army Team Emergency Radio Network (SATERN) is another group that supports Salvation Army operations in local, regional, and international disaster and emergency situations (6).

Early communication with local and regional hospitals surrounding the incident should be established. The number and severity of the injured, the approximate transport times, and the means of transportation required for effective evacuation should be communicated so that these centers can begin their preparations and can gather additional personnel if needed. Hospitals should communicate with the incident commander concerning bed availability, the number of casualties already received, and their capability for receiving additional victims. The incident commander can use this information to divert the transport of victims to centers capable of handling additional patients.

Rescue Operations

The International Commission for Alpine Rescue (IKAR-CISA) is the major search and rescue operation for 26 member countries in Europe. The commission is well organized, and it has impacted standards for a wide variety of rescue-related industries, including rope manufacture and avalanche beacon frequencies, and has made recommendations for standard curriculum for air crews performing search and rescue. Canada also has a central coordinating agency with the National SAR Secretariat (NSS), which oversees ground and maritime SAR. The Search and Rescue Volunteer Association of Canada (SARVAC) unites the volunteers and gives them a common voice. In the United States, SAR operations involve a variety of state and local agencies and volunteers. The services offered by these SAR groups can range from general SAR units with specific scenting canine teams, mounted horse units, snowmobile units, jeep posses, and tracking posses to highly specialized, high-angle technical rescue or diving rescue teams. The federal government lists its responsibilities in the National Search and Rescue Plan. This states that all inland SAR is ultimately the responsibility of the United States Air Force under the Air Force Rescue Coordination Center at Lang-

ley Air Force Base in Virginia and that all maritime and navigable water SAR is the responsibility of the United States Coast Guard. Inland Alaskan rescues are the responsibility of the Air National Guard (7). These agencies are responsible for the coordination of federal resources used in response to SAR incidents.

Other agencies that may be able to assist depending on the type of disaster are the Civil Air Patrol, FEMA, the Office of United States Foreign Disaster Assistance (OFDA), the Air Force Parajumper units, and the Marine/Navy combat SAR crews (8). The Civil Air Patrol is a federally based agency with general volunteer pilots and observers who look for downed aircraft. FEMA typically works through the local fire service to assist with civil and urban disasters. OFDA generally works with other countries or with those families with relatives in trouble in other countries by locating resources that are available. The Air Force Parajumpers and the Marine/Navy combat SAR teams can be used to augment the services of local agencies, but they do not supplant the local resources that can provide the same services.

National organizations that operate SAR groups or provide training include the National Park Service, the National Ski Patrol, the Mountain Rescue Association (MRA), the National Cave Rescue Commission, and the National Association for Search and Rescue (NASAR) (8). The National Park Service has parks with SAR teams staffed by several full-time and seasonal rangers and augments their staff with local volunteer experts. The National Ski Patrol operates teams of volunteer and paid patrollers at ski sites in the United States that provide SAR and medical care on the slopes. The MRA performs mountain and technical rescues. The National Cave Rescue Commission is a nonoperational organization that provides training in cave rescue to existing SAR units. NASAR unites general SAR groups and the state SAR coordinators of most United States emergency management agencies. It also holds a federal contract to provide training for urban search and rescue.

Each state has its own division of emergency management that provides a link between FEMA and the state, directs the management of civil disasters, and may provide some reimbursement of costs incurred in a SAR mission. In most states, SAR is the statutory responsibility of the sheriff of each county in the state. In other states, the state police or another state agency, such as the Fish and Game Division, are given this responsibility. Some sheriffs use a regional team for all counties in the state.

The details of who is responsible for or available for assistance for search and rescue in the United States can quickly become overwhelming, and knowledge of the system of local SAR in a given area is critical before the disaster occurs.

Transfer Issues

In remote areas, the decision of how to evacuate someone from the disaster site must be carefully made. The safety of the rescue team is more important than the ideal management of any single patient. If the patient is able to ambulate, this may be the best method of extrication despite the presence of other injuries. Otherwise, litter evacuation is a labor-intensive, slow, and demanding task. On average, six to eight fresh rescuers are needed for every 100 yards that a loaded litter must be carried, and frequent breaks must be taken to allow the rescuers to rest and to reevaluate the patient. High angle rescues using anchoring systems, ropes, and pulleys are even more time-intensive and labor-intensive. Helicopter evacuation is usually a possibility in most areas of the United States, but knowledge of local helicopter services and their limitations is necessary. Helicopters have various configurations and capabilities, and the skill level of the crews may vary among services. Some services have winching capability, allowing rescue from more rugged terrain; but others require a suitable landing zone free of hazards. Most civilian services are unable to operate in fog, icing conditions, or high winds, which limits their utility during severe storms. Some local rescue services may have specialized vehicles available for patient transport from remote areas, such as snowmobiles, snowcats, and converted four-wheel drive vehicles. These local emergency services may be overwhelmed if large numbers of victims need transportation, and ambulances from other regions may need to be requested.

DEVELOPING WORLD

Natural Disasters and Complex Emergencies

Natural and Technologic Disasters

In the developing world, the effects of natural disasters tend to be amplified compared to those that occur in developed countries. For instance, inadequate or poorly enforced building codes were blamed for the large death toll following the 1999 earthquake near Izmet, Turkey. The 7.5 magnitude quake left over 15,000 dead and nearly 24,000 injured, and it damaged or destroyed over 100,000 homes, leaving 100,000 homeless (9). Poor building design or construction and the lack of adequate shelter are significant risk factors for cyclone-related morbidity and mortality. In the cyclone of 1991 that killed 140,000 people in Bangladesh, 22% of Bangladeshis who did not reach a block or concrete structure perished (10). Those affected mostly lived in low-lying coastal islands and sandbars where 95% of the housing was wood and split bamboo interwoven mesh walls with thatched roofs. Only 3% of the coastal housing withstood the storm surge.

The developing world contains the largest populations at risk for the devastation of disasters. By 2050, the global population is expected to reach 10 billion, with 95% of that increase in developing countries. Not only does overpopu-

lation stress the ecosystem generally, but the concentrated growth and development in low-lying coastal zones and deltas erodes the protective capacity of these systems for floods and storm surges, putting peoples and economies at risk. Half of the world's rapidly growing population lives in coastal zones. Already, one billion people live within 60 to 100 km of coastline. In Indonesia, 110 million of the population of 179.4 million live along the coasts (11). In Bangladesh, where population density is the highest in the world, the poor landless live as tenants on the vulnerable coastal plains described previously. Widespread poverty forces large numbers to live in such disaster-prone areas.

Moreover, urbanization rates are high in developing countries. Of the world's sixty megacities (those with a greater than 5 million population), three-quarters are in developing countries (12). Urban slums now contain more than 50% of the poor in the developing world (13). In places where the economically disenfranchised have left the rural areas for cities, many have had to settle in urban disaster-prone areas, such as washes and flood plains or deforested hillsides. Most of the more than 2,000 killed from the explosive spread of methyl isocyanate in Bhopal, India, in 1984 were poor urban squatters living on land surrounding the plant. In addition, the growth rate of these areas is outstripping that of their water and sanitation systems, leaving the poor vulnerable to public health catastrophes.

Furthermore, the concomitant environmental degradation has placed millions in the Third World at risk. Desertification and deforestation reduce the land's resilience to normal climatic stresses—particularly heavy rains, high winds, and drought—and undermine food production, putting the inhabitants at risk for famine. One-third of the earth's surface, some 45 million square kilometers, is at risk for desertification. This area affects the livelihood of 900 million people in 100 countries, 135 million of whom are living in areas that are already severely degraded (14). On degraded soils, heavy rains fail to absorb, increasing the run-off and erosion. Deforested and eroded mountains and hills are also home to the vulnerable urban poor. After a week of torrential rains soaked the Andes in September 1987, a massive mudslide wiped out half of Medellin, Colombia's shantytown of Villa Tina, killing 500. Five months later, following a 3-week, 18-inch drenching, the once forested mountains around Rio de Janiero, which since had been covered with slum dwellings of scrap metal and wood, gave way, killing 300, injuring 1,000, and leaving 18,000 homeless (15). The denudement of the watershed area of the Blue Nile in Ethiopia reduced its holding capacity. As a result, a heavy storm sent a torrent of water through the downstream Sudanese capital Khartoum in 1988, leaving 1.5 million homeless. The Sudanese plain, which is not commonly given to flooding, experienced its worst water-related devastation in a century. The worst single disaster from Hurricane Mitch in November 1998 was the mudslide from the deforested slopes of Nicaragua's

Casita Volcano that wiped out several villages, killing 2,000 of the 11,000 total dead of the three countries affected. As a result of deforestation, whatever weather extremes could be readily endured in the past are now causing large-scale catastrophes in developing countries.

Developing countries generally lack the plans and the resources to minimize the effects of disasters. Disaster prevention, a well-funded and well-organized structure in developed countries, is either nonexistent or, at best, piecemeal in developing countries. During a 1996 tornado that struck northern Bangladesh, 88% of indoor victims did not take any protective action due to the lack of public education. Ninety-four percent did not know that a disaster was even imminent because no systematic warning system existed (16).

Complex Emergencies

Humanitarian relief, generated in response to the myriad of international armed conflicts that have blossomed since the end of the Cold War, has become a complex field in its own right. Involving a variety of international, governmental, and nongovernmental agencies, as well as militaries and military alliances, the widespread use of the term "complex emergencies" among planners and responders should come as no surprise. Generally, the term defines an acute event that involves some combination of civil strife, food shortage, and population displacement (17). Most of these complex emergencies occur against a backdrop of abject poverty, a lack of natural resources, environmental degradation, a tenuous public health infrastructure, and an absence of a functional government whose purpose should be to protect its subjects and their basic human rights. Burkle outlines the characteristics of complex emergencies as follows: administrative, economic, and socio-political degradation and collapse; high levels of violence; cultural, ethnic, or religious groups at risk of extinction; catastrophic public health emergencies; vulnerable populations at risk; internal conflicts with flagrant disregard for the Geneva Conventions and the Universal Declaration of Human Rights; increasing competition for diminishing resources among conflicting groups; increased population displacement both across and within borders; and a conflict that is prolonged (13).

Not surprisingly, the delivery of medical care is difficult in these arenas. Civil strife inevitably disables the health care delivery apparatus; and hospitals, clinics, and the public health infrastructure suffer early in conflicts. Moreover, in the face of a lack of medical staff and medical supplies come large numbers of victims such that whatever medical services are left available are easily overwhelmed by the magnitude of injuries. Victims of armed conflicts have a wider array of medical problems versus those who are victims of natural disaster alone; these include trauma, infectious disease epidemics, malnutrition, and psychosocial trauma. The latter is critical as

many armed conflicts are prolonged and the victims may not have an idea of when they can return home and resume life as they had known it. Food is often used as a weapon of war; its shortage exacerbates mass population migration and makes these populations prone to infectious diseases. In the 1990s, roughly 90% of the victims in complex emergencies were civilians, predominantly children, who comprise the most vulnerable segment of the population. Providing health care may prove difficult because natural disasters such as floods, drought, or famine may have precipitated or may be superimposed on top of the ongoing civil strife, thus limiting access to victims or disrupting the supply lines. The condition of anarchy that often exists may prohibit the delivery of medical relief and supplies due to security risks, as was seen with the conflicts in Liberia and Somalia in the 1990s. No formalized government apparatus may exist that can ensure the sustainability or support of the medical relief effort. Land mines—over 100 million in 60 countries still exist—may drain medical resources and delay access to victims (18). Establishing sustainable medical care among a refugee or an internally displaced population is in and of itself an imposing feat.

In these situations, health care providers find themselves working in environments for which they have no formal training or experience. Health care in the midst of armed conflict and refugee movements goes beyond traditional diagnosis and treatment—it requires establishing epidemic surveillance, ensuring potable water and efficient sanitation, documenting human rights abuses, and providing specialized support for psychologically traumatized victims. It also involves interacting with a panoply of international and nongovernmental relief agencies and military forces who have varying levels of involvement and expertise in establishing public health projects and providing medical relief. It often means working with failed communications systems and limited resources.

In addition, expatriate medical providers must deal with the stresses of surviving in a foreign country that requires constant cognizance of their own security. In that setting, they perform physically demanding work for long hours, often in difficult environmental conditions, while separated from friends and family. All of these factors add significant personal stresses, in addition to the natural stress derived from viewing the devastation and injustice of a war environment up close. Medical volunteers are often unprepared for the psychologic stresses they will encounter in relief work. A 1998 World Health Organization report on the lack of training for aid workers from nongovernmental organizations found that, during the time from recruitment to deployment, 53% of the workers surveyed had no medical brief and 20% were not sure of their vaccination status. In most cases, advice on food, water, and parasites was lacking (19). Mental health preparation for the providers themselves is often neglected before, during, and after their stint of relief work.

Despite the formidable task of providing medical relief in arduous conditions, adequate preparation can make the work deeply rewarding. Agencies providing medical care should train providers in understanding logistics, procurement, security, and communications, in addition to public health interventions, such as water, sanitation, vaccination protocols, rapid needs assessments, and disease surveillance. Medical care workers should be aware of field stressors well before deploying. Once in the field, providers should meet regularly with the country's ministry of health, public health authorities, and health coordinating agencies to plan health care delivery and to review surveillance data. Such meetings should involve all agencies providing health care in the field, including humanitarian agencies, United Nations agencies, Geneva-based agencies, and military groups.

REFERENCES

1. American College of Surgeons. *Advanced trauma life support*, 6th ed. Chicago: American College of Surgeons, 1997.
2. Weiss EA, Donner HJ. Wilderness improvisation. In: Auerbach PS, ed. *Wilderness medicine: management of wilderness and environmental emergencies*, 3rd ed. St. Louis: Mosby, 1995.
3. SOLO, Inc. *Wilderness weekend.* Conway, NH: Solo, 1999.
4. Bowman WD Jr, ed. *The National Ski Patrol's outdoor emergency care.* Lakewood, CO: National Ski Patrol System, 1988. Available at: http://www.patrol.org/instructor/oec/index.html. Accessed March 2002.
5. American Radio Relay League, Inc. Amateur Radio Emergency Communication page. Available at: http://www.arrl.org/pio/emergen1.html. Accessed February 2002.
6. Salvation Army Team Emergency Radio Network. Home page. Available at: http://www.satern.net/page1.htm. Accessed February 2000.
7. National Oceanic and Atmospheric Administration. Search and Rescue Satellite Aided Tracking page. Available at: http://www.sarsat.noaa.gov/rcc.html. Accessed February 2000.
8. Kovacs TA. A primer on search and rescue. *AirMed* 2000;6:1.
9. Office of Foreign Disaster Assistance, 1999.
10. Bern C, Sniezek J, Mathbor GM, et al. Risk factors for mortality in the Bangladesh cyclone of 1991. *Bull WHO* 1993;71:73–78.
11. Climate Institute. Rising seas threaten cities, erode beaches and drown wetlands in key developing countries. *Climate Alert* 1995;8.
12. McMichael AJ. *Planetary overload: global environmental change and the health of the human species.* Cambridge: Cambridge University Press, 1993.
13. Burkle FM. Lessons learnt and future expectations of complex emergencies. *BMJ* 1999;319:422.
14. Myers N, Kent J. *Environmental exodus: an emergent crisis in the global arena.* Washington, D.C.: Climate Institute, 1995.
15. Jacobson JL. Environmental refugees: a yardstick of habitability. *Worldwatch Paper 86.* Washington, D.C.: Worldwatch Institute, 1988;November.
16. Kunii O, Kunori T, Takahashi K, et al. Health impact of 1996 tornado in Bangladesh. *Lancet* 1996;348:757.
17. Toole MJ. Complex emergencies: refugee and other populations. In: Noji EK, ed. *The public health consequences of disasters.* New York: Oxford University Press, 1997.
18. Human Rights Watch and Physicians for Human Rights. *Landmines: a deadly legacy.* New York: Africa Watch, 1993.
19. The Center of Excellence in Disaster Management and Humanitarian Assistance. *Combined humanitarian assistance response training, 2000.* Tripler AMC, Hawaii: Center of Excellence in Disaster Management and Humanitarian Assistance, 2000.

PART
III

NATURAL DISASTERS

16

EARTHQUAKES

CARL H. SCHULTZ

Earthquakes are probably the most costly of all natural disasters, both in terms of the lives lost and the property destroyed (Table 16.1)(1). They strike without warning, making mitigation efforts difficult and evacuation impossible. Most other natural disasters capable of inflicting this level of suffering are predictable (e.g., tsunamis after earthquakes, floods) or detectable (e.g., hurricanes, typhoons); or they frequently give warnings before they occur (e.g., volcanic eruptions). The Northridge, California earthquake caused an estimated 20 to 30 billion dollars in damage (2,3), while the Hanshin-Awaji temblor in Kobe, Japan, produced at least twice that amount in damage and killed over 6,000 people (4). These events occurred in wealthy nations with relatively modern seismic building codes. In countries less fortunate, the death toll can be staggering. For instance, the 1976 Tangshan earthquake in China caused 250,000 deaths.

The current theory describing the origin of earthquakes relies on the geology of the earth's crust. Rather than consisting of a smooth sheet covering the planet, the crust is fragmented into several large sections known as tectonic plates. Major faults occur where these plates meet. The San Andreas Fault in California is located at the juncture at which the North American Plate contacts the Pacific Plate. As these plates slowly move against each other along fault lines, they generate increasing levels of stress. When a stress point ruptures, energy is suddenly released in the form of

seismic waves, resulting in an earthquake. Three types of seismic waves exist, but the slower moving secondary wave causes the greatest impact. The energy released by the Northridge temblor (magnitude, 6.7) was slightly less than that produced over 4 months by Niagara Falls (5). Surrounding the major faults are numerous smaller cracks in the crust, or minor faults. These can also give rise to seismic events, as happened in California's 1989 Loma Prieta and the 1987 Whittier Narrows earthquakes. Still, the explanation for earthquakes is incomplete. Tectonic plate theory is attractive for many reasons, but it does not adequately explain all seismic phenomena, such as the significant activity found in the New Madrid zone in the central United States. Large earthquakes have occurred there, over 1,000 miles away from the nearest plate boundary.

The medical challenge posed by earthquakes can be extreme. The potential to reduce significant initial mortality is limited to roughly the first 24 to 48 hours (6). Yet, precisely during this time, the greatest degree of chaos exists. Movement in and out of the disaster zone is difficult, and accurate information is scarce. By the time outside medical care arrives in force, most victims have either received intervention or are dead. Hospitals are the traditional providers of medical care after earthquakes, and they are frequently overwhelmed with patients. Unfortunately, they are also vulnerable to structural and nonstructural damage, which further compromises their ability to provide medical care. Eight hospitals were so badly damaged in the Northridge earthquake that they were forced to evacuate patients (7). Four hospitals ultimately were condemned. For these reasons, hospitals alone cannot meet the entire demand for medical assistance.

The solution to providing an effective medical response to earthquakes is optimizing the use of all available resources. Major challenges to planners and responders in this regard include the following: (a) ways to modify initial responses at the prehospital and hospital level; (b) knowledge of what local options are available to supplement acute hospital care; (c) clinical conditions that will exist and increase in frequency, placing unusual demands on the

TABLE 16.1. EARTHQUAKE MORTALITY

Location	Year	Death toll
Italy	1908	75,000
China	1920	200,000
Japan	1923	143,000
USSR	1948	100,000
Peru	1970	70,000
China	1976	250,000
Iran	1990	40,000

Abbreviation: USSR, Union of Soviet Socialist Republics.

health care system; and (d) reasonable expectations for outside assistance. By understanding these issues, health care providers can maximize the outcome from medical intervention. However, one caveat does exist—most of the material in this chapter applies to industrialized nations with significant resources. Less affluent countries can still use this information, but they will have to tailor it to their needs.

PREHOSPITAL IMPACT

The initial medical response immediately following an earthquake will probably be by paramedics answering 911 calls or reporting to a scene of structural damage. In systems not using paramedics, the first responders are police, fire, or ambulance services. A varying period of confusion follows, depending on factors such as the magnitude of the earthquake, the time of day, the degree to which communications are compromised, and the training and experience of the prehospital providers. Once information clearly shows that the demand on resources may exceed that seen under standard operating procedures, establishing a system of command and control becomes key to effective management.

Events producing few casualties and slight damage may require nothing more than activating previously established mass casualty incident (MCI) protocols. Triage occurs, but it plays a minor role because medical care is not limited. Providers frequently perform triage using a system similar to the Simple Triage and Rapid Treatment (START) protocol (6,8). Hospital contact is possible, so first responders can communicate their patients' conditions to the emergency departments. The emergency operations center (EOC) may activate, but it can manage the event with existing resources. An example of this type of event is the 1987 Whittier Narrows earthquake, which resulted in eight fatalities and 500 million dollars in damage.

Large magnitude earthquakes causing many casualties and heavy damage are quite different. The initial medical response may be delayed as prehospital providers struggle to prioritize conflicting missions. Many paramedics are also firefighters. In situations where fires break out immediately after a earthquake, their first duty is fire suppression. If all available fire departments are needed to fight fires, the paramedic calls will not be answered. Sections of the city of San Francisco went without paramedic support in the early hours following the Loma Prieta earthquake for this reason (9). Management of these complex prehospital situations requires a sophisticated strategy such as the incident command system (ICS).

ICS was first developed by fire departments in California to coordinate all the resources used in fighting large brush fires. Many organizations throughout the United States are now familiar with this system. It provides a standardized system of command and control that is flexible enough to manage many different events involving multia-

gency and multijurisdictional responders. It is extremely useful for managing the unique and chaotic situations arising after an earthquake. A detailed explanation of ICS can be found in Chapter 9 (10).

Once the prehospital response begins, different paradigms are used. The potential exists for the medical needs of victims to exceed the available resources. Therefore, triage becomes very important in casualty management (see Chapter 2). Using a system such as START, providers can begin the process of prioritizing treatment. Moribund victims with agonal respirations or those in cardiac arrest do not receive care. The remainder are transported in the order established by their triage category. Although little data exist supporting the efficacy of START triage, a recent study examining the sensitivity and specificity of START in trauma patients concluded that the methodology could accurately sort these patients (11).

In an earthquake of this magnitude, communication will be severely limited or nonexistent. Hospital notification before arrival therefore is generally not an option. Patients are simply transported to the nearest hospital. With the passage of time and the establishment of an EOC and some form of ICS, prehospital providers begin receiving information on the status of surrounding hospitals. They can then exercise some discretion in selecting the hospitals to receive patients.

The transportation of victims can be problematic. Immediately following an earthquake, significant damage occurs to roads, traffic control devices, and street lighting. Seriously ill survivors who require vehicle transportation to reach medical care will experience delays until responders identify safe and passable routes to hospitals. The early use of police or National Guard members to control important transportation corridors can improve this situation.

Many individuals will not wait for the arrival of paramedics or other providers. Family and friends will drive many victims to the hospital themselves, conditions permitting. This contributes to the all too familiar convergence or geographic effect (the tendency of patients to go to the nearest hospital, overwhelming it and ignoring hospitals just a few miles away). Although this phenomenon is undesirable, it is virtually impossible to prevent in the first hours after an earthquake.

The loss of communication systems is inevitable, and it hampers all aspects of the medical response, including the direction and coordination of EMS activities. Paramedic radios frequently rely on repeaters to transmit radio signals to the dispatcher or base station. These repeaters can fail, which makes contact with paramedics in the field difficult. Cellular telephones can supplement the use of radios, but they also have limitations. One intriguing possibility is the use of ambulance radios. Unfortunately, however, ambulances from different jurisdictions do not use the same frequencies, so communication between a central coordinating body, such as the EOC, and the units in the field is unreliable. Authorities in San Francisco encountered these types of problems in the aftermath of the Loma Prieta earthquake (9). Thus, establishing a universally recognized disaster frequency would make a significant contribution to improving communications after an earthquake.

The problem of urban search and rescue after a seismic event is particularly vexing. Most morbidity and mortality associated with earthquakes results from building collapse (1). Victims who survive the initial event but who are trapped in a collapsed structure die rapidly if they are not quickly extricated. Data from the earthquakes in Tangshan, China (1976); Campania-Irpinia, Italy (1980); and Armenia (1988) demonstrate that 85% to 95% of those surviving entrapment in collapsed buildings were rescued in the first 24 hours (6). In the Italian study, 95% of those who died expired before extrication (12). When Dr. Peter Safar reviewed these data, he concluded that 25% to 50% of the injured who died slowly could have been saved if they had received immediate medical care (13). The unfortunate implication of these data is that most trapped victims will die if they are not extricated in the first 24 hours. A significant improvement in survival could be achieved if sophisticated urban search and rescue (USAR) teams arrived during this period. Unfortunately, a team takes about 24 hours to deploy and begin search and rescue activities. In the Northridge earthquake, 19 hours passed before the Riverside USAR team began operations at the Northridge Meadows Apartments. In the Oklahoma City bombing, state rescue personnel extricated the last survivor approximately 14 hours after the explosion (14). No one was evacuated alive from the damaged building by out-of-state USAR teams. The first United States USAR team took 48 hours to begin operations in Turkey after the 1999 earthquake (15). While USAR teams are successful in recovering live victims, most survivors appear to be extricated by early local search and rescue activity.

HOSPITAL IMPACT

Hospitals remain the medical provider of choice for victims of large seismic events. Therefore, institutional disaster plans must simultaneously prepare hospitals to evaluate their functional status, as well as to receive casualties. Unfortunately, no clear criteria are available for assisting hospitals in making evaluation decisions. Nonetheless, a rapid assessment of an institution's functional integrity by hospital personnel is critical. Guidance for this assessment can be obtained from documents such as ATC-20 and ATC-20-2, which were developed with the support of Federal Emergency Management Agency (FEMA), the National Science Foundation, and the State of California's Office of Emergency Services and Office of Statewide Health Planning and Development (16,17). Facility closure and evacuation are mandated by the identification of significant structural damage (e.g., "X" cracks and partially collapsed buildings) or an environment that is so compromised by nonstructural damage (e.g., severe water damage, loss of all life safety systems, human waste in patient care areas) that patient safety is at risk.

Little data are available regarding hospital evacuation after an earthquake. A common scenario calls for management of this event by the EOC. While this can be effective if time is not critical and communications are intact, it may be difficult under existing conditions after a large temblor. Data from the Northridge earthquake suggest that hospitals can successfully evacuate patients independent of EOC coordination if mutual aid agreements with other hospitals are already in place (7). However, coordination with the EOC is desirable if possible.

Making firm recommendations regarding the actual evacuation process is difficult, but information from the hospital evacuations after Northridge may be helpful. When time is not a factor, the strategy of evacuating the sickest patients first appears to work best. These individuals require extensive resources, and thus they are difficult to manage immediately after a large earthquake. Lessening the burden on the hospital enables the staff to provide better care to the more stable patients who remain and to concentrate on victims arriving from the field. When time is critical, the opposite strategy of evacuating the healthiest patients first may be best. This situation occurs when personnel believe that hospital structural collapse is imminent. This plan permits the staff to evacuate the greatest number of patients in the least amount of time.

The actual techniques for moving patients vary, but, in general, the simpler they are, the better. After Northridge, many special devices such as slides or stair chairs functioned poorly, and they were abandoned. The method of choice is to carry the patients using backboards or just blankets. In one hospital, the cloth litters purchased for hospital evacuation had not been used in years and had to be discarded because the material had rotted.

Evacuation routes should not involve elevators. They usually shut down after an earthquake because they are damaged or because the earthquake switches trip. In either case, the elevators cannot be used until they have been inspected. Stairwells should be used for vertical evacuations.

If the institution is considered capable of providing patient care, then all personnel must prepare for the arrival of victims. This usually involves the activation of a code triage or of the external disaster plan. Effective command and control of the facility's response requires hospital administration to implement a flexible management system that is not dependent on the presence of any specific individual. A proposed model that many hospitals use is called the hospital emergency incident command system (HEICS). It is similar in principle to ICS, but it is designed for use in medical institutions. HEICS has been used successfully in a number of disasters, including the Northridge earthquake and Hurricane Andrew in Florida. A detailed review of HEICS is available elsewhere (18).

After establishing a command post and implementing a system such as HEICS, the initial concerns of hospital administration include personnel, communications, and resources. Like the general population, hospital staff rely on telephones as their primary method of communication. Standard telephones will fail due to physical disruption or oversaturation. Alternate communication methods may be used if they are still functional. Alternate communication methods may include cellular telephones, fax machines, pay telephones, the internet/e-mail, alphanumeric pagers, and portable two-way radios (see Chapter 14). Because telephones do not function, hospital personnel at home cannot be contacted and told to report to work. Therefore, an automatic system is needed. An existing policy should state that hospital staff should report to work in the event of a large earthquake unless they are notified to remain at home. With respect to maintaining the flow of medical goods, notifying suppliers of a sudden increase in demand may be difficult if communication is disrupted. Therefore, an agreement should be negotiated in advance that requires suppliers to deliver a predetermined amount of equipment and material in the event of an earthquake.

Some individuals have questioned whether hospital employees would remain on duty or if they would instead abandon their positions to return to their home and check on family. While this probably occurs to some extent, it did not play a significant role in Northridge, nor does any evidence support this concern in general. Most staff remained on duty until they were relieved by other workers. In addition, most workers who did not immediately report to the hospital cited problems with communication and transportation as the reasons. This is consistent with other studies documenting the volunteer tradition of most United States citizens during times of disaster. Disaster planners should assume that most hospital staff will continue working.

If the hospital is located within an area of moderate-to-extensive damage, some form of convergence behavior due to the geographic effect is likely. Therefore, the emergency department (ED) should prepare for an influx of victims. Utilization of all available space, even areas not designed for patient care, such as auditoriums and parking lots, is important. In both the Loma Prieta and Northridge earthquakes, parking lots provided safe areas for patient care when the indoor space was compromised by structural or nonstructural damage.

In an attempt to get an early estimate of potential patient volume, information on the status of surrounding hospitals is valuable. If other hospitals in the area are damaged or are in the process of evacuation, the burden on remaining facilities will increase. Functioning hospitals can then expect an increase in ED volume above that which is already anticipated, as well as requests to accept patients in transfer from the damaged institutions. A wireless computer–driven hos-pital communication system can provide this type of information. While these systems are not impervious to damage, they do have the potential to give surviving hospitals a rapid crude estimate of the number of functioning facilities. This is especially important in light of the fact that nursing homes are more vulnerable to earthquake damage than hospitals and thus they usually transfer their patients to EDs during disasters.

The first wave of patients usually arrives within 15 to 30 minutes after the earthquake. They generally drive themselves to the hospital, presenting with minor injuries and lacerations. Triage becomes a critical issue for ED management of these patients. Because most do not have life-threatening or limb-threatening conditions, they should be quickly evaluated and should then be placed in an observation area. Emergency physicians must resist the temptation to treat this group in order to avoid the consumption of potentially limited resources. Treatment of conditions such as uncomplicated lacerations and fractures can be postponed until the ED staff has a better estimate of the overall demand for medical care. Because of the risk of missed foreign bodies and wound infection in this chaotic environment, some individuals have suggested that wounds not be closed primarily. They recommend either letting them heal by second intention or using delayed primary closure. Insufficient evidence exists to make a recommendation at this time.

After some delay, victims with more serious problems begin arriving. These individuals generally are transported by paramedics or ambulances, and they suffer from medical conditions as well as injuries. Reasons for delayed arrival include the time lost during extrication and the more critical condition of the patients, which makes transport by lay individuals difficult. This patient group provides the greatest challenge to the ED strategy for overall casualty management. Depending on the scenario, the number and acuity of patients presenting for care may possibly overwhelm the ED's resources for providing that care. Triage decisions must now focus not only on prioritizing patients for medical intervention but also, more importantly, on which patients should receive care at all. This situation has never happened in the United States, so a generally accepted algorithm guiding physician judgment does not exist. START triage provides guidance for selecting the order in which patients receive care but not for selecting which patients should be denied care and allowed to expire (except for the extreme of cardiopulmonary arrest). A proposed algorithm, the Secondary Assessment of Victim Endpoint (SAVE), holds promise.

The SAVE triage algorithm was designed specifically for the mass casualty situation following a large seismic event. It postulates an admittedly arbitrary but reasonable axiom that, given available resources, no person with less than a 50% chance of survival should be treated. Based on this assumption, the SAVE system creates specific triage pathways driven by outcome. Adult head-injured patients with a Glasgow Coma Score (GCS) of 8 or more have at least a 50% chance for a normal or near-normal recovery, and therefore these patients should receive care. Those with a GCS of 7 or less should not be treated. Patients with burns can also be stratified based on age greater than 60, the presence of an inhalation injury, and a total body surface area burn greater than 40%. Any patient with these three markers has a mortality of 50% or more and thus should receive comfort care only. A detailed discussion of SAVE triage can be found elsewhere (19).

Although still a work in progress, SAVE triage or something like it has the potential for improving medical judgment under stressful conditions and optimizing resource utilization. Areas for future development include the use of ultrasound to stratify patients with blunt abdominal trauma. Ultrasound machines have become truly portable (battery powered handheld devices are now on the market), and these will function after an earthquake. These devices could improve the triage of patients with blunt abdominal injuries through the use of methods such as the focused abdominal sonography for trauma (FAST) examination.

NEED FOR OTHER SOURCES OF MEDICAL CARE

Despite an improvement in the seismic durability of hospitals, they remain vulnerable to structural and nonstructural failure after large temblors. The Northridge earthquake effectively illustrates the problem. Eight hospitals in the Los Angeles area sustained enough damage to force the evacuation of at least one patient. Four institutions completely evacuated their facilities in the first 24 hours, including two hospitals that met the more current earthquake construction codes (7). Further structural damage, identified later, forced two additional hospitals to evacuate completely in the next 2 weeks. Ultimately, four of these hospitals were permanently closed and scheduled for demolition. In the aftermath of the Northridge earthquake, the California Seismic Safety Commission issued a report to the governor discussing the reduction of seismic risk through retrofitting. Unfortunately, the commission concluded that the occurrence of a catastrophic earthquake before California could reduce its seismic risk through this approach was a significant possibility (20). Also complicating the retrofitting strategy was the unexpected discovery of failed welds in steel-frame buildings (21). Many modern hospitals constructed to resist earthquake damage share this design flaw. Engineers incorrectly believed that this type of construction could tolerate earthquake forces. A method to repair these welds effectively remains elusive.

Clearly, hospitals cannot meet the entire demand for medical care. High magnitude earthquakes produce large casualty numbers. Many victims with serious but treatable injuries will die if they are not treated in the first 24 to 48 hours. If every hospital remained operational, the number of patients requiring hospitalization would exceed the number of beds. Yet, many hospitals will be rendered partially or completely nonfunctional. A 1981 study by the United States Geological Survey estimated that 25% of all hospital beds in the Los Angeles metropolitan region would be unavailable due to earthquake damage (22). If hospitals are damaged and no back-up plan exists, immediate advanced medical care will not be available, and many people will die.

Therefore, an alternate source of medical care is necessary to reduce early earthquake mortality. The Japanese came to the same conclusion after a review of data from the Hanshin-Awaji earthquake (23,24). Special medical teams, such as disaster medical assistance teams (DMATs), are a potential source of acute medical care and are a valuable resource. However, DMATs may not significantly impact acute survival if they arrive more than 48 hours after the earthquake. Most data to date suggest that deploying the large numbers of DMATs that are necessary after a high magnitude temblor will require at least this much time (25).

The use of local health care providers represents a solution to this dilemma. Because they are at or near the disaster site as soon as the event occurs, they can respond within hours. The most advanced model of this local medical response concept is the medical disaster response (MDR) project. MDR, which was developed by emergency physicians in Southern California, has the following two components: (a) the training of medical personnel in the management of disaster victims under austere conditions and (b) the placement of sophisticated medical supplies at predesignated sites within the community. Under this plan, victims could receive rapid advanced medical care from surviving volunteer health care providers even if hospitals are destroyed. A detailed discussion of the MDR project can be found in other publications (6,26).

EARTHQUAKE-RELATED MEDICAL ISSUES

The majority of patients requesting acute medical care after earthquakes suffers from lacerations, contusions, and simple fractures. Management of such cases is not difficult. However, a significant number of victims will present with more challenging conditions; some of these deserve special mention. The first group consists of individuals with common illnesses that are exacerbated by large seismic events. EDs will experience an increase in patients with these diagnoses. Examples include chronic obstructive pulmonary disease, myocardial infarctions, and possibly childbirth. The second group includes those with conditions or issues more unique to earthquakes, such as crush injury, the need to use ketamine, and indications for hypertonic saline treatment.

Not surprisingly, the number of patients with pulmonary complaints increases after seismic events. Collapsing structures fill the air with dust, as do early search and rescue activity. This dust poses an immediate threat to trapped victims. It can result in early mortality caused by airway obstruction or asphyxiation or delayed mortality from dust-induced pulmonary edema (1). Survivors with chronic lung ailments will also suffer from the dust exposure and will subsequently experience an increase in symptoms.

The number of patients who present with cardiac complaints is somewhat unexpected. An increase in the number of patients presenting with problems related to cardiovascular disease, including myocardial infarction and cardiac arrest, also appears to occur after an earthquake. A 50% increase in cardiac deaths was reported in the first 3 days following the 1981 Athens temblor (27,28). Data from the Northridge earthquake give further support to this phenomenon and suggest that it may be secondary to psychological stress, which precipitates the ischemic event, not to an increase in physical exertion (29). The incidence of sudden death actually decreased in the 6 days following the Northridge earthquake, suggesting that those who died immediately after the earthquake were predisposed to cardiac events. EDs should be aware of the increased incidence of these medical conditions and should be prepared to treat them.

Crush injury with associated crush syndrome and compartment syndrome is frequently found in victims of large-scale earthquakes. Standard therapy for crush syndrome includes vigorous intravenous (IV) hydration, sometimes as much as 12 L per day; bicarbonate; cardiac monitoring; and possible dialysis. In the first 24 to 48 hours following such an event, however, IV fluids will be scarce and the standard therapy cannot be administered. Under these austere circumstances, prevention may be the only alternative to the otherwise inevitable morbidity and mortality resulting from untreated crush syndrome. Prevention is accomplished using amputation and/or fasciotomy.

After a crush injury with elevated compartment pressures, muscle tissue can remain viable for approximately 2 to 3 hours (30). A fasciotomy performed within this time frame may save the extremity and prevent crush syndrome. The double incision technique for decompressing the lower leg is probably best. Use of a simple device consisting of IV tubing, a needle, and a manometer or a commercially available device can augment the clinical assessment of compartment pressures in difficult or confusing cases. After 4 hours, the risk that dead muscle is present increases. A fasciotomy executed at this point may expose nonviable muscle to the environment, thus resulting in sepsis and death; therefore, it should not be attempted. Instead, amputation should be considered. Clearly, the availability of IV fluids and estimated time to definitive care will affect this decision.

Amputations may also be necessary to extricate victims from rubble and to remove hopelessly mangled extremities. The mangled extremity severity score (MESS) is a useful tool in aiding in decisions regarding amputation of the lower extremities in questionable cases (Table 16.2) (31). Under austere conditions, a guillotine amputation performed at the most distal site possible is best. The stump can be revised at a later date. A field amputation was necessary to free a trapped victim after the Loma Prieta earthquake.

To facilitate the performance of major procedures like amputations, fasciotomies, and fracture reduction, a profound state of anesthesia and analgesia is required. This could be accomplished using regional anesthesia, such as axillary, femoral, or sciatic nerve blocks. However, these procedures can be technically difficult, and they can produce variable results. A more reliable option is the use of ketamine.

Ketamine is safe and effective, it has a rapid onset and a short duration of action, and it is easily administered orally, intravenously, rectally, or intramuscularly. In addition, it supports the cardiovascular system, preserves airway reflexes, and does not significantly depress ventilation under most conditions. No other agent currently available can produce the necessary levels of anesthesia and analgesia as reliably and as simply as ketamine can. It has been used safely and effectively by non-medical persons in the unmonitored, austere environments of Afghanistan for years to facilitate field amputations and other procedures (32). In a review of 11,589 patients treated with ketamine, only two otherwise healthy patients required intubation (33). Recent articles in the emergency medicine literature

TABLE 16.2. MANGLED EXTREMITY SEVERITY SCORE

Finding	Points
Skeletal/soft-tissue injury	
Low energy (stab; simple fracture; civilian GSW)	1
Medium energy (open or multiple fractures, dislocation)	2
High energy (close-range shotgun or military GSW, crush injury)	3
Very high energy (above plus gross contamination, soft-tissue avulsion)	4
Limb ischemia	
Normal pulse	0
Pulse reduced or absent but perfusion normal	1*
Pulseless; parasthesias, diminished capillary refill	2*
Cool, paralyzed, insensate, numb	3*
Shock	
Systolic BP always >90 mm Hg	0
Transiently hypotensive	1
Persistent hypotension	2
Age (yr)	
<30	0
30–50	1
>50	2

*Score doubled for ischemia >6 hr.
Abbreviations: BP, Blood pressure; GSW, gunshot wound.

document the safety and efficacy of ketamine (34,35). The currently recommended dose for intravenous (IV) administration is 2 mg per kg; for intramuscular (IM) injection, it is 5 mg per kg.

Since quantities of intravenous fluids may be limited in the first 24 to 48 hours after a large earthquake, typical practice patterns involving the type of fluid chosen and the amount infused must be modified. The optimal IV solution for resuscitation and stabilization of disaster victims remains controversial. However, limited data suggest that hypertonic saline for initial resuscitation and normal saline for maintenance are reasonable choices. These are the fluids recommended by the MDR project (6). At a dose of 4 mL per kg, hypertonic saline appears safe and effective in a variety of trauma patients, including children (36–38). If patients respond to challenges with hypertonic saline, they can be supported with normal saline. The eventual development of hypernatremia is a concern, so this regimen cannot be used indefinitely. However, it can reduce the use of normal saline, and its intent is to buy time until definitive care becomes available.

Complicating this situation is the controversy concerning the extent to which a trauma patient should be resuscitated before establishing control of the bleeding site. Reports by Bickell et al. (39) on the initial fluid management of patients with penetrating trauma and by Pretto et al. (40) on the early management of war casualties in Bosnia suggest that patient prognosis is improved by withholding aggressive fluid resuscitation until hemostasis is achieved. Whether these data apply to patients with blunt trauma is currently unknown. If fluids are scarce, one option is to halt resuscitation when the systolic blood pressure reaches approximately 80 to 90 mm Hg as was done in Bosnia. Until more data are available, making firm recommendations is difficult.

MEDICAL ISSUES DURING RECOVERY

The increased demand for medical services after an earthquake is intense, but the duration is relatively brief. Most evidence suggests that, within 3 to 5 days after the event, hospital case-mix patterns have returned to near normal (1). After 1 week, the arrival of aid directed at treating patients with acute medical illnesses or traumatic injuries related to the earthquake will have less of an impact. The vast majority of patients will have received treatment, died, or been transferred to other hospitals. The issue at this point is reconstitution of the basic medical care system. Earthquakes destroy not only hospitals, but medical offices and clinics as well. Disaster or not, the basic health care needs of the population will continue.

In this situation, DMATs provide their most important function. They can arrive and can begin treating ambulatory patients in 48 to 72 hours, thus helping to decompress overburdened emergency departments. Because they are self-sufficient from both a personnel and medical supply perspective, they can establish temporary clinics without assistance from an already resource-depleted community. DMATs can support the ongoing health needs of the general population until the medical community can reconstitute the healthcare infrastructure. Although DMATs can provide acute medical care, most of their experience has been in the delivery of ambulatory care, and that is where they have enjoyed their greatest successes (see Chapter 13).

A brief discussion about epidemics is indicated as some disaster planners worry about the outbreak of epidemics following earthquakes. While this is technically possible, it does not appear likely, based on recent world experience. Decisions to bury bodies hurriedly or to begin mass vaccination campaigns based solely on the fear of possible epidemics are generally inappropriate. The results of epidemiologic surveillance should guide such decisions.

SUMMARY

The medical management of earthquake victims remains a difficult challenge. However, the amount of data on this subject continues to increase, and making several recommendations is now possible. Implementation of field triage and unified command using systems similar to START and ICS is important in seizing early control of the chaotic prehospital disaster scenes. Hospitals will provide the bulk of medical care in the first 24 to 48 hours, but they cannot do it alone. A back-up plan is necessary to support hospitals in case they are damaged or overwhelmed. Otherwise, potentially salvageable patients will die. Some institutions will likely be severely damaged by the earthquake, so hospitals should have a viable evacuation plan. Furthermore, the number of patients seeking care may exceed the available resources. Therefore, ED personnel should be prepared to implement a system such as SAVE for selecting which patients should receive care. After the disaster, rebuilding the medical infrastructure will require time. DMATs play an important role in maintaining the health of the general population until the medical community is reestablished. Finally, clearly more information is needed on the optimal management of earthquake victims. Research in this area must be funded to build on the medical advances already achieved.

REFERENCES

1. Noji EK. Natural disasters. In: Kvetan V, Carlson R, Geheb M, eds. Disaster management. *Crit Care Clin* 1991;7:271–292.
2. Friedman E. Coping with calamity—how well does health care disaster planning work? *JAMA* 1994;272:1875–1879.
3. Scientists of the United States Geological Survey and the Southern California Earthquake Center. The Magnitude 6.7 North-

ridge, California, Earthquake of 17 January 1994. *Science* 1994; 266:389–397.

4. Associated Press. Kobe damaged, rebuilds. January 13, 1996, V0759.

5. The Los Angeles Times. Images of the 1994 Los Angeles earthquake. *Los Angeles Times*. Los Angeles, 1994;4:31.

6. Schultz CH, Koenig KL, Noji EK. A medical disaster response to reduce immediate mortality following an earthquake. *N Engl J Med* 1996;334:438–444.

7. Schultz CH, Koenig KL, Auf der Heide E. Hospital evacuation after the Northridge earthquake [abstract]. *Acad Emerg Med* 1998;5:526–527.

8. Super G, Groth S, Hook R, et al. *START—simple triage and rapid treatment plan*. Newport Beach, CA: Hoag Memorial Presbyterian Hospital, 1994.

9. Emergency Medical Services Earthquake Project Study of the Emergency Medical Impact of the Loma Prieta Earthquake. *The emergency medical impact of the Loma Prieta earthquake*. San Francisco: Emergency Medical Services Agency, Department of Public Health, City and County of San Francisco, 1993.

10. Irwin RL. The incident command system (ICS). In: Auf der Heide E, ed. *Disaster response: principles of preparation and coordination*. St. Louis: Mosby, 1989:133–163.

11. Garner A, Lee A, Harrison K, Schultz CH. Comparative analysis of multiple-casualty incident triage algorithms. *Ann Emerg Med* 2001;38:541–548.

12. de Bruycker M, Greco D, Annino I, et al. The 1980 earthquake in southern Italy: rescue of trapped victims and mortality. *Bull WHO* 1983;61:1021–1025.

13. Safar P. Resuscitation potentials in mass disasters. *Prehosp Disaster Med* 1986;2:34–47.

14. Hogan DE, Waeckerle JF, Dire DJ, et al. Emergency department impact of the Oklahoma City terrorist bombing. *Ann Emerg Med* 1999;34:160–167.

15. United States Agency for International Development, Office of Foreign Disaster Assistance. *Turkey—earthquake*, factsheet no. 6. Washington, D.C.: United States Agency for International Development, Office of Foreign Disaster Assistance, August 20, 1999.

16. Applied Technology Council. *ATC-20: procedures for postearthquake safety evaluation of buildings*. Redwood City, CA: Applied Technology Council, 1989.

17. Applied Technology Council. *ATC-20-2: addendum to the ATC-20 postearthquake building safety evaluation procedures*. Redwood City, CA: Applied Technology Council, 1995.

18. The San Mateo County Health Services Agency. *Emergency medical services: hospital emergency incident command system*, 3rd ed. San Mateo, CA: San Mateo County Health Services Agency, 1998.

19. Benson M, Koenig KL, Schultz CH. Disaster triage: START then SAVE. A new method of dynamic triage for victims of a catastrophic earthquake. *Prehosp Disaster Med* 1996;11:117–124.

20. California Seismic Safety Commission. *The Northridge earthquake—turning loss to gain: a report to the governor*. Sacramento, CA: California Seismic Safety Commission, 1995.

21. Kerr RA. Bigger jolts are on the way for Southern California. *Science* 1995;267:176–177.

22. Steinbrugge KV, Algermissen ST, Lagorio HJ, et al. Metropolitan San Francisco and Los Angeles earthquake loss studies: 1980 assessment. *U.S. geological survey open-file report 81-113*. Denver: United States Geological Survey, 1981.

23. Tsuboi S, Meguro F. Medical coordination at the time of the disaster. *Japanese J Disaster Med* 1996;1:36–45.

24. Kobayashi H. Revised emergency disaster medical response plan and preparedness of Hyogo prefecture after the Great Hanshin-Awaji earthquake. *Japanese J Disaster Med* 1996;1:73–77.

25. Leonard R, Stringer L, Alson R. Patient-data collection system used during medical operations after the 1994 San Fernando Valley-Northridge earthquake. *Prehosp Disaster Med* 1995;10: 55–60.

26. Schultz CH, Koenig KL. Preventing crush syndrome: assisting with field amputation and fasciotomy. *JEMS* 1997;22:30–37.

27. Trichopoulos D, Katsouyanni K, Zavitsanos X, et al. Psychological stress and fatal heat attack: the Athens (1981) earthquake natural experiment. *Lancet* 1983;1:441–444.

28. Katsouyanni K, Kogevinas M, Trichopoulos D. Earthquake-related stress and cardiac mortality. *Int J Epidemiol* 1986;15: 326–330.

29. Leor J, Poole WK, Kloner RA. Sudden cardiac death triggered by an earthquake. *N Engl J Med* 1996;334;413–419.

30. Vaillancourt C, Shrier I, Falk M, et al. Quantifying delays in the recognition and management of acute compartment syndrome. *CJEM* 2001;3:26–31.

31. Johansen K, Daines M, Howey T, et al. Objective criteria accurately predict amputation following lower extremity trauma. *J Trauma* 1990;30:568–573.

32. Halbert RJ, Simon RR, Nasraty Q. Surgical theatre in rural Afghanistan. *Ann Emerg Med* 1988;l7:775–778.

33. Green SM, Johnson NE. Ketamine sedation for pediatric procedures: part 2, review and implications. *Ann Emerg Med* 1990;19: 1033–1046.

34. Chudnofsky CR, Weber JE, Stoyanoff PT, et al. A combination of midazolam and ketamine for procedural sedation and analgesia in adult emergency department patients. *Acad Emerg Med* 2000;7:228–235.

35. Green SM, Clem KJ, Rothrock SG. Ketamine safety profile in the developing world: survey of practitioners. *Acad Emerg Med* 1996;3:598–604.

36. Bowser BH, Caldwell FT. The effects of resuscitation with hypertonic vs. hypotonic vs. colloid on wound and urine fluid and electrolyte losses in severely burned children. *J Trauma* 1983;23: 916–923.

37. Mattox KL, Maningas PA, Moore EE, et al. Prehospital hypertonic saline-dextran infusion for post-traumatic hypotension: the USA multicenter trial. *Ann Surg* 1991;213:482–491.

38. Younes RN, Aun F, Accioly CQ, et al. Hypertonic solutions in the treatment of hypovolemic shock: a prospective, randomized study in patients admitted to the emergency room. *Surgery* 1992; 11:380–385.

39. Bickell WH, Wall MJ Jr, Pepe PE, et al. Immediate versus delayed fluid resuscitation for hypotensive patients with penetrating torso injuries. *New Engl J Med* 1994;331:1105–1109.

40. Pretto EA, Begovic M, Gegovic M. Emergency medical services during the siege of Sarajevo, Bosnia and Herzegovina: a preliminary report. *Prehosp Disaster Med* 1994;9:S39–S45.

TORNADOES

DAVID E. HOGAN

On May 3, 1999 a significant outbreak of tornadoes occurred throughout the states of Oklahoma and Kansas. One of these tornadoes was one of the largest in the last 50 years to pass through the Oklahoma City metropolitan area. This tornado produced winds of over 316 mph, classifying it as the most intense tornado recorded on the planet (1). The storm resulted in 45 deaths, 637 known injuries, and 140 patients hospitalized throughout the Oklahoma City metropolitan area (2).

Tornadoes generate the most violent winds of any storm on earth. Although the geographic extent of a tornadic storm is much less than that of a hurricane, it can devastate entire communities with little or no warning. Approximately 800 tornadoes strike in the United States annually (3). From 1950 to 1994, over 4,115 deaths and 70,000 injuries have been reported to the National Weather Service due to tornadic storms (4). One estimate is that over $20 trillion dollars has been lost due to tornadic storms during the same period (5). Aside from the death and injury caused, the impact on the health and well-being of the community from a tornadic storm can be devastating. A 1986 storm in Pennsylvania not only resulted in 91 deaths and 800 injuries, but over 3,000 people were left homeless (6). A 1990 storm in Illinois resulted in the loss of electrical power and other basic utilities to 65,000 homes for an extended period (7). The 1999 Oklahoma City tornado significantly damaged or destroyed over 15,000 single-family dwellings, rendering over 10,000 homes uninhabitable (1).

Although almost all regions of the earth are subject to the risk of tornadic storms, the unique landscape and weather patterns of the United States cause it to have the greatest severity of these storms in comparison to anywhere else on earth. Tornadoes are generally created in large thunderstorms known as "supercell" thunderstorms. An unstable environment is created by a cold dry air mass at a high altitude that overlies a warm, moist air mass close to the ground level. Thunderstorms developing in such an environment have the potential to become massive supercell thunderstorms with tops reaching 35,000 to 45,000 feet. The lateral boundary between the dry, cool air and the warm, moist air is known as the dry line. The interaction between these two elements of the atmosphere can result in a spinning stream of air along the dry line. This stream of air in combination with thunderstorm activity is thought to be instrumental in the generation of tornadoes.

Although they are a chaotic atmospheric phenomenon, the behavior of tornadoes still follows some statistical patterns. During each 24-hour period, the frequency of occurrence of tornadoes is predictable; approximately 60% will occur between noon and sunset, 21% from sunset to midnight, and approximately 19% from midnight to noon (5). In addition, a region of high tornado occurrence within the United States has led to the central corridor of the country being nicknamed "Tornado Alley" (Fig. 17.1). This is due to the mixing across this region of high level, cold, dry air from the northern tier of states with the warm, low level, moist air from the Gulf of Mexico. The frequency of tornado occurrence is highest during the spring in Texas, Oklahoma, and southern Kansas. As the year progresses, tornado frequency shifts to the northern states in the central tier, including northern Kansas, Nebraska, and South and North Dakota. All regions of the United States have experienced tornadoes, many of which have been severe. In addition, phenomena such as El Niño may alter the weather patterns of the United States and may temporarily shift the probability of tornado occurrence to other locations.

The severity of tornadoes is graded on the Fujita-Pearson Tornado Scale. This is a scale that ranges from a designation of F0 through F5. Although initially based on the level of structural damage, the scale now primarily reflects the measured wind speed of the tornado. The majority of tornadoes are considered weak (F0, F1) with wind speeds of less than 113 mph. These weaker tornadoes cause minor property damage, but they typically do not result in significant injuries or loss of life. At the other end of the scale, the more violent tornadoes (F4, F5) have wind speeds of greater than 206 mph. Although these severe tornadoes only account for 1% to 2% of the total number of tornadoes on an annual basis, they are responsible for more than 50% of all tornado-related deaths in the United States (8).

The National Weather Service is the sole United States official agency for issuing warnings during threatening

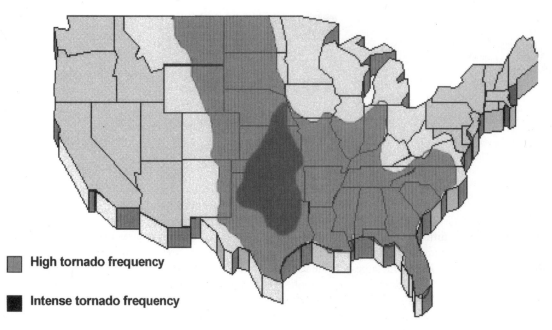

High tornado frequency

Intense tornado frequency

FIGURE 17.1. Distribution of tornado frequency in the United States.

weather situations. Established on February 9, 1870 by President Ulysses S. Grant, the National Weather Service and its divisions have created a set of watch and warnings criteria for tornadic thunderstorms. The responsibility for monitoring, forecasting, and issuing watches and warnings related to tornadic thunderstorms rests with the Storm Prediction Center (SPC) located in Norman, Oklahoma, a Division of the National Centers for Environmental Prediction (NCEP) of the National Weather Service. A *tornado watch* will be issued by the SPC for a specific area of the United States when conditions within that area are conducive to the formation of tornadoes. A *tornado warning* is issued for a specific area when either visual sighting of a tornado occurs or radar indications demonstrate the presence of an active tornado within that region. The United States Weather Service has deployed a "next-generation" radar (NEXRAD) system throughout the United States to improve monitoring, prediction, and warning capabilities. With this new system, providing warning to specific geographic locations of impending tornado strikes is possible approximately 20 minutes or more before impact (1).

PREHOSPITAL CONSIDERATIONS

Tornado disasters provide some unique problems for the prehospital health care provider. As opposed to some disasters that result in a well-localized region of disruption, tornadoes create several linear areas of destruction throughout the community. These zones of destruction average several hundred yards in width, and they may be several miles long. Zones of destruction cut across and destroy utility services,

such as electrical power and communication. In addition, they block usual access routes throughout the city, making entrance and exit into the areas of destruction difficult. Usual routes to emergency departments may also be obstructed, thus altering casualty distribution. Emergency medical services (EMS) units may be at risk when moving into areas of destruction because of lingering elements of the storm, downed power lines, flooding, and adverse traffic conditions. Debris on the road may not only block EMS vehicles, but it can also result in vehicle damage, taking units out of service.

In previous tornado disasters, the majority of victims who die do so at the scene (4). Only small numbers of victims who arrive at emergency departments die after hospital admission (2,6,9). This suggests that, although EMS may have a significant impact on the morbidity of patients, there may be little impact on mortality. Rapid identification of the location of severely injured victims in a tornado strike zone and the delivery of those individuals to an emergency care system may assist in decreasing mortality, as well as morbidity. That the most severely injured victims will be located within the core area of the tornado strike is intuitive, and is illustrated by the report in the 1996 Topeka, Kansas tornado (10). Many tornadoes also are known to exhibit damage patterns within the core zone of damage that are known as multiple vortex suction spots (3). In a 1970 tornado in Lubbock, Texas, Dr. Ted Fujita correlated the location of the fatalities to the location of the multiple vortex suction spots on the ground. Almost all the fatalities in this report occurred within the areas defined by these multiple suction spots (Fig. 17.2) (11). These multiple suction spots are visible both from the air and the ground fol-

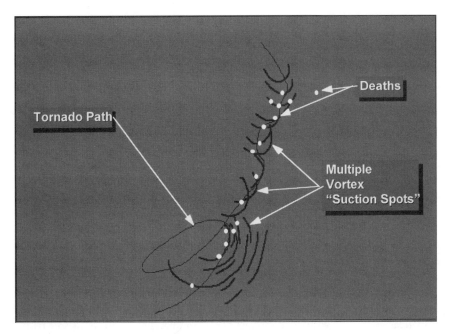

FIGURE 17.2. Deaths and tornado suction spots after Fujita (From Grazulis TP. *A guide to tornado video classics—II: the magnificent puzzle*. Johnsbury, VT: The Tornado Project of Environmental Films, 1994:20, with permission).

lowing a tornado. Additionally, severe injuries have been correlated with increasing degrees of structural damage to dwellings (12–14). If particularly heavily damaged buildings can be identified, they may represent areas for the initiation of search and rescue activities.

Deployment of EMS vehicles to field sites after a tornado strike must be carefully considered and coordinated. Although EMS units should be deployed along areas of significant damage, care should be taken to support initial EMS responders adequately with additional units for the evacuation of triaged patients. EMS units are commonly overwhelmed with casualties at the scene without adequate supplies or evacuation resources. Known radio communication blackout zones should be avoided in the creation of casualty collection or triage points. Medical command and emergency dispatch should keep careful track of the location of each unit to coordinate prehospital teams with casualty collection points.

One previous suggestion has been that air medical units in a metropolitan area may not be particularly useful following a tornado disaster (15). However, more recent indications are that air medical units might provide specific and valuable services. Helicopters have been used to deploy physician and paramedic units to the site of rural tornado disasters. This is invaluable, particularly when disruption of the medical infrastructure has occurred in these communities (16). In addition, reconnaissance may be performed by air-medical units to help delineate the extent of destruction, as well as to identify initial areas for search and rescue. In metropolitan areas, air medical units can be valuable in transporting patients from casualty collection points to definitive care. During the May 1999 Oklahoma City tornado, air medical units were used to transfer patients from

injury scenes and casualty collection points and from hospital to hospital. This was accomplished by coordination among fire, EMS, and air medical elements before the occurrence of the disaster. Well-marked and lighted landing zones were established at most casualty collection points and were manned by knowledgeable ground personnel (17). Interhospital transport of critical victims to specialty hospitals in the city avoided the serious disruption in ground traffic that was caused by the storm.

EMERGENCY DEPARTMENT CONSIDERATIONS

Loss of electrical power is a very real possibility during a tornado disaster. Emergency departments typically have back-up electrical generators available as part of the overall hospital disaster plan. However, these back-up generators often provide limited amounts of electrical energy to the emergency department. They may be inadequate to supply the level of care needed to evaluate the number of tornado victims arriving. Consideration should be given to the location of additional back-up electrical generators, particularly for outside triage areas. Lights of sufficient intensity should be available for the triage area in the event of electrical failure. Large flashlights in sufficient numbers should be provided for the physician and nursing staff to carry in the event of the loss of power. These flashlights should be part of the regular disaster stock in the emergency department, and they should be evaluated for potency of batteries on a regular basis. If outdoor lighting is inadequate, vehicle headlights may provide a short-term remedy.

Communication within the emergency department during a tornado disaster is a problem as well. Coordination between the emergency department arrival areas, triage, the emergency department proper, and the operating rooms is dependent on the ability to communicate. This may be achieved by numerous methods, including hand-held FM radio transmitters, hard-wire technology, or runners. If radio communication methods are selected, these radios should be part of the regular disaster stock, and the batteries must be maintained regularly. Personnel should be trained in radio use procedures.

Traffic control has consistently been reported as a problem in and around emergency departments following a tornado disaster. The hospital and the surrounding access and egress routes should be secured by hospital security or police. Law enforcement agencies should be familiar with the requirements for traffic flow into and out of the emergency department during a disaster. Walking wounded, privately operated vehicles, and EMS vehicles should be directed to the appropriate triage and evaluation areas.

Adequate water supply is also vital for the continued functioning of the emergency department. Many victims of tornadoes present with soil and debris coating their skin. At times, the contamination can be so substantial that primary surveys are difficult to perform with any proficiency (4). Plans should be made to provide a continuous and adequate water supply to emergency departments during tornado disasters. Portable or fixed shower facilities are highly desirable, and they may be used to decontaminate tornado victims as part of overall evaluation and care.

All emergency departments should have access to real-time weather information for their local community. This is necessary not only to prepare during watches and warnings but also to monitor ongoing weather conditions during the time that the emergency department is receiving casualties. The occurrence of other severe weather phenomena, such as hail, lightning, and additional tornadoes, can threaten emergency department operations in the midst of the response to the primary event. Internal storm disaster plans must be in place as a part of each institution's disaster plan.

The majority of victims arriving to emergency departments following a tornado will arrive by privately operated vehicles. Most of these victims will be walking wounded, but some will have serious injuries. Health care providers involved in triage must be cognizant of proper spinal immobilization and vehicle extrication techniques. These are used in an effort to avoid causing additional injury to the victims as they arrive to the emergency department without having had the benefit of prehospital medical stabilization. Education of the emergency department staff in appropriate spinal immobilization and vehicle transfer techniques should be a routine part of ongoing education in the emergency department.

As with most disasters, tornado victims tend to arrive in a two-wave pattern. Initial victims usually arrive within 15 to 20 minutes of the tornado strike. This constitutes the first wave and usually primarily represents the walking wounded with minor injuries. The second wave of more seriously injured victims tends to arrive within 1 to 4 hours following the storm; these will arrive by a mixture of private vehicle and EMS transportation (4).

TORNADO-RELATED INJURIES

A review of the reports and experiences of health care providers responding to tornado disasters provides some insight regarding the type of injuries seen. The most common injuries tend to be complex contaminated soft-tissue wounds. These are various lacerations, contusions, abrasions, and punctures. Over 50% of the cases seen in emergency departments suffer from these wounds. The majority of the soft tissue wounds will be contaminated with soil and foreign bodies. Many wounds will be deep and complex in nature with concomitant blunt trauma. The majority of soft-tissue injuries are seen on the exposed areas of the body, such as the head, neck, and arms. In addition, eye injuries, including ocular rupture, corneal foreign bodies, and abrasions, occur regularly. Up to 50% of the soft-tissue wounds may be sustained during rescue and recovery activities (12,18).

Fractures are the second most common injury typically reported from tornadoes, and they may account for up to 30% of total injuries (4). Fractures are often the most common cause for hospital admission. Up to one-quarter of the fractures reported may be open (19). One small study conducted of the Oklahoma City tornado in May 1999 indicated that 46% of the cases taken to the operating room at a community hospital required operative intervention for fractures (20).

Head injury following tornadoes is commonly reported. Severe head injury usually accounts for less than 10% of the total, but it is reported as the most common cause of death following a tornado (4). The majority of reported head injuries are considered minor concussions. Most cases are discharged from emergency departments with head injury instructions. Head injury is usually the second most common cause of hospitalization.

Blunt trauma to the chest and abdomen accounts for less than 10% of the overall injuries reported in emergency departments. The number of cases needing exploratory laparotomy or other surgical interventions has not been clearly documented in the literature. One community hospital reported that 23% of the cases following a tornado required emergency laparotomy for blunt abdominal trauma (21). The rate of intraabdominal trauma and hemodynamic shock following tornado injury has been suggested to be greater than that for motor vehicle crash victims when the two cohorts are compared (22).

Most patients who arrive in the emergency department will survive (7,9,10,23–26). Those victims who die in the field typically succumb to severe head injury, cervical spine trauma, or crush injury to the chest (6,9,10,19,25,27,28). Admission rates for victims injured by tornadoes typically are about 25% (12,24,25,29–32).

WOUND CARE

The highly contaminated nature of wounds seen in the emergency department following a tornado disaster deserves additional consideration. A wounding phenomenon almost unique to tornadoes has been reported in the medical literature (4). This is a dermobrasive effect caused by fine soil, sand, and mud particles being accelerated by tornadic winds to such a degree that the skin is essentially sandblasted. The types of therapy provided for this abrasive injury and the outcomes of these wounds have not been reported. Therefore, the logical conclusion is that tornado-abrasive wounds might be treated similarly to extensive abrasions from any other mechanism (Fig. 17.3).

Because of the complex nature and the high frequency of contamination of tornado wounds, these injuries have been compared to shrapnel wounds sustained during military conflicts from mortars (22). In addition, extremely high frequencies of wound infections have been suggested, although they have not been statistically documented (33). Most authors in the literature suggest delayed primary closure for the majority of tornado wounds (4). However, few emergency physicians actually do this in practice. No studies are found in the literature to support delayed primary closure over immediate closure in the emergency depart-

ment for tornado wounds. Therefore, the author can make no firm recommendations, but caution is advised due to the perceived likelihood of wound repair complications. The recommendations are discussed below.

The effect of antibiotics administered at the time of wound closure is unknown. Previous authors in reports from the late 1960s and early 1970s have suggested that antibiotics are ineffective in preventing wound infection following tornado injuries (23,28). What protection the newer generation of antibiotics available to emergency departments today may offer these patients is unknown.

Currently, considering delayed primary closure for all tornado wounds presenting to the emergency department would seem appropriate. Should the decision be made to close wounds primarily, they should be subjected to intense exploration and irrigation to decrease the bacterial count and to remove foreign bodies. Antibiotic coverage should probably be provided for these victims. If a wound is closed primarily in the emergency department, the antibiotic should preferentially be administered at least 1 hour before any significant tissue manipulation. Parenteral routes of antibiotic administration are preferred to allow the rapid accumulation of the antibiotic in tissues. In addition, the antibiotic should be one that is effective against the predicted pathologic contaminants for that wound.

Aerobic gram-negative species, such as *Escherichia coli*, *Klebsiella*, *Serratia*, *Proteus*, and *Pseudomonas* species, are commonly found as wound contaminants in tornado wounds (22,23,34,35). Staphylococcus and streptococcus species have been suggested as the most common causes of wound infections in patients discharged from emergency

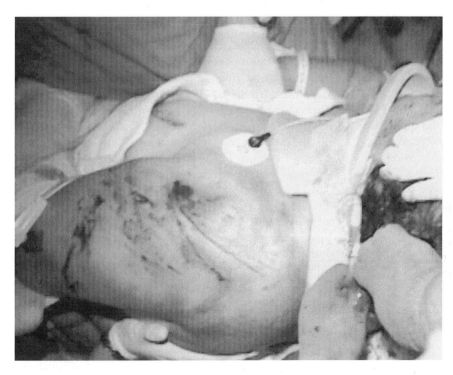

FIGURE 17.3. Abrasive effect on skin due to tornado. Courtesy of Gary Quick, M.D.

department with tornado-sustained wounds, although this has not been confirmed. *Pseudomonas* is also a known tornado wound contaminant, suggesting that antibiotic coverage may need to be extended for this organism as well to patients who are at risk for such infections. Antibiotic coverage should be continued for 24 to 72 hours following wound closure in the emergency department. All patients treated in this way require wound follow-up in 24 to 48 hours.

Patients admitted to the hospital seem to have an increased frequency of *pseudomonas* infections, although gram-negative nosocomial infections were not controlled for in these reports (22,23,34). Infections due to *Clostridium perfringens* and the resultant gas gangrene have been reported in victims with tornado wounds (34). However, that tornado wounds are necessarily more at risk for infections by this organism than wounds sustained by any other traumatic process would be is unlikely (22,34,35). Despite the chaos associated with tornado disasters, careful record-keeping and follow-up are important in wound care.

One death secondary to tetanus in a victim suffering tornado wounds has been reported (14). Tornado injuries generally should be considered as tetanus prone. (Tetanus-prone wounds are generally considered to be those that have a complex or avulsed nature, that are over 1 cm in depth, that are due to a blunt crush, missile-related, or thermal etiology, that have visible contamination, or that have presented to the emergency department more than 6 hours after wounding [36]). If these patients have not received their initial tetanus immunization of three doses, they should receive tetanus immune globulin, 250 U, and tetanus toxoid immunization at separate body sites. All other victims should receive tetanus immunization if more than 5 years have passed since their last tetanus booster. Patients less than 7 years old should receive pediatric diphtheria-tetanus (DT) toxoid, 0.5 mL intramuscularly (IM), and patients more than 7 years old should receive tetanus-diphtheria (Td) toxoid, 0.5 mL IM.

Puncture wounds due to tornadoes also require special consideration. These wounds should not be closed due to the high potential for foreign body and contamination. They should be investigated for foreign bodies by the appropriate radiologic techniques and exploration if possible. Puncture wounds should be irrigated with low-pressure irrigation with normal saline or with 1% povidone-iodine solution. Consideration should be given to debridement or core techniques for these wounds, particularly if foreign bodies are highly suspected or are detected. Such techniques may be performed in the emergency department, but they may be better performed the following day under more controlled conditions in either outpatient or inpatient surgical settings.

SHELTERING ACTIVITIES

Adequate warning of an approaching tornado and appropriate sheltering activities by the population have been demonstrated as the most important factor associated with decreasing morbidity and mortality (12–14,37–39). The population must be adequately educated regarding the appropriate response to take for sheltering during tornado warning. Tornado warnings may be broken into active warning systems and passive warning systems. Active warning systems have been demonstrated to be the most effective (39). These consist of neighborhood storm sirens, weather alert radios, and other systems that do not require the recipient to initiate any activity to receive warning. Passive warning systems consist primarily of the electronic news media, such as television and radio stations, and require that the recipient initiate contact with these media and monitor ongoing events. All public safety agencies and emergency departments should be equipped with both active and passive warning systems. All emergency departments will find having real-time access to the local television and radio media to monitor ongoing events to be valuable.

The population must be adequately educated with regard to the appropriate sheltering activities to take once a warning has been issued. Community education projects in tornado-risk zones are often provided by the local news media as a public service. Additionally, emergency departments and EMS services may be involved. Outreach programs for both EMS and emergency departments into the community may be performed during tornado season as part of a public education program. Public service announcements and newspaper advertisements may not only discuss other health-related issues, but they may also provide sheltering information for severe storms as a public service. Education may also be provided in the form of discharge instructions, both verbal and printed, during discharge from emergency departments in the same manner that other health-related information, such as car seat and seatbelt use, is provided to patients.

Mobile homes are probably the most dangerous structures to be in during a tornado. Facetiously, mobile homes have been suggested to act as tornado magnets, pulling these severe storms to their location. This has not been substantiated by research, but mobile homes have been noted to be excellent tornado-detectors. With even the best known tie-downs for mobile homes, wind speeds of 50 to 55 mph will cause mobile homes to become airborne (14,15,28,29). Injury rates for victims who remain in mobile homes during tornadoes have been estimated at 85.1 per 1,000 versus 3 per 1,000 for victims who shelter in standard constructed homes (14). Communities should install active alert sirens for all mobile home parks. Specific education programs should be targeted for these individuals with regard to appropriate sheltering techniques. Current recommendations are that individuals in mobile homes should leave the mobile homes as soon as possible and should find more substantial shelter. Communal storm shelters have been recommended for all mobile home parks. These shelters should be easily accessible and of sufficient size and number to allow the entire intended population access to them during a tornado warning (9).

Individuals outside during a tornado have also been documented as being at increased risk for death and injury (14). Recommendations are that, during storm season, the individuals maintain communication with at least passive alert mechanisms. At the issuance of a tornado warning, they should seek shelter in a hardened structure, if possible. At minimum, they should shelter in a low ditch or culvert region covered with available materials. Being located in a motor vehicle during a tornado has also been associated with an increased risk for injury and death (14). Although substantially higher injury rates have been reported, these studies have based on vehicle construction before the advent of shoulder and lap restraints, airbags, safety glass, and space-frame construction (4). Recent experiences with tornadoes, however, have clearly documented the ability of these storms to throw even large motor vehicles hundreds of feet into the air and to damage them significantly, as demonstrated in Fig. 17.4. With this in mind, the current recommendation for leaving the motor vehicle to seek more substantial cover or to lie in a ditch or culvert still seems sensible.

Sheltering in a subgrade location (basement) away from windows is the most effective means of decreasing injury through sheltering activities. In houses without subgrade availability, people should shelter in an interior area of the home as low to the floor as possible. Individuals should cover themselves with blankets, mattresses, or pillows, as the exposed areas of the body are at increased risk for injury. The use of protective headgear is recommended and it has been suggested to decrease morbidity and mortality from head injury during tornadoes (28,40). Safe rooms, consisting of concrete and rebar reinforced regions within a standard constructed home, may be built for $2,000 to $5,000.

Some areas of high tornado risk may obtain federally assured loans to assist in the construction of safe rooms. Such structures are likely to protect occupants from all but the most significant tornadoes.

Age has been noted to be a factor associated with increased morbidity and mortality during tornadoes. More importantly, other studies have indicated that the elderly population of a community may be less able to receive and understand tornado warnings. In addition, this older population is more frequently afflicted by medical conditions that diminish its ability to ambulate. These combined conditions result in a population at significantly more risk during a tornado strike. Communities should consider the establishment of target warning and public education programs for these at-risk individuals. Public outreach programs and emergency department discharge instructions might contain information regarding the increased vulnerability of this population and should suggest that family members take steps to ensure that their loved ones are protected during a storm watch.

MENTAL HEALTH IMPACT

As with most disasters, post traumatic stress disorders (PTSD) and increased stress rates have been reported following tornadoes. The rates of severe PTSD following tornadoes have been reported as being from 2% to 59% (41,42). Good support mechanisms and appropriate counseling typically result in a favorable outcome for the majority of victims suffering emotional and psychiatric problems following a tornado. As with any disaster, an appropriately planned and balanced program to deal with these problems should be a key component of the disaster plan.

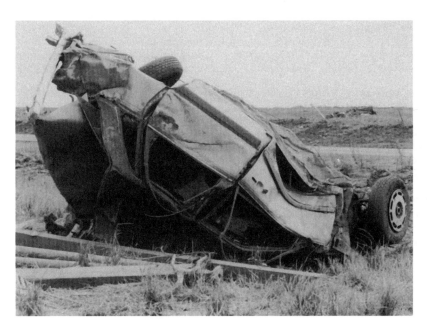

FIGURE 17.4. Vehicle damaged by an F5 tornado. Courtesy of Kurt Feightner, D.O.

SUMMARY

All areas of the United States are at risk for tornadic disasters. Medical planning coordinated with local community planning based on valid assumptions will decrease morbidity and mortality associated with these disasters. Some unique prehospital and emergency department problems are found due to tornado disasters. Soft-tissue injuries and complex wounds are frequently sustained during tornadoes, and they require special consideration to avoid wound complications. Warning and sheltering activities are the most valuable component within a community for decreasing morbidity and mortality. Emergency department and EMS services may fully participate in the tornado education of their local population as part both of outreach programs and of the daily activities of patient education.

REFERENCES

1. National Weather Service. Available at: http://www.nws.noaa.gov/. Accessed November 15, 1999.
2. Injury Prevention Service, Oklahoma State Department of Health. Investigation of deaths and injuries resulting from the May 3, 1999 tornadoes. Oklahoma City, OK: Oklahoma State Department of Health, July 21, 2000. Available at: http://www.health.state.ok.us/program/injury. Accessed March 2002.
3. Grazulis TP. *Significant tornadoes 1680–1991.* St. Johnsbury, VT: The Tornado Project of Environmental Films, 1993.
4. Bohonos JJ, Hogan DE. The medical impact of tornadoes in North America. *JEM* 1999;17:67-73
5. National Severe Storms Research Laboratory. Available at: http://www.nssl.noaa.gov/. Accessed March 25, 2002.
6. Centers for Disease Control. Tornado disaster—Pennsylvania. *MMWR* 1986;35:233-235.
7. Centers for Disease Control. Tornado disaster in Illinois, 1990. *MMWR* 1991;40:33–36.
8. Lillibridge SR. Tornadoes. In: Noji EK, ed. *The public health consequences of disasters.* New York: Oxford University Press, 1997: 228–244.
9. Centers for Disease Control. Tornado disaster—Texas, May 1997. *MMWR* 1997;14:1069–1073.
10. Beelman FC. Disaster planning: report of tornado casualties in Topeka. *J Kansas Med Soc* 1967;68:153–161.
11. Grazulis TP. *A guide to tornado video classics—II: the magnificent puzzle.* Johnsbury, VT: The Tornado Project of Environmental Films, 1994:20.
12. Duclos PJ, Ing RT. Injuries and risk factors for injuries from the 29 May 1982 tornado, Marion, Illinois. *Int J Epidemiol* 1989; 18:213–219.
13. Brenner SA, Noji EK. Tornado injuries related to housing in the Plainfield tornado. *Int J Epidemiol* 1995;24:144–149.
14. Glass RI, Craven RB, Bregman DJ, et al. Injuries from the Wichita Falls tornado: implications for prevention. *Science* 1980; 207:734–738.
15. Saunderson LM. Tornadoes. In: Gregg MB, ed. *The public health consequences of disaster, 1989.* Atlanta, GA: Centers for Disease Control, 1989;127:39–49.
16. Naser RO, Cole WA. 3 April 1974—tornado. *J Kentucky Med Assoc* 1974;72:319–321.
17. Hogan DE, Askins DC, Osburn AE. The May 3, 1999, tornado in Oklahoma City. *Ann Emerg Med* 1999;34:226–226.
18. Beales EH. Tragedy of Topeka tornado tests hospitals' disaster plan. *Hosp Topics* 1966;July:45–47.
19. Rosenfield LA, McQueen DA, Lucas GL. Orthopedic injuries from the Andover, Kansas tornado. *J Trauma* 1994;36:676–679.
20. Brunton BM, Feighner KR, Hogan DE. *The emergency department impact of the May 3rd, 1999 Oklahoma City tornado* [abstract]. Presented at the 1999 meeting of the American College of Osteopathic Emergency Physicians, April 20–24, Scottsdale, AZ.
21. May BM, Hogan DE, Feighner KR. Impact of a tornado on a community hospital. *JAOA* 2002;102:225–228.
22. Ivy JH. Infections encountered in tornado and automobile accident victims. *J Indiana State Med Assoc* 1968;61:1657–1661.
23. Gilbert DN, Sanford JP, Kutscher E, et al. Microbiologic study of wound infections in tornado casualties. *Arch Environ Health* 1973;26:125–130.
24. Harris LF. Hospitalized tornado victims. *Ala Med* 1992;61: 12,14,16.
25. Morris BAP, Armstrong TM. Medical response to a natural disaster: the Barrie tornado. *CMAJ* 1986;134:767–769.
26. Deboer J, Bailie TW. Progressive medical care in disaster situations: a critical evaluation of the current situation in the Netherlands. *JEM* 1984;1:339–343.
27. Eckert WG. Medicolegal aspects of tornadic storms in Kansas, U.S.A. *Am J Forensic Med Pathol* 1991;12:281–285.
28. Mandelbaum I, Nahrwold D, Boyer DW. Management of tornado casualties. *J Trauma* 1966;6:353–361.
29. Leibovich M. The December 2, 1982 tornado of Saline and Pulaski counties: implications for injury prevention. *J Arkansas Med Soc* 1983;80:98–102.
30. Breakey P. Emergency nursing: during the Edmonton tornado. *Can Nurse* 1988;84:36–38.
31. Centers for Disease Control. Tornado disaster—Texas. *MMWR* 1988;37:454–456.
32. Centers for Disease Control. Tornado disaster—North Carolina, South Carolina, March 28, 1984. *MMWR* 1985;34:205–213.
33. Sanford JP. Civilian disasters and disaster planning. In: Burkle FM, ed. *Disaster medicine: application for the immediate management and triage of civilian and military disaster victims.* New York: Medical Examination Publishing; 1984:3–30.
34. Brenner SA, Noji EK. Wound infections after tornadoes. *J Trauma* 1992;33:643.
35. Carruthers WB, Zavela D. A narrative report on the tornado disaster in the Anchor Bay area, May 8, 1965. *Mich Med* 1965;64: 843–844.
36. Stone S, Carter WA. Wound preparation. In: Tintinalli JE, Kelen GD, Stapczynski JS, eds. *Emergency medicine: a comprehensive study guide,* 5th ed. Irving, TX: American College of Emergency Physicians, 2000:284–287
37. Schmidlin TW, King PS. Risk factors for death in the 27 March 1994 Georgia and Alabama tornadoes. *Disasters* 1995;19:170–177.
38. Eidson M, Lybarger JA, Parsons JE, et al. Risk factors for tornado injuries. *Int J Epidemiol* 1990;19:1051–1056.
39. Liu S, Quenemoen LE, Malilay J, et al. Assessment of a severe-weather system and disaster preparedness, Calhoun county, Alabama, 1994. *Am J Pub Health* 1996;86:87–89.
40. Brenner SA, Noji EK. Head and neck injuries from 1990 Illinois tornado. *Am J Pub Health* 1992;82:1296–1297.
41. North CS, Smith EM. Post-traumatic stress disorder in disaster survivors. *Comp Ther* 1990;16:3–9.
42. Madakasira S, O'Brien KF. Acute posttraumatic stress disorder in victims of a natural disaster. *J Nerv Ment Dis* 1987;175:286–290.

18

HURRICANES

JOHN T. MEREDITH
SHARON BRADLEY

"Do you hear anything about Galveston?"
   —Willis L. Moore, Chief, United States Weather Bureau,
September 9, 1900

On September 8, 1900, a hurricane that was estimated to be a level 4 storm on the Saffir-Simpson scale struck Galveston, Texas. Informal estimates placed the number of dead at 8,000 to 12,000 persons, not including the thousands who died in the flooded, low-lying towns surrounding Matagorda Bay and Houston, Texas. The Galveston hurricane of 1900 has been recorded as the most devastating hurricane in terms of the number of lives lost in modern United States history. The most catastrophic tropical cyclone in the world that has been recorded was the November 1970 Bangladesh storm, which killed 300,000 to 500,000 people. Hurricanes and tropical cyclones can be equated with earthquakes as the major geophysical causes of loss of life and property in the world (1,2).

HURRICANE MECHANICS

Hurricanes are uncommon weather phenomena. Technically, a hurricane is a tropical cyclone originating in the Atlantic Ocean, eastern Pacific Ocean, or the Gulf of Mexico. In the western Pacific Ocean and the Indian Ocean, this weather phenomenon is known as a typhoon. Large portions of the tropical oceans present for much of the year with the potential to develop hurricanes. This potential is a result of a thermodynamic disequilibrium between the atmosphere and the underlying ocean. Both the ocean and the atmosphere are typically at or near the same temperature; however, the exchange of entropy from the ocean to the atmosphere drives this thermodynamic disequilibrium. Hurricanes do not arise spontaneously even under favorable conditions, and relatively few hurricanes develop in the world each year (2).

What is required to initiate the development of a hurricane is a strong atmospheric starting disturbance. For the North American continent, this starting disturbance is provided by a macroscale wave that arises from the instabilities of the east-to-west atmospheric flow over sub-Saharan Africa during the northern latitude summer. These atmospheric waves are a result of a heat-induced region of low pressure over the sub-Saharan that is moving westerly; it then collides with a region of moist air off the west coast of Africa. Similar waves can form over Central America and the Gulf of Mexico. Known as tropical waves, these waves of unstable air frequently run as far west as Florida without developing into hurricanes. Often, in a single hurricane season, 50 to 60 such tropical waves emanate from West Africa (2,3).

What causes one tropical wave to develop into a hurricane while another tropical wave does not is an area of intense research. What is known is that a number of empiric conditions are necessary for hurricane formation. One of the most significant conditions is for the ocean temperature to be at least 26°C down to a depth of 60 m (2). Another important condition is the absence of significant upper atmospheric tropospheric windshear. A myriad of other climatic-based and ocean-based conditions influence hurricane evolution. Ocean temperature, however, and tropospheric wind shear are two of the more significant ones.

Crucial for a mature hurricane is its energy source, which is the ocean temperature (2). The greater the difference in ocean temperature and the overlying atmosphere, the greater the degree of thermodynamic disequilibrium and the transfer of entropy to hurricane. Thus, the greater the potential is for a severe hurricane. Additionally, a strong correlation is seen between summertime monsoon rainfall in the sub-Sahara and hurricane intensity. Heavier seasonal rainfall in the sub-Sahara is strongly correlated with better-organized and stronger tropical waves. As such, the most severe hurricanes (Saffir-Simpson scale 3, 4, and 5) typically occur during periods of heavy sub-Saharan precipitation. This association has been noted as a multidecadal climate cycle. Over several cycles of wet periods in the sub-Sahara, a recorded two to four times increase in the potential destruction of hurricanes making landfall in the United States has been observed. This climatic cycle is thought to be responsible for the increase in destructive hurricanes

TABLE 18.1. WIND SPEED AND STORM SURGE CRITERIA FOR SAFFIR-SIMPSON (S-S) HURRICANE INTENSITY CATEGORIES AND HURRICANE POTENTIAL DESTRUCTION SCALE

S-S category	Range of central pressure (mbar)	Maximum sustained wind speed (mph)	Storm surge (ft)	PD value
1	≥980	74–95	3.28–6.56	1
2	965–979	96–110	6.56–8.2	4
3	945–964	111–130	8.2–13.12	9
4	920–944	131–155	13.12–18.04	16
5	<920	155	≥18.04	25

PD is assumed to increase with the square of the Saffir-Simpson category.
Abbreviation: PD, Potential destruction. From National Oceanic and Atmospheric Administration.
National Hurricane Center home page. Available at: http://www.nhc.noaa.gov/. Accessed March 27, 2002.

striking the United States from 1947 to 1969 and 1988 to present (3). From 1970 to 1987, the sub-Sahara experienced a drought, and the frequency of intense Atlantic hurricanes was diminished (3). Also statistically significant is the fact that most intense North American hurricanes occur during August and September. A level 3 to 5 Saffir-Simpson scale hurricane strikes the continental United States every 1.5 years.

As the tropical wave emerges off the West African coast and becomes more intense, it organizes to form a tropical depression. A tropical depression is the first organized stage in the evolution of a hurricane; it is a system of clouds and thunderstorms with a defined circulation pattern. By definition, the wind speeds of a tropical depression are of 38 mph or less. With continued organization and time spent over the warm tropical water of the Atlantic, the tropical depression develops into a tropical storm. A tropical storm is defined as an organized system of strong thunderstorms with a defined circulation pattern and a maximum sustained wind speed of 39 to 75 mph. With progressive intensification and definition of the circulation pattern, a tropical storm becomes a hurricane when sustained wind speeds of 74 mph and higher are obtained (3).

Five classes of hurricanes are defined by the Saffir-Simpson scale (Table 18.1). As was noted above, hurricanes draw their energy from warm ocean waters. The warmer the water is that underlies a hurricane, the greater the potential is for a well-organized strong hurricane with a high Saffir-Simpson rating. As the hurricane grows stronger with the

winds at the core increasing in velocity, a dome of water is drawn up under the core of the hurricane. This dome of water is known as the storm surge; it is often 50 to 100 miles in diameter and 10 to 20 feet above normal sea level. This surge of high water accompanied by storm waves is very devastating. The core is referred to as the eye of the hurricane; it is a central clearing with rotating counterclockwise winds of high velocity forming a cylindrical wall (Fig. 18.1). This counterclockwise rotation is unique to the Northern Hemisphere, and it results from the direction of the earth's rotation and the conservation of the angular momentum of the air flow inward to the hurricane. In the Southern Hemisphere, the direction of rotation is clockwise. Although the Saffir-Simpson scale is based on sustained winds, winds at the eye wall of a hurricane can gust up to 200 mph. The higher the Saffir-Simpson rating and the more shallow the offshore region is, the higher the oncoming surge is (3).

Of importance is the fact that the storm surge is the most dangerous part of a hurricane. If the storm surge of an approaching hurricane occurs at the time of high tide, the combination is known as a storm tide, and the effects are even more devastating. In both the Galveston hurricane of 1900 and the Bangladesh hurricane of 1970, the tidal surge with the compounding factor of the relatively low depth of the Bay of Galveston and the Bay of Bengal combined to result in the devastating loss of life (4).

A hurricane watch, by definition, is announced for a region when a hurricane is scheduled to approach within 24

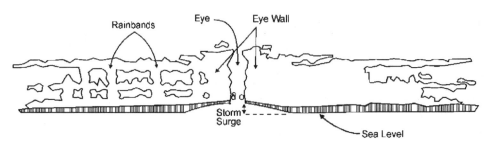

FIGURE 18.1. Cross section of a hurricane.

to 48 hours. A hurricane warning is announced for a region when the hurricane is scheduled to approach within 24 hours or less.

HURRICANE-RELATED DEATHS

Unfortunately, present day terms do not give a universally accepted standard or definition of hurricane-associated death. Often, the determination of a hurricane-associated death is determined by a local medical examiner's office for each respective district of the hurricane impact. Basic categories include, but are not limited to, drowning, electrocution, environmental exposure, falls, fire, natural causes, motor vehicle trauma, and jumping. Nevertheless, since the discovery of the Americas in 1492, an estimated 300,000 to 500,000 deaths due to hurricanes have occurred in the North American hemisphere (5). Of these deaths, the estimation is that 74,800 occurred in the past century (Fig.18.2) (5,6). Numerous hurricanes have resulted in more than 1,000 fatalities, and one recorded hurricane, the Lesser Antilles Great Hurricane of 1780, resulted in 22,000 deaths. Five hurricanes in the 20th century have resulted in more than 8,000 reported deaths per storm. These hurricanes are Galveston hurricane, 1900; Dominican Republic hurricane, 1930; Hurricane Flora, 1963; Hurricane Fifi, 1974; and Hurricane Mitch 1998 (Table 18.2) (5).

Coastal deaths from hurricanes, in general, have diminished over the past 100 years. In large part, this decrease is the result of accurate weather reporting and scientific forecasting allowing for timely evacuation of threatened coastal regions. (The exception is the Galveston hurricane of 1900.) Additionally, in the past century, the continental United States has been extremely fortunate as it has not sustained a direct landfall of a significant hurricane—Saffir-Simpson level 3, 4, or 5—on a major metropolitan area. However, with the rapid growth of many coastal communities and the increasing economic infrastructure of such regions, the potential for catastrophic loss of life and property on a large scale is a real possibility for North America.

TABLE 18.2. FIVE DEADLIEST ATLANTIC HURRICANES IN THE TWENTIETH CENTURY

Year	Hurricane	Saffir-Simpson level	Deaths (estimated)
1900	Galveston hurricane	4	8,000–12,000
1930	Dominican Republic hurricane	4	4,000–8,000
1963	Hurricane Flora (Haiti and Cuba)	4	7,200–8,000
1974	Hurricane FiFi (Honduras)	4	8,000–10,000
1998	Hurricane Mitch (Central America)	5	11,000

From National Oceanic and Atmospheric Administration. National Hurricane Center home page. Available at: http://www.nhc.noaa.gov/. Accessed March 27, 2002.

As such, the societal vulnerability to hurricanes has increased mostly as a result of an increased population at risk, the degree of complacency, and the recent increase in the incidence of intense category 3, 4, or 5 hurricanes (5).

For coastal communities, the greatest threat to life is from the storm surge. In fact, 90% of all hurricane-related deaths in the United States have been from storm surge and flooding, with drowning being the principal mechanism of death (Table 18.3). For instance, in the Galveston hurricane of 1900, 6,000 deaths were attributed to the storm surge. More recently, in 1957, Hurricane Audrey produced a storm surge of over 20 feet that extended as far inland as 25 miles, resulting in 390 deaths in Louisiana (5). Despite numerous technologic advancements in communications and weather forecasting, many of the coastal communities in the Americas are at risk for the effects of storm surge. The reason for this increased risk is multifactorial. First, the ability to predict the rapid storm intensification that can occur is limited, as was evidenced in Hurricane Andrew in 1992. Second, the present infrastructure of many coastal communities lacks the foresight in disaster planning, communica-

TABLE 18.3. FIVE DEADLIEST HURRICANES IN THE UNITED STATES DURING THE TWENTIETH CENTURY

Year	Hurricane	Saffir-Simpson level	Deaths (estimated)
1900	Galveston hurricane	4	8,000–12,000
1919	Florida Keys and Texas hurricane	4	600
1928	Lake Okeechobee hurricane	4	1,836 (actual)
1935	Florida Keys hurricane	5	408 (actual)
1938	New England hurricane	3	600

From National Oceanic and Atmospheric Administration. National Hurricane Center home page. Available at: http://www.nhc.noaa.gov/. Accessed March 27, 2002.

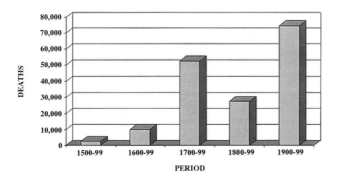

FIGURE 18.2. Mortality due to hurricanes in the North American and Central American continents.

tions, and mitigation activities that is required to evacuate quickly and to limit the loss of life and property. Third, a high level of apathy has developed in many of the coastal areas of the United States with regard to storm potential. This has resulted from the fortuitous absence of a major hurricane striking a major metropolitan area in the United States.

Inland deaths from hurricanes are directly related to the accompanying excessive rainfall and freshwater flooding. Most of these deaths are a result of flood victims drowning or of being caught in landslides or mudslides. Over 1,000 fatalities occurred in Haiti from landslides brought about by the severe rainfall from Tropical Storm Gordon in 1994. Storm surge can also occur on inland bodies of water. Most notably, this type of a storm surge occurred on Lake Okeechobee in 1928, killing 1,836 people in the inland lowlands of Florida (5). In contrast to inland deaths associated with hurricanes, ocean deaths from hurricanes have dramatically decreased in the past century as a result of accurate weather forecasting and improved communications, navigation, and ship technology. However, in the 17th and 18th centuries, populations on the ocean were the most vulnerable to hurricanes. In the 17th century, over 1,000 Spanish sailing vessels were estimated to be lost to hurricanes.

HURRICANE-RELATED INJURIES

The injury patterns most often associated with hurricanes cannot be adequately discussed in statistical terms. Currently, no reporting system exists for defining methods of documenting hurricane-related injury patterns. The required approach should be to manage disaster-related injuries as an illness or disease process. Only through a systematic method can injury prevention be undertaken with regard to hurricane-related injuries. Much of the literature on hurricane-related injuries is variable, and it lacks a consistency in injury classification. A recognized international standard for documenting hurricane-related injuries is not available either, although an elegant classification system has been proposed by Noji (7).

INJURY AND ILLNESS PATTERNS IN GENERAL

The major determination in reference to most hurricane-related injuries is that the majority of injuries are lacerations, accounting for up to 80% of all injuries incurred. Of these lacerations, the majority occur in the poststorm clean-up phase. After lacerations, the next most common injury is blunt trauma (18.2% to 36.5%) as a result of crush injury, flying missile impact, and falls. Puncture wounds account for the third most common injury (14.5% to 31.8%), also in concurrence with clean-up operations.

TABLE 18.4. WOUND MANAGEMENT GUIDELINES FROM DARWIN HOSPITAL

1. Most wounds are clean-cut lacerations less than 12 hr old.
2. Most of the outpatients are essentially homeless, and regular dressing or other supervision of wounds if delayed suture is intended is out of the question.
3. Bleeding is best controlled by sutures.
4. All patients receive tetanus toxoid and antibiotics.
5. No primary nerve or tendon suture is undertaken.

Modified from Gurd CH. The health management of Cyclone Tracey. *Med J Aust* 1975;1:641–644.

Overall, the majority of all injuries (80%) are confined to the feet and lower extremities as a result of stepping on debris or of self-injury during clean-up operations (7).

As a result of these observed coarse injury patterns and the experience of Darwin Hospital, Darwin, Australia (8), a wound care protocol of meticulous wound cleaning, primary suturing of the skin only, and tetanus toxoid update in addition to prophylactic antibiotics is recommended for hurricane-related laceration. This recommended protocol excludes primary tendon and transected nerve repair. These two types of wound repair can be delayed. This wound management philosophy results from several important aspects of hurricane-sustained lacerations as follows: (a) most of the incurred lacerations are less then 12 hours old on presentation to the emergency department or clinic; (b) most of the patients seen after the storm can be assumed to be homeless, and thus regularly scheduled wound care may be difficult; and (c) suturing is an effective way to control bleeding (Table 18.4) (8).

After the storm, one area that is often overlooked in disaster planning is routine medical care. Several reports of a tremendous increase in routine medical needs after a hurricane have been made. Most of these medical needs pertained to individuals who had lost their medications and thus needed refills. Concurrent with this group are those patients with special needs, such as homebound patients, diabetic patients, spinal cord injury patients, and home oxygen or ventilator-dependent patients. These patients often have a significant disruption in the home health care services on which they depend on. Special hurricane shelters may need to be established with additional medical support and supplies, particularly oxygen and ventilator supplies, to care for these patients until home health care services are restored within the community.

INPATIENT ADMISSIONS

Historical data from cyclone Tracy in 1975, a category 4 hurricane that struck the city of Darwin, Australia (population of 45,000), convey the following with reference to inpatient admissions. Darwin Hospital received 145 cyclone-related admissions. Approximately 41.4% of the inpatient admissions were for severe lacerations, and 34.5% were for blunt trauma to the chest, head, and limbs. Closed blunt abdominal trauma accounted for 2% of the admissions. Some crossover occurred among these groups. This demonstrates that the hospital admission rate for a modern city sustaining a direct major hurricane is approximately 0.3% of the population. This percentage is expected to be increased in third world countries with less stringent building standards (8).

PREHOSPITAL CONSIDERATIONS (EVACUATION AND EMERGENCY MEDICAL SERVICES)

Prestorm evacuation along predetermined routes is an extremely important aspect of disaster mitigation. Such evacuations limit the causalities sustained during a storm phase of a hurricane strike. However, in many coastal communities of North America, the necessary road infrastructure to support a timely evacuation and to return citizens to areas under the threat of a hurricane is lacking. Hurricane Floyd in 1999 resulted in the largest peacetime evacuation in the United States, with an estimated 2.6 million people evacuated from Florida, Georgia, and the Carolinas (9). This evacuation also resulted in the largest peacetime traffic jam. Concern stems from the congestion of evacuation routes, which prevents EMS traffic from functioning adequately. As a result, an increase in air-transport requests for patients, particularly from scene runs, may be seen. Coupling EMS transport services with police escort or highway patrol escort can facilitate ground transport to a limited degree.

Air transportation services are often grounded before hurricane landfall because of weather conditions. During the storm phase, transport services are extremely limited. As a result, the time after the storm is the most critical phase for any EMS transport system, and this is when a high volume of transportation requests are received. Obstacles, such as downed power lines, flooded roadways, and road debris, are significant impediments to patient transport. Air services may take time to return to full service after the storm, and they may have sustained damaged during the storm. One method to overcome many of the ground transportation limitations is to pair ground ambulances and EMS crews with electrical utility trucks manned with the appropriate personnel. The utility personnel have the training and equipment to clear road debris, particularly downed electrical power lines. The brunt of patient transportation is then borne by the present ground transportation services. Ensuring that a redundancy of adequately trained personnel for ground EMS services exists is an important component in any community or region's hurricane plan.

HOSPITAL CONSIDERATIONS

Hurricanes do afford a degree of warning before landfall. For a hospital within an area at risk, the coastal United States, storm preparation should commence months, if not years, before the landfall of a hurricane. A hospital can take specific initiatives to weather a major hurricane successfully. Although many areas of preparation must be addressed, in brief, the necessary groundwork consists of an annually updated, well-organized, brief disaster plan based on the hospital emergency incident command system (HEICS); a near turnkey hospital command center; adequate emergency power generators; and an emergency water plan (10). A hospital at risk should plan to be on internal electrical power (generators) for at least 3 days and on alternate water for at least 4 days after the storm. Addressing these four components allows enhanced flexibility and adaptability in coping with most of the contingencies that might be faced by a hospital.

Many hospitals in North America have adopted HEICS in order to carry out their individual disaster plans. Its adaptation has created a degree of similarity in the quality, content, and details of individual hospital disaster plans. The leadership structure of HEICS requires representatives from among physicians, nursing services, hospital administration, and hospital support personnel. Hallmarks of HEICS consist of the following:

- A responsibility-oriented chain of command that provides a manageable scope of supervision for all functions and positions within the HEICS nomenclature;
- Wide acceptance through the commonality of mission and language;
- Prioritization of responsibilities through the use of job action sheets;
- Application to a wide range of different disasters and emergency operation events;
- A format for the systematic documentation of the actions taken in response to the crisis;
- An organized, systematic transfer of resources (internal and external) within a particular hospital system or from one facility to another;
- Flexibility in implementation of the individual sections and subdivisions of HEICS;
- Minimal disruption to existing hospital departments by virtue of parallel job qualifications and responsibilities.

These important hallmarks allow for a flexible and rapid response to events before the storm, during the storm, and after the storm and to the needs that a hospital will face in the event of a major hurricane. However, the actual application of HEICS in a real-time crisis depends on a hospital's facility resources as they apply to command, control, and communications. Specifically, what is required is a physical environment that allows the HEICS leadership to operate. This environment is the hospital command center (HCC).

Hospital Command Center

Ideally, the HCC is a conference room with multiple and redundant communication adjuncts that can comfortably accommodate the HEICS staff. This center is the focus for coordinating all hospital activity though all phases of the hurricane or disaster and into the postrecovery period. The communication adjuncts consist of several landline telephones, including direct telephone lines to the county emergency operations center, operating room, blood bank, and emergency department. Additionally, cellular telephones, Internet access, hospital data system access, local and national television network access, and weather information access should be available in the HCC. Two-way, battery-powered radios, such as the MTX series from Motorola, and runners are another integral component of any HCC. An in-hospital amateur radio station with 24-hour coverage can be extremely beneficial, but it should be located close to the HCC. Any hospital using a HCC should have an alternate site in case the HCC is damaged or becomes inoperable. In summary, the concept of the HCC is that of a communications funnel that provides the HEICS staff with the best information on hospital operations and the community status before hurricane landfall, during a hurricane, and through the postrecovery phase.

Finally, one area of hospital preparation that is often overlooked is the education of hospital personnel as to how to weather a hurricane successfully. This can be accomplished through a carefully developed employee hurricane preparedness manual. Coupled with an annual hurricane preparations seminar and new employee orientation, such a program becomes invaluable. Of all the resources that are critical to hospital operations during any disaster, the employees of a hospital are its most valuable resource.

Electrical and Water Resources

Emergency electrical power for a hospital at risk is often a critical issue in successfully weathering a major hurricane. Before any storm landfall, a complete assessment of the emergency power system should be undertaken. This assessment includes identifying which systems and departments are on the emergency electrical grid, determining whether the grid is a series grid or parallel grid, and fuel and generator status. Most hospitals do not have power generation capabilities for running the entire hospital. Rather, most emergency electrical systems power selected critical systems and areas of the hospital and are not designed to operate for an extended time. Knowing what services can by provided by the laboratory, radiology, surgery, and emergency medicine departments and by the ancillary support on emergency generators is important in determining the level of overall hospital services that can be provided after the storm. An often-overlooked aspect of hospital emergency power systems is the location of the generators and the type

of grid system. Generators in an easily flooded hospital basement are a prelude to compounding the disaster. Ideally, emergency generators should be placed in a secured area of the hospital that is not prone to flooding or disruption. In addition to appropriate generator placement, an electrical grid system that is in parallel and that can have sections easily isolated is necessary. Adequate and safe fuel storage is a major issue; storaage should be in a secure area within the hospital complex. Moreover, hospital generators are often never tested for an extended period of time. Long-term running and testing of the hospital's generators is critical because most component failures occur only after a generator has sustained a supersatuarion of heat throughout the manifolds and cylinder heads. The time required for this to occur is more than 1 hour. Finally, the emergency grid cannot be fully tested unless it is tested completely off-line with a full generator load.

Emergency water supplies and contingencies are just as critical as emergency power generation. A plan should be in place for water conservation and for the utilization of an alternative water supply for every hospital and dialysis unit. With local flooding after the storm, functional water treatment facilities can be inoperable. A plan for backfilling the hospital's water system and maintaining pressurization is important. Backfilling can be accomplished with the conversion of a large swimming pool into a holding and particulate settling tank or with large portable water blivets. Additionally, water tanker trucks, onsite well water, and internal water storage may be required for maintaining pressurization. Limiting internal water usage can be accomplished by using bottled water for cooking and drinking, handwashing with a waterless solution, curtailing flush toilet use, and setting up portable outdoor toilets. Laboratory testing can be limited to routine chemistry and complete blood cell counts. Radiology can be confined to routine radiographs. Computed tomography and magnetic resonance imaging, which require water for cooling and film processing, should be restricted. Primary chemotherapy and radiation therapy can be also curtailed to further restrict hospital water consumption. Once an emergency water system is operational, these restrictions can be reduced.

Of special note are dialysis centers that use large volumes of ultra-pure water. Restricting patient access is impractical because renal dialysis is both time-dependent and date-dependent. Fortunately, most cities have more than one dialysis center. One solution to this problem is to focus resources, both electrical and water, at one dialysis center, which then operates on a 24-hour basis. Support personnel for this extensive operation can be consolidated from other dialysis centers. However, this solution takes resourceful coordination and strong leadership from all the physicians involved in the care of dialysis-dependent patients. Another solution is to transport patients to nearby, out-of-disaster zone, operational dialysis units. However, this particular solution can put an enormous strain on an already compromised transportation system and infrastructure. A modification of this approach is the establishment of collection points for dialysis-dependent patients for transport to an identified or prearranged poststorm dialysis unit. Such collection points can be hurricane Red Cross shelters or even private medical clinics.

Medical and Personnel Logistics

The availability of sufficient medical supplies after the storm is a critical issue because many hospitals operate on a limited stocked warehouse system. Medical supply resources should focus on additional blood products, suture kits, tetanus toxoid, crotalid antivenom, broad-spectrum antibiotics, and general trauma surgical supplies.

Adequate personnel for hospital and emergency department operations is another major issue. Before a hurricane, critical personnel may evacuate with the general population. During the storm, hospital personnel often want to be at home with their families. Furthermore, hospital personnel may not be able to travel to the hospital after the storm because of impassable roads and flooding. One solution is to sequester critical personnel with family members in the hospital before hurricane landfall. This is an unpopular action but, at times, a very necessary one; however, it does place an additional burden on hospital resources. Areas within the hospital or safe areas outside of the hospital need to be established for additional family members and childcare and as sleeping quarters for off-duty staff. Hospital food services need to be enhanced so that they are well stocked before landfall to be able to handle the additional influx of people.

One recurrent phenomenon after a storm is the large number of people from the community that come to the hospital in order to eat and seek shelter. In a community without electrical power or with a compromised clean water system, often the hospital food services provide the only open cafeteria. Thus, restricting hospital food services to inpatient and employee use is unethical. Furthermore, hospitals often become a source of refuge for hurricane victims. As such, the typical daily food services require significant enhancement for poststorm recovery.

Emergency Department Preparations

During the storm, a lull in emergency department patient admissions is seen. Immediately after the storm is when the bulk of the causalities present to the emergency department. Personnel resources should include enhanced emergency department coverage and trauma surgical service coverage during this period. These personnel should include extra physicians, physician extenders, nurses, and ancillary support personnel. Often, an overflow clinic that is organized to take care of minor lacerations and injuries is sufficient. This can consist of a modified family practice clinic with the emergency department as the main triage point. With the majority of hurricane-related injuries confined to lacerations, especially those involving the lower extremities, additional medical supplies for either the emergency department or overflow clinic should focus on extra suture kits and/or carts, tetanus toxoid, and broad-spectrum antibiotics. An overflow clinic should plan to be active for at least 1 week after the storm or until the emergency department can adequately process and treat the influx of storm-related injuries. Additionally, social services and psychiatry services should be enhanced to manage the numerous social and psychiatric problems that occur after the storm. Concurrent with the enhanced psychiatry services, crisis teams for stress debriefing should be established specifically for medical personnel who find themselves overwhelmed in the storm recovery phase.

COMMUNITY HEALTH NEEDS ASSESSMENT

Rapid assessment of a community's health needs following a hurricane is an important first step in guiding relief efforts. The cluster sampling methods have been very useful; they were used for Hurricane Marilyn in 1995, Hurricane Opal in 1995, and Hurricane Andrew in 1992 (11). These methods provide early object data that can be used in determining community health care needs. Survey teams dispatched to hurricane shelters and temporary living facilities with a specific epidemiologic survey can provide the necessary data in a timely and reliable manner in order to assess the full health impact of the hurricane. Such teams were deployed in the recovery phase from Hurricane Floyd in 1999. Objective data from health needs assessments and morbidity surveys allows for the conservation of medical and monetary resources. Even more importantly, these data are critical in decision-making and resource prioritization by disaster management and health care professionals. The Centers for Disease Control gives the following four recommendations for enhancing surveillance in a disaster (11):

1. Use a refined statistical method for population size estimate.
2. Employ a cadre of trained surveillance workers to collect the data.
3. Establish and use a standardized assessment tool.
4. Clearly define whether an illness or injury is disaster-related.

COMMUNITY HURRICANE SHELTERS

The medical aspect of community hurricane shelters is very important. Often, the health care for hurricane shelter refugees is a function of the Red Cross with nurse volunteers. Nevertheless, this responsibility may be tasked to other medical personnel. Additionally, careful consideration must be given to the type of structure in which the shelter is located and whether the wind loads are within the limits defined by the approaching hurricane. Adequate potable water, food provisions, and personal hygiene resources are critical to shelter operations. Some simple guidelines for facilitating shelter health care include the following:

- Sick patients or patients with debilitating disease processes should not be maintained in a community hurricane shelter. At the earliest opportunity, these patients should be evacuated to a hospital or a special needs shelter with an appropriate medical care environment that meets their specific health requirements. Community hurricane shelters are for relatively healthy refugees and not sick or debilitated patients.
- Nursing protocols for the care of routine medical problems should be established when the shelter opens. These protocols should be approved by a supervising physician, often the local public health officer or another responsible physician.
- Prepositioning routine medical supplies and first aid equipment at designated community shelters is not only prudent, but it is also good resource management. If these supplies are time sensitive, they will require routine monitoring.
- Telemedicine links to a primary care hospital can be invaluable in the health care management of shelter refugees. Telemedicine with a physician or specialty physician can provide for the health care needs of a patient on a real-time basis. Additionally, telemedicine can facilitate the heath care needs assessment of a shelter population.

CONCLUSION

Hurricanes are one of nature's most devastating weather phenomena. Planning for a major hurricane takes place months to years before storm landfall. With the increasing population growth along coastal regions, the lack of adequate mitigation planning and infrastructure, and the level of complacency of a population at risk, a tremendous potential for a catastrophic disaster exists. Through careful meticulous preparation, attention to appropriate and timely mitigation strategies, and a flexible but simple hurricane plan, a community or hospital can survive the devastating effects of a major hurricane.

REFERENCES

1. Gross EM. The hurricane dilemma in the United States. *Episodes* 1991;14:36–45.
2. Emanuel KA. Toward a general theory of hurricanes. *Am Sci* 1988;76:371–379.
3. Gray WM. Strong association between West African rainfall and U.S. landfall of intense hurricanes. *Science* 1990;249: 1251–1256.
4. Sommer A, Mosley WH. East Bengal cyclone of November, 1970: epidemiological approach to disaster assessment. *Lancet* 1972;1:1029–1036.
5. Rappaport EN, Fernandez-Partagas JJ. History of the deadliest Atlantic tropical cyclones since the discovery of the New World. In: Diaz HF, Pulwarty RS, eds. *Hurricanes: climate and socioeconomic impacts.* New York: Springer-Verlag, 1997:93–108.
6. North Carolina State Medical Examiners Office. *Preliminary report.* Chapel Hill, NC: North Carolina State Medical Examiners Office, October 1999.
7. Noji EK. Analysis of medical needs during disasters caused by tropical cyclones: anticipated injury patterns. *J Trop Med Hyg* 1993;96:370–376.
8. Gurd CH. The health management of Cyclone Tracy. *Med J Aust* 1975;1:641–644.
9. Franklin JA, Wiese W, Meredith JT, et al. Hurricane Floyd: response of the Pitt County medical community. *NCMJ* 2000; 61:384–389.
10. Division of Emergency Medical Services. *HEICS manual.* Orange County, CA: Division of Emergency Medical Services, 1993.
11. Centers for Disease Control. Surveillance for injuries and illnesses and rapid health—needs assessment following Hurricanes Marilyn and Opal, September–October 1995. *MMWR* 1996;45: 81–85.
12. Hlady WG, Quenemoen LE, Armenia-Cope RR, et al. Use of a modified cluster sampling method to perform rapid needs assessment after Hurricane Andrew. *Ann Emerg Med* 1994;23:719-725.

19

FLOODS

KIM D. FLOYD

On that day all the Springs of the great deep burst forth, and the floodgates of the heavens were opened. And rain fell on the earth forty days and forty nights.
—Genesis 7:11–12. The Bible

Most civilizations have stories of a great flood in the past that have been passed down. The earliest records of this flood are the epics of Gilgamesh and Noah. Similar stories are found in the Mayan and Aztec cultures. Recent archeologic evidence suggests that a massive flood did indeed overwhelm regions around the current location of the Black Sea, probably inundating early human populations around 7,000 BC (1). The most frequent of all natural hazard–related disasters are those due to devastation caused by flooding (2). Flooding has been estimated to account for 40% of all disasters worldwide, with the preponderance of deaths in the modern era occurring in India and Bangladesh (3,4). The Chinese have watched the Yangtze River flood more than 1,000 times in the last 2,000 years. In 1887, over two million lives were lost during a single episode of flooding on this river. Since the third century BC, the Chinese have attempted to control the Yangtze River through a series of dikes and dredging operations.

In the United States in 1889, one of the most costly disasters in terms of lives lost occurred when a 40-foot wall of water crashed through Johnstown, Pennsylvania killing more than 2,200 individuals (5). Another United States river, the Mississippi River, courses approximately 2,400 miles and receives tributaries from thousands of smaller rivers. In 1993, the Mississippi experienced a massive flood. During this flood, the majority of the federal levies that had been built survived; however, 80% of the privately created levies collapsed, flooding the surrounding areas. Excluding the major disruption of services and human lives, this flood is estimated to have cost over 20 billion dollars (6). This 1993 flood has since been followed by several other floods causing billion dollar damages within the borders of the United States. Adjusted dollar flood losses in the United States from 1990 to 1999 are shown in Fig. 19.1.

EPIDEMIOLOGY OF FLOODS

Heavy, constant rains from a slow-moving front, flash floods from a sudden storm, rivers overflowing their banks, and levy breaks are the most common precipitants of flooding. Significant damage may occur from flooding due to other disaster mechanisms. Hurricane Floyd brought with it substantial rains, resulting in flooding inland from the hurricane force winds. Suboceanic earthquakes or volcanoes may trigger tsunamis, causing massive and rapid flooding of costal areas. Growing populations have caused the relentless advance of paved surfaces, which results in less ground absorption of rainfall. This has created virtual death traps out of areas that previously possessed good water runoff patterns. In addition, sudden releases of water trapped by ice floes have been noted to cause flash flooding (7).

Gradual rises in water levels associated with constant rains over time are fairly predictable, and little mortality is associated with these events. However, a fair increase in morbidity may be anticipated. Flash flooding causes the vast majority of deaths associated with flooding (7). The Centers for Disease Control (CDC) estimates that 146 deaths in the United States each year can be attributed to

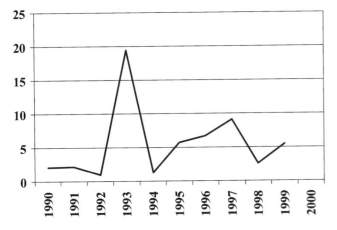

FIGURE 19.1. Flood fatalities in the United States, 1903–2000. (From Hydrometerological Prediction Center. Available at: http://www.hpc.ncep.noaa.gov/. Accessed on March 1, 2001, with permission.)

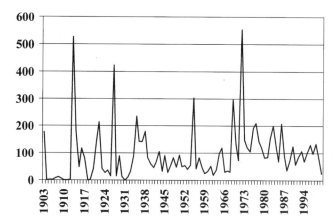

FIGURE 19.2. Flood Fatalities in the United States, 1903–2000. (From Hydrometeorological Prediction Center. Available at: http://www.hpc.ncep.noaa.gov/. Accessed on March 1, 2001, with permission.)

floods (8). The leading cause of death in floods is drowning, and more than half of all drownings in flash floods are related to motor vehicles (9). The peak time for flash flooding generally falls from July to September (10). The total fatality rates for the United States from floods from 1903 to 2000 are depicted in Fig. 19.2.

FLOOD PREDICTION

The National Weather Service in conjunction with its National Centers for Environmental Prediction (NCEP) monitors environmental factors and issues flood watches and warnings. These watches and warnings are based on known and estimated precipitation within specific areas associated with various methods of measuring the saturation of runoff areas, as well as of lake and river levels. In association with the Hydrometerological Prediction Center of NCEP, improvements are being made in the manner of flood prediction in the United States. In 1977, using Des Moines, Iowa as a test site, the Advanced Hydrological Prediction Service (AHPS) was initiated. The goal of this service is to provide better and more timely information about flood (and drought) risk. The information is given in a real-time manner based on actual measurements, radar precipitation analysis, remote satellite sensing, and computer modeling. Rather than providing information in a database table format, the AHPS provides a graphic representation of flood risk and predictions. These graphics are available over the Internet to anyone with Internet access. To date, experience with the AHPS has demonstrated highly accurate predictions of flood zones, as well as of the time and levels of river crests. Such information allows the early evacuation of populations and material goods, as well as the strategic placement of flood-fighting resources during a flood emergency. Although it is not currently available nationwide, the AHPS system is being expanded to include all the major hydrometerologic landscapes in the United States (11).

THE FLOOD LIFE CYCLE

Perhaps one of the simplest methods for evaluating a flood disaster is to study it more thoroughly by separating it into its distinct life cycle segments. During the quiescent phase, the fertile land, low cost, and flat expanses of flood plains attract people to build on them. Many years or generations may pass between significant floods. Populations become complacent, and they minimize the risk in their minds. The population at risk places its trust in flood control measures that have often been constructed by local agencies more for political than hydrologic purposes. Disaster plans may or may not be in place, and, even if they are, they generally are not familiar to the vast majority of the population.

The prodrome phase may be heralded by a gradual rise of rivers above their banks over hours to days, or it may be quite rapid, as in a flash flood. During this phase, warnings are issued to seek high ground. The length and abruptness of the prodrome and the capability of the local disaster system to produce adequate warnings determine the amount of warning a population may get. In underdeveloped regions, people may not receive any warning, or they may not have the means to escape in a timely fashion. Even in more highly developed nations, traffic jams or obstructed roads may prevent a timely exodus from a flood zone.

During the event phase, flooding may result in large numbers of refugees. During 1993, flooding of the Mississippi River displaced hundreds of thousands of persons over a nine-state region (12). A total of 75 towns was completely inundated by the floodwaters (11). Although adequate warning for this type of flooding usually exists, many people remain with their property until the last possible moment. As people then try to escape from the flood, they often drive through the water that is covering roadways. Of the 27 deaths that occurred in Missouri during the 1993 flood, 75% were related to motor vehicle crashes (13). The majority of these were due to driving on roadways that were overwhelmed with water. Drivers must be made aware that as little as 2 feet of water across a road is sufficient to carry most cars away (14).

The recovery phase is heralded by the onset of water recession. Recovery from a flood may take weeks to years. One of the primary health activities during the recovery should be public health surveillance. According to Malilay (2), the following three primary activities should be undertaken: (a) morbidity surveillance for diseases endemic to the affected area, (b) monitoring for infectious disease outbreaks, and (c) injury monitoring and public advisories.

MECHANISMS OF INJURY

Injury prevention is one of the major methods health care providers may use to decrease the human impact of floods. Understanding the mechanisms associated with injury during a flood disaster allows injury prevention efforts to be focused where they may do the most good. Although the emergency department (ED) may not see mass casualties, an increase in the number of visits for illness and minor trauma is observed (15). The most common cause of death associated with floods is drowning. Following drowning as the cause of the death are various combinations of traumas and hypothermia either with or without submersion (12,13,16). One study in Georgia in 1994 indicated that 71% of the overall flood deaths were due to driving a motor vehicle into high water (17). The high rate of death via this mechanism has been further substantiated by a recent study in Texas indicating that 77% of the deaths associated with a storm-related flood were due to drowning and that 76% of this total were related to driving a vehicle into high water (18). These statistics are dramatically demonstrated by Fig. 19.3.

According to Noji, most of the injuries requiring urgent medical attention will be minor; these include lacerations, skin rashes, and ulcers (4). One CDC report listed 524 flood-related injuries during a 48-day time span following the flooding in the Midwest in 1993 (12). This flood resulted in a crude admission rate of 12%, with injuries and illnesses approximately equal in frequency. The summary statistics from this study are depicted pictorially in Fig. 19.4. Medical personnel should exercise caution when performing primary closure of flood-associated wounds due to the risk of contamination (4). No evidence has also been found to indicate that the risk for tetanus is increased, so standard immunization practices do not need to be changed (19). Floodwater in and of itself is not generally considered a toxic or bacteriologic risk. The risk of entities such as possible estuary-associated syndrome (PEAS) from *Pfiesteria piscicida* has even been suggested to be decreased during periods of costal flooding (20).

Electrical Hazards

Electrical hazards exist in both the event phase, as well as in the recovery phase. Appropriate personnel should be notified of downed power lines. Under no circumstances should an untrained person attempt to move, cut, or touch downed power lines. Floating or displaced batteries may still carry a charge and therefore must be handled with care using insulated gloves (21).

Chemical / Gas Hazards

Chemical hazards are also of concern both during and after a flood. Floodwaters may contain agricultural and industrial byproducts. According to the CDC, skin contact with floodwater does not, by itself, pose a serious health risk (21). Open wounds should be protected and should be kept as clean as possible. One should be alert for signs of infection in exposed wounds. Natural gas or propane tanks should be shut off to avoid fire and explosions. Where possible, an area at risk should be entered during daylight hours. When this is not possible or feasible, the use of candles, gas lanterns, and torches should be avoided. Battery-powered flashlights and lanterns are recommended (21). Propane tanks are of special concern. Movement of these should not be attempted due to their propensity to rupture and ignite.

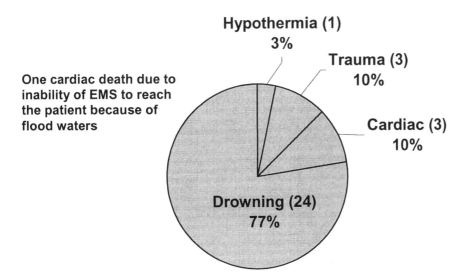

One cardiac death due to inability of EMS to reach the patient because of flood waters

Hypothermia (1) 3%

Trauma (3) 10%

Cardiac (3) 10%

Drowning (24) 77%

FIGURE 19.3. Storm-related mortality from a Texas flood. (From Centers for Disease Control. Storm-related mortality—Central Texas, Oct 17–31, 1998. *MMWR* 2000;49:133–135, with permission.)

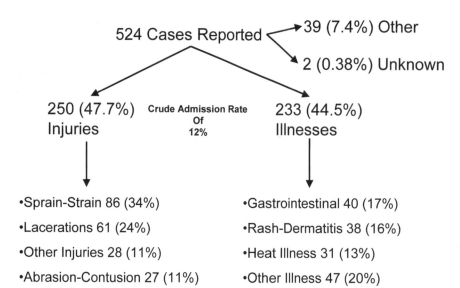

FIGURE 19.4. Morbidity surveillance from Missouri during the 1993 flood. (From Centers for Disease Control. Flood related mortality—Missouri, 1993. *MMWR* 1993;42:797–798, with permission.)

High Water and Swift Water

The general habit of most people is to attempt to cling to their motor vehicles no matter what the cost. As was discussed above, the majority of drowning cases associated with floods is related to motor vehicles. To prevent this, education and injury prevention programs appear integral. Education of the public about not driving into water-covered roadways, even if they do not appear dangerous is the key goal of prevention. Emergency medical services (EMS) personnel must also be properly instructed in not attempting to traverse high water crossings in EMS vehicles. In these situations, reliance should be placed on marine and air medical EMS units.

Water Potability

Potable water is a constant concern in many disasters. Flood disasters, for obvious reasons, expose wells and reservoirs to chemicals, fecal material, and runoff from unusual sources of contaminants, such as fertilizers and matter from holding areas for animals such as hogs and cows. Nonsanitary water has been shown to contribute to an increase in some communicable diseases (22). Therefore, only safe drinking water should be used. Water is considered safe only if it is bottled, boiled, or treated. If viability of a water supply is in doubt, state or local health departments may provide guidance. The CDC recommends that, unless the source of bottled water is known and that source is known to be safe, it should be avoided as well. Water may be made potable by boiling it for 5 minutes at a rolling boil. Chlorine or iodine tablets may also be used to treat water, although this will not always kill parasitic organisms (21). Additionally, immune-suppressed members of the community (e.g., those with human immunodeficiency virus, chronic illness) are particularly sensitive to some water parasites that may

not be killed by chemical treatments or by short-term boiling. Public service announcements regarding water treatment need to state this risk clearly.

Public water supplies must be carefully protected during flood disasters. In 1993, the city of Des Moines, Iowa lost the use of the only water treatment plant for 17 days when it became submerged in the rising flood. This resulted in a citywide water emergency, causing a major impact on the function of municipal and medical agencies (11).

Public service announcements are often beneficial for many reasons. They can educate the public about the dangers of using nonpotable or questionable water supplies. They can warn the public of a dangerous supply of water or inform them of a safe source. Information regarding the treatment of questionable water can be disseminated as well.

Questionable water supplies have the potential to affect all areas of life, including medical and dental facilities, as well as food service (12,19). Close monitoring of water supplies is essential for detecting signs of contamination and taking appropriate action. Any question of contamination should prompt the immediate cessation of use of a given supply of water until the safety of the supply has been verified or treated appropriately.

Waste disposal is closely tied to the issue of water potability. A system whereby food waste can be disposed of should be formulated and implemented before the disaster. Fecal matter and other solid wastes may become a problem at overcrowded shelters for displaced citizens. Plans for solid and liquid waste disposal should also exist.

Other Risks

Displaced wild or domestic animals may be a hazard. While the risk of rabies is always present in populations of wild animals, the actual risk is fairly low if these animals are avoided. Displaced domestic animals may not necessarily carry a rabies threat, but they will be stressed and confused, causing the possibility of them harming someone to escalate greatly. Animal control experts should be contacted to contain any animal, domestic or wild. Increases in human contact with rat, reptile, and insect populations have been noted following floods, although these encounters do not generally cause substantial increases in human injury or illness (23). Food stores should be protected from wild animals and rats.

Toxic exposures increase following flood disasters. In particular, carbon monoxide poisoning from the use of gasoline-powered electric generators has caused death and illness. Increases in pediatric ingestion of cleaning substances (especially chlorine bleach) have also been reported. Other injuries and exposures associated with clean-up and recovery activities are observed. Active public education programs regarding the risks of injury and illness from these mechanisms and others will reduce the incidence for the population at large.

In the aftermath of the flood, environmental concerns such as heat-related illnesses or cold injury often become manifest. Obtaining care for displaced citizens is an obvious need, but many will have routine medical requirements that will need to be addressed as well, such as obtaining and administering cardiac or diabetic medications. Satellite clinics may be a viable option for addressing this concern. Travel for displaced citizens may be an issue, so medical care may need to be undertaken in temporary housing, rather than requiring those persons to come to clinics.

Unearthed caskets, while a grim reminder of the destructive power of floods, typically have not been associated with any health risk as long as they remain sealed. Disaster mortuary teams (DMORTs) are skilled in the management of unearthed remains and the identification of such remains. These units are part of the National Disaster Medical System response program, and they are an invaluable resource during a flood disaster.

COMMUNICABLE DISEASES

Vector-Borne Illnesses

Flood disasters always raise the specter of vector-borne illnesses. In particular, concerns regarding the risk of mosquito-carried illnesses are prevalent. Although malaria is not endemic in the United States, outbreaks of Western equine encephalitis and St. Louis encephalitis are of specific concern. In 1993, vector surveillance for the mosquito *Culex tarsalis* (the major vector for western equine encephalitis) detected an extreme increase in the population of this insect in the flood zone during the summer. However, sentinel chicken flocks being monitored did not experience any positive seroconversions for the virus (23). Under usual circumstances, public health surveillance and routine mosquito control mechanisms are the mainstay of prevention for these entities. However, in 1983, extensive flooding throughout the Midwest stressed mosquito control with a cost in excess of 10 million dollars. At the same time, increased surveillance resulted in a dollar expenditure of $390,000 (24). Augmented surveillance mechanisms and the improved dissemination of public health information can significantly decrease the risk of vector-borne illnesses. If indications point toward mosquitoes as a problem, the population should be warned to avoid mosquito exposure during the twilight hours, to use insect repellents regularly, and to install mosquito netting in sleeping areas.

Non–Vector-Borne Illnesses

Flooding commonly disrupts water purification centers and sewage treatment plants. These events, along with mass shifts of displaced citizens into often-overcrowded conditions, generate fear of an abrupt increase in communicable diseases. Rates of typhoid, paratyphoid, malaria, hepatitis, gastroenteritis, and measles have been monitored, and the occurrence rates of all but malaria were found to increase (22). However, the rates of increase are primarily due to overcrowding; they are not necessarily directly flood-related. The impact of these disease peaks is often felt several months after the initial event. Noji (4) points out that sacrificing and diverting precious resources and manpower for the purpose of mass immunizations does not significantly reduce these problems and that these are not feasible from a managerial and financial aspect. During flood disasters, epidemics of infectious diseases that are not already present in the affected population will not occur. As an example, no outbreaks of cholera were observed during the 1993 Mississippi flood because cholera was not present in the target population.

The outbreak of waterborne illnesses during flood disasters (particularly gastroenteritis) is, however, a concern. Strict adherence to water purification protocols and the distribution of potable water should be mandated. Local health departments should carry out epidemiologic monitoring for outbreaks of enteric illnesses, as well as of other waterborne diseases, during a flood disaster with the assistance from state or national agencies. Strengthening regular public health activities during a flood disaster is more advantageous than devising and implementing new systems (25). Good handwashing techniques and appropriate sanitation methods will diminish the risk of enteric illnesses during a flood disaster. Food-handling practices must be monitored by public health agencies. Refugee shelters and recovery teams should be instructed to refuse donated home-prepared foods because preparation methods cannot be properly monitored (19).

PREHOSPITAL CONSIDERATIONS

Mass casualties from floods are unlikely to burden the EMS and hospital systems. Typically, victims are dead on the scene, or their injuries are generally less catastrophic than those with other disasters due to natural hazards. This pattern may differ in settings where flooding is rapid, such as in a dam or levee rupture. In addition, where flooded regions incorporate substantial areas (square miles), the destruction of the local medical infrastructure may place increased demands on prehospital personnel. Search and rescue teams may be activated; however, typically, bystanders will rescue most stranded victims.

The usual transport routes will often be obstructed by water, converting a previous transport or response time of minutes into hours by alternate routes. Modification in transport and referral patterns may be needed to overcome this problem. Swift water rescue and marine units may be used to assist in the rescue of a stranded population and the provision of emergency medical care to them. As always, adequate safety measures and training are needed for prehospital personnel performing these tasks. Consideration and planning is necessary to support the homes and families of prehospital personnel whose own property and loved ones may be at risk while they are expected to work long hours during the initial flood. Increased reliance on air medical services will alter staffing and mission characteristics and will require the modification of usual activities.

Communication is a consistent problem in any disaster (see Chapter 14). Communication with victims, hospitals, EMS units, and other agencies is rife with potential and expected problems. Land lines may be out of order, and the typical mechanisms for contacting EMS systems (911 systems) may be inaccessible. EMS may be unable to contact local hospitals as well, resulting in ambulances arriving at local EDs unannounced. Response, scene, transport, rescue, and extrication times will likely be increased. Victims also will arrive by non-EMS modes. Normal routes may be blocked, and the nearest facilities may be inaccessible or accessible only by air. Once flooding occurs, routes of evacuation normally used by EDs may be cut off. Hospitals that were once only minutes away may now be hours away by alternate ground routes. In addition, the use of air medical transportation for critical patients may be the only viable means left to some rural EDs.

In some communities, alternate locations for health care may need to be created. In 1977, when floodwaters separated east Grand Forks, North Dakota from its neighboring city, the availability of medical care in east Grand Forks was cut off. The medical community converted a technical college in east Grand Forks to a temporary medical clinic complete with laboratory facilities, radiologic facilities, and other ancillary care (26).

EMERGENCY DEPARTMENT CONSIDERATIONS

Effects felt by the ED may vary widely. If the hospital and ED are in the actual flood zone, most efforts will revolve around the evacuation of patients and rerouting of EMS. The decision to close an ED, however, is an extremely difficult one, because some victims still manage to arrive at a local facility no matter what the environmental concerns are. As this is the case, the ED may have to be moved to a safer part of the hospital or city in an effort to prevent the disruption of patient care. Temporary facilities may need to be opened or erected, depending on the availability of surrounding medical systems. Disaster medical assistance teams may be called in under the federal National Disaster Medical System response program to assist in providing alternate locations for basic and emergency medical care (see Chapter 13). If the ED is functional, it may serve as the only access point within a community for routine medical care, including access to pharmaceutical agents. Plans should take into account the need for increased staffing if the patient census increases. Additionally, they should include access to follow-up care once patients are discharged from the ED.

Simple items that may have an impact on ED management include the oft seen but often unnoticed items such as mops, buckets, flashlights, batteries, and alternate means of communication, both for inside the facility as well as with the outside world. A disaster preparedness plan should include supply lists accounting for these items (see Chapter 8).

As with any disaster, an increase in mental illness and substance abuse has been noted following the impact of floods. One study indicated that suicide rates increased 13.8% over predisaster rates, similar increases in domestic violence and alcohol consumption were observed (6). In addition, preparations should be made for special populations, such as hospitalized patients, nursing-home patients, home health patients, and the elderly. Specialized shelters may be necessary for such populations.

REFERENCES

1. Ballard and the Black Sea: the search for Noah's flood. *National Geographic website*. Available at: http://www.nationalgeographic.com/blacksea/ax/frame.html. Accessed on March 1, 2001.
2. Malilay J. Floods. In: Noji EK, ed. *The public health consequences of disasters*. New York: Oxford University Press, 1997:287–301.
3. French JG. Floods. In: Gregg MB, ed. *The public health consequences of disasters*. Atlanta, GA: United States Department of Health and Human Services, Public Health Service, Centers for Disease Control, 1989:39–49.
4. Noji EK. Natural disaster management. In: Auerback PS, ed. *Wilderness medicine: management of wilderness and environmental emergencies*, 3rd ed. St. Louis: Mosby-Year Book, 1995:644–663.

5. Floyd C. *America's great disasters*. New York: Mallard, 1990.

6. Axelrod D. Primary health care and the midwest flood disaster. *Public Health Rep* 1994;109:601–605.

7. Federal Emergency Management Agency. *United States Senate Appropriations Subcommittee report*. Washington, D.C.: United States Government Printing Office, 1992.

8. Centers for Disease Control. Viral gastroenteritis associated with consumption of raw oysters—Florida, 1993 [editorial note]. *JAMA* 1994;272:510–511.

9. Frazier K. *The violent face of nature: severe phenomena and natural disaster*. New York: William Morrow, 1979.

10. French J, Ing R, Von Allmen S, Wood R. Mortality from flash floods: a review of National Weather Service reports, 1969—81. *Public Health Rep* 1983;6:584–588.

11. Hydrometerological Prediction Center. Available at: http://www.hpc.ncep.noaa.gov/. Accessed on March 1, 2001.

12. Centers for Disease Control. Flood related mortality—Missouri, 1993. *MMWR* 1993;42:797–798.

13. Centers for Disease Control. Flood related mortality—Missouri, 1993. *MMWR* 1993;42:941–942.

14. National Weather Service, American Red Cross, and Federal Emergency Management Agency. *Flash floods and floods...the awesome power! A preparedness guide*, report no. NOAA/PA 92050, ARC 4493. Washington, D.C.: United States Department of Commerce, National Oceanic and Atmospheric Administration, National Weather Service and American Red Cross, 1992.

15. Hogan DE. *Disaster–EMS study guide*. Oklahoma City: University of Oklahoma and MorningStar Emergency Physicians, 1999.

16. Centers for Disease Control. Medical examiner/coroner reports of deaths associated with hurricane Hugo—South Carolina. *MMWR* 1989;38:754,759–762.

17. Centers for Disease Control. Flood related mortality—Georgia. *MMWR* 1994;43:526–530.

18. Centers for Disease Control. Storm-related mortality—Central Texas, Oct 17–31, 1998. *MMWR* 2000;49:133–135.

19. Leitheiser AT. Public health response to the 1997 Minnesota flood. *Minnesota Med* 1997;80:25–28.

20. Centers for Disease Control. Surveillance for possible estuary-associated syndrome—six states, 1998–1999. *MMWR* 2000;49:372–373.

21. Centers for Disease Control. Current trends: flood disasters and immunizations—California. *MMWR* 1983;32:171–172,178.

22. Bissell RA. Delayed impact infectious disease after a natural disaster. *JEM* 1983;1:59–66.

23. Centers for Disease Control. Public health consequences of a flood disaster—Iowa, 1993. *MMWR* 1993;42:653–656.

24. Centers for Disease Control. Rapid assessment of vectorborne diseases during the midwest flood—United States 1993. *MMWR* 1994;43:481–483.

25. World Health Organization. The risk of disease outbreaks after natural disasters. *WHO Chronicle* 1979;33:214–216.

26. Stensrud KM. Floodwaters bring docs to the front. *Minnesota Med* 1997;80:14–19.

FIRESTORMS AND WILDFIRES

ROBERT R. FRANTZ

On August 25, 1949, an elite smokejumper crew responded to a small forest fire approximately 20 miles north of Helena, Montana. Smokejumpers had been used by the Forest Service for years and, as a corps, had never experienced a fatality. The winds in Helena were reported to be 6 to 8 miles per hour, and the general feeling was that the fire would be easy to suppress in its early stages. After a routine jump and landing, the firefighters proceeded to confront the fire, which was located near a minor drainage to the Missouri River known as the Mann Gulch. After walking down the gulch in an attempt to flank the fire near the river, the squad found that spot fires breaking out at the mouth of the drainage were blocking their route to the river. The spot fires started in a heavily treed area, and crown fires soon followed. The winds at the mouth of the gulch were estimated at 30 miles per hour. The 16 men turned up the canyon and started a retreat from the intensifying fire that was now just 150 yards behind them. The fire was burning uphill with a following wind, and the grade worked against the men while accelerating the fire. The crew continued up the 18% grade as quickly as they could travel. As they continued upward, the timber thinned, exposing more brush and cured grass. Within 8 minutes, the fire was spreading at a rate of 250 feet per minute. The terrain was littered with loose rock, and no trail was availabe. The smoke must have been choking for the crew who had no special breathing apparatus. The temperature, which was near 100°F outside of the fire area, was probably much hotter in the gulch. After 8 minutes, the crew foreman told the men to drop their heavy tools. At this point, the fire was only 75 to 100 yards behind them, a distance that would be easily covered in under a minute. The wind increased as it climbed the slope, causing the fire to accelerate to almost 610 feet per minute. Ironically, as the crew climbed away from the fire, they moved into more danger. The thinning of the trees allowed more wind to drive the fire, and more easily ignitable grass and light brush was present. The crew split into three separate groups at this point in their desperation to avoid the pursuing firestorm. One group of three men fled up a steep area toward the rim of the canyon, confronting slopes as steep as 70 degrees. Another group of four men continued to run up the canyon ahead of the main group at an incredible 500 feet per minute, while the foreman stayed behind and lit the

surrounding grass in an escape fire. He survived by lying down in the burning grass while the wildfire raged around him. In the end, only three men survived the Mann Gulch fire. The remaining 13 men were caught by the pulsing 10-foot to 40-foot flames that were burning at temperatures as high as 1,800°F and spreading at a rate of nearly 700 feet per minute. The foreman of the crew later said that the extremely high winds from the firestorm lifted him from the ground several times as they passed over him (1).

The Mann Gulch fire has had long-lasting repercussions for the Forest Service, and it serves as a tragic reminder of the extreme dangers associated with forest fires. Many advances in fire safety, training, and an improved understanding of fire behavior have occurred since 1949. However, fatalities in association with the suppression of wildland fires continue today. More recently, the South Canyon fire in Colorado in 1994 trapped and killed 14 firefighters, making it one of the most tragic wildland fires to occur in the United States in this century (2). This only serves to underscore the fact that, even with all the recent advances in fire safety, fighting wildland fires continues to be extremely hazardous.

SCOPE OF THE PROBLEM

In the United States, about 70,000 wildland fires per year burn almost 2 million acres and require the efforts of approximately 80,000 firefighters (3). Wildfires continue to be an ongoing problem in large part because people are moving into the wilderness areas at an unprecedented rate. The area where the private citizen meets the wildland has been called the urban/wildland interface, and it is the zone of greatest concern for contemporary firefighters. As urban residents move their homes into the wilderness, many take with them the expectation for continuation of urban emergency services (4). More demands are being placed on the wilderness for recreational and casual use as well. Attendance at United States parks and recreational areas has been steadily increasing for years. Ironically, in an attempt to get away from the dangers and troubles of an urban lifestyle, many place themselves at greater risk for loss of life and property through wildland fire. Most people do not see their cozy cabins in the woods or their new homes in the hills of California in this light. However, the risk is not just for those people living in the western United States or in the mountainous regions traditionally thought of as having the greatest risk of forest fire.

In early 1996, Texas, a state known more for its expanses of prairie land, became one of the first states to be hit hard by a rash of wildland fires. On February 10th of that year, a fire ignited in the LBJ National Grasslands area in Wise County, Texas. The fire complex was fought over a 3-month period. An unfortunate combination of weather, dried fuels, fire ignitions and urban/wildland interface situations provided a fire suppression situation that appeared, at times, to be insurmountable. During the 3-month period of fire suppression, various teams controlled 1,742 wildfires involving approximately 170,000 acres across Central and East Texas. One hundred thirteen structures were destroyed by the fires, and an additional 3,170 structures valued at $158 million were threatened but were saved. No lives were lost during this lengthy event. Of the 254 counties in Texas, the Federal Emergency Management Agency (FEMA) issued an emergency declaration covering 47, or almost 20%, of the counties. Total costs of the Texas Fire Siege amounted to $7,817,522 (5).

Nearly every state has experienced fires in the urban/wildland interface that have resulted in significant losses (6). While we may have become accustomed to the annual wildland fires in California, fires have ranged from Florida to Maine to Washington State. The National Fire Protection Agency (NFPA) estimated that, from 1985 to 1995, wildfires destroyed more than 9,000 homes and resulted in many deaths of firefighters, as well as of civilians, with untold numbers of injuries (6). In 1994 alone, between $250 to $300 million of the federal wildland suppression dollars were estimated to be spent on the urban/wildland interface (4).

While no one is prepared to estimate the future losses both in property and lives due to wildfire, the general consensus is that both will continue to grow as people go on moving from urban to rural areas (4). Another major factor in rising injuries is the lack of public education. In general, the public has a tendency to underestimate the risk from fire in the urban/wildland interface (7). After the Yellowstone complex fires in the early 1980s, the zealous fire prevention and suppression practices within the park were clearly shown to have allowed an accumulation of more fuel, thus setting the stage for an intense fire. This scenario is common to other wildland areas within the United States, thus increasing the threat to people from fast-moving, high-intensity fires similar to those experienced in the Yellowstone complex (8). The Forest Service, using lessons learned from the Yellowstone fires, has now adopted the policy of prescribed burning in some national parks and wilderness, which will further increase the likelihood that the general public will encounter fires (8).

Wildfire management, particularly at the urban/wildland interface, is complex. Barriers, such as jurisdiction, mutual aid agreements, zoning, legal mandates, building codes, insurance, and environmental concerns, can be overwhelming. Not surprisingly, the federal government has always maintained an active role in the suppression of wildfires. The United States Department of Agriculture (USDA) Forest Service has collected almost all the data that exists concerning wildland fire behavior, injuries, and fatalities. They also maintain research stations to study and estimate risks for wildland fires. The Forest Service has a long history of fire suppression as well, one that began long before the Mann Gulch fire (1).

Wildland fire fighting is a high-risk endeavor with serious injury or death possible in every phase from response to suppression. While no good data are available concerning injury from wildland fire suppression, the Forest Service follows fatality information closely. Examining these data may be helpful because they illustrate the most dangerous aspects of wildland fires. From 1990 to 1998, 133 fatalities were associated with wildland fire activities (9). This is demonstrated in Fig. 20.1. These deaths occurred in 94 separate events caused by two significant wildfires involving

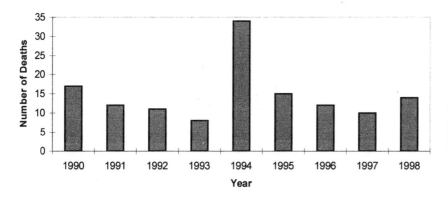

Total Wildland Firefighter Deaths 1990 to 1998

FIGURE 20.1. One hundred thirty-three total deaths in persons involved in fighting wildland fires from 1990 to 1998. (Adapted from Mangan R. *Wildland fire fatalities in the United States 1990 to 1998*. United States Department of Agriculture Forest Service, 1999, with permission.)

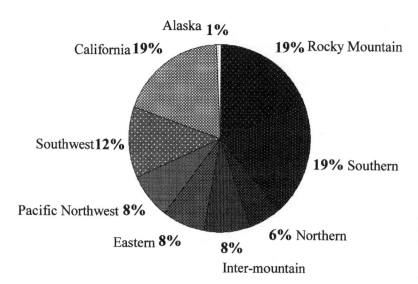

FIGURE 20.2. Fatalities by geographic location of those involved in wildland fire suppression activities. (Adapted from Mangan R. *Wildland fire fatalities in the United States 1990 to 1998*. United States Department of Agriculture Forest Service, 1999, with permission.)

multiple fatalities. Wildland fatalities occurred in 33 different states, 13 of which experienced three or more deaths (9). Of note is the fact that wildland firefighter fatalities occurred in every region of the country, as Fig. 20.2 illustrates. California had the highest number of fatalities and was followed by Colorado, which experienced 14 fatalities on 1 day during the South Canyon fire of 1994. The individuals killed while fighting wildland fires belonged to seven different groups, and the fatalities have been categorized by the activity being performed that led to death.

Figure 20.3 demonstrates that, by far, the most common cause of death was burnover (9). This occurs when a firestorm burns over the individuals in the path of the advancing fire front. This was the cause of death for the smoke jumpers mentioned in the Mann Gulch fire. Burnover can lead to a significant number of fatalities during a single fire because it usually involves a number of firefighters caught

in an explosive or rapidly changing fire. This is the true firestorm with incredibly high temperatures and winds and a rapidly advancing fire front. In the most recent period studied by the Forest Service, burnovers were responsible for 29% of the fatalities, with 39 firefighters dying in 15 separate events (9). The only documented private citizens to die as a direct result of wildland fire suppression also died as a result of a burnover event in Montana (9).

Burnover was also the leading cause of death for the 14 firefighters in the South Canyon fire of 1994, which was one of the largest number of fatalities in a single event in the past century (2). An executive summary evaluating the fires identified several points that contributed to this large loss of life. It noted that topography, vegetation, and smoke all have the potential to reduce visibility, thereby decreasing the ability to sense changes in fire behavior. The summary also noted that the transition from a slow-spreading, low-intensity fire to a high-intensity, blowup situation can occur rapidly, thus catching firefighters by surprise and cutting off their safety zone and means of escape (2).

The next leading cause of fatality in wildland fire fighting activities was aircraft accidents (23%), followed closely by heart attack (21%) and vehicle accidents (19%). The last significant fatality-causing event was falling snags, dead trees that have begun to burn. This amounted to 5% of fatalities in the reported period. As a group, volunteers experienced the most fatalities, with heart attack as the most common cause. This is demonstrated in Fig. 20.4. Members of federal agencies along with members of state fire organizations were the next largest group to experience fatalities. Fatalities following burnover events were responsible for the most deaths in both of these groups, with heart attack being the second most common cause of death for both (9). This is demonstrated in Fig. 20.5. The high prevalence of myocardial infarctions associated with wildland fire

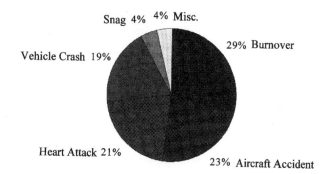

FIGURE 20.3. The causes of death for all 133 persons who died while fighting wildland fires from 1990 to 1998. (Adapted from Mangan R. *Wildland fire fatalities in the United States 1990 to 1998*. United States Department of Agriculture Forest Service, 1999, with permission.)

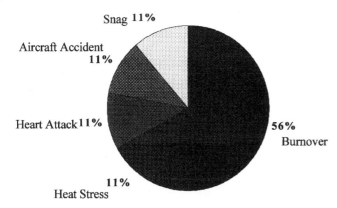

FIGURE 20.4. Causes of death in firefighters from state agencies during wildland fire fighting activities from 1990 to 1998. (Adapted from Mangan R. *Wildland fire fatalities in the United States 1990 to 1998.* United States Department of Agriculture Forest Service, 1999, with permission.)

deaths is not surprising. Fire fighting is an extremely physically demanding endeavor. A smokejumper, for instance, begins suppression activities by parachuting into the fringes of the building fire and hiking to the fire front while carrying packs and tools. The attack on the fire is often made with hand shovels and chain saws. Often, wildland firefighters are required to work in the forest for several days with little rest. The imperative need for appropriate levels of physical fitness has been noted by the Forest Service, which developed a physical training program and fitness test that wildland firefighters working for federal agencies must pass on an annual basis (8,9).

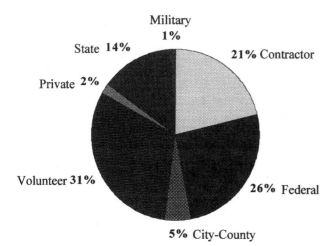

FIGURE 20.5. Fatalities grouped by the organizations of persons who died while fighting wildland fires from 1990 to 1998. The high proportion of contractors is due in large part to aircraft accidents. (Adapted from Mangan R. *Wildland fire fatalities in the United States 1990 to 1998.* United States Department of Agriculture Forest Service, 1999, with permission.)

EMERGENCY DEPARTMENT IMPACT

In October1992, a fire in Oakland, California in the urban/wildland interface resulted in a major uncontrolled blaze that eventually killed 25 people and injured 150 others. The fire was so intense that it consumed 790 homes in the first hour (10). In the greater Yellowstone area fires, over 30,000 medical visits were made by firefighters over 4 months. Forty percent of these visits were for respiratory problems, and more than 600 of those seeking medical attention required more intense medical care than that which could be provided by an aid station (8).

While no comprehensive data are available concerning wildfire injury, clearly many more injuries than fatalities are seen in each event. Those with underlying medical conditions are at a higher risk of death or disability while fighting or escaping from a wildland fire. All the potentially injurious events that one normally associates with the outdoors are magnified for those closely associated with wildland fires. Rough terrain, altitude, poor visibility, and exhaustion increase the risk of trauma. Snake bites, stings from poisonous insects, poison ivy and poison oak exposure, cuts, scrapes, lacerations, and fractures are all examples of additional conditions commonly experienced by those involved with wildfire suppression. The most serious injuries from wildland fires are smoke exposure, respiratory problems, heat stress, burns, or thermal injury. These are a direct result of the heat, flames, and smoke associated with wildland fires. Wildland firefighters generally do not wear the same level of protective equipment as their urban counterparts due to the unusual circumstances related to the fire environment. What the wildland firefighter loses in protection, he or she gains in mobility. A self-contained breathing apparatus or traditional bunk-out gear would be cumbersome at best, and it is dangerous in most circumstances. Therefore, the risks of burning and smoke inhalation are somewhat magnified for these fire personnel as compared to their urban counterparts. Their risk of injury from heat stress, however, is decreased (11).

Thermal Injury

The most common cause of thermal injury is direct contact with flames. While a significant amount of radiant heat can also be created in a wildland fire, clothing is usually enough to offset serious burns. The temperatures generated by a forest fire can be extreme, but they are often of short duration. This depends largely on the nature and quantity of fuels within the fire. Firefighters reduce their risk through constant observation of the fire. A basic tenet of wildland fire fighting is to be where the fire is going, not where it already is. The worst burning events typically involve civilians who are inexperienced with wildland fire behavior or with rapid, unanticipated changes in the fire behavior. Burns can be partial thickness or full thickness. Immediate death is due primarily to hypovolemia or frank incineration.

Airway Injury

Contact with superheated air brings the risk of respiratory tract injury. Respiratory tract involvement should be suspected with burns around the face, neck, and upper body. Physical findings that have a high correlation with upper respiratory tract burns include facial burns, nasal hair singing, facial edema, stridor, and early respiratory distress (12,13). Serious respiratory burns are most often seen in those patients whose history includes being trapped in the burning area. These people have no other choice but to breathe the smoke and hot air. The level of injury is directly correlated with the amount of time spent in the burning area and the actual temperature of the air being breathed. Air is a poor conductor of heat, and the upper airway is very efficient in thermal exchange. For this reason, a person can breathe air at a temperature of 199°F for 30 minutes and of 482°F for 3 minutes without serious injury (8). While most of the injuries to the respiratory tract are mild and they involve only the upper airways, anyone with a significant history of exposure should receive a medical evaluation as soon as possible. Thermal injuries to the respiratory tract can be insidious, with a delayed onset of respiratory distress after contact with superheated air. Significant respiratory distress may present as late as 24 hours after the exposure. Medical personnel should maintain a high degree of suspicion with individuals who report a history of exposure to flames and hot gases in an enclosed space. When thermal injury to the airway is suspected, most experts advocate direct visualization of the larynx and early intubation if injury is noted (14). Thermal airway injury is almost always associated with edema, which can rapidly occlude the airway. Early visualization of the bronchial tree may be a useful predictor of complications and the hospital course after intubation (15).

Heat Stress

All persons involved with the wildland fire are at an increased risk for heat-related illness. This is due primarily to the prolonged nature of the typical wildland fire situation and the physical exertion required to extinguish a fire in the environment. While deaths from heat stress due to heat stroke are rare in firefighters, heat illness in the form of heat cramps and heat exhaustion are common, and these are probably grossly underreported. Obviously, significant exogenous and endogenous heat generation can occur in wildfire events. Individuals working in the heat rarely replace fluids at the same level of that lost through exertion (14). This dehydration ultimately leads to hypovolemia and, if untreated, can eventually trigger heat exhaustion and ultimately heat stroke.

Signs and symptoms of heat exhaustion are variable and nonspecific. They include fatigue, dizziness, weakness, nausea, vomiting, headache, muscle cramps, and sometimes impaired judgment. Obviously, these symptoms pose an even greater risk for the individual involved in wildland fire suppression. Initially, core temperature is not significantly increased and signs of central nervous system involvement are absent. As heat exhaustion becomes more severe, the core temperature rises and the central nervous system signs develop. Heat stroke is the endpoint of this continuum in which all heat control mechanisms for the body fail. Core temperature rises to dangerous levels, central nervous system depression is present, and multisystem organ failure is possible. Heat stroke is a catastrophic, life-threatening medical emergency requiring immediate intervention.

If symptoms are mild, treatment may consist of removing the patient from the environment and providing oral repletion of fluids. As the severity of symptoms increases, so does the level of care. Volume depletion at higher levels should be managed with the use intravenous fluids over time. As long as 24 to 48 hours may be required to correct the water deficit safely, especially if comorbid illnesses exist (16). Patients with heat stroke must have rapid cooling and intense supportive care. Patients in whom heat stroke develops in the context of exertion may have rhabdomyolysis and acute renal failure, in which hepatic injury is present in almost 100% of the cases (14).

Smoke Inhalation

Asphyxia is always a risk when an individual is exposed to smoke. As has been noted, many wildland firefighters do not use a self-contained breathing apparatus. Although many use particulate masks, some use little more than a wet bandanna over the mouth and nose (17). Private citizens trapped in a wildfire may not have access to any airway protection. As was stated previously, significant differences between urban and wildland firefighters' job risk are observed. While both groups experience smoke exposures, wildland firefighters have exposures to different airborne contaminants when compared to their counterparts fighting structural fires. Wildland firefighters are not as likely to experience the extreme, acute exposures that structural firefighters encounter. However, they are often exposed for 12-hour shifts over days at a time in base camps that may be located in areas that fill with smoke as well. The greater Yellowstone Park fires of 1988 were associated with a large number of firefighters and civilians who sought medical care for respiratory problems (14,17). In 1988, several large wildfires in central Florida burned almost 500,000 acres throughout the state. During that time, emergency department visits for asthma increased by 91%, acute exacerbation of bronchitis increased by 132%, and chest pain increased by 37%. However, the increases in admission rates were minimal (18).

The chemical composition of the smoke from wildland fires has been examined. Common compounds include carbon monoxide, sulfur dioxide, particulate carbon and silica (probably from ground dust), polyaromatic hydrocarbons, aldehydes, and benzene (19). Data suggest that firefighters who spend prolonged periods working in visible smoke may be at risk for exceeding the recommended full-shift occupational exposure limits of all of these compounds. In the short term, the agents of greatest concern are the aldehydes and carbon monoxide. Aldehyde exposure results in a local irritation, which can serve as a warning sign. However, carbon monoxide exposure is not associated with warning properties, thus increasing the possibility that dangerous levels of exposure may remain undetected. Firefighters who work at high altitude are at an even greater risk with this exposure, and they require closer monitoring (19).

While the long-term effects of respiratory contaminants are not fully known, studies have shown decreased short-term pulmonary function in wildland firefighters (19,20). The decreased pulmonary function is strongly correlated with recent wildland fire-fighting activity and the number of hours of exposure. Decreased pulmonary function has been shown to be at least partially reversible with reduced contact with smoke; however, this is still being investigated, and no long-term controlled studies have been performed to date. In the short term, the greatest concerns are local airway irritation, carbon monoxide exposure, and the exacerbation of underlying pulmonary conditions, such as asthma or emphysema.

SYSTEMS PLANNING

Fire and Emergency Medical Services

For wildland fires, as in almost all disasters, planning is essential for reducing the loss of life and property. Almost every state in the country is at serious risk for wildland fires. This impacts almost every community, not just those with heavy timber and mountainous topography. Proper planning begins and ends with education.

Fire personnel are usually at the greatest risk of injury due to wildfires. Wildland fire suppression has significant differences from structure fires, and the training should reflect those differences. The National Fire Protection Association has produced a wildfire training course that helps both volunteer and professional fire departments plan for and safely fight wildland fires. While fire departments should be equipped with the proper gear to fight wildland fires, the most important piece of equipment the wilderness firefighter possesses is his or her brain. Instruction in entrapment procedures, wildfire behavior, communications, and escape protocols, at a minimum, should be given.

Mutual aid agreements are also vital to combat wilderness fires. Almost all wildland fires are fought with the help of several municipal, state, and federal agencies. Because the typical wildfire requires several days to suppress, municipalities involved in wildland fire activities will need to ensure adequate coverage to meet their baseline demands for service. This is typically accomplished through agreements with other agencies, perhaps those in neighboring municipalities, and it should be a part of the planning for any disaster. This also provides a good forum for addressing issues such as communication and chain of command to avoid confusion during an actual disaster situation.

Rescue protocols, including the equipment needed, the personnel responsible, and the evacuation procedures to be used if necessary, should also be formulated well in advance. Rescues can become multiple day affairs that tax resources and require a dynamic response to a changing situation. Many serious injuries and a large percentage of the fatalities seen in firefighters are due in part to poor physical conditioning. Federal firefighters must pass a strenuous physical fitness test before they are allowed to work on federal land. Similar standards should be adopted for state and municipal firefighters in order to reduce the risks of death due to myocardial infarction during the strenuous activity of wildland fire fighting.

Minimum safety equipment for the wildland firefighter should include a hard hat, safety goggles, brightly colored clothing made of closely woven natural fabric, long sleeves and pants, leather boots, and gloves. A personal fire shelter should also be carried. These devices, worn on the belt in a pack, are essentially an aluminized one-person tent. They are intended to be deployed in the face of an imminent burnover. They are constructed of an aluminized fiberglass cloth laminate that has the capability of reflecting up to 95% of radiant heat. Such shelters have been in use since the 1960s, and they have been credited with saving at least 220 lives and preventing many more serious injuries (14,21). A wilderness firefighter should also carry a canteen and should drink from it frequently to offset volume loss through sweat. In fire fighting, water losses as high as 2 L per hour have been reported in extreme conditions (14). If the fluids that are lost are not replaced by drinking, heat illnesses almost certainly will occur. During the strenuous work, little opportunity is available for taking a break; therefore, because thirst is a poor indicator of fluid volume status, forced water breaks may become necessary. One of the signs of heat exhaustion is poor judgment, which can be fatal in a wildfire.

Emergency medical services (EMS) can play a critical role in wildland fire safety. The support of a well-prepared EMS system cannot be overestimated. A wildland fire is an ongoing disaster lasting for days or weeks. One positive point from a planning standpoint is that the patients present from a predictable location. Typically at or near the fire front, EMS can play a pivotal role in triage and field treatment of those injured in these events. A mobile command post with the capabilities to treat several patients simultaneously for heat-related illness, trivial trauma, and respiratory complaints is able to reduce morbidity and the emergency department visits of fire personnel. A converted bus with air conditioning, stretchers, oxygen, and personnel trained at least at the paramedic level is ideal. This could also serve as a medical command post or a mini-emergency department for the more mobile EMS units working in the area. Triage and treatment may occur simultaneously with stabilization, and the units must have the ability to move from the area rapidly if this is required by the changing fire environment (22).

At a recent convention of the International Association of Fire Chiefs, fire chiefs were asked about their perception of medical support for their departments. Only 14% of the chiefs asked thought their level of medical support was adequate, 39% thought it was inadequate, and 46% did not respond to the question (23). A good predictor of the chief's satisfaction was the presence of a physician who had a good understanding of emergency operations and the standard operating procedures (SOPs) within the department. Efforts to address this issue have been made. Current recommendations are that physicians who are willing to work closely with departments within the SOPs be identified to serve as Fire Medical Officers (FMO). A physician with knowledge of prehospital emergency medicine, fire fighting, and occupational medicine can reduce the risk and liability of fire personnel and can serve as a health and safety advocate (23). In a wildland fire situation, a FMO serves as a liaison to other medical specialists who will be required, such as the EMS medical director, emergency department physicians, and the medical examiner, while also providing scene oversight.

During a wildland fire, the emergency departments should maintain close contact with medical support at the scene of the fire. This will help to assess civilian risk and will guide resource use. Most emergency visits during wildland fires are comprised of relatively nonserious respiratory complaints (14,18.) Emergency visits increase during these events, but hospitalizations do not appear to be significantly higher (18). Because wildland fires may take weeks or even months to suppress completely, emergency departments should plan and staff accordingly.

The importance of public education cannot be overstated. As more people move into the rural environment, the urban/wildland interface continues to grow. People living in these areas continue to underestimate their risks of wildfire, and they demonstrate even less knowledge about what to do in the event of a wilderness fire (7). Both of these facts contribute to the increasing possibility of injury or death in this group. Commercial companies are marketing equipment, such as swimming pool pumps, to homeowners in these urban/wildland interface areas to allow them to combat wildfires themselves. Without adequate education or training, these people may placing themselves in extremely hazardous situations. Armed with a false sense of security, they may become more likely to ignore evacuation warnings until too late, thus endangering not only themselves but also those who must come to their aid.

Planners and developers should design housing developments with more than one ingress and egress. They should also ensure that adequate water supplies exist in developments and that homeowners in the area understand the risks. Homeowners should clear a defensible area around their homes and should opt for homes made of less flammable materials. They should also be educated about the fuels surrounding their homes and basic fire safety principals.

SUMMARY

Wildfires burn more than 2 million acres each year in the United States. As people move from the cities and into the wilderness areas seeking recreation or permanent homes, these fires are increasingly associated with potential injury and loss of life. The general public tends to underestimate existing fire hazards, and it is usually not experienced in avoiding fire threats.

Past fire exclusion practices have left some areas with large amounts of an unhealthy accumulation of dead and highly flammable fuels. This creates the risk of intense, fast-moving fires in these areas. To reduce these fuels, prescribed burning in national parks and wilderness areas is becoming more common. While this reduces the risks associated with an accumulation of dangerous wildfire fuels, it increases the likelihood that the general public will encounter a wilderness fire.

Fighting these fires is extremely hazardous, and injury is common among these firefighters. Indeed, around 20 firefighters lose their lives each year combating wildfires. The most common injuries seen are respiratory complaints, heat stress, burns, and minor trauma. However, serious trauma associated with responses to these events, heart attack, and heat stroke are possible as well. Emergency department visits increase during these events, which can last as long as months, depending on the situation. Proper planning, as well as with firefighter, EMS, and public education, is vital in order to reduce injury and loss of life.

REFERENCES

1. Rothermel RC. Mann Gulch fire: a race that couldn't be won. General Technical Report INT-299. Washington, D.C.: United States Department of Agriculture Forest Service, 1993.
2. Butler BW. Fire behavior associated with the 1994 South Canyon fire on Storm King Mountain, Colorado. Research paper RMRS-RP-9. Washington, D.C.: United States Department of Agriculture Forest Service, 1998.
3. Ward DE, Rothman N, Strickland P. The effects of smoke on firefighters: a comprehensive study plan. Missoula, MT: United States Department of Agriculture Intermountain Research Station, 1989.
4. United States Department of Agriculture Forest Service, Inter-

mountain Research Station. Protecting people and homes from wildfire in the interior west: proceedings of the symposium and workshop. General technical report-251. Missoula, MT: United States Department of Agriculture Forest Service, Intermountain Research Station, 1988.

5. United States Department of Agriculture Forest Service. *Findings from the Wildland Firefighters Human Factors workshop: improving wildland firefighter performance under stressful, risky conditions—toward better decisions on the fireline and more resilient organizations.* Washington, D.C.: United States Department of Agriculture, Forest Service, Fire and Aviation Management.

6. United States Department of Agriculture Forest Service. Federal wildland fire policy, wildland/urban interface protection. Available at: http://www.fs.fed.us/land/wolfire7c.html. Accessed March 2002.

7. Hubert J. Fire problems in rural suburbs. *Am Forests* 1972;78:24.

8. Davis MK, Mutch RW. Wildland fires: danger and survival. In: Auerbach PS, ed. *Wilderness medicine, management of wilderness and environmental emergencies*, 3rd ed. St. Louis: Mosby-Year Book, 1995.

9. Mangan R. *Wildland fire fatalities in the United States 1990 to 1998.* United States Department of Agriculture Forest Service, 1999.

10. National Fire Protection Association. *The OaklandBerkeley Hills fire.* Quincy, MA: National Fire Protection Association, 1991.

11. Sharkey BJ. *Heat stress.* Missoula, MT: United States Department of Agriculture Fire Service, 1979.

12. Moylan JA. Smoke inhalation and burn injury. *Surg Clin North Am* 1980;60:1533–1540.

13. Wrobelewski DA, Bower GC. The significance of facial burns in acute smoke inhalation. *Crit Care Med* 1979;7:335–338.

14. Yarbrough B, Bradham A. Environmental disorders, heat illness. In: Rosen P, Barker T, eds. *Emergency medicine*, 4th ed. St. Louis: Mosby-Year Book, 1998.

15. Moylan JA, Smoke inhalation and burn injury. *Surg Clin North Am* 1980;60:1533–1540.

16. Schrier RW. Disorders of water metabolism. In: Schrier RW, ed. *Renal and electrolyte disorders.* Boston: Little, Brown, 1980.

17. Sutton PM, Castorina J, Harrison RJ. *Carbon monoxide exposure in wildland firefighters.* Field investigation FI-87-008. Berkley, CA: California Department of Health Services, 1990.

18. Centers for Disease Control. Surveillance of morbidity during wildfires—central Florida, 1998. *JAMA* 1999;281:789–790.

19. Harrison R, Materna B, Rothman N. Respiratory health hazards and lung function in wildland firefighters. In: Orris, et al., eds. *Occupational medicine, firefighters' safety and health.* Philadelphia: Hanley and Belfus, 1995.

20. Large AA, Owens GR, Hoffman LA. The short term effect of smoke exposure on the pulmonary function of firefighters. *Chest* 1990;97:806–809.

21. Putnam T. *Your fire shelter: a facilitator guide.* Missoula, MT: Missoula Technology and Development Center, United States Department of Agriculture Forest Service, 1991.

22. Moore KA. Director of Emergency Medical Services, Norman, Oklahoma. Personal discussion, 1999.

23. Bogucki MS. Medical support for the fire service: current priorities and roles of physicians. In: *Prehospital emergency care.* Philadelphia: Hanley and Belfus, 1997.

WINTER STORM DISASTERS

S. BRENT BARNES

On May 12, 1986, four adults and 14 students began a summit ascent of Mt. Hood in Oregon. Thirteen members of the party ascended to within a few hundred feet of the summit before weather deteriorated as a late winter storm moved in. Five members of the party turned back before the arrival of the storm. Temperatures dropped, ranging from 15°F (−9°C) to 25°F (−4°C) with winds of 20 to 60 miles per hour. More than 4 feet of snow fell on the party within 48 hours. The group was dressed warmly, but it lacked advanced survival gear. At approximately 9,000 feet, the group constructed a small snow cave for survival. The next morning, two individuals from the group successfully descended and joined a search and rescue operation already in effect. On May 14th, three members of the group were found exposed at 8,800 feet and were transported by helicopter to a hospital. The remaining eight people were found in the snow cave buried under an additional 4 feet of snow on May 15th. Only two had signs of life. All were transported to Portland hospitals where a coordinated treatment protocol, including rapid core rewarming with cardiopulmonary bypass was instituted. Core temperatures of the victims on presentation ranged from 3°C (37°F) to 23.4°C (74°F). Of the 11 victims found by rescuers, only the two with signs of life upon discovery survived (1).

The Mt. Hood tragedy is a good example of the severe impact of cold weather on man. Despite the remarkable ability of humans to adapt to harsh environmental conditions, man is still a tropical creature that has better adaptations for losing heat than gaining it.

WINTER STORMS IN THE UNITED STATES

The first major winter storm recorded in the United States was the 1888 blizzard. During this storm, over 22 inches of snow fell on New York City, 26 inches on Brooklyn, and 32 inches on White Plains. More than 400 people lost their lives from this storm, making it the cause of the most significant known mortality of any winter storm in United States history. In late January 1967, a severe winter storm hit the city of Chicago, delivering 24 inches of snow in just

over 29 hours. The city lay paralyzed for several days below 24 million tons of snow. Another storm in 1969 covered the metro areas of New York City and Boston with an average of 25 inches of snow. Winter storms continue to occur with regularity, including, for example, a massive storm in 1993 that essentially paralyzed the nation east of the Mississippi River for days. Winter storms and cold-related fatalities reported to the National Weather Service (NWS) in 1997 accounted for 141 deaths and over 573 injuries, which was second only to the total for tornado injuries for the year (2). Most of the reported deaths were due to motor vehicle crashes, carbon monoxide poisoning, and hypothermia.

FORMATION OF WINTER STORMS

A specific combination of weather conditions must be present to trigger a winter storm. These conditions most commonly exist in the United States from November through April, but they may occur as early as October and as late as May. The jet stream typically begins to dip south across the states during this time. This southerly meander can allow extremely cold polar air to expand into the United States. At the same time, tropical moist air continues to feed north into the states from the Gulf of Mexico. Along the boundary of these two air masses, the warm moist air at a low altitude begins to flow up and over the denser, dry polar air. This results in condensation, the formation of clouds, and precipitation. Depending on what the surface temperatures are, precipitation may fall as snow, ice, or rain. Such storm systems may be expansive, extending from the southern Gulf States to the Great Lakes region.

Although this phenomenon is uncommon, winter storms occasionally extend well into the southern United States. On January 7th and 8th in 1973, north Georgia and the Atlanta region experienced a winter storm. More than 2.25 inches of freezing rain and sleet blanketed the area over a 2-hour period, with the surface temperatures remaining at 32°F (0°C). This resulted in electrical power failure for over 300,000 people for longer than 1 week. Storms of this nature may be particularly dangerous in regions of the country that are unprepared to deal with ice, snow, and frigid temperatures.

COMMUNITY PREPARATION AND PUBLIC EDUCATION

The NWS issues winter storm warnings in the United States. Collections of historic and current data are used in computer models to create long-range winter weather predictions. Short-range predictions are made by coupling these models with real-time data from surface and air measurements, as well as with radar and satellite imaging.

Perhaps nothing has had a greater impact on preventing the dangerous effects of a winter storm on a community than educating the public in what measures they can take to protect themselves. This must be done before the arrival of the storm to allow time to prepare.

Various advisories and warnings may be issued by the NWS. A *frost or freeze warning* means that temperatures below freezing are expected and that damage to plants or trees can result. A *winter storm advisory* implies that winter weather conditions can be expected to cause inconveniences and delays, especially for motorists. A *winter storm watch* implies that a winter storm is likely. A *winter storm warning* implies that a storm is moving into the area and that the public should take protective action. A *blizzard warning* means that significant snow and strong winds will produce deep drifts, poor visibility, and life-threatening cold. The public should seek protection immediately.

Specific measures should be stressed before the arrival of a winter storm. The emergency department (ED) and emergency medical services (EMS) may provide patient education to the public about winter storms during high-risk seasons. These measures include the following (3).

1. Monitor a National Oceanic Atmospheric Administration (NOAA) weather radio, local radio, and/or the local TV station for forecasts and information including emergency instructions.
2. Avoid going outside unless it is absolutely necessary.
3. Dress appropriately when going outside, including several layers of loose-fitting, lightweight dry clothing. Hats minimize heat loss through the head, and covering the mouth with a scarf can minimize respiratory heat loss.
4. If leaving or evacuating, tell others the destination and follow routes designated by local officials.
5. Conserve fuel by keeping homes cool but not cold.
6. Shut off heat temporarily to rooms in the house that are not used.
7. Keep heaters away from flammable objects.
8. Maintain ventilation to avoid toxic fumes when using kerosene heaters.
9. Check on neighbors, especially the very young and the elderly, and pets.
10. Beware of overexertion and recognize that shoveling snow in extreme cold can induce a heart attack.
11. Report any downed power lines and gas leaks.
12. Be cautious of structural damage to homes and buildings due to snow and ice build-up.
13. Winterize your house in advance, including the installation of storm shutters and roof repairs.
14. Develop an emergency survival kit for the home and car.
15. Have an adequate supply of home staples, including canned foods.
16. Remember that community shelters are available for those who need assistance.

Becoming caught in a stranded car during a winter storm can turn into a deadly experience. If one is stranded in a car by a winter storm, the following guidelines should be stressed (3):

1. Pull off the road and turn on flashing hazard lights.
2. Hang a distress flag from the antenna.
3. Remain in the car as rescuers will be most likely to find you there. Do not attempt to walk to safety during a storm unless a building is within sight and is open for shelter.
4. Run the engine and heater for 10 minutes every hour to conserve fuel (open window slightly to prevent carbon monoxide toxicity).
5. Huddle together to maintain heat if other people are in the car,.
6. Keep blankets in the car during the winter season.
7. Use seat covers, maps, paper, or any extra clothing for covering if a blanket is not available.
8. Turn on the inside dome light periodically for rescuers to see, but avoid running the battery down.
9. Spread a large cloth or blanket on top of the snow to attract rescuers by air if in a remote area.
10. Stay on the road and use distant points as landmarks if, after the storm is over, you need to leave the car by foot.
11. Carry a cellular telephone.

PATHOPHYSIOLOGY OF COLD INJURIES

The primary mechanism for conserving heat in humans is behavioral. Individuals with normal sensorium and mental alertness will seek a warm environment if it is available. If they are unable to do so and the loss of core body heat progresses, mental alertness rapidly deteriorates to the point that further protective actions will no longer be taken.

Heat is lost through the following four mechanisms: radiation, convection, conduction, and evaporation. Radiation, in which heat is transferred by electromagnetic waves, accounts for almost two-thirds of heat loss in a cold environment. Radiant heat loss can be minimized by wearing warm clothing and by positioning the body in a curled-up position. This minimizes the body surface area that is exposed to the cold environment. Conduction is the transfer of heat from warmer to cooler objects by direct contact. Heat loss through conduction is usually minimal, but it becomes a major source of heat loss in wet clothes or with cold-water immersion. Conductive heat losses can be increased by five times in wet clothing and 25 times in cold water (4). Convection is the loss of heat to surrounding air and water vapor. Heat loss by convection is dependent on a combination of wind velocity and environmental temperature. Seeking shelter from the wind will reduce heat loss by convection. The *wind chill* index is a combination of the ambient temperature and the wind velocity. This index estimates the equivalent temperature effect on exposed skin. It is a more important consideration than the actual temperature. This index and the time required for skin damage are demonstrated in Fig. 21.1. Evaporation is the heat lost when a liquid is converted to gas. Evaporative heat loss increases on dry days. Sweating and an increased respiratory rate with physical exertion increase heat loss in the cold.

In addition to minimizing heat loss through the previous mechanisms, the body may increase heat production in response to cold. This occurs primarily through the mechanism of shivering. In addition, vasoconstriction of the peripheral and superficial vasculature occurs, shunting warm blood away from the skin and to the body core. These mechanisms are controlled by the hypothalamus, and they appear and disappear at specific degrees of hypothermia. When the core body temperature falls below 35°C (95°F), vasoconstriction and shivering occur. As the core body temperature falls below 32°C (89.6°F), shivering discontinues and vasoconstriction is the only method of heat conservation. Below 24°C (75°F), all heat conservation mechanisms fail. (4)

Cold injuries can be divided into local cold injuries and the systemic state of hypothermia. Hypothermia is further classified as mild, moderate, or severe. The local cold injuries are divided into the freezing injuries of frostbite and frostnip and the nonfreezing injuries of chilblains and trench foot. The pathophysiology of frostbite injury generally occurs according to the following four phases, although these phases may overlap (5,6).

1. **Pre-freeze phase**. In this phase, arterial constriction with venous dilation occurs, leading to transendothelial plasma fluid leakage. Tissue temperature ranges from 3°C (38°F) to 10°C (50°F).
2. **Freeze-thaw phase**. Actual extracellular and then intracellular ice crystal formation occurs. This is observed when the tissue temperature drops below the freezing point.
3. **Vascular stasis phase**. This phase involves further arterial vasospasm and plasma leakage with stasis, coagulation, and shunting resulting in tissue hypoxia.
4. **Late ischemic phase**. This stage is produced by thrombosis and ischemia, and it progresses to gangrene and neural damage.

Nonfreezing cold injuries include trench foot and chilblains or pernio. Trench foot is seen when wet feet are continually exposed to cold temperatures developing slowly over hours to days. Initially, the patient has burning and

APPARENT WIND CHILL

	45	40	35	30	25	20	15	10	5	0	-5	-10	-15	-20	-25	-30	-35	-40
4mph	45	40	35	30	25	20	15	10	5	0	-5	-10	-15	-20	-25	-30	-35	-40
5mph	43	37	32	27	22	16	11	6	0	-5	-10	-15	-21	-26	-31	-36	-42	-47
10mph	34	28	22	16	10	3	-3	-9	-15	-22	-27	-34	-40	-46	-52	-58	-64	-71
15mph	29	23	16	9	2	-5	-11	-18	-25	-31	-38	-45	-51	-58	-65	-72	-78	-85
20mph	26	19	12	4	-3	-10	-17	-24	-31	-39	-46	-53	-60	-67	-74	-81	-88	-95
25mph	23	16	8	1	-7	-15	-22	-29	-36	-44	-51	-59	-66	-74	-81	-88	-96	-103
30mph	21	13	6	-2	-10	-18	-25	-33	-41	-49	-56	-64	-71	-79	-86	-93	-101	-109
35mph	20	12	4	-4	-12	-20	-27	-35	-43	-52	-58	-67	-74	-82	-89	-97	-105	-113
40mph	19	11	3	-5	-13	-21	-29	-37	-45	-53	-60	-69	-76	-84	-92	-100	-107	-115
45mph	18	10	2	-6	-14	-22	-30	-38	-45	-54	-62	-70	-78	-85	-93	-102	-109	-117

Unpleasant | Frostbite likely. Outdoor activity dangerous. | Exposed flesh will freeze within half a minute for the average person.

FIGURE 21.1. Apparent wind chill from a chart provided by the National Weather Service.

numbness of the feet, followed by erythema, swelling, mottling, and numbness. Ice crystal formation does not occur. Anesthesia and cold sensitivity can persist for weeks, or they can be permanent. The prognosis of trench foot is better than that of frostbite.

Chilblains or pernio is characterized by localized erythema, plaques, nodules, or vesicles caused by chronic intermittent exposure to damp, nonfreezing cold temperatures. It is most commonly seen in the hands, feet, ears, and lower legs, and it is more common in women than men. The skin lesions appear 12 to 14 hours after exposure to cold, and they are accompanied by pruritus and paresthesias (5,7).

Frostnip is an early stage in the continuum of frostbite, and it is a superficial cold injury without ice crystal formation or tissue damage. Clinically, the involved area is pale from vasoconstriction, and mild burning or stinging is usually felt. Symptoms improve with rewarming, and no long-term tissue damage occurs.

Frostbite can occur anywhere, but it is most commonly observed on the nose, ears, face, hands, and feet. It can be divided into superficial and deep injuries. Erythema, mild edema, and no blisters characterize first-degree frostbite. Typically, it is accompanied by mild stinging or burning. Second-degree frostbite is characterized by erythema and edema, followed by the formation of clear blisters in 6 to 12 hours. The blisters may desquamate into black eschars over several days. Initially, the patient will have numbness, which is followed by a deep throbbing. First-degree and second-degree frostbite injuries usually portend a good prognosis.

Deep frostbite injuries are those that extend beyond the epidermis. Third-degree frostbite results in dark hemorrhagic blisters and skin necrosis. Often, a blue-gray discoloration of the skin is seen. Initially, the area feels numb and heavy, but the sensation progresses to intense burning and throbbing. Fourth-degree frostbite is characterized by the extension of the injury into the muscle, bone, or tendons. Little edema is present. The skin is mottled and cyanotic, and it will be transformed into a dry, black mummified eschar. The patient suffers from a deep, aching pain. The prognosis of deep frostbite injuries is poor (7).

Hypothermia is defined as a core temperature of less than 35°C (95°F). While hypothermia can affect virtually any organ system in the body, the most prominent effects are on the neurologic and cardiovascular systems. The clinical manifestations of the various stages of hypothermia are well defined. Mild hypothermia is a core body temperature between 32°C (89.6°F) and 35°C (95°F). In this range of core temperature, the body undergoes an excitation stage in which attempts are made to generate heat. Shivering is accompanied by an increase in the metabolic rate. The heart rate, blood pressure, and cardiac output all increase. Moderate hypothermia is seen with a core temperature between 27°C (80.6°F) and 32°C (89.6°F). As the temperature drops below 32°C (89.6°F), progressive slowing of all bodily functions is observed. Shivering ceases between 30°C (86°F) and 32°C (89.6°F). Decreased mentation develops, and atrial fibrillation or other arrhythmias may occur. Below 28°C (82.4°F), the irritability of the myocardium increases, making the patient susceptible to the development of ventricular fibrillation with minor cardiac stimulation. At 25°C (77.°F), voluntary motion stops, loss of reflexes occurs, and cardiac output drops to less than 50% of normal. The lowest reported accidental hypothermia survivor thus far has been an infant whose initial core temperature was 15.2°C (59.4°F). The signs and symptoms of progressive hypothermia are summarized in Table 21.1.

Certain individuals are more susceptible to hypothermia in winter storms. Neonates and infants lose heat more readily due to their larger surface area to volume ratios. The elderly may lose their ability to sense cold. Those with altered sensoria may neither take protective actions nor remove themselves from the cold. Accidental hypothermia will be obvious in some scenarios, such as when a lost hiker was found unconscious in a winter storm. An elderly woman found with altered mental status inside a cool, unheated home may, however, be less obvious. Measuring the core temperature in every patient in whom hypothermia is suspected is crucial. Thermometers that can measure low temperatures must be used, as most commonly available thermometers will not read below 35°C (95°F).

TABLE 21.1. SIGNS AND SYMPTOMS ASSOCIATED WITH PROGRESSIVE HYPOTHERMIA

Core temperature in °C (°F)	Clinical findings
37 (98)	Normal oral temperature.
36 (96)	Hyperexcited state; increase in metabolic rate.
35 (95)	Maximum shivering temperature.
34 (93)	Amnesia, altered level of consciousness, poor judgment, maximum respiratory stimulation.
32 (89)	Stupor, shivering slows, oxygen consumption decreased.
31 (87)	Shivering stops.
30 (86)	Atrial fibrillation common; marked slowing of pulse and respirations.
28 (82)	Ventricular fibrillation threshold markedly lowered; pupils dilate, muscle rigidity.
27 (80)	Clinically appears dead; loss of deep tendon reflexes and voluntary motion.
24 (75)	Severe hypotension.
20 (68)	Cardiac standstill with electrochemical activity.
19 (66)	EEG flatline.
18 (64)	Asystole.

Abbreviation: EEG, electroencephalogram.

PREHOSPITAL CONSIDERATIONS

Proper winterization and maintenance of EMS vehicles are necessary during winter storm conditions. Good engine and electrical maintenance are essential, as well as that of cabin heat and environmental support systems. Additional winter supplies, such as water, food, lights, and warm clothing, should be placed in the vehicles in the event that crews become stranded. Although snow tires and chains may be placed on vehicles, no vehicle performs well on ice. Under such conditions, vehicle contact incidents will be common. Consideration should also be given to alteration of normal posting positions to avoid external postings in frigid temperatures.

Storage of medications in ambulances or helicopters in cold weather can be a problem. The United States Pharmacopoeia recommends storage of most medications between 15°C (59°F) and 30°C (86°F). A recent study measuring temperatures inside a drug storage box carried by paramedics on helicopters indicated that medications are exposed to extremes of temperature well outside the recommended range in periods of inclement weather (8). The impact that the extreme temperatures have on the degradation of the drugs is unclear. However, a strong recommendation is that medications should be removed from the ambulance or helicopter and stored in a room temperature environment when they are not being used.

EMS personnel should be properly equipped with protective equipment against the cold weather. The mnemonic *COLD* may be used in reference to insulation against cold weather. This includes *Clean*, *Open* clothing during exertion to avoid sweating, *Loose* layers to retain heat, and *Dry* clothing to minimize conductive losses (4). Gloves are necessary, but they may need to be temporarily removed for some procedures, such as starting an intravenous (IV) line or intubation. In extreme cold and blizzard conditions, eye protection may be needed to prevent cold-induced or ultraviolet-induced keratitis. EMS personnel should have access to heated areas when they are not directly involved in patient care. Shifts may need to be shortened as cold stress has been shown to reduce an individual's working ability (9). EMS personnel should be educated in how to recognize the early symptoms of cold injuries in themselves and their coworkers. They should immediately seek medical treatment when such symptoms arise.

Prehospital Localized Cold Injury Interventions

Optimal treatment of cold-related injuries must begin before hospital arrival. All EMS systems should have protocols for the care of patients with localized and systemic cold injuries. Prehospital care of the patient with local cold injuries such as frostbite should focus on preventing further damage to the injured tissue. Although the degree of tissue injury has been shown to correlate with the length of time the tissue is frozen, aggressive wound management in the field should be avoided. Thawing of frozen extremities can be performed best in the ED. The primary concern with regard to thawing tissue in the field is the risk that the tissue may be exposed to further cold and refreezing. The repetition of the freeze-thaw cycle causes substantially more tissue damage than a single freeze-thaw cycle (5). Reperfusion of an area with frostbite results in increased leakage of fluid into interstitial areas through damaged capillaries, increased intracellular swelling, platelet aggregation, vasoconstriction, and the release of oxygen free radicals. One exception to the guideline of not thawing frozen tissue in the field is when transport to the ED will take more than 2 hours. In this situation, field thawing may need to be considered. Great care should be taken, however, to prevent any further exposure of the injured tissue to cold.

In general, the prehospital approach to localized cold injuries should follow the simple guidelines detailed in the following (3,5).

1. Remove wet or constrictive clothing.
2. Elevate the affected extremity, and wrap it in dry sterile gauze or other dressings. Carefully separate the fingers and toes if they are involved.
3. Avoid a constricting wrapping, if splinting the area for comfort. Splinting is not necessary, but it may be used for comfort.
4. Avoid rubbing, massaging, or other mechanical stimulation to the injured areas.
5. Keep the area away from heat sources, such as a campfire or car heater, to prevent partial thawing.
6. Leave blisters intact.
7. Transport as quickly as possible to an emergency department.
8. Judicious amounts of parenteral analgesics may be given during transport.

Rewarming is a complicated process, and it should only be attempted in the field if the appropriate equipment and trained personnel are available and if transport to an ED will require more than 2 hours. Basic guidelines for field rewarming are similar to the requirements for ED rewarming (5,7). No wound debridement should be performed prehospital. Adequate analgesia should be provided during rewarming as parenteral morphine or meperidine because the process is often intensely painful. Elevate the extremity, and splint as needed for comfort. Avoid constrictive wrapping or bandages, but do cover the area with sterile bandages or gauze. Transport the patient to an ED as soon as this is feasible.

All patients with suspected frostbite should be transported as soon as possible. The severity of frostbite is difficult to assess in the field. Even patients who appear to have only mild frostbite should be transported. All patients with frostbite should be suspected of having hypothermia.

Prehospital Hypothermia Interventions

Treatment of suspected hypothermia should begin as soon as possible. Field treatment depends on the severity of the hypothermia. A general summary of prehospital care of hypothermia is to rescue, examine, insulate, and transport. Rapid assessment of the patient's mental status, vital signs, and possible traumatic injuries should be implemented. The patient should be removed from the cold environment and sheltered from the wind. Wet clothing should be taken off. A low-reading thermometer should be used to measure the core body temperature. The patient should be hooked up to a cardiac monitor and should be closely watched for ventricular fibrillation. The patient should be transported in a horizontal position and should be handled carefully to avoid the induction of ventricular fibrillation. For a patient with mild hypothermia who is awake and alert, the prognosis is good regardless of the method of rewarming. These patients need simple, external passive rewarming using blankets or active external rewarming by applying hot water bottles to the axilla and groin. Warmed humidified oxygen and IV fluids are usually adequate. These methods can increase the patient's core temperature by 0.5°C (0.9°F) to 1.0°C (1.8°F) per hour (10).

Treatment of patients with moderate-to-severe hypothermia in the field is more controversial. All patients should be placed on a cardiac monitor and observed for ventricular fibrillation. Patients with a pulse should be treated with external core rewarming. This is accomplished primarily with warm humidified oxygen administration. In the patient with spontaneous respiration, warm oxygen administration via mask is adequate. If the patient requires intubation, the concern about induction of ventricular fibrillation is real. However, a recent prospective study of hypothermic victims suggests that intubation will not induce ventricular fibrillation (11). Warmed IV fluids may also be administered, with a 250-mL to 500-mL bolus of warmed normal saline. Care should be taken to insulate the IV line to prevent cooling to room temperature (although this likely will still be warmer than the patient). Altered mental status protocols, including naloxone and thiamine administration and fingerstick glucose measurement, should be part of the routine. Active external rewarming methods, such as warmed water bottles, hot packs, or heating blankets, should be avoided in the patient with moderate-to-severe hypothermia. These methods of warming may cause peripheral vasodilation, resulting in the return of cold, lactic acid–rich blood to the core of the body from the periphery. This has been termed core after-drop. It should be avoided by attempting to warm the core, while avoiding active external rewarming of the extremities (10).

The patient with severe hypothermia and cardiac arrest presents unique problems. A patient who is in cardiac arrest and who is hypothermic should not be considered dead until he or she has been warmed. Case reports of patients with hypothermia and prolonged periods of cardiac arrest who have survived with no long-term sequelae are found. The pulse can be difficult to palpate in the severely vasoconstricted, bradycardic patient. One should palpate for a pulse for more than 45 to 60 seconds. If no pulse is detected, cardiopulmonary resuscitation (CPR) should be started. If ventricular fibrillation is present, defibrillation should be attempted three times at 200, 300, and 360 J. If this is unsuccessful, further defibrillation is unlikely to be effective until the core temperature is increased to at least 30°C. No further defibrillation attempts should be conducted until the core temperature is raised. Standard advanced cardiac life support cardiac drugs have an unpredictable action in the hypothermic patient. Thus, CPR should be continued, and the patient should be rapidly transported to an ED where active core rewarming can be attempted. An approach to the hypothermic patient in cardiac arrest is presented in Figure 21.2.

The treatment of hypothermic patients in a mass casualty incident or disaster situation follows the recommended protocols. However, triage decisions vary depending on the number of victims and the resources available. If resources are overwhelmed, triage should focus on providing the greatest good for the greatest number of people. Thus, hypothermic patients in cardiac arrest may need to be triaged as expectant, as they have a much poorer prognosis than do those with vital signs.

Aeromedical transport of hypothermic patients warrants special consideration. Aeromedical transport of hypothermic patients has not been well studied, but it may have advantages. Concerns have been raised about the increased wind-chill factors due to helicopter downdraft and the cool temperatures in the helicopter. However, a retrospective review of hypothermic patients transported by helicopter indicated the presence of no adverse consequences from helicopter transport (12). Attempting to load patients should be done after engine shutdown when possible to avoid the rotor downdraft. Aeromedical transport becomes a good option for the transport of the hypothermic patient when the environmental circumstances prohibit or retard ground transport.

Helicopter transport may be impossible due to adverse weather conditions. The most common condition that precludes helicopter transport is icing. Federal aviation regulations prohibit any pilot from taking off in icing conditions unless the aircraft has been equipped with deicing equipment. As this type of equipment is rare in helicopters, icing conditions usually prohibit such flights. In these circumstances, fixed-wing transport may be an alternative. Aeromedical systems must abide by federal flight safety reg-

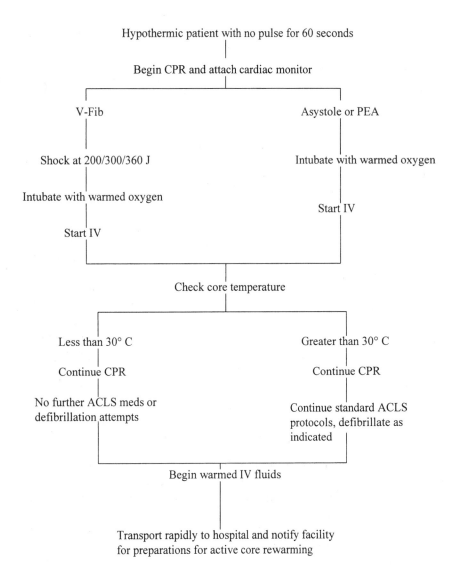

Hypothermic patient with no pulse for 60 seconds

Begin CPR and attach cardiac monitor

V-Fib

Asystole or PEA

Shock at 200/300/360 J

Intubate with warmed oxygen

Intubate with warmed oxygen

Start IV

Start IV

Check core temperature

Less than 30° C

Greater than 30° C

Continue CPR

Continue CPR

No further ACLS meds or defibrillation attempts

Continue standard ACLS protocols, defibrillate as indicated

Begin warmed IV fluids

Transport rapidly to hospital and notify facility for preparations for active core rewarming

FIGURE 21.2. The prehospital approach to the hypothermic patient in cardiac arrest. (Temperature equivalent for 30°C is 86°F.)

ulations for flying in extreme weather, even in the instances of a mass casualty incident or disaster.

EMERGENCY DEPARTMENT CONSIDERATIONS

Winter storms have a direct impact on the ED. Emergency electrical power generators should be in good working order. Equipment to maintain the access and egress routes to the ED should be available. Sufficient facility maintenance, support, and administrative staff should be available to meet hospital needs. ED equipment required for treating cold-related injuries should be inspected and readied for potential cases.

At the time a winter storm warning is issued for a specific area, each ED should have a plan to augment staffing before the storm impact. Staff may become stranded at the hospital, and the relief staff may not be able to travel in. The staff stranded in the ED may be required to work for the next 24 to 48 hours. Work–rest cycles should be used to reduce fatigue. In addition, the staff will likely be concerned about their families if they are unable to get home. Efforts should be made to help staff tend to personal matters in order to ease their fear and stress. Plans to accommodate stranded ED staff members should also be implemented. Sleeping quarters need to be available, in addition to nourishment, hot beverages, showers, and fresh scrubs (most hospitals provide this service free during a disaster).

Depending on the severity of the weather conditions, consultant staff (e.g., surgeons, intensivists, and pediatricians) may not be able to reach the hospital for some time. Alternate modes of transport may need to be arranged through law enforcement or other public service agencies that have vehicles that are able to traverse the weather.

Aeromedical units have been used in the past to pick up staff and transport them to the hospital when a critical need has arisen.

Emergency Department Local Cold Injury Interventions

The treatment of frostbite and local cold-related injuries in the ED centers on rapid rewarming. Although rapid rewarming of local cold injuries is important, this should not delay the identification and treatment of systemic hypothermia. A rapid but thorough history should be obtained as treatment is started. The length of exposure, an environmental temperature estimate, wind velocity, the presence of clothing (including whether it was wet or dry), prehospital treatment, and the underlying medical conditions are important pieces of information.

With local cold injuries, the injured extremity should be placed in water warmed to 40°C (104°F) to 42°C (107.6°F). The water temperature must be kept in that range for optimal thawing and the prevention of burning. The extremity should be left in the warmed water for 10 to 30 minutes, at which time the distal areas of the frostbite injury should begin to be pliable and erythematous. This process is extremely painful, and parenteral analgesics or conscious sedation may be necessary. Efforts should be made to minimize hospital transfers because these might expose the patient to extreme cold again, resulting in refreezing. If transfer is necessary, the patient must be protected from the cold.

After rapid rewarming, attention is focused on preventing further ischemia by minimizing the production of local and systemic thromboxane, which contributes to localized ischemia in damaged tissue. A suggested protocol for treatment to minimize further ischemia includes the following guidelines (13).

1. Debride white blisters after rewarming because they have a high concentration of thromboxane. Apply topical aloe vera, which helps block the arachadonic acid cascade, and leave hemorrhagic blisters intact.
2. Elevate and splint the extremity, keeping fingers and toes separated by cotton or gauze.
3. Apply aloe vera every 6 hours.
4. Administer tetanus prophylaxis.
5. Use parenteral analgesics, such as morphine or meperidine, as needed.
6. Administer ibuprofen, 400 mg, orally every 12 hours.
7. Administer penicillin G, 500,000 U, intravenously every 6 hours for 2 to 3 days.
8. Perform hydrotherapy for 30 to 45 minutes at 40°C (104°F). The following solutions are recommended with hydrotherapy:
   For a large tank of 425 gallons, the fill level is 285 gallons. Use NaCl, 9.7 kg; KCl, 282 g; and 95 mL of calcium hypochlorite solution.

For a medium tank capacity of 270 gallons, the fill level estimate is 108 gallons. Use NaCl, 3.7 kg; KCl, 107 g; and 36 mL of a calcium hypochlorite solution. For a small tank capacity of 95 gallons, the fill level estimate is 72 gallons. Use NaCl, 2.5 kg; KCl, 71 g; and 24 mL of a calcium hypochlorite solution.

9. Photograph injured areas for documentation on admission, again at 24 hours, and then every 2 to 3 days until the patient is discharged.
10. Instruct the patient to avoid cold exposure when discharging him or her. Ibuprofen and aloe vera should be continued. The patient should be observed weekly until the wounds are stable.

Interest has been shown in the use of low molecular weight heparin, hyperbaric oxygen, and intraarterial reserpine for treatment of frostbite. No studies have indicated a clear benefit with the use of these agents. One must emphasize that surgery has little role in the early management of frostbite, but it may be necessary later in the course if gangrene is present.

Almost all patients with frostbite should be admitted. No patient with even minimal frostbite should be discharged from the ED unless the assurance is present that they will not go back into the cold. Frostbite victims need consultations with social workers to make sure that they have adequate transportation, a warm environment, proper clothing, and an ability to keep follow-up appointments before they can be discharged.

Emergency Department Hypothermia Interventions

The treatment of systemic hypothermia in the ED is based on the severity of the symptoms and the degree of hypothermia. As in the field, the initial treatment of all patients should be to prevent further cold injury, which includes the removal of wet garments and the prevention of further heat loss by protecting from air movement, covering the patient, and establishing the ABCs. Evaluation for other traumatic injuries should be conducted. The patient's core temperature and underlying cardiac rhythm should be evaluated. If the patient has an altered mental status, naloxone and thiamine should be administered, and bedside blood glucose should be obtained. For mild hypothermia (34°C [93°F]–36°C [96°F]), passive rewarming with blankets with warmed humidified oxygen and IV fluids heated to 43°C (109.4°F) is usually adequate.

For patients with moderate hypothermia (30°C [86°F] – 34°C [93.2°F]) who are hemodynamically stable, active external rewarming should be added, with heat applied to the truncal area only. This is accomplished by water bottles or electric warming devices (10). Active external rewarming of the extremities should be avoided because it promotes core after-drop due to peripheral vasodilation. Observation for core after-drop, which manifests with hypotension, acidosis, and arrhythmias, should be a priority.

For patients with severe hypothermia (less than 30°C [86°F]) or for those who are hemodynamically unstable, active internal rewarming must be conducted. Several techniques of active internal rewarming are used. Endotracheal intubation and the application of warm humidified oxygen are usually the first step. Lavage of the gastrointestinal tract and bladder can be done with normal saline warmed to 40°C (104°F). The saline is placed into the stomach via the nasogastric tube or into the bladder by Foley and is left for 15 minutes. The fluid is then aspirated or drained and is replaced by more warmed fluid. Aspiration is a risk during this procedure, and caution is required if the patient is not intubated. Pleural rewarming can be done with two thoracostomy tubes in each hemithorax: one tube is used for inflow and the other for outflow of warmed sterile saline. Input and output must be monitored carefully to prevent an iatrogenic tension hydrothorax (14). A left thoracotomy can be done, and the cold heart can bathed in warmed sterile saline in patients with pulseless electrical activity. Peritoneal lavage or dialysis with warmed isotonic dialysate or normal saline may also be used. This approach is similar to a diagnostic peritoneal lavage. Two L of isotonic dialysate or normal saline warmed to 40°C (104°F) to 45°C (113°F) is used, is retained for 20 to 30 minutes, and is then removed through aspiration or drainage (4).

The best technique for active core rewarming is cardiopulmonary bypass. The advantage is not only rapid core rewarming but also the maintenance of blood flow and oxygenation even without cardiac output, which is due to the severe hypothermia. The most common approach is to use the femoral vein and artery for vascular access. Pump-assisted cardiopulmonary bypass is initiated, and the blood is warmed and oxygenated. The core temperature can be increased by 9.5°C (49°F) per hour with this technique. This method is the active core rewarming technique of choice when the patient is in cardiac arrest or when the patient has a core temperature of less than 25°C (77°F) (15). However, cardiopulmonary bypass requires special equipment and trained personnel, it is not universally available, and it usually cannot be done immediately on arrival to the ED.

Emergency Department Triage Considerations

The treatment of multiple hypothermic patients in a mass casualty incident during a winter storm follows the same principles of treatment as those for a single patient. However, with a large number of victims, attention must be focused on resource utilization. Several hypothermic patients presenting in cardiac arrest will represent a significant problem for any ED. Generally, a hypothermic patient is never considered dead until the core temperature is increased to 28°C (82.4°F) to 30°C (86°F). Therefore, the presentation of multiple

hypothermic patients to the ED can create a profound triage dilemma with regard to the choice of who to warm first. One study concluded that, in patients in cardiac arrest from severe hypothermia, serum potassium, activated clotting time, and pH drawn from a central venous source can assist in triage by determining which patients are the most salvageable. If venous pH is less than 6.50, the potassium level is greater than 9.0 mmol per L, or the activated clotting time is greater than 400 seconds, then death likely preceded hypothermia. Spontaneous circulation will probably never be restored under these circumstances (16). Although these findings are the result of a small study, they may provide some guidance for triage in this situation.

SUMMARY

Disasters related to winter storms are uncommon, and large numbers of victims from winter storms or cold injuries have generally been limited to military campaigns. The potential for a large number of victims to sustain cold injuries is increasing as the popularity of outdoor recreational activity increases. The EMS treatment of localized cold injuries emphasizes rapid transport and the avoidance of potential thawing-refreezing circumstances. Systemic hypothermia should be treated at the prehospital stage with rapid transport and interventions based on the severity of the exposure. Specific protocols for treating frostbite should be developed in areas where these injuries are commonly seen. Core afterdrop is a potential complication of hypothermia that should be avoided. Severe hypothermia is treated through various mechanisms accomplishing active core rewarming. The best technique involves cardiopulmonary bypass with hemodialysis. Aggressive education of the public in areas that are at high risk for winter storms can limit the injuries and the impact of the storms on that community. Planning for a uniform response to a winter storm disaster will decrease the adverse effect of such events on EMS and EDs. In addition, patient morbidity and mortality will be reduced.

REFERENCES

1. Hauty MG, Esrig, BC, Hill JG, et al. Prognostic factors in severe accidental hypothermia: experience from the Mt. Hood tragedy. *J Trauma* 1987;10:1107–1112.
2. National Weather Service. Available at: http://www.nws.noaa.gov. Accessed November 30, 1999.
3. Surviving old man winter. *Occup Health Saf* 1998;67:186–187.
4. Danzl DF, Pozos RS, Hamlet MP. Accidental hypothermia. In: Auerbach PS, Geehr ED, eds. *Management of wilderness and environmental injuries*, 2nd ed. St Louis: Mosby-Year Book, 1989: 35–78.
5. Smith DJ, Robson MC, Heggers JP. Frostbite and other cold-induced injuries. In: Auerbach PS, Geehr EC, eds. *Management of wilderness and environmental injuries*, 2nd ed. St. Louis: Mosby-Year Book, 1989:101–118.

6. Pulla RJ, Pickard LJ, Carnett TS. Frostbite: an overview with case presentations. *J Foot Ankle Surg* 1994;33:53–63.
7. Rabold R. Frostbite and other localized cold-related injuries. In: Tintannelli JE, Ruiz E, Krome RL, eds. *Emergency medicine: a comprehensive study guide*, 4th ed. New York: McGraw-Hill, 1996:843–846.
8. Madden JF, O'Connor RE, Evans J. The range of medication storage temperatures in aeromedical emergency medical services. *Prehosp Emerg Care* 1999;3:27–30.
9. Anttonen H, Virokannas H. Assessment of cold stress in outdoor work. *Arct Med Res* 1994;53:40–48.
10. Weinberg AD. Hypothermia. *Ann Emerg Med* 1993;22:370–377.
11. Hall KN, Syverud SA. Closed thoracic cavity lavage in the treatment of severe hypothermia in human beings. *Ann Emerg Med* 1990;19:204–206.
12. Fox JB, Thomas G, Clemmer TP, et al. A retrospective analysis of air-evacuated hypothermia patients. *Aviation Space Environ Med* 1988;59:1070–1075.
13. McCauley RL, Hing DN, Robson MC, Heggers JP. Frostbite injuries: a rational approach based on the pathophysiology. *J Trauma* 1983;23:143–147.
14. Bessen HA. Hypothermia. In: Tintannelli JE, Ruiz E, Krome RL, eds. *Emergency medicine: a comprehensive study guide*, 4th ed. New York: McGraw-Hill, 1996:846–850.
15. Vretenar DR, Urschel JD, Parrott JC, et al. Cardiopulmonary bypass resuscitation for accidental hypothermia. *Ann Thorac Surg* 1994;58:895–898.
16. Mair P, Kornberger E, Furtwaengler W, et al. Prognostic markers in patients with severe accidental hypothermia and cardiocirculatory arrest. *Resuscitation* 1994;27:47–54.

HEAT WAVE DISASTERS

JAMES S. WALKER
MICHAEL CHAMALES

A heat wave is a meteorologic term rather than a medical term, and it is defined as a prolonged period of excessive heat and humidity. This obviously is a relative or conceptual term without any threshold criteria for the minimal ambient temperature or the absolute duration or time span. A heat wave is comparative to the normal seasonal temperature and humidity for a given geographic region. Accordingly, heat waves in various parts of the country can vary greatly in intensity and duration. Usually, heat waves occur in the summer; however, rarely, they can transpire in the spring or fall. Although precise conditions are lacking for accurately defining a heat wave, the Centers for Disease Control recommends caution when a daytime heat index of 105°F (40.6°C) or higher and a nighttime minimum temperature of 80°F (26.7°C) persists for at least 48 hours (1).

EPIDEMIOLOGY

Throughout the history of the world, heat waves have had an enormous impact on human morbidity and mortality. Heat waves have been known to increase the incidence of heat stroke and other heat-related illnesses markedly. When the environmental heat stress is high, strenuous exercise is not required to produce heat illness. In 1743, a heat wave in Beijing resulted in 11,000 deaths. During the summer of 1987, a heat wave in Greece and Italy precipitated the deaths of approximately 3,000 elderly people. In the Middle East each year, approximately two million Muslims undertake the Hadj, the pilgrimage to Mecca. During this pilgrimage, over 1,000 will be treated for heat stroke, and hundreds may die before reaching treatment facilities (2). In 1998, scorching temperatures (116°F) killed more than 2,500 during India's worst heat wave in 50 years.

In the United States, a major heat wave can cause literally thousands of deaths over a given summer. In the past 40 years (1936 through 1975), nearly 20,000 Americans died as a result of heat-related illnesses. Comparatively, in a normal or non-heat wave year, approximately 175 Americans die as a consequence of heat-related illnesses, whereas, during a heat wave year, this mortality rate increases by fivefold. Between 1975 and 1995, a total of 6,615 deaths in the United States were attributed to the effects of heat and excessive heat exposure. In July 1995, a protracted heat wave settled on Chicago, causing more than 600 deaths and 3,300 emergency department (ED) visits (4,5). During the summer of 1998, a severe heat wave and subsequent drought extended from Texas and Oklahoma eastward to the Carolinas, culminating in $6.9 billion dollars of damage and at least 200 deaths. During the summer of 1999, a heat wave and drought located in the eastern United States was responsible for 256 deaths and over $1 billion in damages. In the United States, estimations of the annual heat-related deaths have been as high as 4,000 persons (6).

When one analyzes heat waves from a disaster-oriented approach, the topic breaks into two categories—heat waves of relatively short duration and heat waves that are comparatively long. The immediate impact of the heat wave is a high incidence of heat stroke and other heat-related injuries in the population. Over greater periods, individual physiologic acclimatization to the heat develops, and a decrease in direct heat injury morbidity and mortality is observed. The long-term and often more consequential impact of heat waves involves drought, wildfires, and firestorms. This chapter will primarily address the management of heat waves as it relates to heat injuries. Drought and its consequences will be briefly discussed. Wildfires and firestorms are presented in Chapter 20.

MECHANISMS OF INJURY

In addition to death and injury from heat stroke, analysis of the causes of injury associated with heat disasters have detected the following three primary organ system manifestations: cerebrovascular, cardiovascular, and respiratory (7). Although many deaths are reported as being associated with heat injury, significant increases in cerebrovascular infarction and hemorrhage, myocardial infarction and associated cardiovascular complications, pneumonia, asthma, and respiratory failure are noted. One report from the Philadelphia heat disaster of 1993 indicated a 100% increase in cardiovascular deaths during the event (7). These increases have not been found to be consistent, but they are thought to be related to the effects of heat stress on pathologic conditions in the underlying organ systems.

PREHOSPITAL CONSIDERATIONS

Prehospital personnel face additional hazards from heat when providing routine care during the summer. During a heat wave, even greater stress is placed on both personnel and equipment. Vehicles must be maintained for heat stresses to prevent breakdowns. Stationary running of vehicles may need to be curtailed or may need to be done with the hood up to prevent overheating. Air conditioning is a necessity, not a luxury, because it provides not only the relief of heat stress for the crew but also a more stable temperature environment for medications and equipment. In addition, air conditioning provides an important cooling mechanism for patients suffering from heat-related illnesses. Emergency medical services (EMS) personnel should use lightweight uniforms, drink plenty of fluids, and avoid sun exposure. Work–rest cycles should be observed, and breaks within air-conditioned areas should be provided on a periodic basis. Evaporative cooling protocols should be available, and personnel should be well trained in the recognition of heat-related illnesses. EMS should be involved in community outreach programs during heat waves, especially those targeting high-risk populations and high-risk areas of the city.

EMS and search-and-rescue teams deploying to a long-term rescue and recovery mission during a heat disaster face additional problems. True acclimatization to a hot environment takes 2 weeks to achieve, and it usually is not practical in disaster response. Strict monitoring and water discipline are needed to prevent rescue crews from becoming additional heat casualties. Personnel should understand that feeling thirsty is equated with dehydration, and therefore they must adhere to drinking fluids before they experience the sensation of thirst. In addition to water, the initial fluids should consist of a balanced electrolyte solution (0.05% to 0.1% NaCl or half-strength commercial sports drinks), as sodium depletion occurs during the initial phase of heat exposure. Provision of shade and shade gear, as well as sunscreen, will diminish the impact of radiative energy on the team. Work–rest cycles providing frequent breaks are as important as water discipline in preserving the effectiveness of the responders.

EMERGENCY DEPARTMENT CONSIDERATIONS

ED preparations during a heat wave should be undertaken at the first alert. The EDs should monitor the ongoing weather conditions regarding the heat index and other factors posing a risk to the population at large. Cooperative involvement with municipal disaster planners and EMS should be undertaken to educate and monitor high-risk populations and areas. Equipment, such as large fans, spray bottles, and cooling packs, should be readily available for the treatment of serious heat injuries. Cool, balanced electrolyte oral rehydration solutions should be on hand for less serious heat illnesses. ED visits have been noted to increase up to 14% during a heat disaster, although high variability in this effect is observed (8).

COMMUNITY PLANNING POINTS

Municipal disaster planners should have specific protocols for monitoring and care of populations during a heat disaster. Urbanization alone has long been acknowledged to be a risk factor for heat injury. Early studies have indicated substantially higher rates for heat-related deaths in urbanized areas when compared to those in rural regions (9). In 1966, high death rates in St. Louis, Missouri, were reported during a heat wave for populations located in crowded alleyways and high towers in the inner city lacking air conditioning and adequate ventilation (10). During the 1978 heat disaster in Texas, the high cost of maintaining air conditioning for many elderly individuals on fixed income caused them to shut the service off. A number of these elderly individuals then died of heat stroke (10). Municipal planners should use city employees to provide monitoring of such high-risk city locations and populations as they carry out their normal duties. In addition, community volunteer programs may be initiated to reach these individuals. When the heat index reaches critical levels, ventilation and fans will not be adequate to protect some of the population. They will need to be given the opportunity to go to an air-conditioned location, such as a mall or public building, for a period of time during the hot part of the day. Providing even a brief relief from the heat may be life-saving (7). Transportation to such locations should be provided free of charge to high-risk individuals via public or volunteer agencies. Educational programs should be initiated even before the first heat warning. Some general recommendations are given in Table 22.1.

TABLE 22.1. SAFETY INSTRUCTIONS TO AVOID HEAT ILLNESS

Safety tips for the community during a heat-related disaster	
Slow down.	Decrease strenuous activity or postpone or reschedule it for the cooler parts of the day (4:00 AM to 7:00 AM).
Dress for summer.	Wear lightweight loose-fitting clothing of light color.
Diet.	Eat fewer proteins and increase carbohydrate intake to reduce endogenous heat production.
Fluids.	Drink fluids even when not noticeably thirsty.
Alcohol.	Do not drink as it dehydrates the body.
Salt tablets.	Do not use salt tablets.
Air conditioning.	Seek an air-conditioned place for at least a few hours every day.
Sun exposure.	Avoid direct sun exposure as it causes heat gain.
Shades.	Use shades to protect living areas from morning and evening sun.

From the National Weather Service. Available at http://weather.noaa.gov/weather/hwave.html. Accessed July 28, 1999, with permission.

PATHOPHYSIOLOGY OF HEAT-RELATED HOMEOSTASIS

The human body maintains a narrow core temperature range through the interactions of various heat-producing and heat-dispersal mechanisms. The primary form of heat production in the body is the basal metabolic rate (BMR), which is a thermal expression of the many biochemical reactions that occur at the cellular level. Although individual BMRs vary, they average 50 to 60 kcal per hour per m². Without the intervention of cooling mechanisms, the BMR can result in the body temperature increasing by 1.1°C (1.9°F) each hour (11). Any modality that increases the basic metabolic rate or decreases the physiologic cooling mechanisms is a risk factor for heat illness.

The body uses the following four important physical mechanisms to diffuse or dissipate heat: conduction, convection, evaporation, and radiation. Conduction is the transfer of heat from warmer to cooler objects by direct physical contact. Under normal circumstances, only 2% of the body heat load is dispersed by conduction because air is a good insulator. However, if the body is immersed in water, potential exists for significant conductive heat loss because water has a 32-fold higher degree of conductivity that air. Accordingly, submersion of a hyperthermic body in cold water results in rapid heat loss. Convection is the loss of heat to the surrounding air. Heat loss by means of convection is highly dependent on air temperature and wind velocity. Tight-fitting clothes decrease heat loss through convection. Evaporation is the loss of heat due to the conversion of a liquid to a gas. This results from the principal of physics that evaporation is a cooling process. The primary mechanism of heat loss through evaporation in the human body is sweating. Up to 58 kcal of body heat can be dissipated per mL of sweat excreted under ideal evaporative conditions (13). Heat loss via this mechanism can be markedly attenuated by volume depletion, high ambient humidity, or any condition (physical or drug-induced) that impairs the body's capacity to perspire. Radiation is the transfer of heat by electromagnetic waves. Under normal circumstances, this is the primary mechanism by which the body dissipates heat. However, if the ambient temperature exceeds skin temperature, radiation can be a source of significant heat gain.

Conduction and radiation are sensible or dry heat exchange mechanisms by which the body can gain or lose heat depending on the relationship of the ambient temperature to the body's temperature. For example, on a hot day when the ambient temperature is greater than the skin temperature, these mechanisms may become a source of heat gain. Evaporation, however, is a wet or insensible heat exchange mechanism, and therefore, it is unidirectional. Heat can only be lost through evaporation and not gained. This is an important thermal homeostatic concept, especially on a humid day when evaporation becomes the only source of heat loss for the human body.

METEOROLOGIC VARIABLES OF HEAT STRESS

Four primary atmospheric conditions associated with heat waves greatly influence the body's ability to regulate thermal homeostasis. These meteorologic variables are the temperature of the air, the humidity of the air, the movement of the air or the wind speed, and heat energy derived from solar radiation. Although air temperature is extremely important, it is not the sole determinant of environmental heat stress. None of these preceding four atmospheric conditions exist in isolation; they are all present simultaneously in the form of a thermal environment.

Temperature

A high ambient temperature not only increases the potential for heat production, but it also impairs heat dissipation. The impact of air temperature on thermal regulation is best appreciated when it is compared to the body's temperature. When the air temperature is lower than the body temperature, radiant heat loss accounts for 65% of the body's cooling. However, when the ambient temperature approaches or exceeds body temperature, heat loss by radiation stops and the body may begin to gain heat by radiation. To facilitate heat loss by radiation in a hot environment, the peripheral blood flow to the skin can increase by a factor of 20. Also, as the ambient temperature increases, the amount of heat dispersion by convection decreases. Once the air temperature exceeds the skin temperature, the body gains heat.

Humidity

The humidity of the air is of paramount importance in temperature regulation. In humans, the primary means of evaporative heat loss is sweat from the skin. The magnitude or degree of humidity determines the ability of a person to disperse heat by sweating. Conditions of high humidity impede heat dissipation by preventing the evaporation of sweat. Conditions of low humidity are conducive to sweating, and thereby they facilitate the body's cooling. Respiratory evaporative heat loss is significant for panting mammals; however, this is insignificant in humans. The combination of high ambient temperature and high ambient humidity results in a significant accumulative heat load due to increased heat production and impaired heat loss.

Wind Speed

The effect of air movement on thermal regulation is small when compared to temperature and humidity. The heat exchange between the surface of the body and vaporized water molecules circulating in the air around the body is an example of convection. Convection accounts for approximately 10% to 15% of heat loss by the body. It is greatly influenced by wind velocity. Obviously, as the wind speed increases, so will the amount of heat loss by means of convection.

Radiation

Radiation is the heat transfer by electromagnetic waves. Radiation is the primary mechanism of heat loss when the air temperature is lower than body temperature. Conversely,

when the ambient temperature is greater than body temperature, radiation can be a major source of heat gain. The effect of radiant heat from buildings, the pavement, or other such sources on thermal homeostasis can be substantial (14). To facilitate heat loss in a hot environment, the peripheral blood flow to the skin can increase by a factor of 20.

Heat Index

Based on the preceding discussion, one can readily recognize that taking atmospheric conditions and apply them in a singly in an attempt to determine if the weather is conducive to the development of a heat-related illness is difficult. Historically, the wet-bulb globe temperature was the primary tool for determining the total environmental heat stress. The wet-bulb globe temperature was used extensively by the military for a number of years to dictate or limit the amount of physical activity permitted in training during hot weather. The drawback of the wet-bulb temperature was that it was cumbersome to determine and that it only took temperature and humidity into consideration. However, now the National Weather Service (NWS) has devised the *heat index*, which gives the relative temperature for how hot the weather actually feels (15). This index takes into consideration all the relevant atmospheric variables, not just the temperature and humidity. The heat index is usually calculated on a computer because of its many variables and is then broadcast over the weather segment of television newscasts. The heat index is initially calculated with the assumption that the atmospheric conditions are shady with a light wind. Corrections for bright, sunny conditions result in an increase of 15°F (8°C) in the heat index. Just as the military used the wet-bulb globe temperature to limit physical activity levels, the NWS has made similar recommendations for activity levels based on the heat index. The heat index chart is depicted in Table 22.2. The relative risks of heat illnesses based on the heat index are demonstrated in Table 22.3.

TABLE 22.2. THE HEAT INDEX CHART

| Relative humidity (%) | Air temperature (°F) | | | | | | | |
| | 70 | 75 | 80 | 85 | 90 | 95 | 100 | 105 |
	Heat index (°F)							
0	64	69	73	78	83	87	91	95
10	65	70	75	80	85	90	95	100
20	66	72	77	82	87	93	99	105
30	67	73	78	84	90	96	104	113
40	68	74	79	86	93	101	110	123
50	69	75	81	88	96	107	120	135
60	70	76	82	90	100	114	132	149
70	70	77	85	93	106	124	144	—
80	71	78	86	97	113	136	157	—
90	71	79	88	102	122	150	170	—
100	72	80	91	108	133	166	—	—

From the National Weather Service. Available at: http://www.erh.noaa.gov/er/lwx/wxcalc/heatindex.html. Accessed March 31, 2002, with permission.

TABLE 22.3. HEAT INDEX AND HEAT ILLNESS RISK

Heat index	Possible heat illness at various heat index levels
130°F or higher	Heatstroke/sunstroke highly likely with continued exposure.
105°–130°F	Sunstroke, heat cramps, or heat exhaustion likely; heatstroke possible with prolonged exposure and/or physical activity.
90°–105°F	Sunstroke, heat cramps, and heat exhaustion possible with prolonged exposure and/or physical activity.
80°–90°F	Fatigue possible with prolonged exposure and/or physical activity.

From the National Weather Service. Available at: http://www.weather.noaa.gov/weather/hwave.html. Accessed July 28, 1999, with permission.

THE SPECTRUM OF HEAT-RELATED ILLNESS

Heat Edema

Heat edema presents as a transient swelling of the hands, feet, and ankles during the first few days of heat exposure. Heat edema is generally secondary to increased aldosterone secretion, which enhances water retention. When combined with peripheral vasodilatation and venous stasis, the excess fluid accumulates in the dependent areas of the extremities. A thorough history and physical examination are usually helpful in establishing the diagnosis and in ruling out more serious causes for the edema (congestive heart failure). Extensive diagnostic testing is generally unnecessary. The heat edema usually resolves within several days after the patient becomes acclimated to the warmer environment. No treatment is required, although wearing support stockings and elevating the legs helps minimize the edema. Diuretics should be avoided.

Heat Rash

Known also as prickly heat, this maculopapular rash is accompanied by acute inflammation and blocked sweat ducts. The sweat ducts may become dilated and may eventually rupture, producing small pruritic vesicles on an erythematous base. Heat rash frequently affects areas of the body covered by tight clothing. Continued heat exposure can result in deeper blockage of the sweat ducts and recurrent rupture into the dermis. This can lead to the development of chronic dermatitis or a secondary bacterial infection. Prevention is the best therapy; advise patients to wear loose-fitting clothing in the heat. However, once heat rash has developed, the initial treatment involves the application of chlorhexidine lotion to remove any desquamated skin (talcum powder is not effective). The associated pruritus is treated with topical or systemic antihistamines. Vesicles may subsequently form in the deeper layers of the dermis, and a secondary *Staphylococcus aureus* infection can be common. If infection occurs, the patient is treated with any of the following:

- Erythromycin (250 mg four times a day);
- Cephalexin (250 mg four times a day);
- Dicloxacillin (250 mg four times a day);

- 2% Mupirocin ointment (apply to the affected area three times a day).

Heat Cramps

Heat cramps are painful, often severe, involuntary spasms of the large muscle groups used in strenuous exercise. Heat cramps tend to occur after intense exertion. They usually develop in people performing heavy exercise in the heat while sweating profusely and replenishing fluid losses with nonelectrolyte-containing water. This triad is believed to lead to hyponatremia that induces cramping in stressed muscles. Patients who suffer from heat cramps generally have hypochloremic hyponatremia and low urinary levels of sodium and chloride. Rehydration with salt-containing fluids provides rapid relief. Patients with mild cramps can be given oral 0.2% salt solutions, while those with severe cramps require intravenous isotonic fluids (6). Interestingly, the mandated consumption of salt-containing liquids has eliminated heat cramps among workers at several steel mills. Encourage patients who are predisposed to heat cramps to maintain adequate hydration with salt solutions. The many sports drinks on the market are a good source of electrolytes, and they are readily accessible. Patients should not use salt tablets for the following two reasons: they provide inadequate fluid volume replacement, and they are gastric irritants that may cause nausea and vomiting (6,12).

Heat Tetany

Severe carpopedal spasm, paresthesias, and tetany may occur in previously asymptomatic persons who experience a short period of intense heat stress. Heat stress induces hyperventilation, which leads to respiratory alkalosis and subsequent symptoms. In general, heat cramps do not precipitate heat tetany. The recommended therapy consists of removing the patient from the hot environment and either decreasing the ventilatory rate or instituting carbon dioxide rebreathing.

Heat Syncope

Heat exposure may produce postural hypotension, which can precipitate a near-syncopal or syncopal episode. Heat syncope is believed to result from intense sweating, which leads to dehydration, followed by peripheral vasodilation and reduced venous blood return in the face of decreased vasomotor control. Management of heat syncope consists of cooling and rehydration of the patient using oral rehydration solutions (e.g., commercially available sports drinks) or isotonic intravenous fluids. The history and physical examination should identify any underlying neurologic, cardiovascular, or metabolic abnormalities that may account for the episode. In addition, evaluate the patient for injuries that may have resulted from the associated fall. Warn patients who experience heat syncope to avoid standing in the heat for long periods. Advise them to move to a cooler environment and to lie down if they recognize the initial symptoms. Wearing support stockings and engaging in deep knee-bending movements can help promote venous blood return.

Heat Exhaustion

Many experts consider this condition to be a forerunner of heat stroke. Heat exhaustion may resemble heat stroke, but neurologic function remains intact. Heat exhaustion is marked by excessive dehydration and electrolyte depletion. Symptoms may include headache, nausea and vomiting, dizziness, tachycardia, malaise, and myalgia. The body temperature may be normal but generally is elevated (although it rarely rises above 104°F [40°C]). The laboratory test results almost always show dehydration, which is indicated by an increased hematocrit and hemoglobin value. Typically, sufficient time will not have elapsed for a high blood urea nitrogen level to develop. Various electrolytes abnormalities may be present, depending on whether the patient has been drinking plain water or salt-containing liquids to replenish the lost fluids. Mild to moderately elevated liver enzyme levels are commonly seen. Definitive therapy consists of removing patients from the heat and replenishing their fluids. Although mild episodes can be treated with oral fluids, most patients require intravenous fluid replacement. Isotonic fluids should be used initially; the salt content is then adjusted as necessary once the electrolyte levels are known. Volume replacement and a few hours of observation are often sufficient for most patients unless marked laboratory abnormalities are seen (hypokalemia, hypocalcemia, and/or hypoglycemia). Patients who remained stable during observation can be discharged. They should be instructed to rest, to drink plenty of fluids for the next 2 to 3 hours, and to avoid the heat for several days. Patients who are elderly, who have unstable vital signs after 2 hours of treatment, or who have cardiovascular disease may need to be hospitalized for extended observation (16,17).

Classic Heat Stroke

Classic heat stroke occurs during a period of sustained high temperature and humidity (e.g., a heat wave). Epidemics are common. Sweating is absent in from 84% to 100% of those affected. Typical victims are the elderly or the chronically ill who may have no access to air conditioning. These persons often are taking prescription medications (e.g., diuretics, anticholinergics, antipsychotics, and antihypertensives) that interfere with their ability to dissipate heat.

Exertional Heat Stroke

In contrast to the classic heat stroke, exertional heat stroke is not necessarily linked with heat waves. It usually develops in healthy young persons whose mechanisms of heat dispersal are overwhelmed by endogenous heat production. Athletes and military personnel are frequently affected. In contrast with classic heat stroke, marked sweating, rhabdomyolysis, acute renal failure, severe hepatic damage, and disseminated intravascular coagulopathy characterize this condition. The distinction between classic and exertional heat stroke is academic because both forms are treated in the same manner. The differential diagnosis of heat stroke is depicted in Table 22.4.

Widespread organ system injury may ensue, and central nervous system effects may be extensive because the central nervous system is extremely sensitive to heat. The cardiovascular system generally is hyperdynamic, which is manifested by an increased heart rate, cardiac index, and central venous dilation. Heart failure, pulmonary edema, myocardial infarction, hypotension, and cardiovascular collapse may develop. The presence of hypotension and decreased cardiac output and index indicate a poor prognosis. Hepatic damage almost always occurs. Liver transaminase levels may be markedly increased, peaking within 48 to 72 hours. Jaundice sometimes develops after 24 to 48 hours. Most survivors of heat stroke, however, suffer no permanent liver dysfunction. Coagulopathy, as indicated by reduced levels of platelets, fibrinogen, and clotting factors is common, suggesting a poor prognosis and an increased risk of death. Pulmonary symptoms nearly always include hyperventila-

TABLE 22.4. DIFFERENTIAL DIAGNOSIS OF HEAT STROKE

Anticholinergic toxicity
Cerebral hemorrhage
Diabetic ketoacidosis
Encephalitis
Infectious hepatitis
Malaria
Malignant hyperthermia
Meningitis
Neuroleptic malignant syndrome
Sepsis
Status epilepticus
Tetanus
Thyroid storm
Typhus

tion and respiratory alkalosis; pulmonary edema sometimes occurs. Renal function abnormalities are common and likely are a consequence of hypokalemia and hypoperfusion. However, disseminated intravascular coagulopathy and direct glomerular damage from heat may also contribute to renal dysfunction. Acute renal failure is seen in 25% to 30% of patients with exertional heat stroke. Rhabdomyolysis may impart a machine oil appearance to the urine. Although acute renal failure may necessitate dialysis, most patients recover full renal function.

The key to prompt diagnosis is maintaining a high index of suspicion because numerous conditions can lead to hyperpyrexia and neurologic dysfunction. Although the diagnosis may not be confirmed until other entities are ruled out, immediate treatment is mandatory when heat stroke is suspected. Further diagnostic testing to investigate alternate causes can be carried out during therapy. The initial management of both classic and exertional heat stroke includes immediate assessment of the airway, breathing, and circulation (the ABCs). Oxygen therapy is indicated, and immediate endotracheal intubation may sometimes be needed to remedy respiratory distress or to secure control of the airway. Cardiac monitoring is also necessary. Administration of intravenous isotonic fluids is mandatory, but rapid fluid replacement should be avoided because it may worsen pulmonary edema. Potassium should not be administered until urinary output has been ensured. Laboratory tests, including a complete blood cell count, comprehensive metabolic studies, and a hepatic panel, are indicated. In addition, measurements of arterial blood gases, prothrombin, and partial thromboplastin times, as well as of fibrinogen and fibrin degradation products, are useful. A quick bedside check of the blood glucose level for all patients with altered mental status is advisable. A Foley catheter should be used to monitor urinary output. Order an electrocardiogram and chest radiograph.

Rapid cooling is the crux of therapy. Evaporative cooling is the easiest method for reducing body temperature. Other techniques include cold-water submersion, complete body ice packing, strategic ice packing at the axilla and groin, and cold gastric and peritoneal lavage. An effective method for the induction of evaporative cooling is the placement of fans around the undressed patient who has been sprayed with tepid water. Cold water should be avoided because it causes peripheral vasoconstriction and diminishes the heat loss. Likewise, the patient should not be covered with sheets. Ice packs can be placed in the axilla and the groin regions. When possible, a nasogastric tube can be inserted in order to perform cold gastric lavage. Immersion cooling involves setting the patient in a tub of cold water deep enough to cover the trunk and extremities. Cardiac monitoring is difficult when this procedure is used, and defibrillation cannot be performed while the patient is submerged. Cold peritoneal lavage is the most rapid cooling technique. However, it is highly invasive, and it is not always available.

Studies in humans are somewhat limited, and the risk presented to the patient may not be worth the benefit that is gained (6). No matter what cooling method is chosen, the patient's temperature should be measured frequently (every 5 minutes) with a rectal or esophageal monitor until the core temperature reaches 102°F (39°C). Additional cooling beyond this point may lead to hypothermia. A common detrimental effect of rapid cooling is shivering, which increases endogenous heat production. Intravenous diazepam (5–10 mg) or chlorpromazine (10–25 mg) can abolish the shivering reflexes; however, the latter's anticholinergic effects impair heat loss. One should note that neither aspirin nor acetaminophen is useful for decreasing the temperature in patients with heat stroke. Therefore, both medications should be avoided because they may worsen hepatic damage. Finally, close supportive care must continue during cooling. Persistent hypotension or hemodynamic instability may necessitate invasive cardiovascular monitoring. All patients with heat stroke warrant admission to the hospital.

DROUGHT

A drought is a natural disaster that does not have the notoriety of volcanoes, earthquakes, tornadoes, hurricanes, or floods. However, a drought can be just as catastrophic when the economic, environmental, social, and medical consequences are examined. Historically, man's reaction to drought has been crisis intervention rather than risk management. The points that drought is unavoidable and that it is found at some time in every region on the earth must be emphasized. Furthermore, as the human population continues to increase, man's susceptibility to water deficits and drought increases accordingly. Therefore, governmental decision-makers must recognize the imperative need to plan for drought and to develop coordinated policies for regulating water and other natural resources. The medical profession should also be involved in this preparation in order to facilitate the health and well-being of the population served. Drought can induce famine, malnutrition, diseases, and significant morbidity and mortality. Thus, certain medical nuances are uniquely associated with drought.

Definitions

Drought may be defined as a period of abnormally dry weather that is sufficiently prolonged so that the lack of water causes a serious hydrologic imbalance in the affected area. Although it is classically envisioned as a lack of rainfall, drought may be precipitated solely by increased water utilization. Thus, drought may often be ill-defined. In fact, no single definition of drought works in all regions or under all circumstances. Drought is a normal and repetitious (almost rhythmic) feature of climate. It is a transient variation of climate and is not synonymous with aridity because aridity is confined to low rainfall regions and it generally is permanent. Ironically, very few people die of thirst or dehydration during a drought, even in Third World countries. Drought-related deaths generally occur secondary to the agricultural, economic, and medical side effects of drought, such as famine, malnutrition, poverty, poor public health practices, contamination of existing water supplies, infectious diseases, social strife, and heat-related illnesses. Drought then is not just a meteorologic or climatologic occurrence. It represents a cascade of events that illustrates how a natural climate variation can impact the environmental, economic, social, and medical qualities of a given region and a given population (18).

Consequences of Drought

Economic Effects

Throughout human history, the most feared impact of drought has been the shortage of food. As water tables drop, causing wells, rivers, and lakes to become low or even to disappear, a corresponding decline in the amount of vegetation is observed. The lack of rain causes farm crops, legumes, and rangeland grasses to wither and die, especially in farmlands that are not irrigated. Consequently, the reduction in rangeland and crop productivity increases the morbidity and mortality of livestock. The same effect is also noted in the fish and wildlife populations.

If drought strikes an agricultural region, one immediate effect is a significant increase in food prices (19). All consumers have experienced this effect at the local supermarket at one time or another. Therefore, a drought can have catastrophic effects on the regional or national economy, as well as on the individual consumer. Drought-related farm industry losses often run into the billions of dollars. The drought and heat wave that struck the eastern United States in the summer of 1999 resulted in extensive agricultural losses that were estimated to be over $1 billion. The southern drought extending from Texas and Oklahoma to the Carolinas during the summer of 1998 was responsible for between $6 billion and $9 billion in losses to the regional economies and for a loss of more than $40 billion dollars nationally (10). A similar drought occurred in Oklahoma and Texas from the fall of 1995 through the summer of 1996; it accounted for $5 billion in losses (19).

Excluding the consumer, the real economic victims of the drought are farmers and ranchers (20). Only if the government is willing and able to provide emergency low-interest loans, to pay for crop insurance, or to provide government subsidies are farmers able to survive economically during a drought. In some areas, government aid may not be enough. A sustained drought can result in repeated losses. In this situation, governments may need to reevaluate their role in disaster aid for farmers. Otherwise, the eco-

nomic result is the existence of fewer and fewer farmers and ranchers to feed the respective populations (18).

Environmental Effects

As the drought induces a decline or deterioration of local flora, the local fauna are likewise affected. Reduced water levels obviously decrease the habitat for fish and other aquatic animal life. The local wildlife is forced into human-occupied areas to search for food and water. These animals start to compete with man and livestock for edible plants and crops. Under such circumstances, the invasion of neighborhoods and even of homes by rodents, deer, and coyotes is quite common (19). Rodents are notorious for destroying stores of grain and food. The intrusiveness of these wild animals brings many diseases that may be contracted by humans, including Lyme disease, Hantavirus, plague, and typhus.

Medical Effects

The medical consequences of drought consist of an increased incidence of malnutrition and infectious diseases, many of which are zoonotic in origin. As was stated earlier, the most dreaded consequence of drought is a famine. A food shortage of this magnitude and the subsequent increase in food prices restrict the availability of food. The people who occupy the lower socioeconomic strata are not able to afford many foods. The resultant lack of nutrition for many people can ultimately lead to the classic states of marasmus (lack of caloric intake) and kwashiorkor (lack of protein intake). Collectively, the states of inanition are referred to as protein-energy malnutrition (PEM). PEM has been shown to affect the human immune system adversely by impairing T-cell function, as well as antibody production by B cells. This impaired immune system makes those who are affected more susceptible to infection and creates a higher mortality rate. Depending on the severity and the duration of malnutrition, virtually every organ system in the human body can be compromised. Conceivably, a resurgence of the nutritionally related diseases of the 17th and 18th centuries would be possible. These include endemic goiter, ariboflavinosis, scurvy, rickets, beriberi, pellagra, and PEM.

One other direct consequence of drought is the contamination of the existing water supply with waterborne pathogens. The normal circulation of natural water serves to cleans and purify it and to provide a habitat for fish and other aquatic life. As the surface water level recedes, the normal movement and flow of water are interrupted, and it becomes stationary and stagnant. Warm, brackish water is not able to clean itself of contamination, and it thus serves as an abode or medium for unusual parasites and opportunistic bacteria. Under these circumstances, an increase in the incidence of zoonotic and parasitic infections in man is observed. Primary amebic meningoencephalitis (PAM) is a life-threatening infection caused by the facultative parasitic free-living amoebae *Naegleria fowleri* (21). PAM results from inhaling contaminated water while swimming. The organisms penetrate the mucosa of the nose and travel along the olfactory nerve branches through the cribiform plate to the meninges, and they eventually ingest cerebral tissue. The signs and symptoms are similar to those of bacterial meningitis. Leptospirosis is a bacterial febrile illness acquired by contact with water that is contaminated with infected rat urine. More recently, this disease has been described as increasing among those who participate in recreational water sports. The bacteria enter the body through the mucous membranes or fresh cuts in the skin. Jaundice and renal failure with an acute febrile illness suggests the diagnosis of leptospirosis. Enterotoxigenic *Escherichia coli* (ETEC) has a worldwide distribution, and it is a major health hazard in developing countries (22). ETEC spreads by the fecal-oral route via food or water sources. It is a major cause of gastroenteritis and traveler's diarrhea.

The drought-induced migration of wildlife that are in search of food and water to areas inhabited by man can also result in the exposure of man to a number of diseases. In this situation, either the animal is the vector, or the parasites on the host animal serve as the vector for the illness. Tick-borne diseases, such as Rocky Mountain spotted fever, ehrlichiosis, tularemia, and Lyme disease, are prime examples. Flea-borne diseases include the plague and the Hantavirus pulmonary syndrome.

Social Effects

The predominate social response to a drought focuses on the decreased quality of life, the major changes in lifestyle, and an increase in conflict. Many disagreements are generated over water use, the management of water resources, and political philosophies. Sometimes, the easiest solution is to move to a nondrought area. An example of such a population migration is the flight of the Okies from the "Dust Bowl" in the 1930s to the luscious state of California. The agricultural and economic consequences of this mass exodus significantly changed the futures of both states. Strife generally is endured as litigation or armed conflict centered on the control of water and food resources. The degree of social strife may be at the international, interstate, community, or individual level. At the individual level, drought increases the incidences of homicide, domestic violence, and suicide.

Forecasting Drought

To be able to prepare adequately for the consequences of natural disasters, such as drought, the ability to predict its occurrence is extremely beneficial. Superficially, forecasting drought may appear to be based predominantly on the ability to predict temperature and precipitation. In reality, however, drought prediction is extremely difficult because the meteorologic phenomena resulting in drought are highly complex and interactive. Air–sea interactions, topography, soil moisture, the jet stream, infiltration runoff, percolation rates, and groundwater recharge rates are just a few of these variables. Despite the technologic advances in meteorology and climate, the capability to forecast drought remains in its infancy. In the United States, the National Drought Mitigation Center (NDMC) provides predictions for drought occurrence and stresses risk management rather than crisis intervention (23). The NDMC is one of several associated groups of the Climate Prediction Center that covers all major meteorologic phenomena in the United States. Climate prediction capabilities for many developing countries are inconsistent or absent.

CONCLUSIONS

Droughts are important natural disasters that have far-reaching effects on the economic, environmental, social, and medical aspects of society. All of these aspects are interrelated, and one cannot be present without involving the other three. Because of increasing population and the ever-changing climate of the world, droughts remain inevitable. To react to a drought by the philosophy of crisis intervention causes chaos, strife, suffering, disease, and death. Clearly, the proper response to a drought is through prior preparation and advanced planning. The medical community must become involved in this preparation in order to be able to address the health and medical facets of this natural disaster adequately. The central theme for such preparation is a unified governmental policy for the regulation of water and other natural resources during a drought.

A relative paucity of information exists on drought in the disaster-oriented literature. Two agencies have been particularly active in addressing the issues of drought-related disasters. The first agency is the National Drought Mitigation Center. Researchers and students of disaster medicine are referred to this organization for further information. Contact information is provided below[1]. Current projects of the NDMC include developing new drought monitoring and impact assessment methods and creating a network of drought planners. The NDMC helps organize and conduct workshops and conferences on drought. Additionally, it conducts research on the economic, environmental, and social impacts of drought. The second agency is the National Oceanic and Atmospheric Administration (NOAA). NOAA maintains an online drought information center[2] that is a

---

[1]Contact by mail at National Drought Mitigation Center, University of Nebraska-Lincoln, 239 L.W. Chase Hall, P.O. Box 830749, Lincoln, NE 68583-0749; by telephone at 402-472-6707; by fax at 402-472-6614; and by e-mail at ndmc@drought.unl.edu.

[2]The URL address for the NOAA drought information center is http://www.drought.noaa.gov/.

compilation or collection of various NOAA websites, as well as a good source of information on climate conditions and drought. In response to the private and public concern for the preparation for drought, the Interim Drought Council was established in September, 2000. This council is an attempt to integrate and coordinate the drought services between the various levels of federal government until Congress authorizes and funds a permanent council. This agency can be found at http://www.fsa.usda.gov/indc/about_us.htm.

REFERENCES

1. Centers for Disease Control. Heat related illnesses and deaths—Missouri, 1998, and United States, 1979-1996. *MMWR* 1999; 48:469–473.
2. Khagoli M. Heat-related illnesses. *Middle East J Anesthesiol* 1944; 12:531.
3. Centers for Disease Control. Heat-related mortality: United States, 1997. *MMWR* 1988;47:473.
4. Semenza JC, Rubin CH, Falter KH, et al. Heat-related deaths during the July 1995 heat wave in Chicago. *N Engl J Med* 1996;84:335.
5. Whitman S, Good G, Donoghue E, et al. Mortality in Chicago attributed to the July 1995 heat wave. *Am J Public Health* 1997; 87:1515–1518.
6. Walker JS, Barnes SB. Heat emergencies. In: Tintinalli JE, Kelen GC, Stapczynski JS, eds.*Emergency medicine: a comprehensive study guide*, 5th ed. New York: McGraw-Hill Professional Publishing, 2000:1235–1242.
7. Kilborne EM. Heat waves and hot environments. In: Noji EK, ed. *The public health consequences of disasters*. New York: Oxford University Press, 1997:245–269.
8. Jones TS, Liang AP, Kilborne EM, et al. Morbidity and mortality associated with the July 1980 heat wave in St. Louis and Kansas City, Missouri. *JAMA* 1982;247:3327–3331.
9. Shattuck GC, Hilferty MM. Causes of death from heat in Massachusetts. *N Engl J Med* 1933;209:319.
10. National Weather Service. Available at: http://weather.noaa.gov/weather/hwave.html. Accessed July 10, 2000.
11. Knochel JP. Heat stroke and related heat stress disorders. *Dis Mon* 1989;35:301–378.
12. Barnes SB, Walker JS. Summertime emergencies: how to stay cool as summer heats up. *Consultant* 1999;39:2011.
13. Tak O, Olshaker JS. Heat illness. *Emerg Med Clin North Am* 1992;10:299.
14. Buechley RW, Van Bruggen, Truppi LE. Heat island = death island? *Environ Res* 1972;5:82–92.
15. Jarling A. *Current weather—heat wave heat index*. Silver Spring, MD: National Weather Service, Office of Systems Operations, 2000.
16. Fish PD, Bennett GCJ, Millard PH. Heat wave morbidity and mortality in old age. *Age Ageing* 1985:243–245.
17. Sprung CL. Hemodynamic alterations of heat stroke in the elderly. *Chest* 1979;75:362–366.
18. Wilhite DA. *Drought mitigation technologies in the United States: with future policy recommendations*. International Drought Information Center technical report series 93-1, 1993.
19. Wilhite DA, Smith KH, Hayes MJ. The national drought mitigation center. In: *The Proceedings of Conserve '96' American Waterworks Association*, Orlando, FL, January 4–8, 1996:795–799.
20. Wilhite DA. *Planning for drought: a process for state government*. IDIC technical report series 90-1, 1990.
21. Barwick RS, Levy DA, Craun GF, et al. Surveillance for waterborne disease outbreaks–United States, 1997–1998. *MMWR CDC Surveill Summ* 2000;49:1–21.
22. Hogan DE. The emergency department approach to diarrhea. *Emerg Med Clin North Am* 1996;14:673–694.
23. Hayes MJ, Wilhite DA, Sovoboda MD, et al. Drought management crisis vs risk management. In: *The Proceedings of the 1996 International Conference and Exposition on Natural Disaster Reduction*, American Society of Civil Engineers, Washington, D.C., December 3–5, 1996:371–372.

VOLCANIC ERUPTIONS

RALPH FORD
DAVID E. HOGAN

At 8:32 AM on May 18, 1980, a magnitude 5.1 earthquake struck the northwestern United States with an epicenter below the volcano of Mount St. Helens. Seconds later, the north flank of the mountain slid away in the largest landslide ever recorded. With the weight of the north side of the mountain relieved from the volcanic cone, a lethal lateral blast of gas, steam, and rock debris spewed forth in a massive pyroclastic flow at 1,100 km per hour. Temperatures in the jet that was released from the mountain exceeded 300°C (572°F). Snow and ice instantly melted, resulting in kilometer-size flows of volcanic debris and mud through the river valleys. Within minutes, a plume of volcanic ash reached 19 km into the atmosphere, where the winds carried 540 million tons of ash over 57,000 square miles of the United States.

Between 1980 and 1990, volcanic activity in the world has killed over 26,000 people and has forced the evacuation of over 450,000 more [1]. The largest eruption on the planet in the 20th century occurred in 1912 at Novarupta Mountain in the Alaskan peninsula. Fifteen cubic kilometers of magma explosively erupted over a 60-hour period. This resulted in a volume of material that was 30 times greater than that ejected during the Mt. St. Helens eruption. Fortunately, this eruption occurred in an isolated area in Alaska, thus minimizing human effects. The United States ranks third behind Indonesia and Japan for the number of historically active volcanoes within its borders. Over 10% of the 1,500 volcanoes that have erupted in the past 10,000 years are located within the boundaries of the United States.

Volcanoes throughout the world are distributed primarily along the edges of continents, as well as along island chains and undersea mountain ranges. This ring of volcanoes correlates roughly with the intersections of the Earth's tectonic plates. Fifty percent of the known active volcanoes on Earth are along a circular region around the Pacific Ocean known as the "Ring of Fire."

GEOPHYSICAL EFFECTS

Numerous geophysical effects that occur during volcanic eruptions either individually or in combination may result in physical injuries and illnesses to exposed populations. Two major types of volcanic eruptions are observed. In the most common type, molten rock (magma) flows down the volcanic slopes covering vast expanses of land and creating a volcano type known as a shield volcano. This volcanic variety is typified by Mauna Loa volcano in Hawaii. Such volcanoes eject large volumes of relatively viscous magma that flows slowly enough to allow evacuation of the immediate area. This causes a slowly expanding area of burned property as the lava field creates new land and reclaims old. However, lava has been known to pool, forming large lakes around the volcano. Volcanic dams sequestering these molten lakes may rupture, spewing lava rapidly down the slope. One such event occurred in 1977 in Zaire (now the Democratic Republic of Congo), killing 300 people [2].

The second major type of eruption is associated with explosive force from within the chimney of a volcano variety known as a composite volcano. Eruptions of this type commonly occur in the Cascade Mountains of the American West. These volcanoes erupt less frequently than the Hawaiian-type volcanoes, but their eruptions are characterized by significantly more violence. Air shock waves from these volcanic blasts have broken windows up to 18 km away in some cases. Shrapnel-like rock projectiles may be produced in these sudden, explosive eruptions. In 1979, rocks ejected from the Mt. Etna eruption struck nine tourists [2]. Rocks up to 1 inch in diameter were blown as far as 19 km away in the Mt. St. Helens eruption, and much larger rocks were hurled as far away as 6 km. Many of these projectiles maintain high thermal energy for days following the eruption. These hot rocks may start fires over an extensive area surrounding the eruption.

Pyroclastic flows and mudslides are the most common direct cause of death associated with volcanic eruptions. Pyroclastic flows are associated with volcanoes producing viscous magma; they are extremely hot mixtures of gas, ash, pumice, and rocks. These flows may travel for great distances in excess of 100 km per hour. Pyroclastic flows have been associated with the majority of volcano-related deaths over the past 400 years, including at least 70% of the deaths from eruptions this century. In 1908, 28,000 people, nearly the entire population of St. Pierre, Martinique, were killed within minutes when a pyroclastic eruption occurred at Mt. Pele, 6 km away. The pyroclastic effect from Mt. St. Helens was estimated to contain 8 megatons of energy and 4 cubic kilometers of ash and rock, resulting in the devastation of over 200 square miles of forest. Death from pyroclastic flows can result from the blast effect itself, intense heat, or asphyxiation (3).

Mud flows, or lahars, are a deadly volcanic phenomena that contribute to the destruction from volcanic eruptions. Water from rain, crater lakes, melted snow, or steam mixes with volcanic debris to form mud flows. The mud, approximating the consistency of fluid concrete, is heavy and gravity-dependent. It may travel rapidly for many kilometers. Mud flows follow the contour of the land as they descend the volcano slopes. Victims may be overcome and buried under tons of fluid mud. These flows may also be quite hot, and they can result in fatal thermal injury even if the victim is not totally buried. Victims partially trapped in mud that dries to a concrete consistency require long and difficult extrications. These persons are at risk for crush syndrome and sudden death upon release from the mud (4). The mud may hamper rescue for many days by staying too soft to allow either foot or vehicular travel. Bridges and roadways are easily destroyed. Additionally, flooding due to water displacement in rivers, lakes, and reservoirs results in the disruption of normal routes of escape and rescue.

One of the most impressive effects of volcanic eruptions is the amount of ash ejected into the atmosphere. Ash and dust may cause substantial visibility problems for many days following an eruption. Ground accumulations of ash can make vehicular traffic nearly impossible. Even small amounts of wet or dry pumice, ash, or dust make road surfaces extremely hazardous. When combined with the low visibility, road and bridge damage, and the panic, this culminates in an increased risk for motor vehicle crash–related injuries. In addition, ground emergency medical services (EMS) transport evacuations are hampered (2).

Ash may settle on buildings at a rate of 5 tons per m² in an 8-hour period. This buildup, especially when coupled with rainfall, may lead to roof collapse. Locations, such as school gyms, churches, bowling alleys, and other public facilities that may be designated as evacuation centers, often have large, flat roof spans. Such buildings are at high risk for roof collapse secondary to ash collection. Periodic removal of the dry ash from the roofs is necessary but difficult because of the respiratory and eye irritation it causes. The dry ash becomes easily airborne with manipulation. Ash may be distributed over an extensive region, resulting in significant deterioration in air quality. The long-term health effects of such ash contamination are not clear (5).

Air filters in motor vehicles, electrical generators, and other critical machinery may quickly become clogged and inoperable. The abrasive effect of the ash can permanently destroy sensitive motors and mechanisms. In addition, rain-soaked ash acts as a conductor, and it may short out exposed electrical insulators, causing widespread power failures and scattered electrical fires.

Electrical storms often accompany volcanic eruptions. These result from particles of charged ash in the atmosphere. Electrical storms may cause fires, may damage electrical equipment, and may result in death or injury by lightning strike. In large volcanic eruptions, the storm effects are not limited to the immediate area; they can follow the cloud of ash hundreds of miles downwind (6). Communications, including EMS radio and telemetry transmission, may be significantly hampered by electrostatic discharge and lightning storms.

Volcanic eruptions may cause interruption of fresh water and sewage facilities. Mud and lava flows follow riverbeds and cause flooding, thus blocking fresh water sources and sewage outlets. Sewage may back up and overflow, mixing with and contaminating fresh water sources. Electrical outages result in water pump failure. Ash fall may overwhelm water-filtering and pool reservoir sources. In addition, water waste treatment machinery may fail due to the abrasive effect of the ash (2).

Toxic gases may be produced by volcanic eruptions. In 1979, toxic gases killed 149 people from the Dieng volcano in Java. Over 1,700 people were killed by a toxic gas eruption of the Lake Nyos volcano in Cameroon, West Africa in 1986 (7). Carbon dioxide, sulfur dioxide, hydrogen chloride, hydrogen sulfide, hydrogen fluoride, and carbon monoxide are among the more important gases emitted. Carbon dioxide and hydrogen sulfide pool in low-lying areas and represent a serious threat to individuals located within those regions. Hydrogen fluoride and hydrogen chloride become extremely corrosive when they make contact with water. Sulfur dioxide mixed with steam from the volcano or atmospheric water has resulted in acid rain with a pH as low as 2. Such acid rain may contaminate surrounding agricultural lands, resulting in long-term crop failure. In addition, wet ash can deposit toxic and corrosive chemicals into the environment. The major toxic gasses from volcanic eruption and the associated risks and therapy are depicted in Table 23.1. As a result of the acid rain mentioned above and other effects of the volcano, previously fertile lands may become unproductive for years, resulting in local famine conditions. In addition, volcanic eruptions can produce substantial effects on worldwide climates. Mt. Pinatubo ejected massive amounts of sulfate aerosols into the upper stratosphere. This resulted in a significant decrease in sunlight penetration across the affected area. Events such as this have resulted in diminished crop productivity and additional food source problems (8).

Minor earthquakes accompanying volcanic eruptions are common, but they are usually of no significance. Tidal waves or tsunamis, however, can be produced by submarine volcanic eruptions or landslides into coastal areas, killing many more people than the volcano itself. In addition, mas-

TABLE 23.1. MAJOR HAZARDOUS GASSES FROM VOLCANIC ERUPTIONS

Substance	Risk	Therapy
Carbon dioxide	10K ppm/8 hr TLV allowed 20–30K ppm: loss of consciousness, seizures CNS stimulant, vasodilation	Avoidance SCBA Oxygen supplementation Supportive therapy
Hydrogen sulfide	<10 ppm/10 min allowed >50 ppm: evacuation of area 200 ppm: respiratory irritant >1,000 ppm: lethal Cellular asphyxiant Binds to cytochrome oxidase Sulfhemoglobin produced	Avoidance SCBA Hyperbaric oxygen therapy Nitrates to produce methemoglobin if administered early
Sulfur dioxide	40 ppm produces severe symptoms Respiratory irritant Inflammation, edema, bronchospasm, and hypoxia	Avoidance SCBA Oxygen and respiratory support Beta agonists Steroids
Hydrogen chloride	Respiratory irritant Inflammation, edema, bronchospasm, and hypoxia	Avoidance SCBA Consider HCO_3 nebulizer treatment Beta agonists Steroids

Hydrogen fluoride	Topical and respiratory irritant
	Airway inflammation, edema, bronchospasm,
	   and hypoxia
		Avoidance
		Hydrofluoric acid burns treated with calcium gluconate
		   therapy
		Supportive care for airway problems

Carbon monoxide	35 ppm TLV/8 hr 100 ppm × 1 hr causes symptoms Binds to hemoglobin and cytochrome Displaces oxygen Cellular asphyxiant	Avoidance SCBA Oxygen therapy Hyperbaric oxygen

Abbreviations: CNS, central nervous system; SCBA, self-contained breathing apparatus; TLV, threshold limit value.

sive landslides have been documented with volcanic eruptions, thus adding to the list of hazards causing human death and suffering that can be associated with a volcano.

VOLCANIC RISK IN THE UNITED STATES

Alaska and the continental United States have 35 volcanoes considered likely to erupt in the future. These include a substantial number of major volcanic craters in the Cook Inlet region of Alaska where 60% of Alaska's population resides. Of greatest concern are those volcanoes that have a history of erupting every 200 to 300 years. The most hazardous volcanic mountains in the lower United States include the Cascade volcanoes of the American West—Mt. St. Helens, the Mono and Inyo craters, Lassen Peak, Mt. Shasta, Mt. Rainier, Mt. Baker, and Mt. Hood (1). The location of the cascade volcanoes is depicted in Fig. 23.1. The combined 50-mile population density surrounding these seven volcanoes exceeds 2.2 million people. Mt. Rainier is the largest volcano in the Cascade Range, and it is probably the most dangerous volcano in the United

States. Its last eruption occurred 200 years ago, resulting in a mud flow that reached all the way to Puget Sound. It is expected to erupt again within the next 100 to 200 years, but it could erupt at any time. Current hazard predictions by the United States Geological Survey place much of the dense metropolitan areas of Tacoma, Washington and suburbs at significant risk. The predicted channelized flow zones of Mt. Rainier are shown in Fig. 23.2.

PREDICTING ERUPTIONS

Monitoring the activities of volcanoes and attempting to predict eruptions in the United States is the task of the United States Geological Survey. In some settings, an eruption may be accurately predicted within a range of 24 hours, allowing warnings to be issued. The Nevada del Ruiz eruption in Mexico exemplified this as a warning was provided more than 24 hours before eruption. Unfortunately, the warning was not widely distributed and the order to evacuate was largely ignored. The eruption that followed caused massive debris slides and more than 20,000 deaths

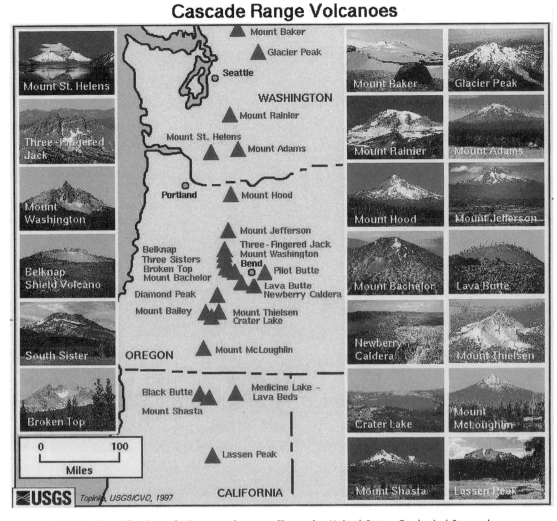

FIGURE 23.1. The Cascade Range volcanoes. (From the United States Geological Survey home page. Available at: http://vulcan.wr.usgs.gov. Accessed November 11, 1999, with permission.)

within the slide zones. Despite some recent successes, great difficulties remain in accurately predicting the time of volcanic eruptions. For the most part, geologists are only able to predict eruptions within a time frame from a few to several hundred years (1). Because monitoring of all potentially active volcanoes by geologists is impossible, communities in the vicinity of volcanic features should be aware of the local risk for eruption. All such communities should have plans for volcanic eruption integrated into their overall community disaster plan.

PREHOSPITAL CONSIDERATIONS

Municipalities and local EMS services must begin implementing their volcanic eruption disaster plans at the first sign of warning. Although explosive eruptions cause the most damage, low-lying areas and river valley regions draining the volcano are at significant risk for mud and pyro-

clastic flows for many kilometers. The only protection against these hazards is the evacuation of areas at risk.

Public health information should be provided to prehospital health care providers. When working in areas of accumulated volcanic ash, activity that would lead to significant airborne exposure should be avoided if possible; this would include dry cleanup of fallen ash. Individuals who must work in dusty conditions should wear a respiratory mask that has been recommended by the National Institute for Occupational Safety and Health. Goggles or other eye protection should also be used. Fallen ash may be wetted before cleanup to prevent it from becoming easily airborne with the remembrance that wetting the ash adds weight and provides electrical conductivity. Caution should be exercised when walking or driving on either wet or dry ash in order to avoid falls or motor vehicle collisions. Unnecessary driving should be avoided.

Indications from Mt. St. Helens show that automobiles offer little protection from volcanic hazards, with several

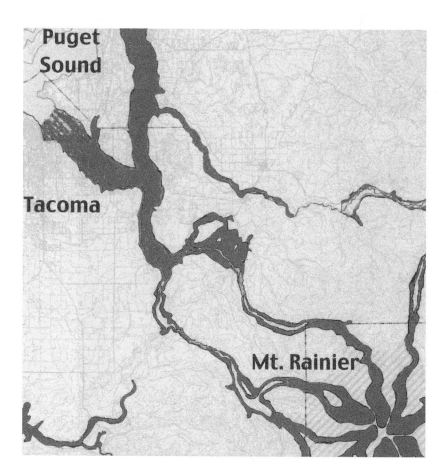

FIGURE 23.2. Volcano hazards from Mount Rainier. (From Hoblitt RP, Walder JS, Dreidger CL, et al. *Volcano hazards from Mount Rainier.* Washington, D.C.: United States Geological Survey, 1998, with permission.)

known incidents of victims having been asphyxiated from the ash while in their automobile (9). Outside air intakes in homes and offices should be covered immediately at the onset of an eruption. During the acute phase of the eruption, airtight buildings have been shown to be protective against some toxic gases as long as survivors open them to the fresh air as soon as the gas plume has passed. Air handling systems should temporarily be shut down, and filters should be regularly maintained.

Volcanic ash and electrostatic effects disrupt air medical operations. In 1989, during the eruption of the Redoubt volcano in Alaska, a commercial jet airliner encountered the ash cloud while descending into Anchorage. All four engines lost power and the aircraft dropped 4,000 m before they could be restarted. After landing, inspection found over $80 million dollars in damage due to ash abrasion (1). With factoring in the considerations of decreased visibility, ash swept up by rotor wash, and electrostatic communications blackout, air medical operations become highly hazardous.

SPECIFIC PLANNING POINTS

The overall planning process for volcanic eruption disasters generally includes the following three major points:

1. Establish a lahar monitoring, evacuation, and warning system.
2. Provide relocation plans for the population within flow and other risk zones.
3. Develop and install engineering countermeasures to redirect lahar flows, if possible, to protect the population.

Which of these planning points is the most effective or the most economical is not clear. The best approach is probably a combination of all three (10).

In addition to routine prehospital disaster planning, specific planning points should include the following:

- Relocation and support of evacuees from high-risk areas for many months;
- Emergency warning and evacuation plans for communities at risk for floods and flows along the rivers draining the volcano;
- Search and rescue plans for isolated survivors and the dead;
- Sites of emergency field morgues and appropriate staffing;
- Rehearsal with local hospital emergency plans for evacuation and the sudden influx of victims with blunt trauma, burns, and pulmonary problems from the inhalation of ash and gas;

- Education of local communities as to the actions to take when an eruption becomes imminent or after it has occurred;
- Regular practice of overall community volcano disaster plans;
- Advice and supplies for EMS personnel and other agencies who are temporarily permitted to work in restricted areas. This includes devising an alert system for emergency evacuation if an eruption is imminent and survival measures in the event workers become marooned;
- Equipment for emergency air monitoring for sulfur dioxide, hydrogen disulfide, carbon dioxide, carbon monoxide, hydrogen fluoride, and other gasses should be available although ground-level release toxic gases are rare;
- Plans for alternate communication methods if radio communication becomes impossible due to electrical storms;
- Provision for increased maintenance for EMS vehicles and equipment against the abrasive effect of ash;
- Ash-removal protocols for EMS buildings, as well as access and egress routes
- Respiratory and eye protection guidelines and equipment;
- Protocols and training for hazardous driving conditions due to volcanic debris and ash;
- Public health and safety surveillance of EMS and other workers for stress and ash exposure.

EMERGENCY DEPARTMENT CONSIDERATIONS

Mt. St. Helens eruption is currently the only major volcanic eruption in the United States for which physical injury reporting and medical impact studies have been undertaken. This eruption occurred in a relatively remote area with a low population density. As a result, the number of immediate victims requiring care was relatively low, with injuries consisting primarily of burns and inhalation injuries (3). In an eruption close to a more populated area, such as Mt. Rainier, emergency departments (EDs) should anticipate higher numbers of survivors with more diverse injuries.

Some observations have been made that are applicable to EDs functioning in and around a volcanic eruption. During the Mt. St. Helens eruption, EDs became the predominant source of medical care in smaller communities where local physician offices had been closed. In addition, a transient increase was seen in visits to emergency departments (EDs) for asthma and other respiratory ailments. The two largest hospitals near the Mt. St. Helens eruption were studied for the respiratory effects associated with the eruption. These hospitals experienced a fourfold increase in the number of asthma patients and a twofold increase in the number of bronchitis patients attended to in the ED when com-

pared to the previous year (11). Although motor vehicle crash frequency and morbidity increased, no indication of increased mortality from this mechanism was observed. No increases in eye injury problems were noted (12).

In vitro tests have suggested that ash is mildly fibrinogenic. This has been supported by *in vivo* tests with animals and by autopsy on some human victims. Ash may impair bacterial resistance by interfering with alveolar macrophage activity. Reactive airway disease in chronic obstructive pulmonary disease (COPD) may be exacerbated secondary to ash exposure. The potential for the delayed onset of ash-induced pulmonary fibrosis should be a consideration for both victims and rescue workers. Silicosis is a potential problem for outdoor workers if they are exposed to large amounts of ash in the form of crystalline silica (3). High-risk groups are individuals with prior asthma or COPD and those exposed to large amounts of ash at work.

Volcanic eruptions have been known to release significant amounts of radon gas in the volcanic plume. Typically, these radionuclides pose no threat to health or property as they are distributed over a wide area throughout the atmosphere. However, in some eruptions, ash has been found to contain substantial amounts of radon and radon-related particles. Volcanic rocks in some regions also contain sizeable amounts of active radionuclei. Incidences have been detected where such material has been used for building homes, thereby increasing the risk for radon exposure to the inhabitants. Ash fall during volcanic eruptions should be monitored on an ongoing basis for the presence of radionuclide content.

Fluoride poisoning also has occasionally been associated with ash from volcanic eruptions. Although the majority of ash particles are within the respirable range (less than 10 μm), most fluoride poisoning results from the ingestion of contaminated food and water (13). Fluoride toxicity commonly presents with symptoms similar to those of phosgene poisoning. High doses may result in a rapid loss of consciousness and the development of pulmonary edema. Most early symptoms from lower exposures present with shortness of breath; tightness in the chest; productive cough; nose and eye irritation; and, almost universally, headache, nausea, and vomiting. Fluoride levels can be measured directly in the laboratory, and they should be considered in patients presenting with such symptoms after having been exposed to volcanic ash. Gastric lavage has been indicated in large oral exposures, but it is not likely to be of benefit for patients exposed to fluoride by volcanic eruptions. Milk, oral calcium salts, and aluminum-based or magnesium-based antacids bind fluoride in the gastrointestinal tract. Some severe cases may require hemodialysis. The fluoride content of ash fall should be monitored on an ongoing basis during eruptions. Other substances, such as mercury and various hydrocarbons, have also been detected in ash fall, and their presence should be monitored; these, however, typically present no major hazard.

Infectious diseases in exposed populations are generally not a prominent feature of volcanic eruptions (14). One noted exception occurred following an eruption in Armero, Colombia in 1985. This eruption resulted in 23,000 deaths and over 4,500 injuries. Significant numbers of the seriously injured victims who were transported out of the region to Bogota were found to have necrotizing fasciitis or mucormycosis (15). The mortality rates for these cases ran as high as 80%. The exact reasons for this outbreak have never been clearly elucidated, but the austere conditions at the disaster scene were thought to be a contributing factor. Enteric illness and respiratory infections have been noted to increase significantly in underdeveloped areas following a volcanic eruption. This phenomenon is thought to be associated with a breakdown in the usual public heath measures and the contamination of water supplies (16).

The displacement of a population following volcanic eruptions may create problems associated with mass refugee care. Indications in some less-developed nations are that elderly members of the community may be left behind. Thus, special planning is needed for these individuals (17). Large refugee populations in and around a volcanic eruption zone are difficult to monitor. Mobile refugee camps may inadvertently move to lahar risk zones without the knowledge of disaster responders. Such population movements and relative volcanic risk zones can be monitored more accurately by community leaders via the use of low orbit satellites by remote sensing (18).

SUMMARY

Death and destruction from volcanic eruptions are increasingly becoming a reality. Specific criteria demarcate areas that are at risk for volcanic eruption. Phenomena related to these eruptions might cause injury and may hamper search and rescue activities in manners peculiar to the volcanic eruptions. Established methods can prevent morbidity and mortality and aid in the management of injuries that have already occurred. Evacuation teams and prehospital and ED personnel must be prepared to respond to these disasters.

Increasing population density around active and potentially active volcanoes worldwide has increased the probability of significant volcano-related disasters. Although health effects from volcanic eruptions may extend over a wide region, direct death and injury tends to occur in localized, predictable zones of destruction. Some specific health effects from these disasters do exist, but they usually have a minor impact on the local population. Preeruption evacuation plans and reasonable posteruption response plans will decrease the adverse impact of volcanic eruptions on local populations.

REFERENCES

1. United States Geological Survey home page. Available at: http://vulcan.wr.usgs.gov. Accessed November 11, 1999.
2. Baxter PJ, Bernstein RS, Falk H, et al. Medical aspects of volcanic disasters: an outline of the hazards and emergency response measures. *Disasters* 1982;6:268–276.
3. Baxter PJ. Medical effects of volcanic eruptions. *Bull Vulcanol* 1990;52:533–544.
4. Noji EK. Acute renal failure in natural disasters. *Ren Fail* 1992; 14:245–249.
5. Nania J, Bruya TE. In the wake of Mount St. Helens. *Ann Emerg Med* 1982;11:184–191.
6. Bernstein RS, Baxter PJ, Buist S. Introduction to the epidemiological aspects of explosive vulcanism. *Am J Pub Health* 1986;76: 3–9.
7. Baxter PJ, Kapila M, Mfonfu D. Lake Nyos disaster, Cameroon, 1986: the medical effects of large scale emission of carbon dioxide. *BMJ* 1986;298:1437–1441.
8. McCormick MP, Thomason LW, Trepte CR. Atmospheric effects of the Mt. Pinatubo eruption. *Nature* 1995;373:399–404.
9. Baxter PJ, Bernstein RS, Buist S. Preventative health measures in volcanic eruptions. *Am J Prevent Health* 1986;76:84–90.
10. Tayag JC, Punongbayan RS. Volcanic disaster management in the Philippines: experience from Mt. Pinatubo. *Disasters* 1994; 18:1–15
11. Bernstein RS, Baxter PJ, Falk H, et al. Immediate public health concerns and actions in volcanic eruptions. *Am J Pub Health* 1986;76:25–37.
12. Fraunfelder FT, Kalina RE, Buist AS, et al. Ocular effects following the volcanic eruptions of Mount St. Helens. *Arch Ophthamol* 1983;101:376–378.
13. Baxter PJ. Volcanoes. In: Noji EK, ed. *The public health consequences of disasters.* London: Oxford University Press, 1997: 179–203.
14. Toole MJ. Communicable diseases and disease control. In: Noji ER, ed. *The public health consequences of disasters.* New York: Oxford University Press, 1977:79–100.
15. Patino JR, Castro D, Valencia A, et al. Necrotizing soft tissue lesions after a volcanic cataclysm. *World J Surg* 1991;15: 240–247.
16. Malilay J, Real MG, Ramirez-Vanegas A, et al. Public health surveillance after a volcanic eruption: lessons from Cerro Negro, Nicaragua, 1992. *Bull Pan Am Health Organ* 1996;30: 218–226.
17. Cooper R, Tuitt J. Montserrat. Managing health care in a volcanic crisis. *West Indian Med J* 1998;47:20–21.
18. Oppenheimer C. Satellite observations of Lava Lake activity at Nyiragongo volcano, ex-Zaire, during the Rwandan refugee crisis. *Disasters* 1998;22:268–281.

TSUNAMIS

DAVID L. MCCARTY

The giant Inugpasugssuk waded into the ocean to hunt seals. His penis stuck up out of the water so far away that he thought it was a seal putting its head up, and he struck it by mistake. He fell backwards in pain, and that raised a wave that flooded the whole district of Arviligjuaq.

— Netsilik Eskimo myth (1)

Tsunamis, which are commonly but incorrectly called tidal waves, have inspired superstitious awe and fear among coastal peoples for many centuries. Although today man has a more scientific understanding of the phenomenon, tsunamis remain an awesome and deadly natural disaster. Since 1945, more people have been killed by tsunamis than by direct effects of earthquakes. With coastal populations that are continuing to increase, especially in the tsunami-prone Pacific region, more tsunami disasters are inevitable. Minimizing the toll of injuries and deaths requires (a) the assessment of potential tsunami hazards, (b) public education and awareness, (c) effective and timely warnings, and (d) prompt and complete evacuation of threatened areas. Protective measures such as seawalls and reinforced construction are of limited benefit. No manmade structure can be relied upon to resist the incredible power of a large tsunami. Medical care after the disaster has little influence on mortality. The vast majority of tsunami-related deaths occur immediately. Emergency care providers in tsunami-prone areas should be familiar with this phenomenon and should especially recognize the need for advance tsunami hazard assessment, early warning, and appropriate response for their communities.

THE PHYSICS OF TSUNAMIS

A tsunami is a series of waves generated by an undersea disturbance. About 90% to 95% are caused by earthquakes; the remainder are primarily due to volcanic eruptions or landslides (2). Events such as oceanic meteorite or comet impacts may produce tsunamis rarely. Tidal forces, however, never cause tsunamis, so the term "tidal wave" should be avoided. Tsunami waves are remarkable for their destructiveness, speed of propagation, and especially their ability to cross thousands of miles of ocean with little or no diminution of their power, thus causing destruction in areas far distant from the original disturbance. Because of great size and depth and the large amount of earthquake and volcanic activity within the "Ring of Fire" in the Pacific Ocean, the vast majority (90%–95%) of tsunamis occur there.

The height of a tsunami wave arriving at a specific shore may be estimated. In order to understand this physical process, some terms must be defined. The *amplitude* of the wave is the approximate height of the wave generated above sea level while in deep water. The *run-up height* is the vertical height of the wave at its farthest point inland following its run up the shore. The *run-up factor* is the run-up height divided by the deep water wave amplitude. This relationship is depicted in Fig. 24.1. Typical run-up factors are 2 to 3 (expressed in meters); however, the average run-up factor for earthquake-generated tsunamis in Japan is 10. Run-up values up to 40 have been observed in Hawaii (3). In some locations, tsunamis do not break on the shore but instead surge onto the land as a massive high tide–like flood covering large expanses of low-lying areas (4,5).

Historic evidence for massive tsunamis exists in many locations of the world. For example, research indicates that the coast of New South Wales in Australia has suffered the impact of six massive tsunamis over the last 6,000 years (6). If such an event with a 10-meter wave would occur in the same location now, the estimated death toll would be 35,000 lives (7). The tsunami phenomenon is divided into the following three phases: (a) generation, (b) propagation, and (c) inundation. The generation phase is the production of the tsunami waves; the propagation phase is the spread of the tsunami away from the disturbance; and the inundation phase is the interaction of the tsunami with the affected coastal areas, resulting in flooding.

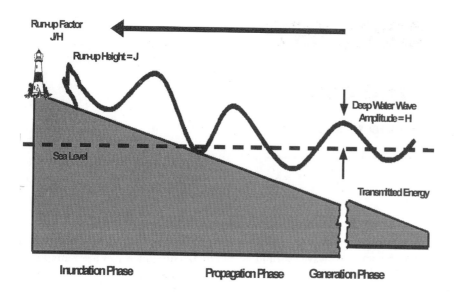

FIGURE 24.1. The physics of a tsunami. (Adapted from Crawford DA, Mader CL. Modeling asteroid impact and tsunami. *Sci Tsunami Haz* 1998;16, with permission.)

Generation Phase

To produce a tsunami, an event occurs that produces a large vertical displacement of the ocean floor. The displaced volume of water represents a large potential energy, which is then transformed to kinetic energy in the form of a series of extremely low-frequency, long wavelength waves called tsunamis. Large earthquakes (usually those of Richter magnitude 6.5 or greater) are the usual cause (5). However, the type of earthquake is as important as its strength in determining whether a tsunami occurs. Generally, tsunami production requires an earthquake occurring at a subduction zone—a fault in which one tectonic plate overrides another. Movement along this type of fault produces vertical displacement. Earthquakes along strike-slip faults (e.g., the San Andreas) produce mainly horizontal motion, and thus they seldom produce tsunamis. For instance, the great San Francisco quake of 1906 failed to generate a tsunami despite an estimated 8.3 magnitude (2). Additionally, the focal depth of the quake must be relatively shallow (<50 km), or its energy may not be transmitted to overlying water effectively enough to cause a tsunami (3). Given these facts, determining whether a tsunami will be generated is not a simple matter, particularly in the first few moments after an earthquake.

Volcanic eruptions produce tsunamis by several mechanisms, including earth tremors, underwater explosions, and large landslides. Landslides, underwater explosions, and meteorite impacts transfer energy directly to the ocean water. Generally, distant tsunamis (i.e., those that can traverse an entire ocean) are produced by earthquakes.

Propagation Phase

Once the tsunami has been generated, waves spread out from the area of disturbance like ripples do from a rock thrown into a pond in a process that is called propagation.

This analogy, however, is misleading—pond ripples (and ordinary ocean waves) are surface waves, while in tsunamis the entire depth of the ocean overlying the disturbance is affected—this represents a tremendous amount of potential energy when the huge volume is considered. Ordinary waves, even huge hurricane-generated waves with crests rivaling those of tsunamis, involve only a small volume of water near the surface and contain relatively trivial amounts of energy by comparison. Therefore, an extremely large volume of water carrying a prodigious amount of energy is disturbed.

Tsunami waves have extremely long wavelength—up to 300 km in the open ocean. By comparison, an ordinary ocean wave is 100 to 200 m in wavelength. This long wavelength and the related long period of time between wavecrests have two important consequences. First, the wavelength greatly exceeds even the deepest part of the ocean; tsunamis act as "shallow-water waves" in which the speed of propagation varies directly with depth. This means that tsunamis can travel extremely fast in deep water—typically 450 to 600 km per hour, which approaches jetliner speeds (8). Because the energy is spread through such a large volume in deep water, a killer tsunami may be only 2 feet high in midocean, making them hard to detect. For instance, a tsunami struck Sanriko, Japan, in 1896, killing 27,000 people. Fisherman from that port who were at sea did not notice the tsunami (which would have been only inches high at their location), and they were stunned to find their home port devastated and many loved ones dead when they returned (3). The second major consequence is that little energy is lost in propagation because energy dissipation is inversely proportional to wavelength. For example, a 1960 tsunami generated in Chile traveled all the way across the Pacific, killing 185 people in Japan 22 hours later (4). Such transoceanic tsunamis fortunately are uncommon, but they do occur about once a decade.

Inundation Phase

This last phase, called the inundation phase, is perhaps the least well understood of the phases. As the wave train begins to encounter shallow water, the wave grows in height and kinetic energy. Because the speed of the wave depends on the depth of the water, the front portion slows while the rear portion piles up against it. Thus, the kinetic energy previously spread through the large volume of deep ocean water is now concentrated in a much smaller quantity of water, resulting in a towering wave of immense destructive potential. Unfortunately, even though the wave is slowed by the shallow water, the wave still moves much faster than humans can run, so the first sighting of a tsunami may already be too late. Usually, the generation phase results in a series of waves that are spread anywhere from 5 to 90 minutes apart (usually 10 to 45 minutes). Predicting whether succeeding waves will be smaller or larger is difficult. Thus, further damage can be inflicted after the first wave strikes. Aftershocks or further landslides may generate additional tsunami trains as well, although typically these are smaller.

The wave is also affected by refraction, a wave phenomenon, around obstacles such as headlands and irregularities of the shallow coastal bottom. This can serve to focus the wave around obstacles. For instance, the tsunami often wraps around a protruding headland, thus concentrating the force on this area. In fact, many areas that are safe from a storm wave may be associated with areas of the shoreline that may produce an even larger tsunami. As this is characteristic of many harbors, the Japanese word *tsunami* means "harbor wave." The end result of these physical interactions is that the tsunami may rush ashore as a breaking wave, a wall of water, or a tidelike flood.

A tsunami can be up to 100 m high, but it is usually from 3 to 15 m high. A 70-m wave was recorded following the great Alaska earthquake in 1964, but waves of only 2 to 3 m are sufficient to cause damage or deaths (9). Barring obstruction, the wave may propagate inland many hundreds of meters, producing a large area of devastation; disrupting utilities, communications and transportation; and complicating search and rescue efforts. It may also disrupt medical care in the immediate area. The physical propagation of an earthquake-generated tsunami is depicted in Fig. 24.1.

TSUNAMI EFFECTS

General Effects

Due to the tremendous amount of mass and energy contained in a tsunami, damages to structures and the affected areas is universal. Multistory, concrete-reinforced structures such as well-built hotels may provide some protection if evacuation is impossible, but they cannot be relied on to resist larger waves. Sea walls may mitigate the effect of smaller waves, but they do little to stop the large tsunamis. Many buildings and all vehicles are likely to be obliterated, and debris of all sorts is propelled along with this wave. Many utilities, such as water, sewage, power lines, and gas lines, may be damaged, leading to subsequent hazards of electrical fires, gas explosions, and septic contamination of water supplies. Surviving dwellings and vehicles may sustain damage from mud and salt water. In short, the devastation is near total.

Mechanisms of Injury

In a large tsunami, deaths frequently exceed the number of injured. Average death rates are believed to be 50% for the population caught by a tsunami, but rates up to 80% have been reported (7). For example, in the 1998 Papua New Guinea tsunami, the death toll was conservatively estimated at 2,200, with approximately 700 injured persons received formal medical care (10). Of course, most deaths result from drowning. Those who are not strong enough to withstand the physical rigor of saving themselves from the tsunami, such as young children, the elderly, and physically infirm, are disproportionately affected. However, the tsunami does not just consist of water; it also contains a great amount of debris, and it is capable of inducing injuries from blunt trauma, as well as abrasions and impalements. One of the initially puzzling features of the Papua New Guinea wave involved bright lights that survivors saw on the crest of the wave, and these were subsequently connected with subsequent burn-type injuries on the survivors. However, these lights were actually due to phosphorescent algae that was activated by the wave; the burns were actually abrasions from being scraped over the sands of the area (10). Many other victims were flung against trees, impaled on bamboo limbs, and so on. Clearly then, a wide spectrum of injury may be encountered. Many of these are more serious injuries, such as those to the head, spine, thorax, and abdomen, making survival virtually impossible when given the force of the tsunami and the likely delays in subsequent rescues. In Papua New Guinea, no survivor with any of these injuries was found (10). Other survivable injuries include near drowning and aspiration pneumonia. Orthopedic and soft-tissue injuries are the most common conditions among survivors (11). Orthopedic injuries include both open and closed fractures, as well as sprains and strains. Wounds are often contaminated with debris and foreign bodies.

Survivors, when located, are likely to suffer from dehydration, hypothermia, and sunburn. Aspiration pneumonia is common. In areas with active wildlife, bites and exposures to wild animals are quite possible. Finally, secondary fires and explosions from disrupted utility lines can occur. Infectious disease from contaminated drinking water and disrupted sewage facilities may arise. The common injuries associated with tsunamis are presented in Table 24.1.

TABLE 24.1. PRIMARY INJURIES ASSOCIATED WITH TSUNAMIS

Tsunami injuries
Drowning (accounts for a significant number of the dead)
Near drowning (in severely injured survivors)
Aspiration pneumonia (complicates multiple trauma cases)
Blunt trauma (significant head, thoracic, spinal cord, or abdominal injury usually precludes survival)
Orthopedic injuries (often multiple fractures of long bones)
Soft tissue injuries (often complex and contaminated)
Toxic exposures (due to fires and clean up activities)
Hypothermia (exposure to water and the elements)
Heat injuries, sunburn, and dehydration
Wildlife exposure (bites and stings)
Infectious diseases (upper respiratory and waterborne, if endemic)
Fires (due to ruptured gas mains and electrical lines)
Explosions (due to ruptured gas mains and fuel storage areas)

MEDICAL CARE AFTER TSUNAMI DISASTERS

Tsunami disasters produce extensive effects. Due to the relatively short warning times and the lack of protective structures, fatalities are high in relation to injuries. Because of the difficulty of timely rescue and the physical effort required to survive the wall of water and debris, the more seriously injured are unlikely to survive even in developed areas. Following the impact phase, the medical care provided depends somewhat on the type of area affected; for instance, urban and developed areas, Third World areas, or rural isolated areas will have varying degrees of devastation and resources available. As with many disasters of significant destructive power, the medical infrastructure of the community impacted by the tsunami may be destroyed, leaving no source of even routine medical care for the victims.

Prehospital Considerations

Search and rescue efforts are complicated by the widespread devastation and the disruption of transportation, as well as by secondary hazards, such as severed utility lines. Aeromedical evacuation may help to save salvageable patients with time-dependent conditions and may also allow leap-frogging of severely affected areas (i.e., overfly nearer, but overburdened, hospitals to distribute serious casualties more efficiently). Therefore, helicopter landing zones should be set up and maintained in safe areas as close in proximity to casualty collection zones as possible. Secondary hazards, such as debris power lines, or additional tsunamis or weather-related phenomena, should be minimized to help with aeromedical evacuation. Search and res-

cue and emergency medical services (EMS) personnel are likely to experience frustration and a loss of morale from the feelings of futility that attend the high fatality-to-survivor ratio, especially as many of the victims are likely to be young children. Search and rescue administrators and EMS personnel should anticipate this and should attempt to incorporate appropriate personnel support into their planning.

Prehospital care should concentrate on ensuring adequate oxygenation as near drowning and aspiration are common and the splinting of injured extremities. If possible, intravenous (IV) fluids for correcting dehydration should be administered, and preventing further wound contamination should be attempted. In addition, the provision of psychologic support should be considered. Many victims are stunned by the overpowering aspects of this awesome phenomenon and the sudden devastation and loss of their loved ones.

Emergency Department Considerations

Emergency department and hospital care will most likely involve wound care and orthopedic procedures. Aspiration pneumonia and secondary effects such as dehydration should be anticipated. Psychologic support should be continued. More serious internal injuries are unlikely to be seen unless the search and rescue and EMS transport is rapid and the casualty load is not overwhelming. In large disasters, the salvage of such cases is unlikely. This is true because, to survive a tsunami, one must first avoid drowning and then must secondarily survive until rescue arrives. Thus, the more seriously injured, especially those with head and spinal cord injuries, do not live long enough to be transported to emergency departments (8).

Late sequelae that can anticipated are systemic and wound infections, pulmonary infections, and enteric infections, such as hepatitis and bacterial dysentery. Burns and carbon monoxide inhalation may be seen along with animal bites and stings. Injuries such as crush syndrome, which is often seen with earthquakes after a tsunami, are unlikely unless the earthquake generating the wave was local.

TSUNAMI PLANNING POINTS

A tsunami is an extremely powerful natural phenomenon that cannot be prevented or modified by any method that is known at this time. Engineering (e.g., breakwaters, seawalls, reinforced construction, and pine tree belts) can provide minimum protection, but no technology can reliably protect a human from a tsunami. Therefore, early warning and evacuation are of primary importance in preventing death and injury. However, early warnings are useless if the public fails to heed them or if they do not know the proper response. In 1994, a survey of National Oceanic and Atmospheric Administration (NOAA) warnings of a tsunami was conducted by the Federal Emergency Management Agency (FEMA). The results showed that, of 14 communities in the warned area, the warning was unheeded in 30% and that it was not timely in 71% (3). Therefore, considerable improvement is needed. The 1960 tsunami in Hilo, Hawaii, following an earthquake in Alaska serves as another example. Several previous warnings had been false alarms, with tsunamis of only 6 inches arriving. Therefore, the population failed to respond in an appropriate manner to this warning, and 59 fatalities occurred (3). Public education in this area is critical. Giving a proper and timely warning is not sufficient if the public is not adequately educated as to the hazards and the appropriate protective response. Disaster physicians in tsunami-prone areas can play an important role in this education process.

Given the importance of warning, knowing how such warnings are generated can be helpful. The current warning system in the Pacific is primarily triggered by seismic alerts. Any earthquake with a magnitude greater than 7 results in a tsunami watch. If this is confirmed by a tidal gauge, then a tsunami warning is distributed to areas likely to be affected by the wave. This is generally adequate for distant tsunamis, which are the biggest threat to the United States. In fact, only one person has been killed by a tsunami in the Continental United States since 1945. This is thought to be due to the adequate warnings that have been provided (3).

Local tsunamis (i.e., those that occur in the immediate vicinity of the tsunami-producing event) provide much less warning and thus may not allow an adequate evacuation time. In Papua New Guinea, an earthquake was felt, but this was not understood by the local population to be a risk factor for tsunami. Some have though that, even if a warning had been given, the population may not have had time to evacuate (10). In Nicaragua in the most recent earthquake, the earthquake waves did not reach the shore; the residents, therefore, had no warning. Local tsunamis will continue to be a significant hazard in some areas, and these are best coped with by community planning and education. Residents should be taught to move to higher ground if an earthquake is felt. Clearly planned evacuation routes and safe areas that are well marked should be available. Aggressive public education campaigns should be undertaken to make the community aware of the risks, the procedures, and the evacuation routes that must be taken even if an alarm is not sounded. In Hawaii, this information is included in the local telephone books.

Hazard signs should be posted in tsunami-prone areas. A tsunami preparedness program has been formulated for Eureka and Crescent City, California by FEMA and NOAA (3). It involved a detailed inspection of the area and the preparation of inundation maps. These areas were then clearly marked with signs. This plan should serve as a model for tsunami-prone communities.

One serious problem continues to be the occurrence of false tsunami alarms. The prediction of exactly where, when, and with how much force a specific tsunami will strike is not as exact as could be desired. As a result, alarms are sometimes given for tsunami events that are less than dramatic. That people will learn to disregard the alarms if they are usually false is a fact of human nature. The complex physical interactions occurring among the tsunami-generating event, the sea, and the shoreline make exact predictions impossible. Currently deployed technology can measure only the magnitude of the earthquake, which is an indirect measure of the amount of force imparted to the ocean water. New sensors that are under development may have the ability to be deployed at the sea bottom to detect very small amounts of water movement. In addition, other sensors under development combine spaceborne radar with global positioning satellites (a GPS system) to achieve a sensitivity with the capability to detect small movements in the sea level and sea floor. These require further research and funding, and disaster physicians can play a role by supporting development of such sensors. Once these sensors are deployed, the percentage of false alarms should drop considerably. The short warning time with the local tsunami will, however, continue to be a problem. Public education will continue to be important in this area.

SUMMARY

Tsunamis are short-term, but devastating, events that occur primarily in the Pacific. They can propagate across thousands of miles of ocean, or they may occur from a local disturbance. Tsunamis are unpredictable in size, but the larger ones are devastating, producing significant fatality rates. Early warning and evacuation are key to reducing the number of fatalities. False alarms are currently a problem, but better technology and improved understanding of the physical nature of these waves will be available in the future. The disaster emergency care provider should be aware of the characteristics of the tsunami-related disaster and should actively participate in planning for such disasters. Communities at risk for tsunamis must provide adequate public education as part of their overall disaster planning. In addition, evacuation routes and safe zones should be clearly researched and marked for public use during tsunami warnings.

REFERENCES

1. Norman H. *Northern tales, traditional stories of Eskimo and Indian peoples.* New York: Pantheon Books, 1990:233.
2. Bolt BA. *Earthquakes: a primer.* San Francisco: WH Freeman, 1978.

3. National Oceanic and Atmospheric Administration. *Tsunami, the great waves*. Washington, D.C.: National Oceanic and Atmospheric Administration, 1994.

4. Souza DM. *Powerful waves*. Minneapolis: Carolrhoda Books, 1992.

5. Steinbrugge KV. *Earthquakes, volcanoes and tsunamis*. New York: Skandia American Group, 1982.

6. Young RW, Bryant EA, Price DM. The imprint of tsunami in quaternary costal sediments of Southeastern Australia. *Bulg Geophys J* 1995;21:24–32.

7. Crawford DA, Mader CL. Modeling asteroid impact and tsunami. *Sci Tsunami Haz* 1998;16.

8. Reed SB. Natural and human-made hazards: mitigation and management issues. In: Auerbach PS, ed. *Wilderness medicine: management of wilderness and environmental emergencies*, 3rd ed. St. Louis: Mosby-Year Book, 1995:580–615.

9. Alaska Division of Emergency Services. *Tsunami! The great waves in Alaska*. Anchorage, AK: Alaska Division of Emergency Services, 1992.

10. Taylor PR, Emonson DL, Schlimmer JE. Operation Shaddock—the Australian Defense Force response to the tsunami disaster in Papua New Guinea. *Med J Aust* 1998;169:602–606.

11. Holian AC, Keith PP. Orthopaedic surgery after Aitape tsunami. *Med J Aust* 1998;169:606–609.

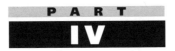

PART

IV

INDUSTRIAL, TECHNOLOGIC, AND TRANSPORTATION DISASTERS

MEDICAL MANAGEMENT OF RADIATION ACCIDENTS

FUN H. FONG, JR.

Radiation accident responses share a great deal of commonality with those of hazardous materials (HazMat) responses. Indeed, the first HazMat response documents were originally derived from modified radiation response documents. Since then, HazMat response has evolved separately so that HazMat doctrine now may seemingly conflict with radiation response doctrine at times. While HazMat response has undergone a period of increased awareness and renaissance, a true consensus has yet to emerge for HazMat response principles, especially within the hospital setting. Radiation does not pose the same potential degree of hazard that some hazardous materials pose for both the victim and personnel; hence, providers for radiation accident casualties have the opportunity to ensure that their patients are medically stable before the definitive radiation accident measures of decontamination and other radiation-related therapy are undertaken. Additionally, radiation is eminently detectable and is much more easily traceable than hazardous chemicals or biologic agents.

The radiation accident victim may be approached, as in a trauma response, with universal precautions. The standard emergency protocols of advanced cardiac life support (ACLS), advanced pediatric life support (APLS), and advanced trauma life support (ATLS) *always* take precedence over radiation issues. Medical stability should be assured before concentrating on the radiation issues. The clinician should determine whether the possible mode of exposure presents a contamination hazard and whether the patient is likely to be locally or systemically affected. If the patient is contaminated, the clinician collects samples from the orifices and the contaminated areas, documenting in much the same manner as in an assault examination. The patient can be definitively decontaminated either inside or outside the emergency department. If the patient is thought to have experienced significant systemic irradiation, conventional disease, or trauma, the patient should be admitted; otherwise, the patient should be referred for follow-up and counseling on the impact of his or her exposure.

In radiation accident history, overexposures on the order of radiation absorbed dose have occurred for site responders and first responders on rare occasions. Hospital personnel rarely accumulate any occupationally significant exposure in the case of caring for a radiation accident victim. However, in radiation accident history, stories are rife with accounts of patients who are turned away or whose care is delayed for fears of contamination.

An earnest effort in preplanning by reviewing radiation response plans will uncover needed revisions in a hospital's radiation accident response plan before such plans can become an embarrassment.

BASIC RADIATION PHYSICS AND RADIOBIOLOGY

Radiation is the transfer of energy through space. Ionizing radiation may be one of many different types of charged or uncharged particles or photons or a mixture of both that can cause ionization to occur (1). The amount of ionizing radiation energy necessary to create a uniform whole-body median lethal dose (LD_{50}) in a human is approximately equal to the thermal energy found in a cup of hot coffee.

Beta particles are high energy electrons emitted from unstable nuclei; they are only able to penetrate a few centimeters of tissue. *X-rays* and *gamma* rays are high energy photons that pass readily into and through tissue; these can be greatly attenuated by thicknesses of lead. Beta, gamma, and x-ray radiations are designated as low linear-energy transfer (low=LET) radiation, and they have approximately equivalent biologic effects per unit of radiation.

Alpha particles are helium nuclei stripped of their electrons. They are heavy particles that have no penetrating power past the keratinized layer of the skin but that may be of medical significance when these particles have been internalized. *Neutron* emission is regarded as highly potent radiation that penetrates deeply, creating denser ionization trails. Few neutron sources exist outside of reactors, nuclear devices, and industrial moisture density gauges. Alpha and neutron emissions are designated high linear-energy transfer (high=LET) radiation. High=LET radiation has the potential for significantly greater biologic effects— by a factor of two to twenty—than does low=LET radiation. The radiation penetration guide given in Fig. 25.1 demonstrates this.

The subject of ionizing radiation has the most relevance when the process of ionization occurs within living tissue. This process causes breaks in chemical bonds that may or may not make a difference in the function of the cell. Cellular repair occurs, and most repairs are successful. The most vulnerable target in the cell is the nuclear deoxyribonucleic acid (DNA). Damaged DNA may cause (a) an impairment of the cellular process of mitosis as either delay or inhibition or (b) genetic mutation, which may cause an alteration in the gene's expression or in cell lines.

Ionizing radiation may cause two discrete effects. The first is *stochastic effects*, or all-or-nothing effects, the severity of which does not vary with dose; however, the probability of occurrence does vary with the dose (2). Examples of stochastic effects are an increased risk for the development of malignancy over an individual's lifetime and inheritable genetic mutations. The second is *deterministic effects*, which have a clinical threshold, so that exposures above the threshold will induce effects in a number of individuals. With these, the severity of the effect increases with the dose (3). Examples of deterministic effects are hematopoietic depression, organ or tissue fibrosis, cataract induction, and the impairment of fertility. A representative dose-response curve for stochastic and deterministic effects is available in Fig. 25.2 (4).

Ionizing radiation is measured either in the English unit, the radiation absorbed dose (rad), or the international sci-

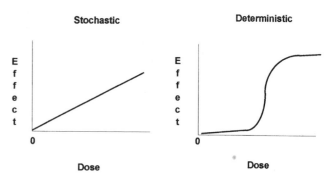

FIG. 25.2. Diagram characterizing the stochastic and deterministic effects of ionizing radiation

entific (SI) unit, the Gray (Gy), in which 100 rads equals 1 Gy. Occasionally, rads may be expressed in terms of centigray (cGy) and, in radiation oncology circles, in terms of measuring units. Differences in the biologic effects are taken into account in the common unit, the roentgen equivalent in man (rem), or the SI unit, the sievert (Sv), where 100 rem equals 1 Sv. In radiations such as alpha or neutrons, ionization may be up to 20 times more effective than the corresponding gamma radiation. In this chapter, SI units will be used and will be followed by the corresponding common unit in parentheses. Table 25.1 shows common representative radiation exposures and places radiation overexposures in perspective.

Organisms are subject to the following three main mechanisms of radiation exposure (Fig. 25.3): (a) irradiation, (b) external contamination, and (c) internal contamination (5). Organisms may be affected by any combination of these mechanisms.

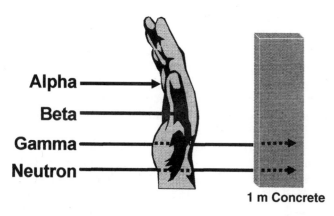

FIG. 25.1. Radiation penetration guide

TABLE 25.1. REPRESENTATIVE RADIATION EXPOSURES

Exposure type	Exposure level	SI units/ Common Units
Sleeping next to someone	0.00005 Gy/yr	5 mRem/yr
Transcontinental flight	0.00005 Gy/flight	5 mRem/flight
Chest radiograph	0.00012 Gy/film	12 mRem/film
Background radiation	0.0025–0.0040 Gy/yr	250–400 mRem/yr
CT head (nonspiral scanner)	0.01 Gy to head	1 rad to head
CT abdomen (nonspiral scanner)	0.02–0.05 Gy to abdomen	2–5 rad to abdomen
Bone scan	0.05 Gy whole body	5 rad whole body
Radiation treatment	2.5–3.0 Gy locally	250–300 rad locally

Abbreviation: CT, computed tomography; Gy, Gray; mRem, millirem.

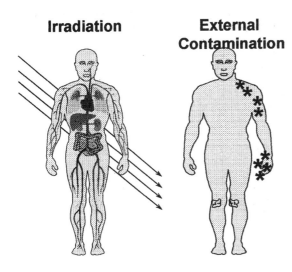

Irradiation   **External Contamination**   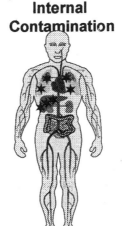   **Internal Contamination**

FIG. 25.3. Three main modes of radiation exposure

TYPICAL SCENARIOS

Events that are immediately recognized as a potential radiation accident usually involve a single individual or smaller numbers of individuals. Radiation accidents that are recognized in a delayed fashion have the potential to involve larger numbers of individuals who are contaminated or exposed. Table 25.2 shows the different origins from which radiation accidents may arise.

DETAILS RELEVANT IN HISTORY-TAKING

Circumstances of Exposure

The mechanism of possible exposure needs to be understood in order to determine whether an exposure took place and if it involved either irradiation, internal contamination, external contamination, or some combination of these. Understanding the circumstances of a victim's exposure is important because the radionuclide involved, the mechanism, and the geometry of exposure may determine the ultimate survivability of a high-dose radiation accident exposure.

TABLE 25.2. TYPICAL RADIATION ACCIDENT SCENARIOS

Radiography
Medicine (nuclear medicine/radiology/radiation oncology)
Radionuclide production-manufacturing (occupational)
Reactors
Research
Military (broken arrows, bent spears)
Transportation
Public domain (including terrorism scenarios)

Corroborating and/or Confirmatory Evidence of Exposure

Radiation exposure allegations occur episodically. The clinician may not be able to confirm true radiation overexposure from a clinical workup because lesser radiation overexposures may have no clinically detectable effects. One investigates an allegation of exposure by verifying the presence of a radioactive source or by obtaining corroborating history (from a coworker or supervisor). If radiation is involved, one should assess the potential for contamination. It may be necessary to request the state radiologic health department or an equivalent agency to send a radiation survey team for field measurements. Most state agencies should be able to field such a team either emergently or urgently (within 24 hours), depending on the situation. If institutional resistance is encountered, issuing a notice to go public to the news media may be effective and necessary if done politely but firmly. This warning usually undermines any resistance to surveillance that the clinician may encounter. In radiation accident history, radiation overexposures also have occurred from contaminated scrap metal or lost sources that unexpectedly appeared in the public domain. Therefore, taking allegations of radiation exposure seriously is important, unless the patient is obviously delusional or some other contradictory history uncovered.

Once true radiation exposure has been verified, one must determine the radionuclide(s) involved, the amounts, and the chemical and physical forms involved. The author has seen some cases in which the radionuclide was listed as a highly insoluble form but was found later either to be a more soluble form or to contain some other unexpected radionuclides. Cases such as these reinforce the point that confirmatory health physics tests for radionuclides should be performed in an emergent fashion to ensure that the specific radionuclides involved and their solubilities are known early.

Form of the Radionuclide

The physical and chemical form of the radionuclide will determine the potential for contamination and whether other chemical hazards might be involved. Radionuclides are frequently dissolved in acids, thus presenting a potential mixed hazard. When they are mixed with acids, radionuclides usually are considered highly soluble. Uranium occasionally presents as uranium hexafluoride (UF_6) as an intermediate step in uranium enrichment. If UF_6 is released into the air, it reacts with moisture to form UO_2F_2 and hydrofluoric acid (HF) (6), an exothermic reaction that has the potential to create thermal burns. The high-fired oxide of plutonium, a common component of transuranic (TRU) waste renowned for its insolubility, should not be as significantly bioavailable. Americium oxide found in common household fire detectors is also highly insoluble, and thus it may not present a significant hazard if swallowed whole (although this is not recommended).

Immediate or Delayed Recognition of the Accident

One might need to classify radiation accidents as an "immediate recognition" accident or as a "delayed recognition" accident. This fact is important for the following two reasons: (a) delayed recognition accidents have the potential for greater numbers of persons to be involved in the accident, either through exposures or contamination; and, (b) in the case of serious systemic exposure, the prodromal phase and the latent phase may be altogether missed in the course of the patient(s)' presentation, leaving the clinician less time and less clinical data for anticipating the complications and prognosis.

Prodrome Onset

The time to onset of the prodromal symptoms is one of the most useful pieces of clinical information. The onset of prodromal symptoms corresponds to the severity of systemic illness. The more rapid the onset of prodromal symptoms is, the shorter the latent period and the more severe the period of manifest illness is in the setting of systemic irradiation. The modified Union of Soviet Socialist Republics (USSR) Chernobyl triage table (see Table 32.3) graphically demonstrates the correlation of prodrome onset and exposure severity. The knowledge of the onset of prodrome may be useful in making triage decisions in the prehospital environment, as well as in the hospital environment.

Geometry of Exposure

Partial or Total Body

Geometry is a very significant factor in the course of radiation exposure. Uniform whole-body exposure is the most potent geometry of exposure. Partial-body exposures have less potential for lethality than do total-body exposures. Partial-body exposure, by definition, spares some portion of stem cells that are not affected by radiation, thus allowing potential stem cell regeneration and proliferation, particularly in the hematopoietic system. Even when total-body exposure is involved, the fact that radiation accident exposures are usually not uniform makes the survival of some fraction of stem cells possible, thus enabling regeneration to some extent. Radiation accidents rarely involve uniform total-body exposure, which is the most lethal geometry.

Prompt Doses Versus Fractionated or Protracted Doses

Radiation doses in radiation accidents should be expressed in terms of *prompt doses* for comparison purposes. Clinicians and health physicists should be aware that stated doses might include fractionated and protracted doses, which, when numerically added together, actually have significantly less biologic effect than the equivalent prompt dose. Fractionated doses may be converted to a prompt dose equivalent by means of the Ellis formula[1]; however, protracted and fractionated doses may be clinically converted to a very rough prompt dose equivalent by dividing the total dose by a factor of two or three. An example of the difference between prompt and protracted doses may be seen by looking at the changes in doses required to develop prodromal symptoms as presented in Table 25.3.

TABLE 25.3. IF CONTAMINATION IS DISCOVERED INSIDE THE EMERGENCY DEPARTMENT

If contamination is discovered after the patient has arrived:
  Continue medical care!
    Secure victim and provider operation areas.
    No one leaves until cleared by the radiation safety officer.
    Establish control lines (perimeter) and prevent contamination spread.
    Assess patient and contamination.
    Assess and mark contaminated areas.
  Personnel should:
    Remove contaminated clothing before leaving.
    Shower and dress in clean clothes before leaving.
    Resurvey before leaving the area.

---

[1]The Ellis formula for dose factionation is Total dose = NSD $\times$ $N^{0.24}$ $T^{0.11}$ where the total dose is in rads; NSD represents the nominal single dose; N, the number of fractions; and T, the time in days (number of hours/24).

PREHOSPITAL IMPACT AND CONSIDERATIONS

Contamination and Medical Issues

Rescue and medical issues typically take priority over radiation contamination issues. Emergency medical services (EMS) field radioactive decontamination should be limited to the removal of the victim's clothes and shoes and then wrapping the victim in two to three bedsheets. A hair cover may be placed as necessary. Most EMS units will not possess radiation survey equipment, but EMS supervisory personnel should be trained in the use of a radiation survey meter. Prehospital personnel should be detained at a radiation checkpoint outside the hospital and should be surveyed to check for the possibility of cross-contamination unless they are urgently needed back at the same incident site. As with other hazardous materials incidents, hot, warm, and cold zones should be established (Fig. 25.4).

If one is confronting chemical contamination or mixed (radiation and chemical) contamination, then the more serious contamination should take priority. Chemicals that may cause severe injury, such as organophosphates, caustics, corrosives, or acids, should receive immediate decontamination. Metallic sodium is occasionally found in conjunction with some radionuclides, and this element should not be exposed to air or water in attempts to decontaminate.

Terrorism Issues

Terrorism events have the following special considerations: (a) the potential threat of secondary devices exists, (b) the incident site is closed for evidence collection, and (c) the mode of radioactive dispersal varies widely. These are discussed in more detail below.

1. The potential threat of secondary devices dictates that victim rescue takes priority over medical care. Victims

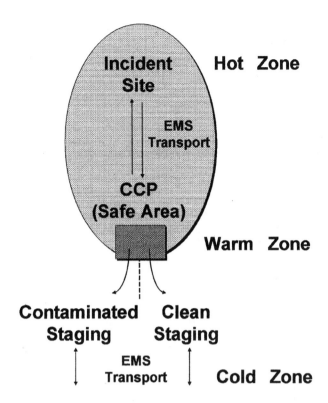

FIG. 25.5. Modification of hazardous materials response in a suspected terrorism incident. (From Mettler FA, Kelsey CA, Ricks RC, eds. *Medical management of radiation accidents.* Boca Raton, FL: CRC Press, 1990:72, with permission.)

should be evacuated to a safe casualty collection point within a designated security zone while a sweep for secondary devices is being done. The minimum safe distance may be quite remote, so victims may need vehicular transport to the casualty collection point (CCP).

2. Security zones set up by the Federal Bureau of Investigation (FBI) and the police tend to be larger than would be expected for most other hazardous materials incidents for reasons of security, population protection, and evidence collection. Therefore, law enforcement officials will have significant concerns for evidence preservation, particularly in fatality cases, especially of shrapnel and with clothing removal. The security zone becomes the boundaries of a *de facto* hot zone. As was stated earlier, the initial CCP would be designated within the security zone, as Fig. 25.5 demonstrates.

3. Potential terrorist uses of radiation are covered in Chapter 32.

Mass Casualty Incident Issues

Some prehospital services have as their guiding principle that all victims remain at the scene until they are decontaminated significantly. Several practical problems are found

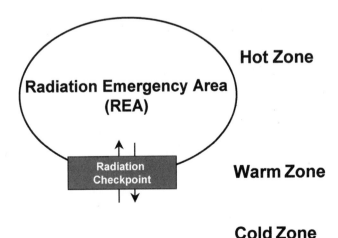

FIG. 25.4. Zones in a radiation emergency area

with this doctrine. Many of the victims at a mass casualty incident (MCI) will self-rescue initially, and they will develop an improvised leadership before an agency response occurs. Self-rescued patients typically arrive at the hospital nearest to the disaster site, and they may not be recognized as contaminated. Planning should take this behavior at the site into account in the process of disaster planning.

National Agency Notification

If an event occurs in a non-private corporation, national agencies should be notified. State radiation health departments or their equivalent agencies will be helpful in giving guidance of which agencies need to be notified. The Nuclear Regulatory Commission (NRC) regulates the reactor use and nuclear by-product material (which is frequently used in hospital environments). The Department of Energy (DOE) is responsible for national radiation research facilities, and it is the actual owner of nuclear weapons in the nuclear arsenal. The Department of Defense (DOD) is the user of the nuclear weapons. The National Aeronautics and Space Administration (NASA) is responsible for their research vehicles and projects. If evidence of criminal or terrorist acts is found, the FBI is legally responsible for locating any nuclear material, weapons, or devices and restoring these nuclear facilities to their rightful custodians; it thus enjoys a special position in the response. The response of national assets is guided by the Federal Radiological Emergency Response Plan (FRERP), which is further elaborated in Chapters 12 and 32.

EMERGENCY DEPARTMENT IMPACT AND CONSIDERATIONS

Medical Issues

Triage

Medical Stability

At the hospital, medical stability takes precedence over all other issues. A given patient will not expire immediately because of radiation exposure issues, but delay in addressing other medical issues, such as airway or shock, could cause either increased morbidity or mortality. Medical issues should never be compromised in radiation accident management. In reality, radiation accident patients initially may be approached in much the same way as any trauma response with standard (universal) precautions.

Conventional Trauma

Conventional trauma is a significant factor in determining the order of medical treatment. ATLS protocols take precedence over radiologic issues. Triaging schemes for nuclear detonation victims take into account the degree of conventional trauma and the systemic radiation exposure, as this

combination is synergistic in causing increased morbidity and mortality. In individuals, the timing of surgery may be dictated by the presence of systemic radiation exposure. In the face of significant systemic radiation exposure, life-saving surgery should occur within 36 to 48 hours, while other elective surgery should take place after hematopoietic recovery, approximately 45 to 60 days later (7).

External Contamination

One of the first radiologic considerations is whether the patient is externally contaminated. If so, emergency personnel must deal with the potential of contamination spread and must devise some sort of plan for personal protective gear and contamination control. This response plan may be either extremely simplistic or very sophisticated, depending on the type of hazard encountered. A radioactive contaminant can be clinically conceptualized to have many of the properties of dirt in its ability to be spread by airborne routes and its potential for cross-contamination among hospital personnel.

Systemic Radiation Exposure

Personnel should understand that irradiation alone will not result in contamination and that no personnel protective

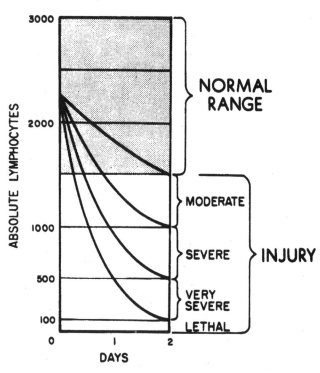

FIG. 25.6. Andrews nomogram. The schematic relationships between lymphocyte levels and radiation dose are conveyed by this graph. (From Andrews GA, Auxier JA, Lushbaugh CC. The importance of dosimetry to the medical management of persons accidentally exposed to high levels of ionizing radiation. In: International Atomic Energy Agency. *Personnel dosimetry for radiation accidents.* Vienna: International Atomic Energy Agency, 1965:13, with permission.)

measures need be taken if the patient has only been irradiated. Time to onset of prodromal symptoms is paramount in the determination of whether a patient has sustained significant systemic exposure. The modified Union of Soviet Socialist Republics (USSR) classification is useful in the initial classification of systemically irradiated patients. The Andrews nomogram verifies the presence of hematologically significant systemic radiation exposure by following the absolute lymphocyte count over several days (Fig. 25.6). Thus, those with *psychogenic* prodromal symptoms can be screened out over time.

Radiation Emergency Area Preparation

The radiation emergency area (REA) is an indoor or outdoor *ad hoc* area which has been designated for treatment of radiation accident victims. In choosing this location, consideration should be given to the preservation of the regular lifesaving functions of the emergency department while still enabling critical care equipment to be available to the REA if the equipment becomes necessary. Emergency departments with advanced designs have an alternate entrance to a closed-off, low-traffic corridor with extra space that can be used as an REA. This corridor should have access to electrical power, oxygen, suction, air, monitoring support, and informatics, should any of these capabilities becomes necessary.

Access to the REA should be easy to control, should require minimal extra personnel, and should have someone who is equipped to perform radiation surveys on personnel with a need to ingress or egress. The floor of the REA may be prepared by placing mats or absorbable paper and taping them to the floor. Absorbable paper makes areas of potential liquid contamination easier to see, and cleaning the REA becomes significantly easier. Equipment and supplies within the REA may be covered with taped bedsheets or plastic sheeting to ensure that important equipment is not compromised by contamination.

Personnel Needs

A radiation accident response, similar to any other trauma code or cardiac arrest, requires significant additional caregiver resources. Ideally, personnel should be assigned and dedicated to the response. On-duty personnel might be assigned to the case, while additional personnel are called in for an expected duty period of 1 to 4 hours. The following treatment team compositions should be considered in the management of radiation accident patients for planning and drill purposes. In actuality, the number of personnel assigned depends on the actual resources that are available. Six personnel should be sufficient to deal with a real radiation decontamination effort involving one victim who requires assisted decontamination.

The early arrival of a medical or health physicist in a response can assist immeasurably with data gathering, determining the specific radionuclides and amount involved, and establishing the mechanism of the accident or incident. The health physicist can assist with the safe disposal of radionuclide waste and can definitively delineate contaminated areas in the emergency department. He or she can aid in the collection of patient samples documenting contamination. Moreover, he or she can generate initial dose estimates that establish the upper bound of a maximum credible event. Health physicists may be affiliated with the radiation shipper, state radiation health department, or another agency. The most helpful person will be the health or medical physicist affiliated with the hospital.

Incorporating environmental and security services to assist with REA preparation, victim, and victim-relative traffic flow are useful as in other disasters. If the hospital has a sizable, active, and engaged security force, this service may be enlisted to do the following:

1. Provide enhanced security for the hospital, especially if high traffic flow is anticipated.
2. Intercept any potentially contaminated victims before they contaminate the interior of the hospital.
3. Assume the responsibility of setting up external decontamination areas and *ad hoc* victim processing patterns.
4. Supply direct assistance with gross decontamination.

SPECIFIC CLINICAL ENTITIES
External Contamination

Isolation of contamination is an important concept and option for health care providers. Any potentially contaminated area (except the head!) may be isolated by covering and taping the contaminated area. The use of plastic bags or plastic absorbent liners (chux) greatly decreases the opportunity for cross-contamination. Once patient stability is assured, the isolated area may be opened and decontaminated at that time. Contaminated areas other than those of the patient may also be isolated to mitigate cross-contamination. For example, any contamination of walls, floors, or equipment that is discovered may be isolated by covering with plastic sheeting, chux, or bedsheets and then taping. The same principle can also be applied to ambulances and air ambulances. Most of the equipment needed to perform decontamination is basic, low-technology equipment. Many hazardous materials doctrines usually do not allow for indoor decontamination, saying that this technique is never desirable. Radiation medicine doctrine, on the other hand, has always maintained that indoor decontamination is the preferred standard of care, particularly if the patient is not medically stable. This doctrinal conflict is confusing for those who are unfamiliar with the concept of all-hazards decontamination.

Outdoor decontamination is expedient and advisable when the victims are awake, alert, and communicative, and they have minimal conventional injuries. Patients who have altered mental status, obvious major external injuries, or unstable vital signs should be stabilized indoors and should undergo definitive decontamination inside the hospital.

In the event of a sizable multiple casualty incident, contaminated patients will self-rescue and will arrive unannounced at the emergency department registration desk, despite the most carefully executed plan. In hazardous material accident history, this scenario is the rule rather than the exception. Thus, a hospital should have contingency plans for radiation accident patient management both inside and outside the hospital.

Decontamination

Open wounds should be decontaminated first because such wounds provide obvious avenues for further internal contamination. Also, they may have some potential for obscuring radioactive foreign bodies that should be removed first to mitigate accumulated radiation exposure better. The contaminated tissue should be debrided as in any conventionally contaminated wound, and exuberance should be avoided in debridement. Leaving some radiation-contaminated tissue in a given wound may be prudent if the alternative is to cause either disfigurement or disability.

Preserve Intact Skin

Intact skin forms a significant barrier to radioactive contamination. Consequently, intact skin should be preserved. Contamination studies comparing various types of skin insult versus intact skin underscore the importance of preserving intact skin. Formerly recommended techniques that worked as superficial desquamating agents, such as household bleach (sodium hypochlorite), potassium permanganate, and tape stripping, are now discouraged as initial techniques, but they should still be available within the clinician's armamentarium.

Perform Multiple Gentle Techniques

The process of decontamination is usually a multistep process in which contamination is progressively removed. Multiple gentle techniques will preserve intact skin, and thus they are preferred over isolated aggressive techniques. The use of multiple gentle techniques may take place over several days as necessary. A patient may be decontaminated on 1 day, and the remaining areas should be isolated with a rubber glove or plastic bag overnight. The process of overnight perspiration will lessen the contamination. The patient can then be brought back the next day for another decontamination attempt.

Application of Time, Distance, Shielding, and Quantity to Clinical Care

The basic health physics principles of time, distance, shielding, and quantity should be used to minimize radiation exposure. Time spent within the REA in which radiation is present should be minimized. In the unlikely event of higher radiation levels (100 mRem per hr or higher at standard patient care distances), personnel rotation may be employed. Distance from radiation sources should be maximized, except when the clinician is providing direct patient care. Shielding is rarely of use in radiation accident response because the commonly used radiation shields provide no significant protection against gamma radiation. The quantity of radiation can be reduced by removing contaminated fluids and trash from the REA as it accumulates. Constant removal of contaminated trash can reduce the ambient background radiation that tends to increase somewhat from the contaminated waste produced as decontamination progresses.

Mixed Contamination

Mixed contamination occasionally occurs, particularly when some radionuclides are dissolved in a solvent, frequently acid solutions. Conceivably, this could also occur when a biologic contaminant is combined with a radionuclide, a situation that is much less likely. In instances in which mixed contamination occurs, the clinician must rapidly determine which is the more life-threatening toxin and must focus treatment toward the more severe toxin. Once the more severe toxin receives emergent treatment, attention can be focused on dealing with the next toxin.

Decontamination Techniques

Survey Techniques

The patient should be first surveyed by a provider functioning as a health physics (HP) technician, who takes an initial total-body survey. The results should be recorded on a human figure diagram (Fig. 25.7). Background radiation counts should be taken initially and periodically as decontamination progresses. Suggested guidelines for survey are as follows:

1. Cover the pancake probe with a glove before beginning the survey. This will not allow alpha radiation detection, but it will prevent the probe from being contaminated. In one case of an altered and combative patient, six probes were contaminated in the course of care. Most hospitals have only one probe available for each survey meter. Once the patient is determined to be cooperative and that a low probability of contaminating the probe exists, the glove may be removed to check for alpha contamination.

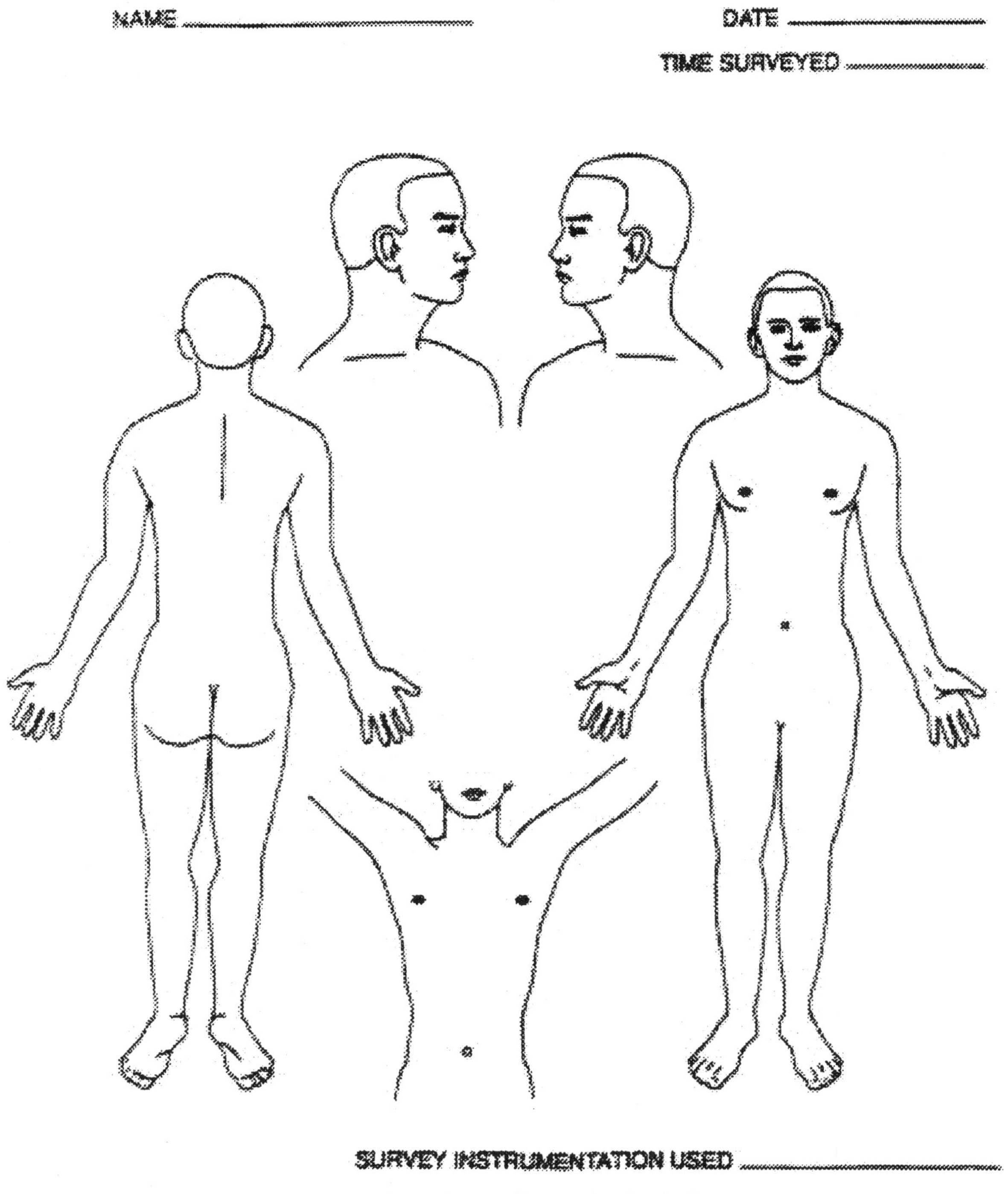

NAME _____   DATE _____
                                     TIME SURVEYED _____

FIG. 25.7. Sample human figure diagram for recording levels of contamination.

SURVEY INSTRUMENTATION USED _____

2. The survey probe should be held approximately 1 inch away from the skin and should be moved no faster than 1 inch per second.
3. The patient should hold his or her extremities in an abducted fashion from the body, so that less confusion will exist as to where contamination might be located and so that a methodical technique of survey can be used

in such a manner that the patient's entire body will be covered (Fig. 25.8).

Plan of Decontamination

After the contaminated areas are identified, these areas should be prioritized and a methodical plan should be

The following procedures are recommended for personnel monitoring.

1. Have person stand on a clean pad.

2. Instruct the person to stand straight, feed spread slightly, arms extended with palms up and fingers straight out.

3. Monitor both hands and forearms to the elbows with palms up, then repeat with hands and arms turned over.

4. Starting at the top of the head, cover the entire front of the body, monitoring carefully the forehead, nose, mouth, neck line, torso, knees and ankles.

5. Have the subject turn around, and repeat the survey on the back of the body.

6. Monitor the soles of the feet.

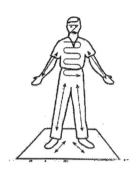

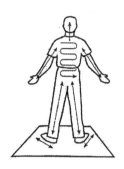

FIG. 25.8. Personnel monitoring. (From Radiation Emergency Assistance Center/ Training Site training material. Oak Ridge, TN: Oak Ridge Associated Universities, with permission.)

developed for decontamination. If the patient is ambulatory, consideration should be given to allowing the patient to shower himself. Self-decontamination is much more rapid than assisted decontamination and is far less labor-intensive. Self-decontamination should be considered a possible initial step in the overall decontamination process in patient care.

If the patient is nonambulatory or he or she has other significant trauma, assisted decontamination will be necessary. If the patient has numerous contaminated areas, a single site should be selected and the other areas should isolated for later decontamination to minimize the opportunity for cross-contamination.

The provider should consider using dry removal or waterless cleansers (e.g., Gojo) before proceeding with water decontamination. Omitting this step may delay the decontamination process unnecessarily. The efficiency of dry removal ranges from 30% to 80%, and it can be performed by practically anyone as it requires minimal training. Dry removal techniques usually consist of *beating*, *brushing*, and *vacuuming* (8). Decontamination of open wounds should take place before that of contaminated areas of intact skin. Debridement should be fairly similar to techniques used for routine debridement. Small amounts of radionuclide contamination will probably remain after debridement, but wound closure should be performed. If, however, contamination is more than these tiny quantities, consideration should be given to leaving the wounds open for delayed closure 4 days later. This procedure might allow the further elimination of radionu-

clide, either through the transudation of fluid from tissues or with later debridement efforts.

Clinicians may wonder when decontamination efforts should cease. Frequently, not all contamination can be removed. The cessation of decontamination efforts should be considered when no additional contamination comes off with the next effort. If National Council for Radiation Protection and Measurements (NCRP) guidelines for patient decontamination have been achieved, then the decontamination efforts may cease. The NCRP no. 65 guidelines state that, from a practical standpoint, cleaning more than the following is difficult (9):

1,000 transformations (formerly disintegrations) per minute using an alpha radiation (air proportional) counter with a 60 cm^2 window.

1 mRem per hour beta radiation.

A quantity that amounts to less than 15 Rem per year to the skin.

Other additional guidelines have been published by agencies such as the DOE for their own radiation workers and naval reactor workers (BUMED guidelines), so one might encounter guidelines other than those recommended by the NCRP.

If the previous guidelines have not been met and no further contamination is removed with an additional effort, consideration should be given for the need to (a) switch to another technique or (b) cease decontamination efforts for this session.

TABLE 25.3. IF CONTAMINATION IS DISCOVERED INSIDE THE EMERGENCY DEPARTMENT

If contamination is discovered after the patient has arrived:
  Continue medical care!
    Secure victim and provider operation areas.
    No one leaves until cleared by the radiation safety officer.
    Establish control lines (perimeter) and prevent
      contamination spread.
    Assess patient and contamination.
    Assess and mark contaminated areas.
  Personnel should:
    Remove contaminated clothing before leaving.
    Shower and dress in clean clothes before leaving.
    Resurvey before leaving the area.

The involved body portion may be isolated, if necessary, and decontamination efforts may be scheduled for the next day. Decontamination efforts may be enhanced by the process of perspiration, and measured radiation levels may be significantly lowered via perspiration alone. One should remember that skin surfaces will completely desquamate over a period of approximately 2 weeks, leaving the skin essentially non-contaminated at that point. Table 25.3 lists actions in the event that contamination is discovered after receiving a patient.

In the course of emergency planning, one should be aware that the hospital nuclear medicine license allows the disposal of a specified amount of radioactive waste in the sewer system. For radioactive decontamination events, the dilution has been calculated to have the effect of keeping radioactive contaminants to levels that will not cause significant health repercussions. Keeping contaminated runoff in a storage tank that can be emptied by alternate methods, particularly for long-lived radionuclides, is preferable, but it is not required. The local jurisdiction should be notified when a contamination event involving potentially radioactive runoff has occurred.

If the waste is collected in a storage tank, the quantity of waste can be greatly reduced by evaporating away the liquids. When dealing with mixed waste, such as a combination of a biologic and radiation waste, converting this combined waste into a single type of waste that can be disposed of more easily is useful.

In radiation accidents, the owner of the radioactive material is responsible for the radionuclide removal costs and its ultimate disposal. The owner should be contacted early in the process to ensure that appropriate financial arrangements are made. If the radioactive material is in the process of being transported, the shipper assumes the prime financial responsibility for cleanup.

Systemic Irradiation

Precise measurements of radiation exposure take considerable time (days or weeks), and they *will not* occur in the timely fashion required by the emergency physician. Estimates of radiation exposure may be available, depending on the type of exposure that is alleged to have occurred. Internal contamination estimates are very difficult to obtain, and, therefore, they will take the longest. Practical clinical estimation of systemic radiation exposure is simple. The first screening tool for the estimation of severity of radiation exposure can be deduced by the time to onset of the prodromal symptoms of nausea, vomiting, and diarrhea. The shorter the onset, the more significant the exposure is. The modified USSR classification of radiation exposure, which takes time to prodrome into account, may be of significant value to the emergency physician. This screening tool may also be used to screen those who are susceptible to psychogenic suggestion. Serial absolute lymphocyte counts plotted on the Andrews nomogram will verify the presence of systemic exposure and will screen out over time those affected by psychogenic vomiting. This clinical determination of systemic exposure forecasts the degree of hematopoietic impairment. Radiation injury to other organ systems, such as the pulmonary, gastrointestinal, and musculocutaneous systems, may be made with more precise dose estimates at a later time after the patient has been admitted. The admitting physician can anticipate additional organ involvement by these dose estimates (Table 25.4).

In cases of delayed recognition of a radiation accident, the patient commonly presents during the period of manifest illness, with affords the clinician no opportunity to witness the prodrome, and thus important clinical lead time is lost.

Acute radiation syndrome progresses through the following four distinct phases:

Prodromal phase. Prodromal symptoms classically consist of nausea, vomiting, and diarrhea. Prodromal symptoms are thought to be mediated by an inflammatory response after radiation insult and by parasympathetic pathways. Other symptoms may include severe abdominal pain, eye burning, and fever, particularly with high-dose exposure.

Latent phase. After prodromal symptoms, the patient will experience a period of relative well-being, particularly after sublethal radiation exposure. This is a period in which inflammatory effects are relatively quiescent and mature cells remain. During this period, however, the replacement of mature cells is impaired, and it will not be sufficient for restore them to the level of the organism's needs.

Manifest phase. In this the period, the cellular deficits make themselves known. In the case of skin, no further skin cells replace the mature layers, and the mature cells slough off naturally, revealing the atrophic dermal elements underneath. Endothelial cells of the microvasculature may not be replaced, causing damaged, leaky blood vessels. Other constantly renewing cell lines, such as the gastrointestinal mucosa and the hematopoietic cells, develop deficits in certain cellular elements, causing special sub-syndromes. Fibrosis of the involved area(s) may begin at any of several different rates.

Recovery/death phase. After a time, the stem cells may recover somewhat and may mount a proliferative response such that the organism reduces the deficits in these cellular elements. If this process is successful so that no life-threatening infection or no critical organ failure develops, then the organism will survive. Otherwise, the organism dies.

SYSTEMIC RADIATION ILLNESS

Systemic radiation illness can be divided into a number of components that occur with certain geometry and certain radiation doses. A summary table of the deterministic effects on selected organs is found in Table 25.4.

Hematopoietic Component

One of the earliest systems that is affected by radiation exposure is the hematopoietic system. Hematopoietic depression tends to appear with doses of 0.25 Gy (25 rads), and depression is generally maximized around 6 Gy (600 rads). With severe doses, a sharp spike in the neutrophil count is observed and is followed by a precipitous fall to neutropenic levels. After several days, an abortive rise in the neutrophil count is seen, and the true nadir in neutrophils occurs at approximately 15 days. Lymphocytes are suddenly and precipitously depressed after 48 hours, as they are one of the most radiation-sensitive cells in the body. Thrombo-

cytes reach their nadir in 30 days with a moderate dose of radiation and in 15 days with severe doses. Levels of mature erythrocytes, which lack a nucleus and have a lifetime of 120 days, decrease slowly (Fig. 25.9).

Immunocompromise from systemic irradiation is somewhat different from the usual immunocompromise encountered by the emergency physician, which usually results from patients with primarily impaired lymphocyte function. In addition to having impaired lymphocyte function, systemically irradiated patients may also be neutropenic. Neutropenia is a potentially life-threatening condition, and, in this patient, it should be treated the same as any other type of neutropenia. Patients with an absolute neutrophil count of 1,000 to 500 cells per mm^3 sustain a slight risk for life-threatening infection, while patients with 500 to 100 cells per mm^3 represent a moderate risk; patients with less than 100 cells per mm^3 are at high risk for developing a life-threatening infection. The emergency physician is unlikely to see patients immunocompromised to this level, except for the case of a delayed-recognition accident.

Patients with neutropenia should be treated for both gram-negative and gram-positive organisms. The inflammatory response in these patients may be muted. Low-risk patients may be treated with oral antibiotics, while high-risk patients should only receive parenteral antibiotics. Enthusiasm for prophylaxis with oral antibiotics in the asymptomatic, neutropenic patient should be tempered by the possibility of the emergence of resistant bacteria. Vancomycin should be considered in symptomatic, nonresponsive patients. Amphotericin B should be considered if a patient remains febrile longer than 5 to 7 days during treatment with antibiotics.

TABLE 25.4. SUMMARY OF THRESHOLD RADIATION EFFECTS

Acute radiation effects	Threshold Gy (rads)	D$_{50}$ Gy (rads)
Lethal bone marrow syndrome (minimal care)	1.5 (150)	3.0 (300)
Lethal bone marrow syndrome (supportive care)	2.3 (230)	4.5 (450)
Lethal pulmonary syndrome	5 (500)	10 (1,000)
Lethal gastrointestinal syndrome	8 (800)	15 (1,500)
Skin erythema	3 (300)	6 (600)
Transepithelial injury	10 (1,000)	20 (2,000)
Ovulation suppression	0.6 (60)	3.5 (350)
Two-year sperm suppression	0.3 (30)	0.7 (70)
Small infant head size	0.05 (5)	0.73 (73)
Severe mental retardation (all gestational ages)		4.1 (410)
Severe mental retardation (8–15 wk gestation)		1.5 (150)
Severe mental retardation (16–25 wk gestation)		7.1 (710)
Embryolethality (embryonic age 0–18 d)	0.1 (10)	1 (100)
Embryolethality (embryonic age 18–150 d)	0.4 (40)	1.5 (150)
Cataracts	1 (100)	3.1 (310)
Acute radiation thyroiditis	200 (20,000)	1,200 (120,000)

Abbreviations: D$_{50}$, effective 50% dose; Gy, Gray.
From NUREG/CR-4214. Health effects models for nuclear power plant accident consequence analysis: low LET radiation. Part II. Scientific bases for health effects models. Bethesda, MD: U.S. Nuclear Regulatory Commission, 1989, with permission.

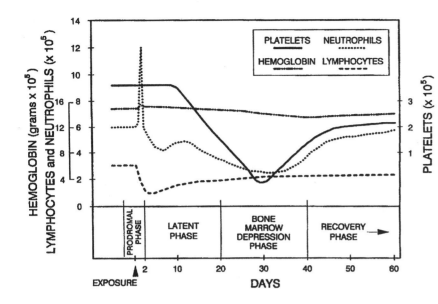

FIG. 25.9. Typical hematopoietic effects with radiation exposure of 300 rads (3 Gy). (Modified from Andrews GA, Auxier JA, Lushbaugh CC. The importance of dosimetry to the medical management of persons accidentally exposed to high levels of ionizing radiation. In: International Atomic Energy Agency. *Personnel dosimetry for radiation accidents.* Vienna: International Atomic Energy Agency, 1965:9, with permission.)

Gastrointestinal Component

The gastrointestinal (GI) threshold begins at approximately 6 Gy (600 rads), in which a significant inflammatory response occurs, and culminates in the desquamation of the GI epithelial lining, thus interfering with nutrient absorption and providing a significant avenue for life-threatening bacterial invasion. Venoocclusive liver disease occurs at doses that affect the GI epithelium, and increases in liver function test values will be observed. Complete sterilization of the entire GI epithelium is believed to occur around 15 Gy (1,500 rads).

Pulmonary Component

Pulmonary effects can be a significant cause of morbidity and mortality. An interstitial pneumonitis can develop; this seems to be worsened in cases of concomitant cytomegalovirus activation. The interstitial pneumonitis will give way to radiation fibrosis, which then occurs at varying times over months to a year, depending on the severity of the dose. The dose-rate dependency of interstitial pneumonitis has been well documented, with prompt doses—doses that are delivered in a single, rapid rate—being more likely to develop radiation pneumonitis. (Table 25.5).

Musculocutaneous Component

Changes begin to occur to hair follicles around 0.75 Gy (75 rads) Hair epilation will occur at 3 Gy (300 rads). Erythema, which occurs at 6 Gy (600 rads), is wavelike, and it occurs more rapidly with more severe doses. Desquamation effects, if they occur, tend to be observed after 2 weeks, which is the time required for mature skin cell elements to live out their normal lives. No further replacement of skin cell elements is seen, and the desquamating lesions are then evident. Dry desquamation occurs at 10 Gy (1,000 rads), and wet desquamation occurs at 20 Gy (2,000 rads). Radionecrosis of deep tissue is evident at 30 Gy (3,000 rads). These numbers may be important if amputation is under consideration.

Neurovascular Component

Neurovascular effects occur at extremely high doses of radiation. The weak link in the neurovascular tissues appears to be located in the stromal and vascular elements, particularly the vascular endothelial cell lining, and thus affects the microcirculation. Dramatic effects, such as *early transient incapacitation* (a period of unconsciousness), is thought to occur following supralethal doses. Gross central nervous system deficits may be witnessed after a short period of latency. Increased intercranial pressure occurs secondary to edema, and death within 2 days can occur in such cases (10).

TABLE 25.5. DEPENDENCE OF RADIATION PNEUMONITIS ON DOSE RATE FOR FORMATION

Dose rate (rad/hr) (Gy/hr)	Threshold (rads) (Gy)
5 (0.05)	31,000 (310)
10 (0.1)	16,000 (160)
50 (0.5)	4,000 (40)
100 (1)	2,000 (20)
1,000 (10)	700 (7)
10,000 (100)	500 (5)

From NUREG/CR-4214. Health effects models for nuclear power plant accident consequence analysis: low LET radiation. Part II. Scientific bases for health effects models. Bethesda, MD: U.S. Nuclear Regulatory Commission, 1989, with permission.

INTERNAL CONTAMINATION

Principles of Decorporation Management

The process of mitigating internal contamination is known as *decorporation*. The clinician should consider decorporation treatment within hours of internal contamination. Treatment may have the potential to reduce the amount of internal contamination by a factor of 2 to 10.

The first useful concept for the clinician is to consider radiation exposure, particularly internal contamination, as he or she would any other toxin of the body and to remember the following dictums espoused by Kent Olson:

1. Treat the patient before the poison.
2. Prevent or reduce the exposure.
3. Enhance the elimination of the agent.
4. Consider specific adjuncts and antidotes.

The process of *incorporation*, or the internal uptake, of a given radionuclide, involves the following four general steps:

1. Deposition along a route of entry.
2. Translocation (changing a given radioactive substance to a transportable mode).
3. Deposition in a target organ (dependent on the chemical properties of the substance).
4. Clearance (naturally occurs with routine metabolism).

During this process, if interception of the radionuclide is possible before the translocation step, a potential time window of enhanced therapeutic effectiveness exists before the radionuclide becomes converted to a biotransportable form. If therapy is successful in this time frame, a large amount of the radionuclide might be prevented from reaching the target organ. Thus, acting within this thera-

peutically enhanced time frame increases the clinical advantage. The Voelz diagram of internal contamination metabolism demonstrates the major compartments of the GI tract, lymph nodes, lung, and skin, into which radionuclides are deposited before they move to the blood compartment, where they are then considered translocatable (Fig. 25.10).

The next step, while keeping the above in mind, is to determine the magnitude of the exposure. In 1992, a European consensus group derived the following criteria as a basis for taking therapeutic action. This criteria is derived from the occupational regulatory construct of the annual limit of intake (ALI) (i.e., the amount of radionuclide that a radiation worker is allowed to accumulate within the space of 1 year). Currently, no other scientific guidelines are used other than those from this consensus group. A few response groups are basing their action levels on the obsolete concept of maximum permissible body burden, but this practice is currently being phased out. The action criteria from the 1992 consensus group is as follows (11):

Less than 1 annual limit of intake (ALI) expected	No treatment necessary
1 to 10 ALI	Consider short-term therapy.
>10 ALI	Initiate therapy.

Treatment decisions should be based on the maximum credible exposure. The final dose estimate should be expected to change dramatically over time, usually to much lower levels and often by several magnitudes. Dose estimates for internal exposure are verified by obtaining periodic body fluid assays (e.g., urine, blood, or feces) over time. Internal dose estimates may take several months in optimal circumstances. Health physics excretion models usually do not account for decorporation therapy, and

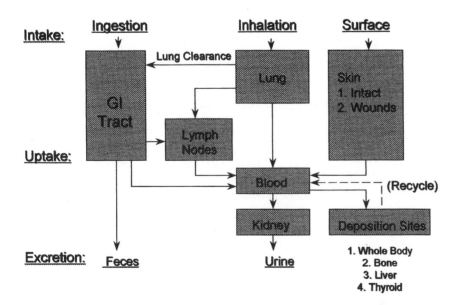

FIG. 25.10. Schematic model for internal contamination. (Based on the work of Voelz.)

health physicists may resist the suggestion of treatment. A few computer programs, such as PuChel, take into account plutonium excretion using diethylenetriamine pentaacetic (DTPA) therapy; some health physicists may not be aware of programs such as these. In these cases, the clinican will need to remind all involverd that patient care comes first and that excretion models have a subordinate role to that.

Consideration of radionuclide chemical solubility is of great importance when making the decision to offer treatment to the patient. Insoluble radionuclide forms may result in only a small fraction of radionuclide being converted to the translocatable form at any given time, so decorporation therapy may not be useful for patients with these forms.

The biologic half-life of a given radionuclide is of some importance in the consideration of whether to initiate therapy. Some radionuclides, such as plutonium, have long residence times in the body (in this case a biologic half-life of 100 years), while other radionuclides, such as tritium in the form of radioactive water, may have a biologic half-life of days. These factors with a few others used in internal dosimetry models help determine the *committed radiation dose* that would eventually ensue over the lifetime of the individual.

Effective half-life takes into consideration both biologic half-life and the radiologic half-life of a given radionuclide. It may be calculated by the following expression:

$$\text{T 1/2}_{\text{effective}} = \frac{\text{T } \frac{1}{2} \text{ biological} + \text{T } \frac{1}{2} \text{ physical}}{\text{T } \frac{1}{2} \text{ biological} \times \text{T } \frac{1}{2} \text{ physical}}$$

The effective half-life is always shorter than the largest term in the formula.

General Routes of Internal Contamination

According to George Poda, the four I's that must be remembered when considering routes of internal contamination are *inhalation, ingestion, injection,* and *infiltration.*

Inhaled Contamination

Inhalation is a common route of exposure, and the solubility of the involved substance plays a great role in radiation management. If solubility of the identified radionuclide(s) is low, chelating agents may be of negligible benefit. Whole lung lavage under anesthesia has been identified as useful when high numbers of ALIs are involved. At best, lung lavage will remove approximately one-half of the radioactivity from the lungs (12,13). The objective of lung lavage is to remove alveolar macrophages from the lung. Macrophages rapidly engulf (usually within 24 hours) particles deposited in the alveoli and alveolar ducts (14). Segmental lung lavage (performed

under no anesthesia; a much more common procedure) has not been investigated due to the rarity of large exposures, and whether this technique has the potential for much less morbidity and mortality and might be useful to the patient remains to be seen.

Ingested Contamination

In the event of radionuclide ingestion, standard toxicologic protocols should be considered. Although gastric lavage has fallen out of favor for most poisonous ingestions, lavage may still be used if the ingestion is quite recent and the patient is highly motivated to remove radioactive contamination. If radionuclides are in the form of simple salts as commonly occurs, activated charcoal will probably not be of any benefit. If the radionuclide is in the form of an insoluble compound, a purgative might be used to decrease GI transit time.

Injected Contamination

Injection implies being stuck with a needle. This can and does happen in the laboratory or testing facilities, thus causing radionuclide contamination within the puncture. Punctures are one of the most common industrial accidents; they often occur on the pads of the finger.

Infiltration

Infiltration occurs through intact skin if radioactive iodine or tritium is placed on the skin. Potassium iodine (KI) is used to block the uptake of radioiodine. Forcing fluids, using other tricks such as hot showers to promote sweating, and administering diuretics to help eliminate tritium are most often used for these types of contamination. However, abrasions, blisters, burns, rashes, and so on that become contaminated allow infiltration to occur, as does overzealous scrubbing of the skin (15).

SPECIFIC RADIONUCLIDE MANAGEMENT
By Radionuclide
Plutonium and Other Transuranic Elements

Plutonium (Pu) and other transuranic elements, such as americium, may be treated in a timely fashion with the chelating agents calcium-dieethylenetriamine pentaacetic acid (DTPA) (Ca-DTPA) and zinc-DTPA (Zn-DTPA). Compound solubility is an important consideration when deciding to give DTPA. Transuranic compounds have a solubility that is precisely known, but they are also classified as D (solubility within days), W (solubility within weeks), or Y (solubility within years). The target organ for plutonium is the skeleton. The skeletal half-life of plutonium is approximately 100 years. The lower the solubility, the less likely DTPA is to be effective. Given soluble transuranic elements, Ca-DTPA is most effective when it is given within 1 hour of exposure. In the case of insoluble transuranic elements, Ca-DTPA will be of minimal or uncertain benefit when it is given promptly. These facts have triggered significant debate as to when DTPA should be given. DTPA has a safety profile with very few side effects, and its use should be considered when the solubility of a transuranic is uncertain. Ca-DTPA will give superior excretion of transuranic radionuclide when it is used initially; subsequent doses should make use of Zn-DTPA to prevent the bodily depletion of zinc. DTPA has been an investigational new drug for decades; it is available through the Radiation Emergency Assistance Control/Training Site (REAC/TS).

Radiocesium

Radiocesium is commonly used in teletherapy sources and other radiation devices. Because ^{137}Cs constitutes an important byproduct of nuclear fission, it is the most commonly encountered cesium radioisotope. For this reason, it must be considered to be present in any fission event. Cesium can be considered a potassium analog, and, therefore, it should be thought of as occupying the same body fluid compartments (mostly the interstitial fluid compartment). Thus, as would be expected, muscle is the primary target organ for cesium. Cesium is eliminated quickly, with approximately 10% of the total systemic burden being cleared with a half-time of approximately 2 days; the remainder is lost with a half-time of 100 days (16).

Insoluble Prussian blue, an ion exchanger, can be given orally to enhance cesium elimination in the feces. Insoluble Prussian blue is not absorbed systemically, and it binds cesium excreted in biliary secretions and that encountered in the GI circulation. Insoluble Prussian blue was administered as 10 g per day in divided doses in the Goiania radiation disaster with significant benefits. Side effects at higher doses are generally reported as GI upset and constipation; 30 g per day is not clinically tolerated. Insoluble Prussian blue is available through REAC/TS.

Radioiodine and Technetium-99m

Radioiodine and technitium-99m radioiodine are most commonly encountered as ^{125}I and ^{131}I because these also are important fission products that are relatively short-lived (days). The great preponderance of radioiodine concentrates within the thyroid. Radiation-stable iodine given within a certain therapeutic window will saturate the iodine receptors and will block its further uptake. Iodine provides the best protection when given prophylactically 1 hour before anticipated exposure. Once exposure to radioiodine has occurred, radiation-stable iodine may have some efficacy up to 3 to 4 hours after exposure. Moreover, stable iodine may be of benefit days later after fallout or reactor release if skin contact with radioiodine has not yet occurred. KI is the traditional form of iodine that is given, but it has a limited shelf life. The United States government had been debating whether stockpiling KI would be useful; it finally agreed to subsidize the state procurement of KI. NCRP publication no. 65 recommends that KI, 300 mg, should be given daily for 7 to 14 days. The World Health Organization published a revision of its iodine prophylaxis guidelines in 1999; these appear in Table 25.6. The dermal application of povidone-iodine has been shown to be extremely effective in animals, and human experiments should be performed to determine the dermal thyroid-blocking dose of povidone-iodine. Povidone-iodine is a potentially superior alternative because it is available in sufficient quantities at all hospitals, it has a proven safety profile for skin contact, and it would not require stockpiling and replenishment on an ongoing basis.

Uranium

Uranium is an actinide that constitutes one of the two common substrates for fission process. It is ubiquitous in the environment, and it has made headlines in times of armed conflict, as modern bullets, projectiles, and armor may all be made from depleted uranium. Longitudinal studies of those injured by uranium shrapnel have begun. Uranium is a common raw material, as well as a product of nuclear production facilities, and occupational exposure regularly occurs.

TABLE 25.6. WORLD HEALTH ORGANIZATION RECOMMENDED SINGLE DOSAGE OF STABLE IODINE ACCORDING TO AGE GROUP

Age group	Mass of iodine (mg)	Mass of KI (mg)	Mass of KIO₃ (mg)	Fraction of 100-mg tablet
Adults and adolescents (over 12 yr)	100	130	170	1
Children (3–12 yr)	50	65	85	½
Infants (1 mo to 3 yr)	25	32	42	¼
Neonates (birth to 1 mo)	12.5	16	21	⅛

Abbreviations: KI, potassium iodide; KIO₃, potassium iodate.
From World Health Organization. *Guidelines for iodine prophylaxis following nuclear accidents.*
Update 1999. Geneva: World Health Organization, 1999:11, with permission.

Weapons-grade or highly enriched uranium contains greater than 90% of the ^{235}U isotope. Many uranium compounds are created in the course of processing uranium, and many different acid solvents have the potential to be used.

Uranium is rapidly removed from the blood into the tissues—25% remains in the blood at 5 minutes, 5% at 24 hours, and 0.5% at 100 hours (17). Volunteers who were injected intravenously with uranyl nitrate typically demonstrated 65% uranium excretion in the urine within 24 hours; an additional 10% was excreted over the next 5 days (17). Within a few days, the kidneys and skeleton accounted for nearly all the remaining systemic content (17). The major source of uranium toxicity is renal toxicity, accompanied by the development of renal tubular acidosis and some degree of renal insufficiency. Alkalinization of the urine has been advocated for decades as a method for increasing the fraction of nontoxic, excretable, complexed uranium compounds by several magnitudes and, more importantly, for the degree of renal protection it affords. Under proper supervision, alkalinization of urine and potassium augmentation display low morbidity and mortality rates. Although no effective chelating agent is available for uranium (18), the practice of alkalinization of urine has recently been called into question (19). The author, however, advocates the use of alkalinization of urine via sodium bicarbonate and supplemental potassium chloride (KCl) in divided doses to achieve an alkaline pH of 7.5 to 8.

Tritium

Tritium is the primary substrate used in fusion reactions, and it is considered to be of great importance to the national defense. It is also a component of self-luminous watch dials, exit signs, and rifle scopes. Tritium is currently processed in the United States, and occupational exposure commonly occurs. It is a weak beta emitter whose half-life is relatively short. Most forms of absorbed tritium occur as a water form. Inhaled tritium gas is less toxic. In radiation accident history, tritium has been used as an instrument of corporate terrorism. Treatment is directed toward increasing the turnover of free water by increasing water intake. NCRP publication no. 65 recommends increasing fluid intake to 3 to 4 L per day in order to reduce residence time to one-third to one-half of the usual values (20).

Foreign Body

Embedded foreign bodies may have potential to be significant radiation sources in their own right. Early examination of wounds that contain foreign bodies will quickly determine any additional radiation hazard that the foreign body possesses. If a foreign body is found to be significantly more radioactive (i.e., exposure rates are in terms of Rem/hr instead of mRem/hr), then the foreign body should be manipulated only with instruments and not with the hands as much as possible.

Overexposure

Overexposure signifies additional unintended exposure (usually over the regulatory levels) that does not have any immediate threshold (deterministic) effects. Overexposures may create an increased risk of developing cancer later in life, depending on the nature of the exposure.

Radiation Exposure Counseling

After an exposure, a patient may be worried about his or her future chances of getting cancer later in life. Thus, some counseling on this subject will be required at a later time. This may be best when conducted by any of the following: an occupational physician who deals with radiation, a nuclear medicine physician, or a radiation oncologist. The patient will need to understand that the background cancer rate for a cancer occurring sometime in life is in the range of 25%. Precise doses will not be known at the time of the accident, so estimates *may* be initially used to provide a framework for the clinician to act. As the dose estimate is refined over time, it frequently changes by a magnitude or two. Several months may pass before the physician and the patient receive a final dose estimate, particularly in cases of internal contamination.

These long-term estimates generally are extrapolations based on the dose estimates of the Hiroshima and Nagasaki bombing survivors and the observations of the long-term effects on these survivors. The basic assumptions used to derive these estimates often change from time to time. The Hiroshima and Nagasaki dosimetry estimates were created in 1965 and were revised once in 1986. Another revision of the Hiroshima and Nagasaki bombing dosimetry is being contemplated; this new dose estimate would likely change risk estimate predictions yet again.

SPECIFIC PLANNING POINTS FOR THIS TYPE OF DISASTER

Health Physics Expertise

A health or medical physicist is commonly assigned to the hospital for the purpose of maintaining radiation hygiene programs for equipment and personnel. Such a physicist should be included in the development of radiation response plans. These plans should identify this individual and should include means for consulting a health physicist in the event of a possible radiation accident. This is the crux of the entire chapter as the health physicist is familiar with a number of other resources that will assist the clinician in the event of a possible radiation accident.

Decontamination Issues

Some hospitals assume that prehospital providers (fire departments and EMS) will decontaminate all victims before their arrival to the ED. Some fire and EMS departments have this doctrine as their standard policy; however, studies show that in any incident scene, survivors self-rescue and improvise a response (see Chapters 1 and 26). These victims usually present to the nearest hospital regardless of its capability. Therefore, for any hospital to labor under the expectation that they will never receive noncontaminated patients is not reasonable.

Large-Scale Decontamination

Within the spectrum of radiation accident response, one scenario is that in which a large number of people believe that they may be contaminated with radionuclides; this would be similar in size and scope to the 1995 Sarin gas exposure in Tokyo. Contingency plans must deal with this possible scenario. The worried well and the minimally injured should be directed to use some type of self-showering procedure, either outdoors or indoors. Another procedure should be available for victims who are incapacitated or who are otherwise unable to perform self-decontamination. A medical officer should supervise this process to ensure that unstable patients are recognized in the process of performing self-decontamination.

If a hospital wants to develop decontamination capabilities, the first efforts toward developing the capability to respond to a radiation accident should be initially directed toward the management of one or two victims as this is the most likely scenario.

Outdoor Decontamination

Outdoor decontamination facilities may be temporary or permanent. An option to decontaminate a large number of individuals should be available depending on the specific hazard analysis of the hospital facility. A supply of hot water allows outdoor decontamination in near-freezing weather, as long as the decontamination occurs in a sheltered area. Separate areas of decontamination should be established for males and females. A procedure for identifying and packaging clothing should be devised. Valuables can be a sensitive issue, so some facilities have devised a technique for handling them in which valuables are placed in resealable plastic (e.g., ziplock) bags and are then tied with a string around an individual's neck. A scheme for providing towels and temporary clothing (usually hospital gowns) to these individuals should be available. Other variants of improvised decontamination schemes under research by fire departments involve the use of generating shower streams for a line of ambulatory individuals simply by using two fire pumper trucks. Whether this technique will ultimately be adopted as an acceptable technique is not clear.

Outdoor assisted decontamination is appropriate if the victim is nonambulatory or altered, if the victim has significant trauma, and particularly if the presumed toxin is highly transferrable to hospital personnel.

Indoor Decontamination

As was discussed previously, hospitals need to have a plan for indoor decontamination because (a) patients frequently are recognized as being contaminated only after they have been checked into the emergency department, (b) critical patients may require the proximity or use of sophisticated emergency department monitoring equipment, and (c) an indoor environment may be more suitable for decontamination due to outdoor conditions. Many emergency departments have some type of fixed indoor facility in which individuals may shower themselves. This is fine for patients with minor injuries and for the worried well. Specialized equipment for indoor decontamination is available, but it is not necessary for decontamination. Areas to be irrigated may be draped with absorbent liners (chux) and taped to make the area water-resistant. Absorbent liners can be used to direct the runoff from a wound into waste receptacles. Temporary cardboard barrels with heavy plastic liners can be used to collect the runoff of any irrigation fluids that are used.

Evaluation Issues
Health Physics Laboratories

These facilities should be identified during the development of radiation response plans. A health physicist may be of great assistance in this identification process. The temptation may exist to send samples for radiologic assay to the conventional laboratory for submission. The conventional laboratory often is reluctant to handle radiation assays for fear of radiation exposure, and, moreover, it may not know where to send these samples, thus causing unnecessary delay. Procedures for the submission of radiation specimens should be laminated and posted within the hospital laboratory for easy reference.

Whole-Body Counters

These detectors, which are somewhat scarce, should also be identified in the radiation response plans. Manufacturers of whole-body counters might, with the permission of their clients, identify those who had purchased whole-body counters. Governmental agencies could then ask these entities if they would be willing to provide their whole body counter in the event of a radiation incident. Whole-body counters are capable of detecting minute amounts of internal contamination if the subject has already been externally decontaminated. Whole-body counters are used to provide follow-up evaluation for those who have possibly been exposed to internal contamination in order to evaluate the committed internal doses.

Laboratory Dosimetry

The gold standard for decades for determining the systemic radiation dose has been the technique of *lymphocyte cytogenetics*. Few facilities in the United States are capable of performing lymphocyte cytogenetics now. The International Atomic Energy Agency fosters development for dosimetry laboratories and standards for them using a variety of techniques, and it maintains lists of worldwide resources. Other techniques for determining the systemic dose are the micronuclei assay of lymphocytes and fluorescent *in situ* hybridization using lymphocytes. At higher dose levels (those greater than 1 Gy [100 rads]), other opportunistic samples, such as clothing items, bone, or teeth, may be used for a technique known as electron spin resonance. These samples can be affected significantly by environmental factors such as heat and cold, so the involved dosimetry laboratory must be consulted about the environmental factors prior to the storage of samples. National dosimetry resources may be identified by REAC/TS and the Armed Forces Radiobiological Research Institute.

Environmental Surveys

In the course of verifying a potential radiation exposure, a radiation survey team may need to be sent to the site in question to determine if a radiation hazard truly exists. This capability will vary from state to state; some states, such as Florida, have radiation survey teams that are available 24 hours a day, while other states with poorly staffed state radiation health departments may have great difficulty activating field teams. In any event, the appropriate state radiation assessment agency will need to be notified of a potential radiation hazard that requires verification. The clinician must be courteous but firm in obtaining this assistance, as encountering resistance to the investigation of a casual allegation of radiation exposure is common. Substantial resistance by state radiation health departments may indicate poor radiation disaster preparedness and planning. The clinician should then make this state of resistance known to state and local political authorities (see Chapters 8 and 10). The clinician then usually obtains cooperation from that state agency with ease.

Internal Contamination Issues

Internal contamination issues include a hazard assessment for which radionuclides a given hospital might encounter, as well as the subsequent sources of needed therapeutic agents. For several decades, a debate has raged over whether potassium iodide should be stockpiled. Most exotic agents for internal decontamination, such as Ca-DTPA, Zn-DTPA, and insoluble Prussian blue, may be obtained through REAC/TS. In view of the narrow time frame in which early treatment may have enhanced effectiveness, stocking these agents in advance of a radiation accident may be advisable.

Terrorism Issues

Nondetonation terrorist incidents involving radiation have already occurred. Common sources of radioactivity, particularly in the medical field, have been made secure against accidental exposure, but they do not necessarily protect against theft. A master's thesis, using a theoretical source of 10 Curie (Ci) of ^{192}Ir dispersed by conventional explosion, calculated that standard radiation survey meters might not be capable of detecting the dispersed levels of radioactivity. Therefore, the initial reports of alleged radiation terrorist events might be dismissed as not involving radiation despite the fact that radioactive sources were actually present [23].

Exercises

Training exercises for radiation incidents should use *no-fault* and *explicit review* concepts. Explicit review should be based on a checklist of major objectives to maintain the standards of objective results. Six major elements of radiation exercise performance have been identified so that objective criteria of evaluation are demonstrated [24] (Table 25.7).

Such exercises should be designed to practice the radiation disaster plan and to familiarize all participants with the elements of the plan. Conducting exercises without outlining the objectives to participants should be avoided as it tends to practice the confusion and chaos of the response, not the plan (see Chapter 37).

TABLE 25.7. OBJECTIVE CRITERIA FOR RESPONSE PERFORMANCE

Hazardous material history and data gathering
  Contact plant supervisor for:
    MSDS sheets.
    Laboratory license to determine radionuclide inventories.
    On-site health physicists to provide further accident details.
  Ability to identify internal and external resource personnel.
Contamination control
  REA preparation.
  Contamination control:
    Patient spread.
    Cross-contamination.
Casualty triage
  Personnel should assess hospital resources available (hospital beds and type).
Treatment and disposition
  Evaluate victims for appropriateness of care, treatment, and referral.
Organizational cohesion
  Response organizational chart should be evaluated.
  Team should be evaluated for effectiveness of its organizational structure.
  Each team member should be tasked with no more than three to five duties.
Decontamination equipment
  Equipment should be evaluated for appropriateness and completeness.

Abbreviation: MSDS, material safety data sheets; REA, radiation emergency area.

SUMMARY

Radiation is a substance of lesser toxicity for both victims and responders on the grand scale of hazardous materials toxicity. Consequently, priorities in care shift so that medical stability using universal precautions should be the first priority before radiation issues are addressed. Radiation has the advantage of being evident by a wide range of detection devices. Responders have the burden of documenting the removal of such radiation because it is easily measured. Radiation exposures are frequently litigated, so good documentation is crucial.

ACKNOWLEDGMENTS

The author would like to recognize his physician mentors, the founding physicians of radiation medicine, Drs. Clarence C. Lushbaugh, Eugene Sanger, George L. Voelz, Neil Wald, Tom A. Lincoln, George Poda, Vic Bond, and Angelique Barabanova for their openness and their willingness to teach; his health physics mentors, Drs. Herman Cember, John Auxier, Michael Stabin, Paul W. Frame, James Stubbs, and Show Fong, for giving him an appreciation for the role of the health physicists; and his REAC / TS coworkers, Dr. Shirley Fry; Ann Sipe, LPN; and Sue Holloway, RT, for instilling in him a sense of discipline and dedication to the subject of radiation medicine.

CONTACT INFORMATION

Radiation Emergency Assistance Center Training Site (REACTS). Telephone at 865-481-1000, or page through the operator at Methodist Medical Center, Oak Ridge, Tennessee at 865- 576-3131. *Provides medical consultation on radiation accidents.*

Chemical Transportation Emergency Center (CHEMTREC). Telephone at 800-424-9300 (in the District of Columbia, 202-483-7616) or 703-527-3887 if outside the continental United States.

Agency for Toxic Substances and Disease Registry (ATSDR). Telephone at 888-422-8737. *Provides 24-hour advice.*

Conference of Radiation Control Program Directors, Inc. (CRCPD). Telephone at 502-227-4543. *Maintains lists of State Radiation Health Contacts for planning purposes.*

Armed Forces Radiobiological Research Institute, Medical Radiation Assistance Team (MRAT). Page at 800-SKY-PAGE (Pin 801-0338) or telephone at 301-295-0316.

Lymphocyte Cytogenetics Evaluation. Four sources.

1. University of Pennsylvania. Contact Niel Wald, M.D.
2. Armed Forces Radiobiology Research Institute (AFRRI).
3. Through REAC/TS referral.
4. Through International Atomic Energy Agency (IAEA) referral

REFERENCES

General Sources

International Atomic Energy Agency. *Diagnosis and treatment of radiation injuries.* International Atomic Energy Agency Safety Reports Series no. 2. Vienna: International Atomic Energy Agency, 1998.

International Atomic Energy Agency. *Lessons learned from accidents in industrial radiography.* International Atomic Energy Agency Safety Reports Series no. 7. Vienna: International Atomic Energy Agency, 1998.

International Atomic Energy Agency. *An electron accelerator accident in Hanoi, Vietnam.* Vienna: International Atomic Energy Agency, 1996.

International Atomic Energy Agency. *The radiological accident at the irradiation facility in Nesvizh.* Vienna: International Atomic Energy Agency, 1996.

International Atomic Energy Agency. *Lessons learned from accidents in industrial irradiation facilities.* Vienna: International Atomic Energy Agency, 1996.

International Atomic Energy Agency. *Accidental overexposure of radiotherapy patients in San Jose, Costa Rica.* Vienna: International Atomic Energy Agency, 1998.

International Atomic Energy Agency. *Planning the medical response to radiological accidents.* International Atomic Energy Agency Safety Reports Series no. 4. Vienna: International Atomic Energy Agency, 1998.

International Atomic Energy Agency. *The radiological accident in Tammiku.* Vienna: International Atomic Energy Agency, 1998.

International Atomic Energy Agency. *The radiological accident in the reprocessing plant at Tomsk.* Vienna: International Atomic Energy Agency, 1998.

Fong F, Schrader DC. Radiation disasters and emergency department preparedness. *Emerg Med Clin North Am* 1996;2:349–369.

Henge-Napoli MH, Stradling GN, Taylor DM, eds. Decorporation of radionuclides from the human body. *Radiat Protect Dosimetry* 2000;1:1–59.

Lincoln TA. Importance of initial management of persons internally contaminated with radionuclides. *Am Indust Hyg Assoc J* 1976;37: 16–21.

Office of Nuclear Regulatory Research CR-4214. *Health effects models for nuclear power plant accident consequence analysis: low LET radiation, part II: scientific bases for health effects models.* United States Nuclear Regulatory Commission, 1989.

Reeves GI. Radiation injuries. *Crit Care Clin North Am* 1999;2: 457–472.

Shull WJ. The somatic effects of exposure of atomic radiation: the Japanese experience, 1947–1997. *Proc Natl Acad Sci* 1998;95: 5437–5441.

Jarrett DG, ed. *Medical management of radiological casualties handbook.* Bethesda: Military Medical Operations Office, Armed Forces Radiobiology Research Institute, 1999. Also available at: http://www.afrri.usuhs.mil/.

Reeves GI, Jarrett DG, Seed TM, et al., eds. *Triage of irradiated personnel.* Bethesda: Armed Forces Radiobiology Research Institute, 1998.

Voelz GL. Current approaches to the management of internally contaminated persons. In: Hubner KF, Fry SA, eds. *The medical basis for radiation accident preparedness.* The Hague, Netherlands: Elsevier, 1980:311–323.

Voelz GL. *A collection of helpful items for medical evaluation of ionizing radiation exposure cases.* Publication LA-UR-80-1105. Los Alamos: Los Alamos Scientific Laboratory, 1980.

Specific Sources

1. Brill AB, ed. *Low dose radiation effects: a fact book*. New York: Society of Nuclear Medicine, 1982:1–5.

2. Kathren RL, ed. *Principles and application of collective dose in radiation protection*, NCRP report 121. Bethesda, MD: National Council on Radiation Protection and Measurements, 1995:65.

3. Kathren RL, ed. *Principles and application of collective dose in radiation protection*, NCRP report 121. Bethesda, MD: National Council on Radiation Protection and Measurements, 1995:64.

4. Nonstochastic effects of ionizing radiation. *Ann ICRP* 1984;41: 1–33.

5. Radiation Emergency Assistance Center/Training Site Videotape. *Hospital management of radiation accidents*. Oak Ridge, TN: Oak Ridge Associated Universities, 1980.

6. Voelz GL. Uranium. In: Sullivan JB, Krieger GR, eds. *Hazardous materials toxicology*. Baltimore: Williams & Wilkins, 1992:1155.

7. Browne D, Weiss JF, MacVittie TJ, et al., eds. *Treatment of radiation injuries*. New York: Plenum Press, 1990:229.

8. Sevara J, Bár J. *Handbook of radioactive contamination and decontamination*. New York: Elsevier, 1991:260.

9. Dunster HJ. *Maximum permissible levels of skin contamination*. United Kingdom Atomic Energy Authority report no. ASHB(RP)R-28. Harwell Birks, England: United Kingdom Atomic Energy Authority, 1962.

10. Walker RI, Cerveny TJ, eds. *Medical consequences of nuclear warfare*. Falls Church, VA: Textbook of Military Medicine Pubications, Office of the Surgeon General, 1989.

11. Gerber GB, Thomas RG, eds. Guidebook for the treatment of accidental radionuclide contamination of workers. *Radiat Protect Dosimetry* 1992;41:25.

12. Muggenburg BA, Felicetti SA, Silbaugh SA. Removal of inhaled radioactive particles by lung lavage—a review. *Health Phys* 1997; 33:213–220.

13. Nolibe D, Métivier H, Masse R, et al. Benefits and risks of bronchopulmonary lavage: a review. *Radiat Protect Dosimetry* 1989; 26:337–343.

14. Gerber GB, Thomas RG. Methods of treatment. Guidebook for the treatment of accidental internal radionuclide contamination of workers. *Radiat Protect Dosimetry* 1992;41:32.

15. Poda GA. *Commonsense decontamination and wound care*. Radiation Emergency Assistance Center/Training Site training handout. Oak Ridge, TN: Oak Ridge Associated Universities, 1991.

16. Taylor DM, Stradling GN, Hengé-Napoli MH. The scientific background to decorporation aerosols. *Radiat Protect Dosimetry* 2000;87:13.

17. International Commission on Radiological Protection. Age-dependent doses to members of the public from intake of radionuclides: part 3. Ingestion dose coefficients. ICRP publication no. 69. *Ann ICRP* 1995;25.

18. Stradling GN, Hengé-Napoli MH, Paquet F, et al. Approaches for experimental evaluation of chelating agents. *Radiat Protect Dosimetry* 2000;87:21.

19. Stradling GN, Taylor DM, Hengé-Napoli MH, et al. Treatment for actinide-bearing industrial dusts and aerosols. *Radiat Protect Dosimetry* 2000;87:46.

20. National Council of Radiation Protection and Measurements. *Management of persons accidentally contaminated with radionuclides*. NCRP Report no. 65. Bethesda, MD: National Council of Radiation Protection and Measurements, 1979:108.

21. Cember H. *Introduction to health physics*, 3rd ed. New York: McGraw-Hill, 1996:277.

22. National Research Council. *Health effects of exposure to low levels of ionizing radiation—BEIR V*. Washington, D.C.: National Academy Press, 1990:6.

23. Aldridge JP. *The role of health physicists in contemporary radiological emergency response*. Master's thesis. Atlanta: Georgia Institute of Technology, March 1998.

24. Fong F, Schrader DC. Radiation disasters and emergency department preparedness. *Emerg Med Clin North Am* 1996;14:365–366.

HAZARDOUS MATERIALS DISASTERS

HOWARD W. LEVITIN
HENRY J. SIEGELSON

A worker collapses while inspecting a chemical storage container. A second worker rescues the first worker and then collapses. Both are assessed by emergency medical services (EMS), placed into hazardous materials (HazMat) body bags, and transported to the local level I trauma center. The patients are admitted to the emergency department (ED). When the body bags are opened, paramedics and nurses become ill. Realizing that the patients are covered with chemicals, personnel in charge make the decision to try to remove the unknown contaminants. The patients are rolled to the showers in the surgeon's lounge adjacent to the operating room to wash off the chemicals. Off-gassing chemicals cause injuries among the transporting paramedics and the nursing staff, and both the ED and the operating room are temporarily closed.

Hazardous materials represent a complex and significant hazard for emergency health care workers. Disasters involving exposures to hazardous materials are relatively rare events, but they still represent one of the most common disasters that occur in the community setting. Unless the ED is prepared to deal with the complications arising from the management of these injuries, a single patient exposed to a hazardous material may overwhelm even a modern, high volume facility.

Victims of HazMat incidents often seek medical assessment and care in the ED. To evaluate and treat these victims safely, policies and procedures that govern contaminated victim assessment and management must be developed.

Although every emergency department has the capacity to offer adequate medical care to these victims, the risk of personal injury due to secondary contamination mandates specific policies and personal protective equipment (PPE) to prevent unprotected contact with the victim. Protecting hospital employees and staff from injury due to hazardous materials is a worker safety issue, and, in the United States, it is covered by federal and state regulations.

An essential component of every hospital ED must be the capacity to assess, decontaminate, and treat victims exposed to hazardous materials safely. The health care facility (HCF) and the administrative staff have the responsibility to provide a safe environment in which to deliver this care. Making this capacity universal will be one of the great challenges for EDs in this decade.

HAZARDOUS MATERIALS

A hazardous material is any substance that is potentially toxic to the environment or to living cells, including microorganisms, plants, animals, and humans. This definition includes not only chemicals but also biologic and radiologic agents. Hazardous materials are used in the production and manufacture of almost every product that man consumes, wears, or uses.

The potential for exposure is significant. In early 1999, the Environmental Protection Agency estimated that approximately 850,000 facilities in the United States were working with hazardous or extremely hazardous substances. Many of these sites are located in urban areas. Approximately 60,500 accidents with hazardous materials occur nationwide annually, with over 2,550 resulting in casualties (1). This number probably underestimates the true scope of the problem. The United States produces over 60,000 chemicals. The Department of Transportation considers many of these chemicals to be hazardous (2,3). The Occupational Safety and Health Administration (OSHA) estimates that 575,000 chemicals can be found in the workplace (4), 53,000 of which are potentially hazardous (5). Over 4 billion tons of chemicals are transported annually by air, surface, and water (Fig. 26.1).

Accurate and reliable data on the public health consequences of hazardous materials releases are difficult to obtain. Few agencies worldwide mandate reporting human exposure to hazardous materials to governmental authorities. In the United States, the Agency for Toxic Substances and Disease Registry (ATSDR) has maintained an active, state-based Hazardous Substances Emergency Events Surveillance (HSEES) system since 1990. This system has generated a great deal of information concerning human expo-

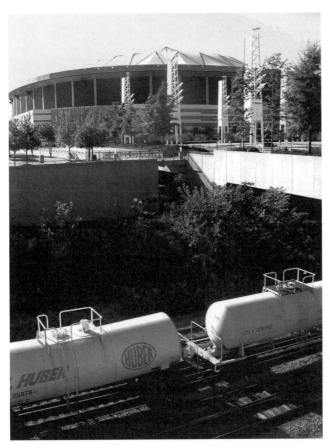

FIGURE 26.1. Chemical rail car near Georgia Dome.

sures to hazardous materials and the public health consequences of these exposures.

The data, however, are limited because the ATSDR must rely on state health departments to collect the information. The number of state health departments participating in the system has decreased to 13 in 1997 from a high of 14 in 1996 (out of a total of 50 state health departments). The data from EDs are particularly scanty because no mandatory reporting requirement exists. In addition, currently little day-to-day communication occurs between hospital EDs and state health departments. Federal support for syndromic surveillance will enable more frequent reporting.

In the 1996 HSEES report (6), the ATSDR data indicated that 5,502 hazardous materials events had been reported in 14 states. Most hazardous materials accidents (70%) occur on weekdays between the hours of 6 AM to 6 PM; only 18% of the accidents occur on weekends. Approximately 68% of these events involve only one or two victims.

ATSDR data reveal that 79% of these hazardous material releases occur at fixed sites (i.e., industrial sites, schools, farms, and manufacturing facilities) and that 21% are transportation-related. A single substance is released in 96% of the events. Volatile organic compounds, acids, ammonia, pesticides, and other organic substances are most commonly involved. The identity of the agent is initially unknown in 25% of the cases.

The victims most frequently are employees of fixed facilities. Among first responders, injuries at fixed facilities are most likely to be among volunteer firefighters (31%), responders of unknown affiliation (22%), and full-time firefighters (17%). In transportation events, first responder victims are primarily police officers (63%) and responders of unknown affiliation (27%). Among the victims, 65% of the employees and 45% of the responders do not wear any PPE. In those cases in which protection was used, the level of personal protection worn was usually insufficient for the responsible agent.

The majority (84%) of hazardous materials accident victims in this study receive definitive medical care at the hospital. Surprisingly, few victims (8%) require admission.

Given the quantity of chemicals handled daily in manufacturing, transportation, and storage, a practicing emergency physician will inevitably be confronted with exposed or contaminated patients. To reduce victim morbidity as well as to ensure the safety of the treating health care providers, the hospital must have the capacity to quickly use PPE and to perform patient decontamination.

A patient is considered contaminated when direct physical contact with a hazardous material has occurred and the substance remains on the body or clothing. Under these circumstances, contaminated victims have the potential of spreading this agent to others (secondary contamination). If the contact is simply an exposure to a toxic vapor or gas, then nearly all of the contaminants will be removed when the clothing is removed (7).

HAZMAT EXPOSURES

HCFs receive victims who are exposed to hazardous materials from numerous sources. Many homes in the United States use insecticides, cleaning agents, and other hazardous chemicals that can be spilled or swallowed by family members. These victims will usually go to the closest hospital for care. Thousands of tons of chemicals are transported in the United States each year. Victims of transportation accidents who are exposed to hazardous materials will be transported to a HCF for definitive care.

Industries that manufacture, transport, and use hazardous chemicals are mandated to develop and exercise a disaster plan. This industry relies on local HCFs to develop the appropriate policies and procedures to enable medical treatment of their employees. Many hospital chief executive officers would be surprised to learn that their HCF is a designated receiving facility that is mentioned specifically in the chemical company's disaster plans. The chemical industry is not required to make certain that the receiving hospital has the capacity to treat their injured employees. Given the low cost of preparedness, equipment, and training, many HCFs could look to the local chemical industry for funds to support this training.

The Superfund Amendments and Reauthorization Act (SARA) title III (Community Right to Know Act) requires most state and local governments to provide planning for chemical emergencies, especially mass casualty events (8). As a component of this standard, the governor of each participating state designates a state and local emergency planning committee (LEPC) to establish procedures for developing and implementing an emergency response plan in the case of a hazardous materials incident. Members of the LEPC include elected state and local officials; police, fire, and public health professionals; environmental, health, and transportation officials; and representatives of health care facilities, community groups, and the media. As part of this planning process, specific hospitals are designated as treatment facilities. The authors of SARA title III hoped that, by creating these designated hospitals, funding and training resources would be concentrated at these institutions and prehospital transfer protocols established (9,10).

Identifying hospitals to receive contaminated patients, in theory, alleviates the hazardous materials preparedness requirements of the other health care institutions in the community. Unfortunately, this concept of designating hospitals as decontamination facilities *falsely* assumes the following (11):

- All contaminated victims will be decontaminated at the scene.
- All patients involved in a HazMat incident will be transported only to designated hospitals.
- Contaminated victims arriving by private vehicle will go only to designated hospitals.
- Victims incorrectly presenting to nondesignated hospitals can be safely transferred to appropriate institutions.

HazMat training, PPE needs, and decontamination requirements do not differ between a designated and nondesignated decontamination facility. Although specific hospitals may be assigned as receiving facilities, this does not alleviate the preparedness requirements of all institutions that might receive emergency patients (12). All hospitals must have a minimum capability to manage chemically contaminated victims safely.

REGULATIONS

Managed care and reduced Medicare reimbursement has strained the financial stability of health care facilities. Thus, unfunded mandates, such as preparedness for HazMat, have been met with incredulity from some and resignation from others. Are these regulations, which are clearly delineated in the United States Code of Federal Regulations published by the United States Government Printing Office

(13), merely an excessive regulation of United States businesses, or are they a reasonable attempt to protect HCF employees?

For health care workers, HazMat preparedness is a matter of worker safety (14). Most hospital administrators, once they are made aware of existing regulations, will attempt to comply. Until the existing OSHA regulations are proven otherwise with rigorous testing and research, they offer a standard upon which hospital preparations for chemical casualties must be based. Extraordinary expenses associated with preparedness for mass casualties from an accidental community HazMat release or an intentional terrorist attack should be augmented with federal and state dollars.

Hospitals are very comfortable with universal precautions designed to protect health care workers from exposure to biologic hazards. PPE that is adequate for biologic and radiologic protection is not adequate for protection from chemicals. Hospitals must support systems that protect ED personnel and other health care workers who are caring for contaminated patients. Because many contaminated patients receive initial care (i.e., decontamination) at the hospital, ED personnel, as well as the facility, are at risk of secondary contamination if these victims are not treated appropriately. Hospitals must be prepared to treat these individuals quickly without jeopardizing the health and safety of their staff.

OSHA regulations require employers to furnish a place of employment free from recognized hazards that are likely to cause death or serious physical harm to their employees (15). Employers are also required to provide appropriate PPE and training to employees who have the potential of being exposed to hazardous materials (16).

OSHA (17,18), the National Institute for Occupational Safety and Health (NIOSH), and the Joint Commission on Accreditation of Healthcare Organizations (JCAHO) (19), as well as several other regulatory and certifying agencies, have developed regulations and standards specific for HazMat emergencies. Although a fair amount of regulatory duplication is found among these various organizations, the standards developed and enforced by OSHA are the foundation upon which all hazardous materials preparedness decisions are based. OSHA's regulations specifically address issues of employee safety, personal protection, decontamination, and training.

OSHA recognizes that hospital personnel do not require advanced training in control, containment, or confinement operations similar to that required of fire department HazMat response teams. These individuals, however, are still considered members of an emergency response team by OSHA, and they must therefore be trained to perform the duties and functions expected of them (18,20). As a result, every ED must address certain regulatory issues (16) specific to an emergency decontamination operation, including the following:

- **Hospital emergency response plan.** A written plan must be established before a HazMat incident addressing staff safety, incident command, decontamination, PPE, evacuation, air monitoring, post-emergency critique of the hospital's emergency response, and the role of the hospital in a community-wide disaster. In addition, standard operating procedures (SOP), which spell out the roles and responsibilities of each member of the decontamination team, must also be developed.
- **Personal protection.** Every employee designated to wear a respirator must have a thorough medical evaluation to verify his or her current fitness to wear PPE. This includes a medical examination, occupational history, and the completion of the OSHA Medical Evaluation Questionnaire.
- **Training.** Minimally, all hospital personnel (e.g., physicians, nurses, security, and triage) who have a designated role in a HazMat emergency operation must be trained to OSHA's First Responder Awareness level (Table 26.1). This level of training provides personnel with an understanding of how to recognize a potential hazardous materials problem and to respond accordingly. Personnel designated to wear PPE to provide patient care must be trained to the First Responder Operations level (Table 26.1) and must then receive additional training in decontamination (21). This level of training includes instruction on decontamination, PPE, incident command, and HazMat emergency response. Individuals indirectly involved in the operation should be trained to the level of their responsibility (i.e., site security). These

individuals are classified by OSHA as skilled support personnel, and they require only an initial briefing at the time of the incident, including instruction in the wearing of appropriate PPE, what chemical hazards are involved, and what duties are to be performed. Retraining must be provided on an annual basis.

The JCAHO refers directly to the training and preparedness of health care personnel with regard to the management of patients exposed to hazardous materials in its environment of care standard. For the management of contaminated patients, the standards refer directly to OSHA's 1910.120 (q) standards (19).

Some will argue that the hospital can simply refuse to care for contaminated patients. Federal law, however, may make this option to be neither viable nor legal. The Consolidated Omnibus Budget Reconciliation Act (COBRA) was passed in 1986 (22). Also referred to as Emergency Medical Treatment and Active Labor Act (EMTALA), this law addresses patient dumping and mandates a medical screening examination of all patients presenting to an ED. The Health Care Financing Administration is responsible for enforcement of this statute. The purpose of the medical screening examination required by EMTALA is to identify the presence of an emergency medical condition. If present, EMTALA also requires stabilization of the emergency medical condition. If the hospital does not have the capabilities to stabilize, then an appropriate transfer should be arranged in accordance with EMTALA. In this case, stabilize means to provide medical treatment so that, within reasonable

TABLE 26.1. HAZARDOUS MATERIALS TRAINING LEVELS

Level 1: First responder awareness
  Witnesses or discovers a release of a hazardous material; is trained to notify the proper authorities. Training includes the recognition and identification of hazardous materials, proper notification procedures, and the employee's role in the ERP.
Level 2: First responder operations
  Responds to the release of hazardous substances in a defensive manner without actually trying to stop the release. Requires level 1 competency and 8 hours of additional training in basic hazard and risk assessment, PPE selection, containment and control procedures, decontamination, and standard operating procedures.
Level 3: Hazardous materials technician
  Responds aggressively to stop a release. Requires 24 hours of level 2 training and competencies in the following: detailed risk assessment; toxicology; PPE selection; advanced control, containment, and decontamination procedures; air-monitoring equipment; and the ICS.
Level 4: Hazardous materials specialist
  Responds with and provides support to hazardous materials technicians, but has advanced knowledge of hazardous materials. Requires 24 hours of level 3 training and proven competencies, along with advanced instruction, on all specific hazardous material topics.
Level 5: On-site incident commander
  Assumes control of the incident beyond what is required for level 1. Requires 24 hours of training equivalent to level 2 with competencies in the ICS and ERP, hazard and risk assessment, and decontamination procedures.

Abbreviations: ERP, emergency response plan; ICS, incident command system; PPE, personal protective equipment. Infection control practices advisory committee. Guideline for isolation procedures in hospitals. *Infect Control Hosp Epidemiol* 1996;17:53–80; with permission.

medical probability, no material deterioration of the patient's condition is likely to occur during the transfer of the individual (23).

With regard to the management of chemically contaminated victims, if the HCF does not have adequate protocols, procedures, and PPE, then performing an adequate screening examination safely will be difficult. A contaminated patient will require decontamination before entry to the HCF. Initial triage is performed at that time. Secondary triage and final assessment will be performed after decontamination. Stabilization of the medical condition will certainly require adequate decontamination and may require further medical intervention. Transferring a contaminated patient to another facility may be difficult because it may lead to further patient injury. Failure to provide a medical screening examination and adequate treatment to this patient may result in a violation of EMTALA, and failure to use adequate PPE with appropriate training will violate OSHA regulations. To date, a test case for this theoretical catch-22 has not occurred.

Hospital administrative personnel have responded with vigor in a review of existing hospital disaster plans after the September 11, 2001 terrorist attack on the World Trade Center and the Pentagon and the subsequent anthrax attacks. Many hospitals are working with their state hospital associations to develop reasonable minimum levels of preparedness to meet the terrorist threat. The JCAHO and the American Hospital Association have recommended policies and procedures for mass casualty and bioweapons planning and response. These can be found on their respective websites (http://www.jcaho.org/ and http://www.aha.org/).

Mass transfer of patients to alternate HCFs or off-site treatment centers may be reasonable during a mass casualty event in which hundreds of victims may present with minimal exposure and a lack of clinical symptoms. Hospital transfer during mass casualty events should be prearranged with memoranda of understanding consistent with the community disaster plan. Before transfer, however, the victims should have the opportunity to remove contaminated clothing to prevent further exposure to the hazard. Triage decisions that lead to transfer should follow prearranged protocols. State legislatures should indemnify triage officers from malpractice and civil suits if the transfer is made during a response to a disaster or a mass casualty incident.

PERSONAL PROTECTIVE EQUIPMENT

PPE shields personnel from contact with hazardous materials. PPE is required of all employees who have the potential of being exposed to any hazard capable of causing injury through absorption, inhalation, or physical contact. Typical hospital universal precautions, such as paper or plastic gowns, paper masks, and surgical gloves, while adequate for most biologic and radiologic hazards, are inadequate for protecting personnel from chemical hazards.

The typical HazMat PPE ensemble includes a chemical-resistant suit, gloves, boots, and a respirator that work in unison to shield an individual from a variety of chemical and physical hazards. Choosing the proper level of protection depends on a variety of factors, including the type of hazard, its chemical properties, and the risk of inhalation and skin contamination posed by the agent (24). Although no combination of PPE protects against all hazards, the equipment selected should provide as much protection as possible to the skin, eyes, face, hands, feet, and respiratory tract.

Fire and HazMat personnel working in environments immediately dangerous to life and health (IDLH) require the highest level of protection. Level A gear, which includes a totally encapsulating suit with very thick gloves and boots, is impractical for the ED (Table 26.2). These suits limit movement, patient assessment, and time in the garment due to heat exposure and a limited air source. This level of threat is rarely encountered in the hospital ED. If an event occurs, such as an attack on a medical facility with chemicals or a spill of chemicals that exceed IDLH levels, the incident should be treated as a 911 emergency. The local fire department or HazMat team should be notified, and the area of the spill should be cordoned off.

Any valid discussion on the appropriate selection of PPE for hospitals must address applicable state and federal regu-

TABLE 26.2. LEVELS OF PERSONAL PROTECTIVE EQUIPMENT

Level A	Provides the maximal amount of vapor and splash protection. This suit is fully encapsulated and chemically resistant. It requires the use of a self-contained breathing apparatus, along with chemical protective gloves and boots.
Level B	Chemically resistant suits that guard against splash exposures and offer less protection against skin, eye, and mucus membrane exposure as compared to a level A. This type of suit requires the use of a positive pressure, full-faced respirator, along with chemically resistant gloves and boots; it is the minimum level of protection required for unknown contaminants.
Level C	Protection is used when the identity of the chemical hazard is known and its exposure risk is below the concentration that will cause ill effects. An air-purifying respirator is required to filter out contaminants.
Level D	Only used when no danger of chemical exposure exists. This ensemble includes work clothes without a respirator.

lations that deal with worker safety issues for general industry and hospitals. Although various levels of protection are available, an atmosphere-supplied (positive pressure) respirator may be required when the agent is unknown and/or it poses a potential inhalation hazard (13). According to OSHA, the level B protective clothing ensemble and atmosphere-supplied respirator is the minimum level of protection allowed under those circumstances (25). Level B protective gear provides the broadest protection from the chemicals and radioactive materials that are most commonly encountered in the ED setting.

In industrial settings in which the contaminant is identified and known to be present at an air concentration below the maximum level for which the respirator is recommended, an air-purifying (mask and filter) respirator may be appropriate (level C). After years of research and discussion, OSHA and NIOSH approved modified level C protective gear (i.e., the use of a powered air-purifying respirator and appropriate air-filtering canister) for use by first responders in the event of a release of chemical agents from United States military chemical weapons depots (26,27). This recommendation refers specifically to the use of level C for identified chemical warfare agents (sarin, agent VX, and mustard) at appropriately low air concentrations that safely allow this level of equipment to be used. This recommendation, however, cannot be extrapolated to all potentially toxic agents that may be involved in hazardous materials incidents or terrorist events.

As more advanced filters are developed and approved for the protection of first responders against unknown chemical exposures, then level C may be appropriate for the hospital (28). However, until the advent of research results prove differently, the current standards require a higher level of respiratory protection (level B).

The level of PPE required for health care providers and support staff varies depending on their risk of exposure and their assigned responsibilities during a HazMat incident. Hospital personnel directly involved in the decontamination of patients will find that level B protective gear (including an atmosphere-supplying respirator tethered via an airline hose to an external air source) is sufficient for such tasks. The proper level of protection, however, must be tailored to the hazard involved. Level C protection may be used if the chemical is identified and its air concentration has measured and determined to be below a level determined to be IDLH. Level D protection is sufficient for security and other support personnel who are responsible for constructing and securing the decontamination area and for assisting designated personnel to don PPE. All other personnel should follow standard (universal) precautions when interacting with patients who have already completed the decontamination process.

The use of PPE may create hazards to the wearer. The equipment can produce heat stress and can impair visibility, mobility, and communication, along with causing a variety of psychological stresses (e.g., claustrophobia). These problems are more commonly associated with higher levels of personal protection in which the responder is totally encapsulated within the protective gear (e.g., level A). The proper selection of equipment, appropriate training (and periodic retraining), and familiarity with the gear will significantly reduce these problems. Because of these potential hazards, the employer must keep accurate training and medical records for all workers who use PPE.

In addition, according to OSHA's respiratory protection policy, employers must provide the following to all employees who are designated to wear a respirator (either atmosphere-supplying or air-purifying):

- A comprehensive medical examination, which includes the completion of a respiratory medical evaluation questionnaire (a sample questionnaire is included in the regulation);

TABLE 26.3. RECOMMENDED PERSONAL PROTECTIVE EQUIPMENT FOR POTENTIAL BIOLOGIC AGENTS

Disease	Type of Precautions Required*	Negative Pressure Required?	Gloves Required?	Gowns Required?	Surgical Masks?	N95 or HEPA Filter?
Anthrax	Standard	No	Yes	As needed	As needed	—
Pneumonic plague	Droplet/standard	No	Yes	As needed	Yes	—
Pulmonary tularemia	Standard	No	Yes	As needed	As needed	—
Brucellosis	Standard	No	Yes	As needed	As needed	—
Smallpox	Airborne/contact	Yes	Yes	Yes	—	Yes
Lassa fever	Airborne/contact	Yes	Yes	Yes	—	Yes
Ebola	Airborne/contact	Yes	Yes	Yes	—	Yes
Marburg virus	Airborne/contact	Yes	Yes	Yes	—	Yes

HEPA, high-efficiency particulate air.
From APIC/CDC Bioterrorism Task Force. APIC/COC bioterrorism readiness plan: a template for healthcare facilities. *Assoc Prof Infect Control* 1999; Garner J. Hospital infection control practices advisory committee: guideline for isolation procedures in hospitals. *Infect Control Hosp Epidemiol* 1996;17:53–80; with permission.
*From Here's mud in your eye. *Health Care Hazard Mater Manage* 1997;11:1,3–4, with permission.

- Mandatory (qualitative or quantitative) fit testing of all employees wearing a respirator;
- A selection of respirators of different sizes and styles; these must be made available to ensure proper employee fit.
- Annual respirator training (or sooner if necessary) of all employees who are designated to wear this equipment.

Victims of contagious biologic infections pose a significant risk to health care workers. Personal protection from potential biologic exposure to contagious illness begins with the aggressive and frequent use of standard precautions. Advanced measures, such as surgical masks, N95 or HEPA filter masks, and negative pressure rooms, are recommended for some potential biologic agents (Table 26.3).

A new recommendation from Seminole County, Florida, suggests that first responders are entering a biologic hot zone when they are within 10 feet of a potentially ill patient. Current recommendations include eye protection, disposable gloves, and a filtration mask. The recommended facial mask is moisture resistant, and it has a minimum bacterial filtration efficiency value of 95% for particles 0.3 μm and larger (N-95 mask) (32).

DECONTAMINATION

Decontamination should be performed whenever known or suspected contamination has occurred with a hazardous substance either through contact with aerosols, solids, or liquids. Patient decontamination is an organized method of removing residual contaminants from the victim's skin and clothing. It is accomplished initially by removing the victim's garments, rinsing the patient with large quantities of water, and collecting the decontamination runoff. Gently scrubbing the skin with soap and a soft brush removes any remaining fat-soluble chemicals and solid materials. Eliminating chemicals from a victim's skin and clothing is important for two reasons. This reduces the risk for further absorption or inhalation and the subsequent toxicity caused by the offending agent. In addition, it helps to prevent others from becoming secondarily exposed or contaminated.

The degree of decontamination performed depends on the situation. In general, removing and bagging the victim's clothing removes up to 80% of the contaminants and minimizes the risk of spreading the toxic agent to others (10). This is the minimum level of decontamination that is acceptable after exposure to a hazardous chemical, a radioactive contamination source, or a terrorist attack.

An area should be established that provides the victims adequate privacy for removing their clothing. Men and women can be separated with the use of privacy curtains that are well shielded from onlookers. This will contribute to the effectiveness of this initial decontamination procedure. A readily available supply of disposable paper gowns or blankets should also be accessible for victims to cover themselves with after they have disrobed or completed decontamination. Personal items (e.g., jewelry, wallets, purses) can be placed in ziplock bags and can be subsequently deposited inside the biohazard bag with their clothing or carried by the patient through the decontamination process. A tagging system should be used to mark the bagged items, as well as the patient, in a mass casualty situation. Local law enforcement or security personnel can be used to guard the victim's belongings. Obviously, prior planning in this area will contribute to the success of the decontamination operation

After a large-scale chemical release with mass casualties, if authorities determine that most of the exposure was due to a vapor, then the removal of clothing may be a sufficient decontamination effort, especially when resources are limited (7,14,33,34). When possible, victims should remove their own clothing to enable staff to assist the symptomatic and nonambulatory victims who may require a full soap and water showering. This form of self-decontamination is feasible because the majority of contaminated patients are ambulatory. Once the clothing has been removed and bagged, the patients can be safely moved into the hospital for medical evaluation as needed. This quick procedure eliminates the need to shelter ambulatory patients outside while they are awaiting decontamination.

A high volume, low-pressure shower (possibly with soap) is required for decontamination if patients are exposed to a liquid or visible hazard. A few chemicals have the capacity to react strongly with water or air with the generation of heat. Water is contraindicated, in theory, in only a few rare situations involving metallic sodium, potassium, lithium, cesium, and rubidium, all of which all react with water. Dusts of pure magnesium, white phosphorus, sulfur, strontium, titanium, uranium, zinc, and zirconium will ignite on contact with air (10). If any of these metallic substances is present on the victim's skin, a chemical reaction already is occurring while the proper method of decontamination is being considered. Although the potential for reaction exists, dilution with very large quantities of water minimizes the ensuing harm. When possible, these substances can be physically removed with forceps and stored in a receptacle containing mineral oil.

Phosphorus burns are particularly destructive. The chemically contaminated wounds, which burn on contact with air, must be asphyxiated with water to stop the burn. The phosphorus particles must be surgically removed. This can be accomplished with a Wood's lamp that causes the chemical to phosphoresce, thus making it easier to remove.

The fire service has routinely provided decontamination at the scene of a release of hazardous materials. Although decontamination is preferably performed at the scene of exposure, a variety of factors, such as adverse weather conditions, inherent time delays, technologic constraints, and the lack of prehospital training and equipment, may hinder or prohibit this procedure. In addition, chemically contaminated victims often bypass even the most experienced decontamination attempts when large numbers of victims are injured. Thus, they present to hospitals in a contaminated state.

Relying on the local fire department to decontaminate patients at the hospital may be impractical. Most fire departments in the United States are volunteer services, with financial constraints that may prohibit investing in HazMat emergency response training and equipment. As a result, many communities do not have teams that respond to HazMat emergencies, and therefore they must rely on the local hospital to perform decontamination. In addition, hospitals in communities fortunate enough to have hazardous materials response teams (HMRT) quickly realize that HMRTs are contracted to the city and not to the hospital. During some HazMat accidents, these emergency responders may be occupied at the scene, thus leaving hospitals to care for contaminated patients who reach their ED without prehospital decontamination. This is especially true in circumstances in which victims are unaware of their contamination and present to the ED for related injuries.

In a 6-year review of patients presenting to a community hospital ED for management of exposure to hazardous chemicals, none of the 72 patients received prehospital decontamination (35). Consequently, hospitals must incorporate the necessary training, protocols, procedures, and equipment to become self-sufficient in the care of the contaminated patient.

In addition, most hazardous materials accidents are small-scale events involving only one or two victims that occur at the workplace (36). These contaminated individuals will often arrive at the hospital by private vehicle before any prehospital decontamination.

Limiting the spread of contamination into the ED is accomplished by the following precautions:

■ Identifying the contaminated individual and preventing him or her from entering the medical facility until he or she has been appropriately decontaminated;
■ Maintaining a safe distance between the patient and caregiver;
■ Ensuring that health care personnel wear appropriate PPE;
■ Having the capacity to perform decontamination quickly with a system of wastewater containment.

Hospital decontamination should be performed at a pre-designated location using an appropriate decontamination system. Entry and exit points should be clearly marked with separate flow patterns established for patients and personnel to limit the spread of contamination. This procedure may be performed outside the ED, perhaps with the use of a portable decontamination system (11,37). Decontamination performed in this manner keeps the contaminant outdoors, and it minimizes the risk of spreading the toxic agent

into the hospital. In addition, an outdoor location provides the space necessary for triaging victims of a mass casualty incident (MCI). The decontamination area should be located outside the hospital facility near the ED entrance but away from the normal patient traffic flow of the hospital.

If a permanent shower facility within the hospital is used, it should be large enough to handle at least two victims along with the appropriate support staff (two to four decontamination team members dressed in protective gear). The decontamination room should include a separate entrance from the outside. In addition, it should be engineered to contain the decontamination runoff, it should be plumbed to provide medical air for the respirators, and it should be capable of ventilating air to the outside. The availability of a permanent facility, however, does not alleviate the need for outdoor decontamination capability in a MCI. Under these circumstances, the need for decontamination will quickly overwhelm the inherent capabilities of a permanent decontamination room. In addition, some chemicals, such as sarin or VX are so toxic that they should never be allowed indoors. Permanent internal and off-the-shelf portable decontamination systems have been developed by some commercial and academic entities (38).

All water runoff from the decontamination process should be collected for future disposal. It should not be allowed to freely flow into the city sewer system, parking lot, or surrounding foliage, as this would serve only to contribute to the spread of the contaminant. After the HazMat response concludes, a private contractor, the local branch of the Environmental Protection Agency (EPA), or the fire department can ascertain the type of chemical contaminant. In some cases, the fire department in consultation with local officials will give the hospital permission to pour the decontamination runoff into the sewer. In other cases, a local HazMat contractor is needed to remove the wastewater for proper disposal. This relationship between the hospital and the HazMat disposal service should be contracted in advance to assure rapid and appropriate disposal.

Personnel who will have direct contact with contaminated patients needing assistance through the decontamination process should wear the appropriate protective gear. At least two individuals must suit up and be ready to intervene if a patient requires help. In most cases, victims will be able to remove their own clothing and to shower themselves without the need of any hands-on assistance. Under these circumstances, the two emergency responders in PPE will remain on stand-by at the side of the decontamination corridor.

In the event of a MCI that results in HazMat contamination that poses a threat to life and health, performing emergency decontamination with minimal or no containment of the run-off is possible. According to the Emergency Coordinator of the EPA (39), the Good Samaritan provision of the Comprehensive Environmental Response, Compensation, and Liability Act (CERCLA), 40CFR, limits liability related to the results of actions "taken or omitted in the course of rendering care, assistance, or advice in accordance with the National Contingency Plan... with respect to an incident creating a danger to public health or welfare or the environment as a result of any releases of a hazardous substance or the threat thereof" (36). In fact, section 107 (d) (2) provides that state and local governments are not liable under CERCLA as a result of actions taken in response to an emergency created by the release or threatened release of a hazardous substance (39). Whether this exception applies to hospitals is not known. CERCLA, however, does not preclude private parties (e.g., an environmental interest group) from filing suit.

INITIAL ASSESSMENT

To protect the hospital facility, personnel, and patients, the contaminated patient must be recognized before entering the facility. The triage area is the entrance to the ED. Triage nurses, ED technicians, clerical staff, and security form the personnel of the triage unit. As patients arrive for care in the department, whether by EMS or private vehicle, all must pass through the triage area. All triage personnel must receive awareness training for HazMat or terrorist-associated patient presentations.

Once victims of a HazMat exposure or terrorist attack are recognized, patients should be directed out of the hospital to a designated location near the ED entrance to await evaluation and decontamination. These patients should not be left alone because they may either leave or may attempt to enter the hospital again. Optimally, contaminated patients might read a sign or poster situated outside the department that might instruct those contaminated with chemicals to press a button and to wait on an adjacent bench for assessment (Fig. 26.2). This would enable the patient to participate in their care by announcing their presence and thus avoiding accidental secondary contamination of the department. That most unsupervised patients would cooperate with such a system is unlikely however, so staff must be appropriately trained to cope with this circumstance.

As soon as hospital personnel recognize the presence of a contaminated patient, the hospital HazMat response plan should be activated. This will enable a specially trained team to do the following:

- Determine the extent of patient contamination;
- Assess the possibility of other victims;
- Activate the hospital decontamination plan;
- Instruct the patient to disrobe, while awaiting decontamination, in an environment that maximizes privacy;
- Begin patient decontamination;
- Provide patient care as needed.

In the event of a terrorist attack or sudden event associated with an explosion or the release of chemicals or radioactive materials, one should assume that the victims are contaminated. Proving with certainty in the initial moments after a terrorist attack whether or not hazardous materials have been used by the terrorist to cause harm to the victims and the community is extremely difficult. Although some chemical detection equipment exists, this equipment is not totally reliable, and it measures only a few types of chemicals. In addition, these resources are not readily available to hospital staff. Fire and HazMat personnel have the capacity to detect certain types of chemicals, and many have expanded this capacity to include some military chemical agents.

Patient decontamination should not be delayed while awaiting chemical identification. Although having detailed information about the involved chemical before the arrival of patient(s) is ideal, this is not always possible. In some cases, the identification of the offending chemical is never determined. If the hazardous chemical is identified, product information can be obtained from the fire department or the HazMat response team at the scene of the incident, from the regional poison center, or from the material safety data sheet (MSDS).

An MSDS is an informational document produced by chemical manufacturers that must be made available to all individuals involved in the manufacturing, shipping, and handling of a hazardous chemical or material. It contains information on the chemical's physical properties, health and safety issues, PPE, and decontamination, as well as information regarding safe use, storage, and disposal procedures. Although the information is not specifically applicable to health care providers, it can assist the decontamination team members in selecting the appropriate level of PPE and the decontamination procedure. The MSDS can be obtained from various sources, including the patient, his or her employer, the manufacturer, regional poison control centers, the Internet, and various other computer databases (40).

(in several appropriate languages)
If you believe that you have been exposed
to a hazardous chemical,
Press the red button below and sit on this bench.
A member of the hospital staff will be out shortly
To assess your condition.

FIGURE 26.2. Sample sign that might be located outside the emergency department in order to instruct contaminated patients. (If you believe that you have been exposed to a hazardous chemical, Press the red button below and sit on this bench. A member of the hospital staff will be out shortly to assess your condition.)

Ideally, patients should be decontaminated before medical treatment to protect the caregiver. In some circumstances, however, trained personnel wearing appropriate PPE might offer medical treatment and decontamination simultaneously. Hospitals should have a portable treatment cart for emergent situations that contains an oxygen tank, Ambu bag, oxygen masks and connections, oral and nasal airways, bronchodilators, bandages, splints, and specific antidotes (e.g., cyanide kit, atropine). Some teams might, after exercises and practice, choose to have intubation equipment as well. Appropriate long-handled instruments should be available to handle contaminated or potentially radioactive materials.

Medical treatment for contaminated patients can be symptom-specific as the following illustrates.

- Eye irritation can be treated with irrigation in the showers, followed by Morgan lens irrigation, medical assessment, and cycloplegia (pupil dilation).
- Pulmonary irritation is treated with bronchodilators and oxygen.
- Skin irritation is addressed with soap and water washing and routine burn therapy.

If adequate time is available, contaminated wounds should be treated before decontaminating the rest of the body. This is best accomplished with the patient sitting on a chair inside the collection pool. A handheld sprayer that is adjusted to provide a gentle flow of water should be used. After the wound has been decontaminated, it should be covered with a water-resistant dressing before the surrounding skin is decontaminated. In the case of radiation contamination, the irrigation runoff can be surveyed to assess the effectiveness of the decontamination. Continued evidence of contamination will require repeated washings, and it may necessitate surgical debridement.

Body orifices, such as the eyes, mouth, and nose should be decontaminated immediately to reduce the rate of absorption of the toxin. This can be initiated during decontamination, and it should then be continued in the ED after decontamination. The eyes should first be anesthetized with a topical anesthetic and should then be irrigated with at least 1 L of normal saline or lactated Ringer's solution. Intravenous tubing (or Morgan Lens) can be used to direct the stream from the inner canthus of the eye to the outer canthus to avoid contaminating the tear ducts. In the case of a corrosive (acid or base) substance, the pH of the conjunctival sac should be checked before and after irrigation to determine if it has returned to normal (tears have a pH of 7.3 to 7.7). If not, the irrigation process should be continued.

In the event of radioactive contamination, biologic samples should be obtained from the nostrils and ears with separate (right and left) Q-tips that are appropriately labeled, timed, and dated. Contamination of the mouth, nose, or ears requires frequent rinsing with tap water or sterile saline.

To complete the decontamination process, brushing of the teeth and cotton swabbing of the nose and external ear canal may also be necessary.

Inhaled toxins or irritants may cause mucous membrane irritation, cough, wheezing, or stridor and may lead to airway compromise in severe exposures. These symptoms may be acute (e.g., anhydrous ammonia, organophosphates, sulfur dioxide, or hydrochloric acid) or delayed (e.g., chlorine or phosgene), and they may be compounded by the presence of combustion byproducts or thermal damage. Treatment requires immediate evacuation from the area, removal of clothing, application of oxygen, and bronchodilators for bronchospasm. Under certain circumstances (e.g., soot in the upper airway, facial burns, stridor, hoarseness, rales, or cyanosis), intubation may be required. Minimally, symptomatic patients should be observed in the ED for at least 6 hours.

CURRENT CAPABILITIES

Few emergency medicine residency programs offer comprehensive training with regard to the management of contaminated casualties (41). In addition, extremely few medical school and nursing school curricula include the management of the victims of HazMat exposures. Although nurses, physicians, and paramedics are being trained nationwide regarding the threats of terrorism, few HCFs or EMS providers have adequate PPE or protocols to deal with the threat of hazardous materials or terrorist attacks.

To prepare the country to deal with the threat of a terrorist attack, the Nunn-Lugar-Domenici Amendment to the FY 97 Defense Authorization Act authorized funds to train local community first responders about the consequences of weapons of mass destruction (WMD) and mass casualty management (42,43). In 1997, the United States Department of Defense's Soldier Biological Chemical Command supervised the development of the Domestic Preparedness Program (44). This training is peer-reviewed, and it is supported by six federal agencies. Emergency physicians and subject matter physician experts facilitate the hospital portion of the program. This program is designed to deliver WMD awareness training to nurses and physicians, but it is limited in scope and geographic availability (45).

The United States Department of Health and Human Services Office of Emergency Preparedness contracted with the American College of Emergency Physicians to identify strategies required to prepare target audiences (e.g., emergency physicians, emergency nurses, paramedics, and emergency medical technicians) to respond to WMD incidents. The contract consisted of two phases. Phase I focused on (a) the identification of needs, demands, and feasibility for nuclear, biologic, and chemical (NBC)-related training; (b) the determination of the barriers and challenges related to delivering NBC training; and (c) the development of high-level educational goals and strategies to attain the identified goals. Phase II focused on (a) a review of educational curricula for each of the target audiences and of six existing courses, (b) a definition of the levels of proficiency and development of associated behavioral objectives, (c) the identification of recommendations for integrating WMD content into initial and continuing education, (d) the identification of recommendations for sustainment of WMD knowledge and skills, and (e) the specification of techniques to ensure continuing proficiencies (46).

For HCFs to prepare to support the community reasonably, separating the discussion of HCF preparations for mass casualties from the daily threat of a HazMat exposure is important. Preparedness for terrorist attacks is a matter of national security, while routine hospital HazMat preparedness is a matter of community responsibility. The current discussion regarding hospital response to a terrorist attack with mass casualties should not obscure the focus on the existing responsibilities inherent upon medical facilities with regard to worker safety. The hospital must provide an environment that is safe for its employees.

Should a hospital prepare for mass casualties from a terrorist attack, as has been recommended by federal agencies, or should hospitals merely prepare for local HazMat events? The answer has significant financial and manpower consequences for a HCF. Hospital chief executive officers have heard mixed and confusing recommendations with regard to this matter. For some hospitals adjacent to large population centers, subways, or large sports facilities, preparations for mass casualties is extremely important. The terrorist attack in New York City on September 11, 2001 and the subsequent anthrax attacks mandate hospital preparation for potential terrorist attacks. How should the hospital begin this preparedness? The author suggests that hospitals focus on community chemical preparedness. Doing so is reasonable because of the following:

- Chemicals are a 24-hour threat.
- Chemicals can cause immediate effects.
- Chemicals require the highest level of personal protection.
- Federal mandates require the appropriate training necessary to wear chemical protective equipment.
- In most communities, the risk of a HazMat exposure is greater than that of a terrorist attack.
- A HazMat emergency is a common community emergency.

Every ED should have the capacity to assess, decontaminate, and treat at least one patient exposed to a hazardous material safely (11). This minimum level of preparedness, which can be expanded based on community needs and threats, mandates specific policies and procedures, PPE, decontamination systems, and OSHA-specified training. The vast majority of HazMat exposures involve only one or two victims (36).

This reasonable model of preparedness for the victims of HazMat exposures, augmented by an awareness of the medical consequences of WMD, should be adequate for most HCFs. The need for HazMat and terrorism mass casualty preparedness should be based on regional HazMat and terrorism threat assessments (47). Selected HCFs identified by regional consensus could offer an expanded and more expansive mass casualty response capacity that is supported by state and federal dollars.

Another popular question is, "If terrorists attack using chemicals, which hazardous agents would be most likely?" Information from ATSDR suggests that industrial chemicals could provide terrorists with effective and the most readily accessible materials to develop improvised explosives, incendiaries, and chemical hazards (48). Weapons of war have changed, and so have the tactics. More than 90% of the casualties of war are civilians (49). Attacks on industry during war threaten surrounding civilians. Iraq destroyed the oil wells in Kuwait during the Persian Gulf War, causing an enormous respiratory threat due to burning oil. In Croatia, the Petrochemia plant was attacked on numerous occasions by the Yugoslavian Serbs in an attempt to expose civilians to hazardous chemicals, including anhydrous ammonia, sulfur, nitric acid, sulfuric acid, phosphoric acid, heavy oil, and formaldehyde (50).

Most facilities should be prepared to treat victims of nerve agent attacks. Iraq used these chemical weapons against Kurdish tribesman and Iranian soldiers. In addition, the religious sect Aum Shinrikyo used sarin against Japanese civilians. The antidotes for nerve agents, atropine and pralidoxime chloride, should be available at the HCF. Although patients exposed to a lethal dose of nerve agent will die quite quickly, some survivors may benefit from antidote therapy.

Sulfur mustard, used extensively by both sides in World War I, is stored in large quantities worldwide. No antidote exists for sulfur mustard.

In his book, *Biohazard*, Alibek describes the former Soviet Union's development of chemicals and biologic agents for which currently no treatment or antidote is available (51).

Therefore, due to the varied threat posed by a terrorist attack, the reasonable course for HCFs is to prepare for a generic unknown hazard. This offers HCF personnel the most protection in the event of an attack. Medical assessment for toxindromes and antidote therapy will proceed once the patient has been decontaminated. In some cases, antidotes may be administered before decontamination by appropriately protected medical personnel and EMS (Table 26.4).

Once HCFs develop policies and procedures that meet the minimum standard, how will hospitals expand their capabilities and manage mass casualties? An Israeli model for mass casualty management after a terrorist attack is a commonly cited approach (52). Ambulatory and nonam-

TABLE 26.4. EMERGENCY ANTIDOTES

Chemical	Antidote
Arsenic	BAL
Atropine	Physostigmine
Carbon monoxide	Oxygen, hyperbarics
Cyanide	Amyl nitrite, sodium nitrite, sodium thiosulfate
Hydrofluoric acid	Calcium
Hydrogen sulfide	Amyl nitrite, sodium nitrite
Iron	Deferoxamine
Lead	Calcium disodium edetate, EDTA, BAL
Lewisite	BAL
Mercury	BAL, D-penicillamine
Nitrites, methemoglobinemia	Oxygen, methylene blue
Organophosphates, nerve agents	Atropine, pralidoxime

Abbreviations: BAL, British anti-Lewisite; EDTA, ethylenediaminetetraacetic acid.

bulatory levels of care are managed in an orderly fashion according to triage criteria. Advanced airway management, bleeding control, and antidote therapy are administered by trained practitioners wearing level C PPE in the warm or contaminated zone. Manpower demands for this system are extreme, and they might require a dedicated in-house specialty response team (Fig. 26.3).

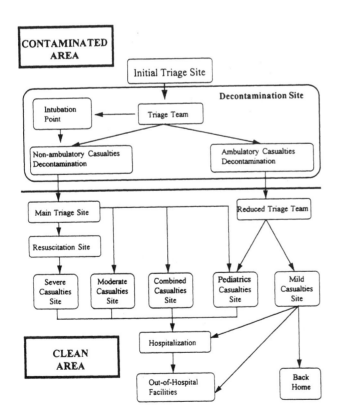

FIGURE 26.3. Hospital deployment plan for the management of mass casualties from a toxicologic event.

A European model using critical care specialists to deliver advanced airway management in the warm zone has been proposed by a number of authors (53–55). In the United States, few programs use anesthesiologists or critical care specialists for airway management in the ED, much less in the field. The Israeli model uses anesthesiologists, as well as other medical specialists, for advanced airway management at the initial triage site.

George Washington Medical Center has developed an in-house chemical mass casualty decontamination system (38). This system was developed due to the proximity of numerous federal buildings in Washington, D.C. and the perceived need for an expanded decontamination capacity.

Several fire departments have developed a system of decontamination using two fire trucks spraying water on an open area.

Commercial systems for the management of contaminated mass casualties are available. These systems are based on portable collapsible shower designs, trailers, and tents (56).

Tur-Kaspa (52) also recommended an Israeli model used to prepare hospitals to respond to a terrorist attack based on the likelihood of the event. These recommendations should be studied for modification in United States hospitals (Table 26.5).

Many of these models assume that large numbers of critically ill survivors will be present. In most studies, however, 80% to 90% of the victims are ambulatory, and they consist of the minimally injured or worried-well. Mass casualty response plans should focus on rapid decontamination (clothing removal) and the evacuation of the ambulatory victims. Then, advanced rescue teams (e.g., fire, HMRT) can use protective gear to evaluate and rescue the nonambulatory survivors from the hot zone. Hospitals should reserve their advanced assessment and treatment modalities for the most critically injured. Ambulatory survivors can be assessed and treated off-site (Fig. 26.4).

TABLE 26.5. LEVELS OF PREPARATION FOR HOSPITAL MASS CASUALTY PREPAREDNESS

Level of preparation*	Action required
I. No threat	Prepare a hospital HazMat deployment plan for a chemical incident. Should be a component of the hospital disaster plan.
II. Minimal threat	1. Review the hospital disaster plan, the HazMat deployment plan, and the principles of chemical agent diagnosis and treatment (once a year). 2. Assign specific tasks in the HazMat deployment plan to hospital personnel. Form HazMat response teams. 3. Enact a partial practice drill as a part of the biannual disaster drills mandated by JCAHO. Coordinate with local fire department (yearly). 4. Consider the need for medical equipment, supplies, and communication systems. Examine yearly for maintenance and equipment review. 5. Set up HazMat decontamination system and review PPE and donning and doffing, every 3 mo.
III. Existing threat	1. Run a full practice drill once in 2 yr; give instruction every year. 2. Prepare appropriate medical equipment, supplies, and communications systems. Examine for maintenance every 6 mo.
IV. Increased threat	1. Organize appropriate shifts of hospital personnel to increase their availability. Activate emergency calling system for the staff and auxiliary manpower according to their assigned tasks. 2. Run a full practice drill once every 1 to 2 yr; give instruction and smaller scale review drills upon receiving the new threat level and as often as possible. 3. Examine maintenance of equipment, protective gear, and communications systems every few months. Increase their availability by storage at or near the sites. 4. Prepare arrangements for shifting patients inside hospital. 5. Review interhospital disaster transfer arrangements. 6. Review contracts with HazMat disposal suppliers and bus companies.
V. Maximal threat	1. Be prepared to receive and treat chemical casualties within minutes to hours. 2. Organize equipment, protective gear, and communication systems at all sites. 3. Arrange patient transfer and discharge when possible. 4. Maintain continuous contact with community authorities.

Abbreviations: HazMat, Hazardous materials; JCAHO, Joint Commission on the Accreditation of Healthcare Organizations; PPE, personal protective equipment.
*Each level should also include the required actions of the previous levels.
Modified from Tur-Kaspa I, Lev EI, Hendler I, et al. Preparing hospitals for toxicological mass casualties events [see comments]. *Crit Care Med* 1999;27:1004–1008, with permission.

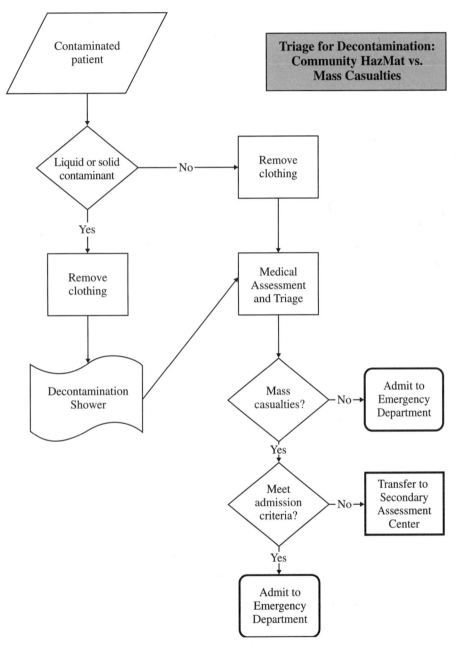

FIGURE 26.4. Triage for decontamination: community HazMat versus mass casualties.

CONCLUSION

Massive quantities of hazardous materials are stored and transported through communities daily. Terrorists have shown the willingness and the capacity to use hazardous chemicals when attacking civilians. Hospitals must be prepared to offer care to these victims. Once a hospital has mastered the technique of decontaminating one victim, they can build on these skills to treat additional victims. The assessment, decontamination, and treatment of mass casualties will require advanced planning, extraordinary resources, and close coordination with local and regional fire, HazMat, and health department assets.

REFERENCES

1. Smithson A. *Ataxia: the chemical and biological terrorism threat and the US response*. Report no. 35. Washington, D.C.: Stimson Center, 2000.
2. Leonard R. Community planning for hazardous materials disasters. *Top Emerg Med* 1986;7:55–64.
3. Leonard R. Hazardous materials accidents: initial scene assessment and patient care. *Aviat Space Environ Med* 1993;June: 546–551.
4. Lerman S, Kipen H. Material safety data sheets: caveat emptor. *Arch Intern Med* 1990:150.
5. Lavoie FW, Coomes T, Cisek JE, et al. Emergency department external decontamination for hazardous chemical exposure. *Vet Hum Toxicol* 1992:34:61–64.
6. Agency for Toxic Substances and Disease Registry. *Hazardous substances emergency events surveillance, annual report*. Atlanta: Agency for Toxic Substances and Disease Registry, 1996.
7. Brennan RJ, Waeckerle JF, Sharp TW, et al. Chemical warfare agents: emergency medical and emergency public health issues. *Ann Emerg Med* 1999;34:191–204.
8. *SARA Title III compliance guidebook*. Washington, D.C.: Government Institutes, 1988.
9. Leonard R, Calabro J, Noji E. SARA (superfund amendments and reauthorization act), Title III: implications for emergency physicians. *Ann Emerg Med* 1989;18:1212–1216.
10. Cox RD. Decontamination and management of hazardous materials exposure victims in the emergency department. *Ann Emerg Med* 1994:23:761–770.
11. Levitin HW, Siegelson HJ. Hazardous materials. Disaster medical planning and response. *Emerg Med Clin North Am* 1996;14: 327–348.
12. O'Toole C. *OSHA standards interpretation and compliance letters*. Washington, D.C.: United States Office of Safety and Health Administration, 1992.
13. Occupational Safety and Heath Administration. Hazardous waste operations and emergency response. In: *Occupational safety and health standards*. 29CFR1910.120. Washington, D.C.: United States Government Printing Office, 1989.
14. Siegelson HJ. Preparing for terrorism and hazardous material exposures: a matter of worker safety. *Health Forum J* 2001:44:32–35.
15. Occupational Safety and Heath Administration. 29 CFR, section 654. Washington, D.C.: United States Government Printing Office, 1989.
16. Occupational Safety and Heath Administration. *Emergency response to hazardous substance releases*. 29CFR1910.120, paragraph q. Washington, D.C.: United States Government Printing Office, 1989.
17. Occupational Safety and Heath Administration. *Hospitals and community emergency response: what you need to know*. Report no. OSHA 3152. Washington, D.C.: United States Department of Labor, Occupational Safety and Health Administration, 1997.
18. Fairfax D. OSHA: emergency response training necessary for hospital physicians/nurses that may treat contaminated patients. In: Occupational Safety and Heath Administration. *Standard no. 1910.120. OSHA standards interpretation and compliance letters: directorate of compliance programs*. Washington, D.C.: United States Department of Labor, Occupational Safety and Health Administration, 1999.
19. Comprehensive accreditation manual for hospitals: the official handbook. In: Joint Commission on Accreditation of Healthcare Organizations. *Environment of care standards, EC.1.5, hazardous materials*. Oak Brook Terrace, IL: Joint Commission on Accreditation of Healthcare Organizations, 1999.
20. Strunk DL. Medical personnel exposed to patients contaminated with hazardous waste [letter]. *OSHA standards interpretations and compliance letters*. Washington, D.C.: United States Office for Safety and Health Administration, March 31, 1992.
21. Clark RA. Training requirements for hospital personnel involved in an emergency response of a hazardous substance [letter]. *OSHA standards interpretations and compliance letters*. Washington, D.C.: United States Office for Safety and Health Administration, October 27, 1992.
22. *Consolidated Omnibus Budget Reconciliation Act* (COBRA). In: Title 42, US Code, section 1395dd. Social Security Act, Section 1867. Washington, D.C.: United States Government Printing Office, 1986.
23. Provider agreements and supplier approval (COBRA, EMTALA). In: *Special responsibilities of medicare hospitals in emergency cases*. 42CFR489.24. Washington, D.C.: United States Government Printing Office, 1986.
24. Occupational Safety and Heath Administration. Personal protective equipment. In: *Occupational safety and health standards*. 29CFR1910.134. Washington, D.C.: United States Government Printing Office, January 8, 1998.
25. Occupational Safety and Heath Administration. Safety and health programs. In: *Occupational safety and health standards*. 29CFR1910.120, section b, paragraph 5-iii. Washington, D.C.: United States Government Printing Office, 1989.
26. Walker L. Comment on CDC recommendations for civilian communities near chemical weapons depots: guidelines for medical preparedness. Federal Register 18191, July 27, 1994. *OSHA standards interpretations and compliance letters*. Washington, D.C.: United States Department of Labor, Occupational Safety and Health Administration, 1995.
27. Lillibridge S, Siegelson H, Levitin H, et al. CDC recommendations for civilian communities near chemical weapons depots: guidelines for medical preparedness—CDC. Publication of final recommendations. *Fed Reg* 1995:60:33308–33312.
28. Siegelson H. Hospitals are on the front lines after acts of terrorism. Are you prepared? *Health Facilities Manage AHA* 2000;13: 24–28.
29. Here's mud in your eye. *Healthc Hazard Mater Manage* 1997; 11(2):1,3–4.
30. Association for Professionals in Infection Control bioterrorism task force and Centers for Disease Control hospital infections program bioterrorism working group. *APICCDC bioterrorism readiness plan. A template for healthcare facilities*. Washington, D.C.: Association for Professionals in Infection Control, 1999.
31. Garner J. Hospital infection control practices advisory committee: guideline for isolation procedures in hospitals. *Infect Control Hosp Epidemiol* 1996;17:53–80.
32. Brown R. Enhanced body substance isolation procedures. Personal communication. Seminole County, FL, 2001.

33. Pesik N, Keim ME, Iserson KV. Terrorism and the ethics of emergency medical care. *Ann Emerg Med* 2001;37:642–646.

34. Lake W. *Guidelines for mass casualty decontamination during a terrorist chemical agent incident.* Washington, D.C.: Chemical Weapons Improved Response Program, Domestic Preparedness Program, United States Soldier Biological and Chemical Command, 2000.

35. Kirk MA, Cisek J, Rose SR. Emergency department response to hazardous materials incidents. *Emerg Med Clin North Am* 1994;12:461–481.

36. Agency for Toxic Substances and Disease Registry. *Hazardous substances emergency events surveillance, annual report.* Atlanta: Agency for Toxic Substances and Disease Registry, 1997.

37. Burgess JL, Kirk M, Borron SW, et al. Emergency department hazardous materials protocol for contaminated patients [see comments]. *Ann Emerg Med* 1999;34:205–212.

38. Macintyre AG, Christopher GW, Eitzen E Jr, et al. Weapons of mass destruction events with contaminated casualties: effective planning for health care facilities. *JAMA* 2000;283:242–249.

39. Makris J. *Impact of contaminated run-off water resulting from mass casualty decontamination.* Washington, D.C.: United States Environmental Protection Agency, EPA Emergency Coordinator, 1999.

40. Greenberg MI, Cone DC, Roberts JR. Material safety data sheet: a useful resource for the emergency physician. *Ann Emerg Med* 1996;27:347–352.

41. Pesik N, Keim M, Sampson TR. Do US emergency medicine residency programs provide adequate training for bioterrorism? *Ann Emerg Med* 1999;34:173–176.

42. United States Congress. *Title XIV: Defense against weapons of mass destruction, subtitle A: domestic preparedness.* Nunn-Lugar-Domenici Amendment to the FY 97 Defense Authorization Act, Pub L, No. 104-201. Washington, D.C.:, United States Government Printing Office, 1996.

43. Socher MM. NBC delta: special training beyond HAZMAT in the USA. *Resuscitation* 1999;42:151–153.

44. United States Department of Defense. *Response to threats of terrorist use of weapons of mass destruction.* Report to Congress. Washington, D.C.: United States Department of Defense, 1997.

45. United States Army Soldier Biological Chemical Command DPO. *Domestic preparedness program, defense against weapons of mass destruction, technician-hospital provider course manual,* 8th ed. Aberdeen, MD: United States Army Soldier Biological Chemical Command Domestic Preparedness Office, 1997.

46. Waeckerle JF, Seamans S, Whiteside M, et al. Executive summary: developing objectives, content, and competencies for the training of emergency medical technicians, emergency physicians, and emergency nurses to care for casualties resulting from nuclear, biological, or chemical incidents. *Ann Emerg Med* 2001;37:587–601.

47. United States Government Accounting Office. *Combating terrorism: threat and risk assessments can help prioritize and target program investments.* Washington, D.C.: United States Government Accounting Office, 1998.

48. Hughart J. *Industrial chemicals and terrorism: human health threat analysis, mitigation and prevention.* Atlanta: Agency for Toxic Substances and Disease Registry, 1999.

49. Levy B. *War and public health.* New York: Oxford University Press, 1997.

50. Hughart J. *Chemical hazards during the recent war in Croatia.* Atlanta: Agency for Toxic Substances and Disease Registry, 1999.

51. Alibek K. *Biohazard.* New York: Random House, 1999.

52. Tur-Kaspa I, Lev EI, Hendler I, et al. Preparing hospitals for toxicological mass casualties events [see comments]. *Crit Care Med* 1999;27:1004–1008.

53. Moles TM, Baker DJ. Clinical analogies for the management of toxic trauma. *Resuscitation* 1999;42:117–124.

54. Moles TM. Emergency medical services systems and HAZMAT major incidents. *Resuscitation* 1999;42:103–116.

55. Kvetan V. Critical care medicine, terrorism and disasters: are we ready? [editorial; comment]. *Crit Care Med* 1999;27:873–874.

56. Institute of Medicine and National Research Council. *Chemical and biological terrorism: research and development to improve civilian medical response.* Washington, D.C.: Institute of Medicine and National Research Council, 1999:239.

MEDICAL CARE OF MASS GATHERINGS

STEVEN PARRILLO

In 1986, Sanders stated that "emergency medical care at public gatherings is haphazard at best and dangerous at worst" (1). In a similar vein, Weaver said, "There are surprisingly few data from which to plan the emergency medical needs for public events and no recognized standards or guidelines for providing emergency medical services at mass public gatherings" (2). Most authorities define a mass gathering as a group exceeding 1,000 people. Realistically, many times that number are likely to be present. Some believe that a mass gathering is better defined as any event that requires its own emergency medical services (EMS) response plan, although that decision may be based on many factors. Much of the relevant medical literature discusses gatherings in excess of 25,000 people. Articles have been published about care during the 1969 United States antiwar demonstrations (3), the Los Angeles Olympics (4), the 1986 World's Expo in Vancouver (1), rock concerts (5–7), National Football League games (8), the Calgary Olympics (9), the Indianapolis 500 (10,11), college football games (12), and papal masses (13). Even the *New York Times* reported in 1969 that 5,000 of the 400,000 people at Woodstock needed medical attention, some for childbirth.

PLANNING BEFORE THE EVENT

A properly planned event will be able to meet the needs of all who ask for help, no matter how minor or how severe the complaint, in an expeditious, cost-effective, and efficient manner. Planners must recognize that, although the majority of complaints will be minor, advanced life support (ALS) and rapid transport must be available for those in need. Typically, event sponsors and designated prehospital and medical personnel meet with a wide array of other agencies months in advance. Hnatow and Gordon identified the following major

Portions of this chapter were previously published by the author in modified form in Parillo SJ. Medical care at mass gatherings: considerations for physician involvement. *Prehosp Disaster Med* 1992;20:141–144, and in Parillo SJ. EMS and mass gatherings. *eMedicine Journal* 2001;2 and are being used with permission.

elements of planning: (a) crowd size, (b) personnel, (c) medical triage and facilities, (d) medical records, (e) public information and education, (f) mutual aid, and (g) data collection (13). Other authors recommend adding discussion and analysis of public access, disaster planning, weather, and event duration to the planning process.

STRUCTURES AND LOCATIONS

Virtually every imaginable structure has served as a venue for mass gatherings. Likewise, reports of mass gatherings come from many countries, but most are set in the United States and the United Kingdom (14). The type of structure and the surrounding geography play a significant role in the planning for the event. Most patients are treated at a predetermined site within the venue, and they must either get to that site by themselves or must be brought there by someone else. Planners must consider the following:

- Transport of patients to treatment sites;
- Routes to treatment sites;
- Routes EMS personnel may need to take to reach patients;
- Optimal number and placement of treatment sites;
- Possible obstructions to patient flow;
- Egress routes to other facilities;
- Availability of other facilities;
- Environmental realities of the location.

Planners may want to consider using regional first aid stations that may then refer the more serious cases to the main treatment facility. Even if this is done, however, some patients will likely bypass the first tier and come directly to the main treatment area.

TYPE OF EVENT

Crowds come to mass gatherings out of specific interest for the event. The nature of the event and the nature of the individuals interested in the event dictate the characteristics of the patient population. The participants for a rock music

TABLE 27.1. CLINICAL ENTITIES ASSOCIATED WITH SPECIFIC MASS GATHERING EVENTS

Event	Associated injuries and illnesses
Rock concerts	Drug and alcohol intoxication
	Minor trauma
Olympic events	Serious trauma (most teams have their own medical personnel)
Civil demonstrations	Moderate to severe trauma
	Riot control agent exposure
Sporting events (professional and collegiate)	Minor trauma
	Alcohol and drug intoxication
	Heat injury
	Cardiac events
Citizen events (e.g., runs, walks, and races)	Heat injury
	Cold injury
	Physical exhaustion

concert are likely to be quite different from those attending the Indianapolis 500. Reports of care at papal masses and rock concerts indicate a high rate of hospital admission among participants (5–7,13,14). While gatherings are commonly a collection of well people, exceptions are seen. Fulde (5) reported on care at a "Concert For Life" in Australia. The event was held to benefit a cardiac research center and an acquired immunodeficiency syndrome (AIDS) service. It attracted large numbers of cardiac patients, including transplant recipients, and sick AIDS sufferers. People of all ages attend sporting events. One author states that the reality of serious cardiac disease in any mass gathering should prompt the strategic placement of automated external defibrillators and the assurance that personnel have had appropriate training in their use (12).

Alcohol or other drug encounters are likely to occur at rock concerts and sporting events. Erickson et al. (15) reported a usage rate of 15% at five concerts. Bowdish et al. (10) reported alcohol as a significant factor in the Indianapolis 500 race. The type of patient encounter is determined largely by the type of crowd and the environment in which the event is held. Most patient encounters are minor occurrences such as headache, minor abrasions, lacerations, burns, and insect stings. Individuals attending papal masses and rock concerts are more likely to suffer serious illness during the event (14). In addition, problems specific to the type of event can be expected. Table 27.1 demonstrates common clinical entities associated with specific mass gathering events.

CROWD CHARACTERISTICS

Bowdish et al. (10) proposed a model using the following seven variables to help predict the use of medical facilities: weather, level of alcohol use, availability of care, the type of event, injury or illness type, crowd mood, and other variables (e.g., audience age and preexisting medical condi-

tions). To assume that longer events with larger numbers of people will generate more casualties makes intuitive sense. In a 25-year review of English language articles, Michael and Barbera demonstrated a strong correlation between crowd size and event duration and the use of medical facilities (14). Usage or casualty rates (the number of people treated per 1,000 attendees) vary widely. At the 1986 Vancouver World's Exposition, the average rate was 3.9% (1). At the 1984 Los Angeles Olympics, the rates varied from a low of 0.68% at the soccer venue to a high of 6.8% at the rowing and canoeing venue (4). When usage is divided into acuity levels as was done at the 1988 Calgary Olympics, the majority was low acuity, with only 0.02% high acuity problems (4). Some authors note that usage rates are generally higher in settings where groups are allowed to move about more freely (14). Such mobility allows for more minor trauma and exposure-related or exertion-related illnesses than in events where spectators are seated for most of the time.

ENVIRONMENTAL INFLUENCES

Warm weather events increase the likelihood of heat-related problems especially among the athletes but also among the spectators. Several years ago, the American College of Sports Medicine issued a position statement that strenuous events be postponed or canceled at certain "wet bulb" temperatures, which are derived from a combination of several environmental factors. Cases of heat cramps are more likely to be seen than cases of heat stroke. However, even well-trained athletes may suffer heat stroke. Insect stings occur primarily in warm weather. A review written by Micheal (14) stated that most cardiac arrests occurred in temperate conditions. Cold weather decreases the total number of injuries, but it does produce a variety of injuries and illnesses that are unique to colder temperatures (18).

Hypothermia may occur in settings that do not necessarily involve cold temperatures. It is especially likely in mass gatherings involving water, such as triathlons or citizen swim meets. The presence of rain in a non-water event markedly increases the likelihood of hypothermia. Miscellaneous environment-related problems may include lightning, flooding, and injuries related to low ambient illumination (e.g., tripping and falling).

PUBLIC HEALTH CONCERNS

Planning for the medical response for mass gatherings requires a multidisciplinary approach that includes emergency medicine, EMS, and public health. The plan must include provisions for drinking water and sanitary facilities (17,18). Shelter may also be a concern, especially with a lengthy or multiday event or in adverse weather conditions.

STAFFING

Micheal points out that a critical analysis of staffing patterns has not been undertaken. The fact that the many reported staffing patterns have worked leads only to the conclusion that staffing was not inadequate (14). Most of the published guidelines are general in nature. The planner must take many variables into consideration. Authors have suggested various staffing models (1,2,14). Most authorities believe that the overwhelming majority of patients can be triaged and treated effectively by registered nurses and paramedics (1,2,4,9–12). The ideal situation is accurate triage by non-physicians with the rapid referral of appropriate cases to physician-level care (9).

Sanders et al. (1) recommend one to two physicians for every 50,000 people and two paramedics or one paramedic or emergency medical technician (EMT) team for every 10,000 people. This group also suggests the following capabilities as the minimum standard: (a) basic first aid and basic life support within 4 minutes; (b) ALS within 8 minutes; and (c) evacuation to a hospital within 30 minutes (1). Several authors have suggested that part of the preparation of the non-physicians should include cardiopulmonary resuscitation (CPR) training and instruction in the use of the automated external defibrillator (2,12).

The question has often been raised about whether the need truly exists for physicians to be present at the site of mass gatherings. There is general agreement that a physician should be the medical director. The complexity and the unpredictability of these events require a physician in the planning process and the availability of a physician for advice during the event (13,19–21). The more likely the chance is that a significant trauma will occur, the more likely the event sponsor will be to demand a physician on the scene. Physicians must be involved in the writing of protocols, policies, and standing orders (19). Some planners suggest that online medical control is sufficient to prevent the unnecessary referral of patients from the event to the hospital (2), while others believe that an on-scene physician does this best (22). Regional medical command requirements will also need to be considered. Advocates of physician presence at mass gatherings note the following as well:

- The likelihood of serious trauma has been the impetus for having physician care available at auto races since the early 1900s (4,10,11).
- The potential of a long distance to definitive care makes the physician's presence valuable (9).
- The event sponsor is much more satisfied with a physician present (9,19).
- Decreased hospital impact, improved disaster response, and improved media coverage will be observed if a physician is present (9).

- The presence of a physician allows competent prehospital personnel to work under protocol with the knowledge that help is immediately available if it is needed (4).
- Much of the research into care at mass gatherings has been done by the physicians who developed and implemented the response plans.
- For special events, many physicians will volunteer their time (8).

The physician at a mass gathering must be able to anticipate and deal with the types of casualties that are likely. Clearly, the services of an orthopedist or sports physician are required at times, but the emergency physician is the most logical choice for an on-site responder, especially because mass casualty incidents may occur. Waeckerle remarks that "emergency physicians are usually the most appropriate for this role, because they are familiar with the system and personnel providing care before hospitalization; they are practiced in rapid assessment, basic treatment, and triage; and they have a good working rapport with other specialists needed during the response" (23).

As the specialty of emergency medicine matures, residency programs are beginning to recognize the value of teaching mass gathering medicine to their residents. For example, the Wright State residency has developed an educational model that includes the following:

- Adequate crowd size to generate useful patient volume;
- Regularly scheduled events;
- Organized medical and disaster preparations meeting local or published standards;
- Didactic instruction on history, principles, and current issues;
- On-site attending physician supervision;
- Degree of responsibility appropriate for the level of training;
- Participation in planning and organizing;
- Postevent briefing (24).

FINANCIAL CONSIDERATIONS

In most cases, the event sponsor will be responsible for the expenses incurred in the planning and delivery of medical care (25,26). Other models depend on care provided by local EMS, hospital personnel, or others, frequently on a voluntary basis (27). Financial arrangements will vary depending on circumstances, but they should be arranged with each venue and service provider well in advance of the event.

COMMUNICATION

Good communication is essential for the successful operation of any large medical activity. Communication techniques used in mass gatherings should closely parallel daily communication techniques used by the health care service providers. Personnel must know how to communicate with each other. As with disaster and mass casualty incidents, radios will provide the bulk of the communications. Land-line telephones are helpful if available. Cellular telephones may also be considered, although their use may be limited by the local infrastructure (28).

DOCUMENTATION AND REPORTING

Most authors admit that a written record probably will not be generated for the vast majority of trivial visits. However, all agree that good records must be kept for all but the most trivial encounters. Standard items include demographic data, brief medical history, type of illness or injury, treatment rendered, and disposition (2). Various databases can be used if they are available. Good records absolutely must be kept for those patients sick or injured enough to be sent to a hospital (1,2,4,8,9,19). Michael suggests that events be categorized not only by their own characteristics but also by the characteristics of the spectators. Good event reporting, therefore, would record age, gender, and socioeconomic status of spectators; the availability of alcohol and other drugs; and any other important variables. When these factors are combined with event characteristics, such as weather, audience mobility, and dangers specific to the site itself, future planners may more logically predict event needs (14). The use of handheld digital devices for medical record documentation during mass gathering events may expedite and improve record-keeping.

TRANSPORTATION

The discussion of transport and patient movement raises several issues regarding mass gatherings. How will the patient access the triage and treatment areas and how will EMS personnel reach patients unable to ambulate? Consideration needs to be given as to what equipment paramedics may use and in what manner that equipment will be carried. The locations of patient litters or backboards should be logical and easy to access. Some authors have suggested the use of a jump bag with appropriate medical supplies (28). Specific routes should be marked to direct patients to medical treatment areas. Deliberation also should be given as to how these routes will be marked and in what languages. Careful selection of the location of patient treatment areas is paramount in increasing their effectiveness.

Ambulance staging areas should be within easy access of the medical treatment stations. Prior consideration as to what roads are available for ambulance traffic as well as what physical obstructions ambulances may encounter

must be part of the planning process. In addition, the plan should consider the number of ambulances that should be kept at the site as opposed to those that are on call. If air medical transportation is necessary, a clear and safe landing zone must be established and maintained. The receiving hospitals for patients should be determined in advance, and mechanisms for notifying these hospitals of incoming patients must be implemented previously.

EQUIPMENT

In addition to transport equipment (e.g., litters and ambulances), a well-stocked basic life support or ALS vehicle, depending on the provider capability, will carry most of the needed supplies. Suggested supplies for a medical response kit are listed in Table 27.2.

INTERAGENCY AND HOSPITAL ASSISTANCE

Essential agencies that should be involved in the planning of care for mass gatherings include emergency medicine, EMS, fire department, police department, local hospitals, and the local chapter of the American Red Cross. As with mass casualty incidents, advance planning is essential to assure the delivery of needed health care. With regard to interagency coordination, anyone who might be involved in an event should help with the planning (19,28). For agencies that may be but that are not likely to be needed, written mutual aid agreements should be obtained (14,19, 28,29).

TABLE 27.2. BASIC EQUIPMENT AND SUPPLY LIST FOR MASS GATHERINGS

Advanced life support	Medications
Automated external defibrillator	Atropine
Cardiac monitors and defibrillators	Morphine
Airway equipment	Dextrose 50%
Laryngoscope and blades	Albuterol
Surgical airway kit	Nitroglycerine
Oxygen administration equipment	Aspirin
Bag-valve masks	Diphenhydramine
Suction devices	Naloxone
Standard equipment	Lidocaine
Bandages	Epinephrine, 1:1000
Immobilization devices	Adenosine
Intravenous fluids, catheters,	Furosemide
and administration sets	Analgesics
Syringes and needles	
Stethoscopes	
Mobile radio sets	
Pneumothorax kit with	
Heimlich valve	

SUMMARY

Mass gathering events present emergency care personnel with complex patient care and transportation problems. Primary variables in planning include the type of event, the characteristics and number of attendees, the location of the event, the presence of alcohol or drugs, and access to local or regional emergency facilities. Available information regarding medical support for such events provides guidelines for future preevent planning. Preparations for mass gathering events should be based on valid assumptions in order to obtain optimal results.

REFERENCES

1. Sanders, AB, Criss E, Steckl P, et al. An analysis of medical care at mass gatherings. *Ann Emerg Med* 1986;15:515–519.
2. Weaver WD, Sutherland K, Wirkus MJ, et al. Emergency medical care requirements for large public assemblies and a new strategy for managing cardiac arrest in this setting. *Ann Emerg Med* 1989;18:155–160.
3. Chused TM, Cohn CK, Schneider E, et al. Medical care during the 1969 antiwar demonstrations in Washington, D.C. *Arch Intern Med* 1971;127:67–70.
4. Baker WM, Simone BM, Niemann JT, et al. Special event medical care: the 1984 Los Angeles Summer Olympics experience. *Ann Emerg Med* 1986;15:185–190.
5. Fulde G, Forster SL, Preisz P. Open air rock concert: an organized disaster. *Med J Aust* 1992;157:820–822.
6. Gay GR, Elsenbaumer R, Newmeyer JA. A dash of M*A*S*H*: the Zep and the Dead head to head. *J Psych Drugs* 1972;5:193–203.
7. Blandford AG, Dunlop HA. Glastonbury Fair: some medical aspects of a rock concert. *Practitioner* 1972;209:205–211.
8. Pons PT, Holland B, Alfrey E, et al. An advanced emergency care system at NFL games. *Ann Emerg Med* 1980;9:203–206.
9. Thompson JM, Savoia G, Powell G, et al. Level of medical care required for mass gatherings: the XV Winter Olympic games in Calgary, Canada. *Ann Emerg Med* 1991;20:385–390.
10. Bowdish GE, Cordell WH, Bock HC, et al. Using regression analysis to predict patient volume at the Indianapolis 500 mile race. *Ann Emerg Med* 1992;21:1200–1203.
11. Bock HC, Cordell WH, Hawk AC. Demographics of emergency medical care at the Indianapolis 500 mile race. *Ann Emerg Med* 1992;21:1204–1207.
12. Spaite DW, Criss EA, Valenzuela TD, et al. A new model for providing prehospital medical care in large stadiums. *Ann Emerg Med* 1988;17:825–828.
13. Hnatow DA, Gordon DJ. Medical planning for mass gathering: a retrospective review of the San Antonio Papal Mass. *Prehosp Disaster Med* 1991;6:443–450.
14. Michael JA, Barbera JA. Mass gathering medical care: a twenty-five year review. *Prehosp Disaster Med* 1997;12:301–312.
15. Erickson TB, Aks SE, Koenigsberg M, et al. Drug use patterns at major rock concert events. *Ann Emerg Med* 1996;28:22–26.
16. Gannon DM, Derse AR, Bronkema PJ. The emergency care network of a ski marathon. *Am J Sports Med* 1985;13:316–320.
17. Carlson L. Spectator medical care. *Physician Sports Med* 1992;20:141–144.
18. Weiss BP, Mascola L, Fannin SL. Public health at the 1984 Summer Olympics: the Los Angeles county experience. *Am J Public Health* 1988;78:686–688.
19. Parrillo SJ. Medical care at mass gatherings: considerations for physician involvement. *Prehosp Disaster Med* 1995;10:273–275.
20. DeLorenzo RA, Gray BC, Bennett PC, et al. Effect of crowd size on patient volume at a large, multipurpose indoor stadium. *J Emerg Med* 1989;7:379–384.
21. Leonard RB, Petrilli R, Noji EK, et al. *Provision for emergency medical care for crowds.* Dallas: American College of Emergency Physicians, 1990:1–25.
22. Ellis DG, Verdile VP, Paris PM, et al. Medical coverage of a marathon: establishing guidelines for deployment of health care resources. *Prehosp Disaster Med* 1991;6:435–441.
23. Waeckerle J. Disaster planning and response. *N Engl J Med* 1991;324:815–821.
24. DeLorenzo RA, Boyle MF, Garrison F. A proposed model for a residency experience in mass gathering medicine: the United States Air Show. *Ann Emerg Med* 1993;22:1711–1714.
25. Lloyd C. Emergency medical services for large crowds. In: Lewis G, Appenzeller H, eds. *Successful sports management.* Charlottesville, VA: The Michie Co, 1985:89–99.
26. Sanders AB, Criss E. Planning medical care for large-scale events. *Emerg Med Serv* 1987;16:33–48.
27. Cohen DL, Montalvo MA, Turnbull GP. Medical support for a major military air show: the RAF Mildenhall medical emergency support plan. *J Trauma* 1994;36:237–244.
28. Leonard RB. Disaster medicine — medical support for mass gatherings. *Emerg Med Clin North Am* 1996;14:383–397.
29. DeLorenzo RA. Mass gathering medicine: a review. *Prehosp Disaster Med* 1997;12:69–72.

MARITIME DISASTERS

THEODORE E. HARRISON

On July 25, 1956, a heavy fog lay 60 miles off Nantucket Island. The Swedish-American liner *Stockholm* with her ice-breaking bow sailed cautiously through the dense visibility. Suddenly at 11:10 PM, the passenger ship *Andrea Doria* appeared directly in front of the Stockholm, seemingly coming out of nowhere. The reinforced bow of the *Stockholm* tore into the starboard side of the passenger liner. The *Andrea Doria* instantly listed 18 degrees to starboard and began to take on seawater though a massive gash in her hull. A missing watertight door to the engine room compounded the flooding. Stability was further diminished by a failure to ballast the empty fuel tanks properly. At the moment of collision, tons of seawater poured into the *Andrea Doria's* still full starboard fuel tanks. With water pouring into her starboard tanks, the empty port side tanks accentuated the dangerous starboard list, dooming the liner.

Within moments of impact, help was summoned, and the order to abandon ship was given. The increasing starboard list made launching half of the lifeboats impossible, thus creating a critical rescue situation. Despite a badly damaged bow, the *Stockholm* provided aid by taking on a number of *Andrea Doria's* passengers. Responding to the SOS, numerous rescue craft quickly arrived and provided the lifeboats necessary for completing the evacuation.

At 6:05 AM on July 26, the last of *Andrea Doria's* 1,662 passengers and crew were evacuated. The primary rescue vessel *Ile De France* circled the *Andrea Doria* one last time, dipping her colors three times in a salute. At 10:09 AM, the *Andrea Doria* quietly slipped to her grave 225 feet below the surface of the Atlantic. The collision resulted in the loss of 52 lives. Only the rapid distress calls and the response of other vessels saved the remainder of her passengers and crew. Fig. 28.1 demonstrates the *Andria Doria* sinking.

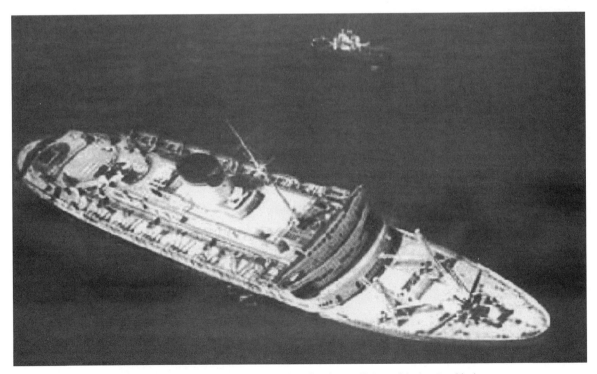

FIGURE 28.1. The *Andrea Doria* sinks after her collision with the *Stockholm*.

OVERVIEW

Mass loss of life is not a common occurrence in maritime incidents. According to the United States Coast Guard (USCG), mass loss of life is defined as an incident in which five or more individuals are killed (1). From 1983 to 1993, 2,559 deaths and 15,778 injuries were reported to the USCG Maritime Mishap System. Almost 50% of the deaths and over 75% of the injuries reported were due to incidents on board the vessel that were not related to the operation of the vessel (e.g., falling overboard, crush injuries, and fires) (1,2). Most of the injuries are associated with ships with a high intensity of industrial activity, such as fishing vessels. The type of vessel and the injury rate based on the reports to the USCG are demonstrated in Fig. 28.2.

Although mass loss of life is generally uncommon, it can be dramatic when a highly populated vessel such as a passenger liner or ferry is involved. The ferry vessel *Estonia* left Tallinn, Estonia on the evening of September 27, 1994 bound for Stockholm, Sweden. Human error resulted in a failure to close the watertight bow loading doors, causing the vessel to take on water quietly during the rough seas. On September 28th at 2:00 AM, the vessel sank in the Baltic Sea, taking 852 lives and leaving only 137 survivors. Worldwide casualty statistics in 1996 indicated that 1,559 individuals lost their lives sailing or working on 180 separate vessels of over 100 gross tons in size (3). Of these deaths, 1,200 (77%) were from two ships. The *Gurita* ran aground and foundered, killing 338; and the *Bukoba*, a ferry that was overloaded with passengers, capsized, killing 869. These densely populated vessels represent a potential for profound loss of life.

The definition of a disaster as an event occurring in which a community's resources are inadequate for coping with an ecologic phenomenon takes on a new meaning when applied to the maritime situation. At sea, the communities are very small and the resources minimal, and ecologic phenomena loom large. Currently, huge freighters may carry a crew of 12 to 24 people; only one or two of these have any knowledge of medical care. A ship's medical chest may be the entire complement of medical resources available. Compared to shoreside catastrophes, not much is required to turn a shipboard emergency into a disaster. Maritime disasters can be roughly divided into the following four groups: collisions, weather-related events, fires, and infectious diseases (4).

COLLISIONS

Collisions between seagoing vessels are relatively uncommon. However when they do occur, spectacular problems are created. The collision of the ocean liner *Titanic* with an iceberg always is evoked as part of this category; however, a far greater number of shipwrecks have been caused by rocks or reefs, such as the *Exxon Valdez* disaster, or by collisions with other ships, such as the *Andrea Doria*. The combination of navigational hazards and bad weather is probably the most common cause of collisions.

Collisions occur with sudden onset and little or no warning. Frequently, damage to the propulsion and steering apparatus occurs. The ship may sink either rapidly or slowly, depending on the hull damage and weather conditions. The first response is signaled by the ship's alarm (usu-

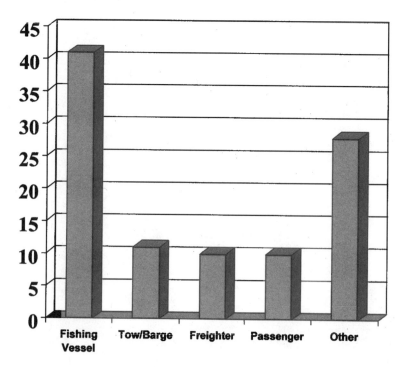

FIGURE 28.2. Reported percentage of injury by vessel type (From data provided by the United States Coast Guard).

ally seven blasts), which indicates that all personnel should don their life vests and proceed to their lifeboat stations. When and if the captain perceives that the situation is hopeless, then the abandon ship alarm will be sounded and the lifeboats will be lowered and boarded. Receiving facilities should be prepared to handle traumatic injuries, hypothermia, and immersion. Many of the fatalities and serious injuries may be due to the force of the collision itself and not as a result of secondary events.

WEATHER

Hurricanes and typhoons in tropical areas and winter storms in the extreme northern and southern latitudes can overwhelm the best-prepared ship. Small and ill-prepared ships frequently founder or capsize when confronted with heavy seas and high winds. Introduce human error (e.g., the Baltic ferry *Estonia*), and the potential for a disaster becomes much greater.

Weather problems generally have a gradual onset with some warning. Heavy weather is usually no surprise, but its effects—capsizing and foundering—usually are. Foundering is often due to some breach of the structural integrity of the ship. Rarely is this something that can be repaired in a timely manner at sea, and it virtually always results in the loss of the ship. As in the case of collisions, the captain will sound the lifeboat alarm when the situation is serious and will proceed to abandon ship when the vessel is determined to no longer be safe. Receiving facilities should be prepared to handle traumatic injuries, hypothermia, and immersion.

FIRE

Except for some sailboats (and even they have engines nowadays), ships are powered by heat-generating engines that consume millions of gallons of flammable liquids. Not surprisingly, fires are common in this environment. As Fig. 28.3 illustrates, about half of all fires start in the engine room. Fig. 28.4 shows the effects of fires on passenger vessel and ferry shipping over the past two decades (5).

Fortunately, systems have been developed over the years by which most fires are easily contained. For instance, the telegenic fire on board the cruise ship *Ecstasy* a few years ago could not be classified as a disaster. It was never out of control, and it never outstripped the resources of the ship. On the other hand, the fire that broke out in the laundry room of the *Universe Explorer* a couple years earlier quickly spread to involve the ship infirmary. This rendered the ship medically helpless at a time when many people were in dire need of medical care.

The classic case in the fire category, however, is that of the *Morro Castle*. This vessel caught fire on the return trip from its maiden voyage to Cuba in 1934. Similar to the *Titanic*, a number of wealthy and famous individuals were on board. Unfortunately, the captain died of a heart attack during the night before the fire. Compounding the problems, neither the crew nor the passengers had rehearsed any fire drills, and the fire hoses were not readily available. In the ensuing confusion, eight of the lifeboats were nondeployable. The ship drifted, smoking and charred, onto the New Jersey shore. Figure 28.5 shows the *Morro Castle* on fire drifting to the New Jersey shoreline.

Fire develops suddenly with no warning. Frequently, damage to the propulsion and steering apparatus occurs due to the fire. A fire may become a disaster without threatening the viability of the ship itself because of its effects on the ship's systems and inhabitants. As soon as a fire is detected, a fire alarm is sounded and the ship's fire control team proceeds to the scene to try to extinguish the blaze. If a cruise ship is involved, the medical team goes to the infirmary and prepares to receive patients. If the infirmary is involved in the fire, the medical team sets up a secondary medical cen-

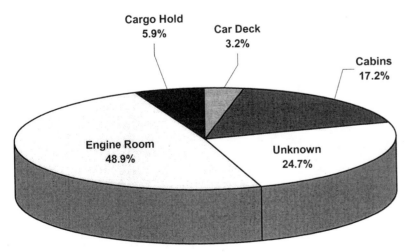

FIGURE 28.3. Starting locations of fires on seagoing vessels.

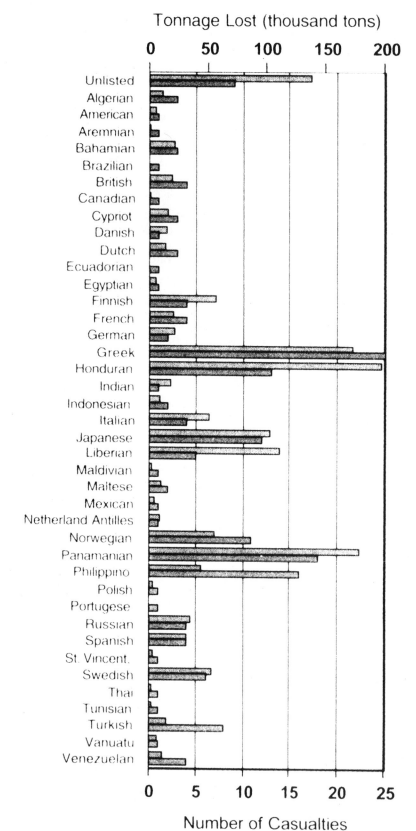

FIGURE 28.4. Casualties and losses on passenger vessels and ferry shipping as a result of fire.

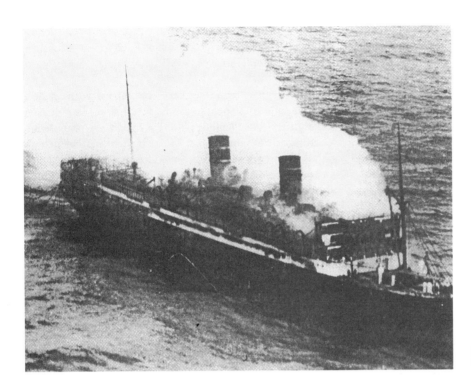

FIGURE 28.5. The hapless *Morro Castle* drifts towards New Jersey.

ter with supplies from the ship's secondary medical space. Occasionally, a fire will become extensive enough to proceed to sounding the lifeboat alarm and then to abandoning ship. More frequently however, the fire will be contained, but many people may suffer from its effects. The onboard medical facilities can easily be overwhelmed. Receiving facilities should expect burns, smoke inhalation, carbon monoxide poisoning, and trauma.

INFECTIOUS DISEASE

On land, infectious disease outbreaks rarely progress to disaster proportions. However, on a ship with limited medical facilities, even a small outbreak can overwhelm the system. According to Centers for Disease Control (CDC) statistics, approximately one in every 400 cruises has an outbreak of diarrheal illness that is significant enough (more than 2%–3% of the crew or passengers) to warrant epidemiologic investigation (6). On a 1,000-passenger ship, which usually carries one doctor and one nurse, 20 to 30 patients with Norwalk virus is definitely a disaster. If one or more of the patients is the doctor or nurse, then the situation is grave indeed. On a Caribbean voyage of the *Regent Sun* in 1994, diarrhea developed in more than 300 passengers, including both the doctor and the nurse. The ship had to be completely evacuated, and a new medical team was flown in.

Infectious outbreaks have a gradual onset with some warning. A few days' incubation period occurs, after which cases build up over 2 to 3 days. Usually passenger liners reach the critical point in patient volume toward the end of

a cruise. Freighters are less susceptible to this kind of problem due to a lower volume of food preparation and handling (7). The onboard medical team will report the outbreak to the captain as soon as it is recognized and will begin to take action to control the outbreak. If the cases are severe, they may be disembarked at ports of call before the end of the cruise, but most passengers elect to stay on the ship to their final destination. If the ship is in or near American waters, the captain will usually report the outbreak to the CDC. The CDC evaluates the situation and decides whether an epidemiology team needs to be sent to investigate. The captain also notifies authorities and the port agent at the final destination so that arrangements can be made for care of the ill who are unable to complete their previously made travel arrangements.

If the CDC decides to investigate, its team will meet the ship at the dock and will begin an exhaustive process of crew and passenger questionnaires, as well as an inspection of the ship. It usually takes a few weeks to analyze the data and come to conclusions. Occasionally, the ship is taken out of service for a short time to undergo extensive decontamination. Shoreside facilities receiving patients from the ship should be prepared to handle mainly dehydration and respiratory and electrolyte problems, depending on the nature of the outbreak.

MARITIME DISASTER PLANNING

All ships are required to have a safety plan that includes a disaster plan in accordance with the International Maritime

Organization International Safety Management code and the Safety of Life at Sea convention. This includes standard procedures and regular drills. The medical department on cruise ships is part of this plan and is included in the drills. They may have their own section of the disaster plan for which they are responsible for maintenance and implementation (8).

On cruise ships, one of the prime disaster-planning responsibilities of the medical department is the establishment and maintenance of a secondary medical space. This consists of two parts as follows:

1. A space (usually a locker) for the storage of medical supplies and equipment that might be needed in a disaster if the main infirmary is inaccessible. This storage space should be located distant from the main infirmary in a separate compartment of the ship. Frequently, it is on or near the bridge.
2. A space where medical care can be rendered when the main infirmary is inaccessible. This space should have emergency power and light. It should also be in a separate compartment of the ship from the main infirmary and relatively close to the disaster supplies. It should be large enough to support both triage and primary medical care.

Communications during a disaster are just as much of a problem on board as they are ashore. Most cruise ship disaster plans call for radios for all officers and the medical team, including the stretcher team. Each group is assigned a separate channel to avoid overload, while the bridge monitors all channels.

Cruise ships frequently carry passengers with medical training, and these people can be very helpful in a disaster. A volunteer management plan that makes use of passenger doctors, nurses, and medics for help in triage and first aid should be prepared. Volunteer health care providers should be able to provide basic documentation (e.g., wallet cards) to verify training. In addition, the medical staff should monitor volunteers when providing care.

For all of the above systems to function effectively in a crisis, practice is necessary. Lifeboat, stretcher team, fire, and basic life support drills should be part of the safety plan and ongoing routine of the ship. The sequence of events in a maritime disaster response is somewhat different than that in shoreside disasters. This is demonstrated in Fig. 28.6.

EVACUATION

In maritime disasters, the hospital is a long way away. Unless the vessel happens to be in coastal waters within a couple hundred miles of a Coast Guard airbase, no chance for rapid air evacuation exists. However, if the ship is within

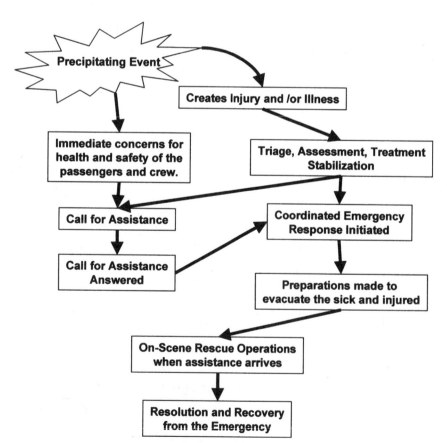

FIGURE 28.6. Maritime disaster flow chart. (Adapted from Ungs TJ, Hogan DE. EMS and disaster medicine at sea. In: Harrison TE, ed. *Cruise medicine*, 2nd ed. Nassau, Bahamas: Maritime Health Systems, Ltd., 1999:29–60.)

helicopter range and patients who are critically ill or injured must be evacuated to a higher level of medical care immediately, the Coast Guard is well equipped to intervene in the situation. Virtually all ships have the radio equipment necessary to communicate with the Coast Guard, and the protocols and procedures necessary to effect a helicopter evacuation are readily available. Obviously, a mass casualty evacuation is not possible, but one or a few victims may be rapidly evacuated.

The more usual method of evacuation is by a military or commercial ship. Vessels tend to travel in sea-lanes, where other ships commonly are relatively close by. The cases of the *Titanic* and the *Andrea Doria* illustrate this as other vessels were able to be on the scene in a matter of hours. Nearby ships will respond to distress calls, and they can take passengers and crew off a stricken vessel. Military ships and the Coast Guard are probably better prepared for this than commercial ships because of operational training and heavy equipment for severe conditions. However, if the number of people to be evacuated is large, military ships may be at a disadvantage because they have little extra space. Cruise ships or even freighters with lots of deck space will be able to take on more evacuees.

If the ship is in critical condition and no outside help is available, the lifeboats serve as the ambulance of last resort. As a matter of international law, all ships have an adequate number of lifeboats that are provisioned with food, water, and medical supplies. The crew should be well trained and drilled in the use of the lifeboats. Cruise ships have a lifeboat drill for both passengers and crew at the beginning of each cruise. If the vessel is not in danger (e.g., an infectious disease disaster), the ship itself can serve as ambulance and can divert to the nearest capable port with adequate resources.

EMERGENCY DEPARTMENT IMPACT AND CONSIDERATIONS

The impact on shoreside emergency departments is small. The population affected by a maritime disaster is, at most, a few thousand people. Air evacuation can bring only a few patients at a time. Evacuation by ship or lifeboat will be slow, and the receiving facilities or system have time to coordinate their approach. The shoreside medical system presumably will not have been affected by the disaster, and it therefore will be operating at full capacity. Casualties can be distributed so as not to overburden any one facility.

While most maritime disasters involve relatively few casualties (although they might produce many evacuees), occasional exceptions may involve the presentation of hundreds or perhaps even thousands of casualties to a shoreside emergency medical services (EMS) system. If the EMS system is small (e.g., a Caribbean island), then it will also have to activate its disaster plan in order to cope with the influx of patients. However, given the generally long time to arrival and the preknowledge of the extent and type of casualties, a shoreside EMS system or emergency department should have enough time to prepare an adequate response.

SUMMARY

A cargo ship, ferry, cruise ship, or drilling platform is a small community where internal resources can be rapidly exhausted and external resources are distant. Disasters usually come in the form of collision, weather-related events, fire, or infectious disease. Because of the remoteness of ships and platforms, shoreside emergency departments and EMS systems usually have time to prepare adequately for the reception of casualties from a maritime disaster. Onboard planning and practice of a disaster plan is part of the safety plan of most ships.

REFERENCES

1. United States Coast Guard. COMDTINST M16465.6. *Marine safety manual*. Washington, D.C.: Department of Transportation, United States Coast Guard, 1992.
2. United States Coast Guard. COMDTPUB P6700.4. *Navigation and vessel inspection circular no. 3-2: recommended program for protection of merchant mariners from occupational health problems*. Washington, D.C.: Department of Transportation, United States Coast Guard, 1992.
3. Ungs TJ, Hogan DE. EMS and disaster medicine at sea. In: Harrison TE, ed. *Cruise medicine*, 2nd ed. Nassau, Bahamas: Maritime Health Systems, Ltd., 1999:29–60.
4. Barnaby KC. *Some ship disasters and their causes*. New York: AS Barnes, 1968.
5. Rushbrook F. *Fire aboard*. New York: Sheridan House, 1998.
6. Koo D, Maloney K, Tauxe R. Epidemiology of diarrheal disease outbreaks on cruise ships, 1986 through 1993. *JAMA* 1996;275:545–547.
7. Addis DG, Yashuk JC, Clapp DE, et al. Outbreaks of diarrheal illness on passenger cruise ships, 1975–85. *Epidemiol Inf* 1989;103:63–72.
8. Watson MH. *Disasters at sea*. Cambridge, England: Patrick Stevens Limited, 1995.

29

AIR CRASH DISASTERS

JULIO LAIRET
DAVID E. HOGAN

On June 1, 1999, at approximately 11:51 PM American Airlines flight 1420 overran the end of runway 4 Right at Little Rock National Airport in Arkansas. The MD-82, which had originated in Dallas, Texas, collided with the approach light stanchion after skidding off the runway. The aircraft carried a crew of six and 139 passengers (1). At 11:55 PM, an initial response of three trucks with four firefighters in each was carried out by Aircraft Rescue and Fire Fighting. At 12:06 AM, the fire captain from Aircraft Rescue and Fire Fighting made a visual of the aircraft and reported to Little Rock central communications that "This aircraft is on the ground off the northern end of runway four right. He's on the ground outside the airport. The aircraft is on the ground; he is burning" (1).

The metropolitan emergency medical service (MEMS) dispatch confirmed the aircraft accident at 12:06 AM. The first three MEMS units arrived on the scene at 12:22 AM. A total of 19 MEMS units responded, along with a number of other support or supply vehicles. The Little Rock fire department's response included a total of 13 engine companies, one ladder company, one heavy rescue unit, one hazardous materials unit, and nine staff vehicles (1).

When the MEMS supervisor arrived on the scene, he found dozens of passengers carrying injured persons from the wreckage. The triage area was set up adjacent to the perimeter road east of the aircraft, and patients were redirected to this area. One patient who was critical was tagged red; air medical evacuation was requested, and this patient was airlifted with another patient that had been tagged yellow. An estimated 40 to 50 patients were triaged and treated on the scene within a 2-hour period. A total of ten patients were tagged red, and 19 were tagged yellow (1). According to MEMS personnel, a great number of lower extremity injuries were seen (1). The final report revealed that, of 145 individuals on board the aircraft, the victims of the accident included 11 fatalities (7.6%), 35 immediate patients (24.1%), 45 minor casualties (31%), and 54 noninjured persons (37.2%) (2).

Since the beginning of flight, crashes involving aircraft have occurred. With the capacity and number of commercial airliners increasing, the risk of a catastrophic event involving an aircraft has multiplied. In United States alone, the total number of commercial air passengers during 1995 totalled 580 million lives in the air. By 1997, the number of commercial air passengers had increased to 630 million, and it is expected to exceed 985 million by the year 2009 (3). Aviation accidents have the potential for the most significant loss of life and the generation of the highest numbers of casualties of any transportation mechanism throughout the world. Essentially, any community that is close to an airport or a major air traffic route is at risk for receiving casualties from an aircraft-related disaster.

Fortunately, keeping safety a primary concern has offset this increased risk. The preliminary data released by the National Transportation and Safety Board (NTSB) for 1999 indicates that 1,908 accidents occurred with a total of 628 fatalities (4). In addition to aircraft crashes, other accidents include ditching, turbulence, rapid decompression, and explosions aboard the aircraft.

PREHOSPITAL CONSIDERATIONS

Scene Access

From a prehospital perspective, the unique considerations that aircraft accidents have must be addressed. The first consideration is how to gain access to the scene. Air crashes occurring in and around the airport will usually occur within the confines of the flight line. An airport flight line is a highly secured and regulated area. Larger and busier airports may need to continue active flight operations near the crash site. Because of this, emergency medical services (EMS) personnel unfamiliar with the regulations and safety protocols of functioning on or near active flight lines must receive prior training or escort from individuals with such knowledge. Clear methods of how the EMS will access the flight line area must be part of the overall air crash disaster plan. Communication links among the responding EMS units and the airport tower, the airport EMS units, and the airport fire and rescue elements must be established.

Reports do exist of EMS units who have attempted to access the flight lines through the planned routes only to find them locked and chained. Carrying a sturdy set of bolt cutters is useful for situations such as this. The dispatcher should confirm access routes and should direct the responding units to the scene accordingly.

When a visual of the scene can be made, it should be surveyed for possible hazards and required resources. When approaching the accident, the units should never drive through the path that the aircraft has taken, in order to avoid fuel spilled by the aircraft during the accident. A priority should be giving an incident intelligence update to the communications center. After arriving on the scene, the initial responding unit should report to the incident command system (ICS) if it has been established. If no ICS has been established, the EMS unit should position itself in an upwind position, and a triage area should be established. As with any other disaster, chaos and confusion will initially reign at the scene.

Identification of the specific location and extent of the crash site either on or off the active flight line area may be difficult. Crashes within the confines of airport property may be easier to contain and regulate. Crashes occurring off regulated areas of the airport may present unique challenges to search and rescue and EMS elements. Access to air crashes occurring in nonsecured areas may be impeded by numerous factors, such as poor roads, poor visibility, and spectator traffic. Use of air medical elements with clear communication channels to ground units may be a significant assistance in these settings. Air medical units may be able to size up the situation more rapidly; they can be used to provide coordinating directions to ground units.

Victim Identification

The identification of the victims from the aircraft may present additional challenges to the disaster responders. Experiences with previous air crashes have indicated that survivors capable of removing themselves from the wreckage will frequently move considerable distances from the crash site. If prehospital disaster response to the site is delayed, these victims may be some distance from the aircraft by the time the response teams arrive, and thus search parties may be required to locate them. This problem is further compounded by darkness. Well-lit triage areas should be established rapidly in an effort to diminish the confusion. Directing all patients to the triage area is important as this improves the process of identifying and assessing all survivors. During the Little Rock accident, many non-triaged ambulatory survivors were transported by bus before the MEMS crews could evaluate them. This complication was solved by creating a separate triage area at the fire department station to which the buses were headed (1).

Hazards for Responders

Additional hazards may be present for the responding units associated with the downed aircraft. Aviation fuel is not only a hazardous substance but also a potential fire hazard. In addition, various aviation and cargo products may give off toxic substances while burning. The aircraft should always be approached from an upwind position to avoid toxic fumes. The damaged aircraft fuselage itself represents a substantial hazard because of its sharp irregular edges. Aircraft debris may be widely scattered, seriously hampering access and egress to the victims.

Necessary Equipment

When establishing the necessary resources for the disaster, the issue of what equipment is necessary should be addressed. If the accident occurs at night, then proper lighting must be established at the scene. The amount of medical equipment should be proportionate to the size of the disaster. With aircraft accidents, the mechanisms of injury mandate a heavy demand for splints, dressings, and backboards. Some services solve this problem by establishing mass casualty incident response vehicles. These vehicles are well stocked with all the equipment needed for handling a mass casualty incident producing 50 to100 patients. The most important aspect in using these vehicles is to deploy them as soon as the need for this equipment on the scene has been established. Alternatively, such equipment may be stored at the airport for use during crashes located on the flight line.

Prehospital personnel should be cognizant of the unique injuries or illnesses that may occur during or as a result of an air crash disaster. In addition to the rapid deceleration injuries, penetrating injuries, burns, and smoke inhalation associated with traumatic mechanisms, EMS personnel should be ready to care for patients with dysbarisms due to rapid altitude changes. The major challenges associated with the prehospital response to an air crash disaster are listed in Table 29.1.

TABLE 29.1. PREHOSPITAL CHALLENGES IN AIR CRASH DISASTERS

Access to the scene of the crash
Flight-line access
Off flight-line access
Communications with the airport tower, EMS, and fire and
    rescue units
Identification of the extent of the crash scene
Identification and collection of the ambulatory victims
Fuel, fire, and hazardous materials
Debris field
Security of the scene (off flight-line crashes)
Evidence preservation (terrorist events)

Abbreviation: EMS, emergency medical services.

TABLE 29.2. MEASURES TO DECREASE RISK DURING AIR MEDICAL MISSIONS

Limit night flights if possible.
Restrict bad weather flights.
Increase pilot proficiency and training.
Decrease pilot and flight crew fatigue.
Limit pilot and flight crew workload.
Use twin engine aircraft.
Eliminate or modify the tail rotor on future airframes.
Establish adequate preventive maintenance programs.

Prehospital care providers and other public agencies should establish a plan for how they will respond if an air crash disaster occurs. This plan should be rehearsed so that problems can be identified and eliminated before an actual disaster.

Air Medical Considerations

Although genuinely concerned with our patients, nothing hits the disaster and EMS community harder than the loss of its own. Air medical units operate in a dangerous environment even during routine operations. Performing air medical operations in the chaos of a disaster generates an added risk. Although no comprehensive studies have been conducted on the risk to flight crews during disaster response, air medical units have traditionally experienced a higher death and injury rate than the general rotary wing aviation community (5). However, the death and injury rate for air medical crews has been steadily decreasing over the past few years (6 deaths/100,000 flight hours in 1986 to 3 deaths/100,000 flight hours in 1991) (6). The vast majority of air medical unit crashes occur due to pilot error (60%–80%) or mechanical failure (20%–25%). In addition, bad weather and night operations, during which 40% of all air medical missions occur, represent additional risks (7). De Lorenzo and others have indicated that, with strict safety protocols, air medical operations could be conducted with a safety profile similar to general rotary wing aviation (8). Additionally, another suggestion is that, with adequate planning and safety protocols, air medical missions may be carried out without undue risk during disasters (9). Table 29.2 indicates some guidelines for decreasing the overall risk for air medical crews.

EMERGENCY DEPARTMENT CONSIDERATIONS

Air crash considerations for the emergency department (ED) begin with planning. That the ED have a well-integrated disaster plan is important, but, in addition, all EDs close to airports should be active participants in the airport's disaster response plan. Coordination of the disaster response and predetermined transport destinations for specific types of patients will improve the overall response immeasurably. Crashes occurring within the airport security area may demonstrate less of a geographic effect because ambulatory victims are less likely to have access to their own modes of transportation.

EDs should plan for multiple blunt and penetrating trauma, burns, hazardous materials exposure, and psychoemotional stress generated by the event. General surgical services and subspecialties will be in high demand. Additionally, ancillary services such as radiology (computed tomography and plain radiography) and blood bank services will be stressed.

Air crash disasters are highly publicized events, thus adding an additional dimension to the ED response. Each ED must be provided with adequate security to protect both patients and staff from unauthorized or unwanted intrusions by news media and other individuals. Regular news media briefings need to be organized and conducted by the public relations officer of each hospital.

MECHANISMS OF INJURY

Rotary Wing

When considering the mechanism of injury of rotary wing aircraft accidents, one must remember that many of the injuries suffered will occur secondary to vertical deceleration forces. In addition, the fact that restraint devices in helicopters are designed more efficiently than those for a passenger aircraft, which relies only on a lap belt, should be taken into account. These restraint systems have decreased the incidence of abdominal injuries seen in helicopter accidents (10).

One study performed on United States Army helicopter crashes showed that head injuries were most frequent (10). This can be explained by both contact injury due to the collapsing structure and the intrusion of high mass items (e.g., rotor system, transmission, and engines) (10).

The lower extremities comprise the next most commonly injured body region, occurring at twice the rate of upper extremities (10). As might be expected, back injuries, specifically those to the lower back, are a concern following a rotary wing accident. The vertebrae most affected with helicopter accidents are T12–L3, with C7 injuries close behind (10). An interesting phenomenon regarding helicopter accidents is the frequent lack of thermal injuries. This can most likely be attributed to the success of the crashworthy fuel systems used in helicopters (10).

Fixed Wing

Fixed wing aircraft accidents have additional considerations in comparison to rotary wing aircraft. For example, the altitude at which airplanes fly is much greater than that of helicopters. Accidents involving fixed wing aircraft can occur both in the air and upon impact with the ground or water.

While in the air, the aircraft can suffer from the loss of cabin pressurization or from turbulence.

Rapid Decompression

Loss of cabin pressurization can be either slow or rapid. Slow decompression is usually insidious, and it does not cause a problem as long as the crew recognizes it. On the other hand, a rapid decompression (RD) occurs abruptly; it can be recognized by flying debris, fogging, and, in many cases, an explosive sound. During a RD, anything that is not secured can become a missile, causing penetrating and blunt trauma to any individual in its path. As the pressure equilibrates within the aircraft, the partial pressure of oxygen will decrease. If the aircraft is above 10,000 feet and the crew and passengers are not on oxygen, they quickly become hypoxic and lose consciousness. The time of useful consciousness depends on the altitude at which the RD occurs.

Other physiologic problems that can occur during a RD include pneumothoraxes, hypothermia, and decompression sickness. Some of the minor problems that occur following a loss of pressurization include sinus and ear blocks. Loss of pressurization does not occur as infrequently as might be expected. Between 1969 and 1990, 205 cases involving United States naval aircraft were reported; 184 of these were accidental (11). Of these 184 accidents, the serious physiologic problems included one pneumothorax, 11 cases of type I decompression sickness, 23 cases of mild-to-moderate hypoxia with no loss of consciousness, and 18 cases of hypoxia with a loss of consciousness (11). Other injuries that were seen included facial cuts, contusions, bruises, and one fractured ulna (11). According to the NTSB aviation accident and/or incident database, six events involving civilian aircraft have been documented during recent decades (12).

Turbulence

Another aircraft emergency that can occur while in flight involves turbulence. If the aircraft encounters severe turbulence, passengers and crew can experience injuries ranging from simple cervical strains to severe closed head injuries. Under high levels of turbulence, the passengers and crewmembers can be thrown about, striking the fuselage and internal aircraft structures. If numerous individuals are not restrained, the number of victims suffering injuries that require evaluation can be quite large. In most cases, the turbulence cannot be predicted and thus can catch the entire crew by surprise.

Several years ago, the primary author was aboard a C-130 H model during a training flight when the aircraft encountered severe turbulence. While carrying out crew duties in the cargo compartment, the aircraft went into a negative 2.5-G drop, so that he was slammed into the roof of the aircraft fuselage. Luckily, only abrasions and bruises resulted from the event. Other individuals have not been so lucky, and turbulence such as this has caused extensive injuries and even death. For this reason, commercial airlines now stress that passengers should remain restrained unless moving about in the cabin is absolutely necessary.

Crash-Related Physical Injuries

The most severe injuries still occur upon the impact of the aircraft with either the ground (crash) or water (ditching). During a crash or ditching incident, the main mechanism of injury is rapid deceleration resulting in blunt trauma (13). During a rapid deceleration, the occupants of the aircraft are at risk for internal organ injury from the deceleration of the body cavity against seat belt restraints. In addition, they may strike the seat in front of them or other structures in the aircraft, resulting in blunt or penetrating trauma. Death usually results from transection of the great vessels or from head or spinal trauma.

Among the survivors of serious aircraft accidents, injuries to the lower extremities occur most often, followed by spinal injuries and head injuries. Of these injuries, fractures predominate (14). Other regions of the body affected by both penetrating and blunt trauma include the thorax and abdomen, with the chest being affected much more often than the abdomen (14). Additionally, environmental factors associated with the crash, such as near drowning during ditching, hyperthermia, or hypothermia, may need to be considered.

Aircraft Fires

One complication that can be experienced both in the air and upon impact is an aircraft fire. A 1980 NTSB review of 22,002 aircraft accidents between 1974 and 1978 indicated that fire was involved in 8% of the accidents (15). In most cases, the cause of the fatality or serious injury was not caused by thermal contact; rather, it was the result of the inhalation of toxic combustion products. Two common toxic gases that are found in the smoke from aircraft fires are carbon monoxide and hydrogen cyanide (16). Hydrogen cyanide will inhibit oxygen use at the cellular level, and carbon monoxide will form carboxyhemoglobin. Both of these mechanisms, especially when added to displaced oxygen concentration, are responsible for the onset of hypoxia in a fire (16).

In addition to its pulmonary toxicity, smoke obscures the vision of the victims, thereby making escape from the aircraft more difficult. The suspended smoke particles may also contain sufficient thermal energy to result in upper airway burns. Although suffering from smoke inhalation during an aircraft accident is more common, this does not mean that burns will not be encountered. Victims with substantial burns may be found, particularly if widespread ignition of aviation fuel occurs. The initiation of prehospital respiratory and burn care should follow the standard guidelines established for such injuries.

PREVENTION AND SAFETY

Since the 1980s, aviation safety has improved remarkably, reducing the number of fatalities by 34% (13). The aviation community has used past experiences to improve safety aspects aboard modern aircraft.

Fire Safety

Although in-flight fires are rare, they can be extremely devastating phenomena. After investigations of fires caused by passengers during the 1970s, the NTSB made recommendations regarding smoke detectors and no smoking regulations for commercial flights that were later imposed. In June 1983, an Air Canada DC-9 experienced an in-flight fire due to a motor in the air-conditioning system that overheated. Although an emergency was declared, 20 minutes passed before the aircraft was able to make an emergency landing. As a result, only half of the 46 persons onboard were able to escape the burning aircraft. The majority of the people who died were overcome by toxic inhalants, and many of the passengers were unable to see the exits due to the smoke. As a result of the investigation of this incident, smoke detectors and automatic fire extinguishers have been installed in all commercial airline lavatories. In addition, floor level escape lighting has been installed, and aircraft throughout the United States have been equipped with fire retardant cabin and seat materials (3). Additional investigations of aircraft fires, such as that of the May 1996 ValuJet DC-9 crash, have led to Federal Aviation Administration (FAA) regulations regarding the installation of fire detection and suppression equipment in cargo holds.

Improvements in emergency breathing devices for passengers in fixed wing aircraft could still be made. More effective emergency breathing devices might prevent survivors from becoming overwhelmed by toxic inhalants in the aircraft. In addition, a cabin water spray system has been proposed. This would slow the spread of cabin fires (16). It would also help to eliminate the particulates and water-soluble fire gases, such as cyanide and hydrogen chloride, from the ambient cabin atmosphere (16).

Wind Shear

Since 1968, the NTSB has issued over 60 safety recommendations regarding wind shear and related weather issues. The August 1985 crash of the Delta Airlines Lockheed L-1011 at the Dallas–Fort Worth airport that resulted in a loss of 135 lives spurred an intense investigation into the phenomenon of wind shear. As a result of this and other investigations, the installation of the terminal Doppler weather radar (TDWR) system throughout the United States is currently in progress. This system detects wind shear phenomena along flight paths, allowing warnings to be given to approaching aircraft. Where it has been installed, the TDWR system has substantially decreased wind-related aircraft incidents.

Icing

The serious effects of icing on aviation have been recognized since the 1930s. Even minimal amounts of icing on the wing can have substantial effects on the aerodynamic performance of modern aircraft. Beginning with the investigations in 1975 with the fatal crash of a USAir Fokker F-28 during icing conditions, substantial changes in the deicing procedures required for commercial aircraft have occurred. The NTSB has even recommended that some aircraft (e.g., the ATR-42 and ATR-72 passenger turboprop) not fly in conditions conducive to icing.

Alcohol

Beginning in 1984, regulations were implemented to assist in identifying pilots who have had their driver's license suspended for alcohol-related offenses. In 1988, the FAA issued regulations requiring the identification of pilots involved in alcohol-related or drug-related motor vehicle offenses. All pilots applying for medical certificate (medical clearance to fly) must now consent to the release of such information to the FAA during the application process. All airlines in the United States now require the performance of preemployment, random, and postaccident drug testing of pilots and flight crew members.

Aircraft Seats

The construction, anchoring, and characteristics of airline seats have also been improved as a result of crash investigations. These investigations identified specific reasons for the failure of aircraft seats and restraint devices. The number of fatalities in fixed aircraft can be decreased dramatically by creating a more effective restraint system (13). Such improvements have resulted in modifications of welding methods and of both seat and seat belt construction.

Cockpit Resource Management

Historic problems due to the hierarchical structure of the pilot and crew relationship have led to catastrophic air crashes (3). These occurrences stimulated the development of cockpit resource management (CRM) techniques during the 1970s. CRM methods have opened up communication lines among all levels of the flight crew, thus improving overall safety and efficiency. The value of CRM techniques was clearly demonstrated during the 1989 United Airlines DC-10 emergency and the subsequent crash landing in Sioux City, Iowa. The interaction of the flight crew and an additional airline pilot who was a passenger enabled them to work through the emergency after a catastrophic engine failure resulted in the loss of all the aircraft hydraulic systems. Although more than 100 people died in the crash landing, almost 200 people survived a situation for which no airline pilot had previously been trained (3).

A similar system, crew resource management, has been implemented within the United States military. Through crew resource management, the barrier between the cockpit crew (front end crew) and the cargo compartment crew (rear end crew) has been eliminated. Crew resource management empowers all crewmembers aboard the aircraft with issues regarding safety matters. For example, if a load master or an aeromedical evacuation technician notices something aboard the aircraft that does not seem right, he or she immediately notifies the aircraft commander. The situation is then investigated, and corrective actions are made as necessary. Crew resource management has been instrumental in decreasing the number of mishaps within the United States Air Force.

MENTAL HEALTH IMPACT

Air crash disasters are one of the most emotionally charged transportation-related disasters. The sudden and massive injury and loss of life take a significant toll on the victim's families, survivors, and rescue workers. Initially, the release of information and often the emotional care of these individuals has been left to the very airline associated with the disaster. In 1996, Congress passed the Aviation Disaster Family Assistance Act, which mandated that the NTSB was required to see to the needs of the bereaved families. In 1998, as part of the overall federal response plan, the NTSB designated the American Red Cross (ARC) as the official agency responsible for consoling and counseling families and victims of air crash disasters.

The ARC has developed regional air disaster teams (ADT) with specialized training that are situated throughout the nation. The first team of 54 members responded to the Korean flight 801 crash on Guam. Each team currently is on call for approximately 2 months of each year. Upon notification of an air crash, these teams deploy to the crash site to initiate and coordinate needed services. Support centers are created for family members close to the site of the crash. The ADT works with the airline to track the status of hospitalized passengers and to provide needed assistance to family members. Although substantially different mechanisms are used, the level and type of support for families and victims have been compared to that following the Oklahoma City bombing.

CRASHES AT SEA

Most crashes at sea result in recovery rather than rescue operations. Recovery of victim's remains from submerged wreckage presents significant challenges for all involved. Medical support for such recovery missions may be quite extensive. Along with routine medical care and emotional support for recovery workers, health care providers may be called on to treat occasional dysbarisms associated with diving activities. Health and occupational monitoring and sanitation become the primary objectives of the medical team in this setting.

SUMMARY

In today's society, more people are flying than ever before. For this reason, aircraft crashes are a reality that require planning. Special preparation must be undertaken by EMS regarding access and operations on or near aircraft flight lines. Unique hazards may confront fire-rescue and EMS personnel responding to the scene of an air crash. Medical personnel must be prepared to deal with the physical and emotional impact of the crash, as well as the substantial media attention it will draw.

REFERENCES

1. National Transportation Safety Board. *Airport and emergency group chairman's factual report of investigation, American Airlines, MD-82, N215AA, Little Rock, Arkansas, June 1, 1999.* Report no. DCA-99-MA-060. Washington, D.C.: United States National Transportation Safety Board, 1999.
2. National Transportation Safety Board. Aircraft accident report no. DCA-99-MA-060. Washington, D.C.: United States National Transportation Safety Board, 1999.
3. National Transportation Safety Board. *We are all safer*, 2nd ed. Washington, D.C.: National Transportation Safety Board Public Affairs Office, 1998.
4. National Transportation Safety Board. *Accidents, fatalities, and rates, 1982 through 1999, US general aviation.* Washington, D.C.: United States National Transportation Safety Board, 1999.
5. Collett HM. Year in review. *Hosp Aviat* 1987;1:3.
6. Preston N. 1991 Air medical accident rates. *J Air Med Transport* 1992;14:102.
7. Isaacs MS, Saunders CE, Durrer B. Aeromedical transport. In: Auerbach PS, ed. *Wilderness medicine: management of wilderness and environmental emergencies*, 3rd ed. St. Louis: Mosby, 1995: 535–565.
8. De Lorenzo RA, Freid RL, Villarin AR. Army aeromedical crash rates. *Mil Med* 1999;164:116–118.
9. Hogan DE, Askins D, Osburn E. The May 3rd 1999 Oklahoma City tornado. *Ann Emerg Med* 1999;34:225–226.
10. Shanahan D, Shanahan M. Injury in U.S. helicopter crashes October 1979–September 1985. *J Trauma* 1989;29:415–423.
11. Bason R, Yacavone DW. Loss of cabin pressurization in U.S. naval aircraft: 1969–1990. *Aviat Space Environ Med* 1992;65:341–345.
12. National Transportation Safety Board. National Aviation safety data analysis center [database]. Available at: http://www.nasdac.faa.gov/internet/. Accessed September 27, 2000.
13. Li G, Baker SP. Injury patterns in aviation-related fatalities. *Am J Forensic Med Pathol* 1997;18:265–270.
14. Chalmers DJ, O'Hare DPA, McBride DI. The incidence, nature, and severity of injuries in New Zealand civil aviation. *Aviat Space Environ Med* 2000;71:388–395.
15. National Transportation Safety Board. *National Transportation Safety Board special study of 1974-8 data, general aviation accidents, postcrash fires, and how to prevent or control them.* Report AAS-80-2. Washington, D.C.: United States National Transportation Safety Board, 1980.
16. Chaturvedi A, Sanders MS. Aircraft fires, smoke toxicity, and survival. *Aviat Space Environ Med* 1996;67:275–278.

FIRES AND MASS BURN CARE

KIM D. FLOYD

At 10 AM on a Monday morning, and the emergency medical services (EMS) phone in the emergency department starts its usual bothersome ringing. A nurse answer it, and the listeners' minds conjure up all kinds of possibilities—a full arrest, a stabbing or a gunshot victim, or even multiple injuries from a motor vehicle collision. Not once does the possibility occur that the nurse is going to turn in horror and exclaim, "The Tower Bank Building three blocks from the hospital is involved in a four alarm fire! The whole fifth floor of the ten story office building is on fire!"

America's fire death rate of 13.1 per million population is one of the highest per capita in the industrialized world (1). In 1999, 3,570 Americans lost their lives and another 21,875 were injured as the result of fire; 112 firefighters were killed in duty-related incidents. Even more tragic, perhaps, is the fact that disasters caused by large structural fires are some of the more preventable disasters. Fire kills more Americans than all natural disasters combined. Of the 1.8 million fires reported in 1999, 82% of all deaths resulting from fires occur in residences. Many others are unreported yet cause additional injuries and property loss. Average

yearly direct property losses due to fires have been estimated at $10 billion. In 1999, an estimated 72,000 incendiary or suspicious structure fires resulted in 370 civilian deaths and $1.3 billion in property damage alone (2,3).

Despite this, America's fire losses today represent a dramatic improvement from more than 20 years ago. In 1971, America lost more than 12,000 citizens and 250 firefighters to fires. Acting to halt these tragic losses, Congress passed Public Law 93-498, the Federal Fire Prevention and Control Act, in 1974; this legislation established the United States Fire Administration (USFA) and its National Fire Academy (NFA). Since that time, through data collection, public education, research, and training efforts, the USFA has helped reduce fire deaths by at least half, making communities and citizens safer (1). The injury and death rates from fire in the United States over the past decade are depicted in Fig. 30.1.

The sad note is that firefighter fatality is not declining. According to the USFA's reports, fatalities among firefighters actually increased in 1999. One hundred and twelve firefighters lost their lives while on duty in 1999. This is the highest total number of deaths since 1989, a year when 119

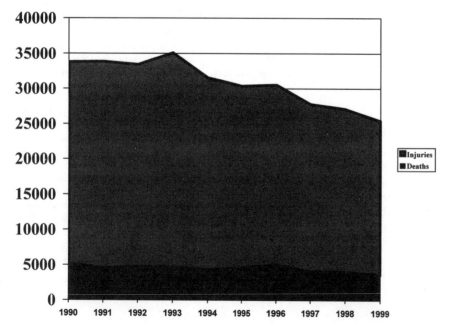

FIGURE 30.1. Injuries and deaths in the United States due to fire, 1990–1999.

firefighters died. This is the first time since 1994 that the number of deaths topped 100, reversing a 4-year downward trend in firefighter fatalities (2).

RESIDENTIAL VERSUS LARGE STRUCTURAL FIRES

The differences between residential fires and those engulfing large physical structures are manifold. One of the most obvious is access to the various areas of a structure. Access to escape routes for victims, as well as routes available to rescuers, become critical in larger structures, while they are often more simple in residential fires. Moreover, the sheer numbers of potential victims increases in larger structures. This increases the risk of EMS system burden and overload as the number of real and potential victims rises, as in any disaster. The potential for collapse resulting in trapped victims is higher with larger structures. Such an event necessitates the use of search and rescue (SAR) teams, thereby endangering more lives in addition to the existing fire and EMS personnel.

Much of the effort in fire prevention, both public and private, has gone into protecting nonresidential structures, and the results have been highly effective in comparison to the residential fire problem. Between 1990 and 1999, non-residential structures represented approximately 4% of fire deaths, 11% of fire injuries, 31% of total fire dollar loss, and 8% of all fires (2,3).

MECHANISMS OF INJURY

Thermal Injury

Direct thermal injury from flame or steam results in coagulation and denaturation of body proteins. This disrupts the function of the skin, which serves to contain and regulate body fluids and temperature, as well as to protect against environmental pathogens. Death rates from burns are highest in the age ranges of less than 5 years and greater than 65 years.

Burns are usually classified by the depth of the burn in tissue and the degree of damage to body structures. First-degree, or superficial, burns involve the epidermis without substantial injury to the underlying cutaneous structures. On examination, the tissue is erythematous, and it blanches with pressure.

Second-degree burns, also called partial-thickness burns, involve the epidermis and parts of the dermis. Hair follicles and sweat glands may be damaged, but the ability to regenerate is usually preserved throughout the area of the burn, thus allowing the healing process to take place. Erythema, blistering, and significant pain are usually seen with this depth of burn. Substantial edema may occur, resulting in an extension of the area of tissue damage due to decreased blood flow and lymphedema. In this setting, a partial-thickness burn may be converted to a full-thickness burn.

Third-degree burns, or full-thickness burns, result in extensive damage to all layers of the skin and to underlying

structures. Charring of the skin or a translucent appearance is noted. The area of the third-degree burn usually is not painful because of the loss of underlying pain sensors. A surrounding area of second-degree or first-degree burns may, however, be quite painful. Third-degree burns result in a substantial loss of the underlying structures and function. Healing results in scarring without the regeneration of the missing skin elements. Extensive skin grafting and surgical revisions are usually required to restore a level of function.

Inhalation Injury

Thermal

Thermal damage of the airway is usually restricted to the upper airway. Heat is dissipated rapidly from the dry air to tissue once it is inhaled. Studies have indicated that extremely hot air is cooled to near body temperature by the time it reaches the carina. Steam or very moist hot air has more ability to cause deep burns in the trachea and bronchi due to the heat energy carried by the vapor droplets. Early and aggressive airway management is indicated if thermal airway injury is suspected, or tissue swelling will result with subsequent airway obstruction.

Toxic

Smoke inhalation accounts for a large majority of the injuries from fires. It is considered the leading cause of mortality in burn treatment centers (4,5). Airway management is perhaps the most critical factor in patient care. Early and aggressive utilization of optimal and appropriate oxygen therapy is needed to provide adequate oxygen supplies for injured tissues, as well as to displace the carbon monoxide that may be bound to the victim's hemoglobin. Definitive airway management should be early and aggressive. Tracheal intubation should be considered not only in the case of obvious respiratory compromise but also in the patient who is expected to deteriorate from a combination of injuries, respiratory damage, toxins, and medications.

Hypoxia may occur due to the fire's consumption of atmospheric oxygen. Carbon monoxide (CO) poisoning is also a significant risk for burn victims, particularly those who have been in an enclosed structure for any period of time with a fire. CO binds to hemoglobin with greater affinity than it does oxygen, thus decreasing the oxygen-carrying capacity of the red blood cells. High flow oxygen and/or hyperbaric oxygen therapy may be needed.

The combustion of various substances (plastics, silk, wool, nylon, and rubber) under the right circumstances results in the generation of cyanide compounds. Cyanide interferes with cellular oxidation through the cytochrome A3 system and acts as a cellular asphyxiant. Any victim presenting from a fire in cardiac arrest or with a substantial metabolic acidosis should raise the suspicion of cyanide toxicity. Immediate therapy with a protocol of amyl nitrite, sodium nitrite, and sodium thiosulfate should be considered. Fires may also generate hydrogen sulfide gas with similar asphyxiant effects on oxygen-carrying abilities. The approach to therapy is similar, including the use of sodium nitrite.

FIRE RESEARCH AND INJURY PREVENTION

Shared information from government agencies, such as the Federal Emergency Management Agency (FEMA), as well as other agencies such as the National Institute of Standards and Technology, have created an electronic-based media in an attempt to bolster the meager, and sometimes difficult to find, written data. FIREDOC is a bibliographic database devoted to the subject of fire research and related areas of interest, such as combustion toxicology, arson, and fire modeling (6). In addition, the Building and Fire Research Laboratory has a searchable database that is quite comprehensive (7). In an effort to help define and chart the future course of the nation's fire services, FEMA released the final report of America Burning Recommissioned titled *America at risk: findings and recommendations on the role of the fire service in the prevention and control of risks in America* (8).

Education is key in the prevention of fire injury, as in any other injury. This involves not only public education but also education at the higher levels of government. The Congressional Fire Services Institute is a nonprofit, nonpartisan policy institute charged with educating members of Congress on fire and life safety issues (9). Fire safety education programs for the public starting in primary school have been effective in increasing the awareness of fire risk, as well as injury prevention actions, in some residential areas (4,10). Placement of smoke detectors in residential areas by public health, fire, and EMS programs may reduce the morbidity and mortality from fires in these locations. Engineering mechanisms, such as smoke detectors, sprinkler systems, fire doors, emergency lighting, and fire alarms, in both public and residential structures have also been suggested to decrease morbidity and mortality from fires (11).

BURN ESTIMATION

Burns are classified by the depth, type, and extent of injury. Factors such as prognosis, burn center referral, and fluid resuscitation of the burned victim are directed by a combination of the involved body surface area (BSA) and the depth of the burn. BSA classically is determined by using the Lund and Browder diagrams or the "rule of nines" or by estimating the victim's palm surface area to be approximately 1% of the BSA. This is depicted in Fig. 30.2. Tradi-

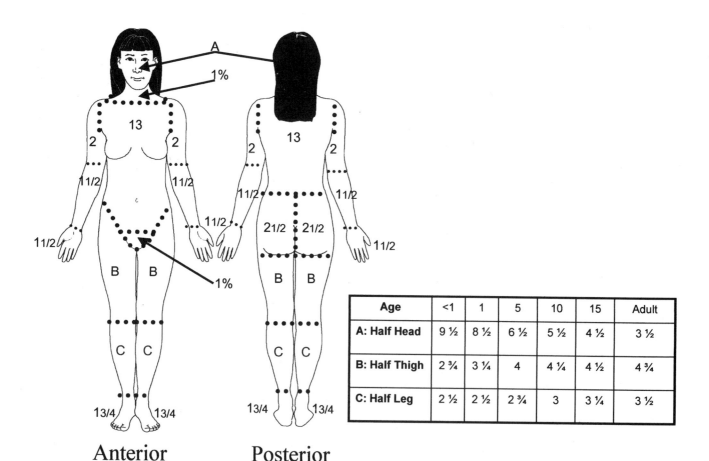

Age	<1	1	5	10	15	Adult
A: Half Head	9 ½	8 ½	6 ½	5 ½	4 ½	3 ½
B: Half Thigh	2 ¾	3 ¼	4	4 ¼	4 ½	4 ¾
C: Half Leg	2 ½	2 ½	2 ¾	3	3 ¼	3 ½

FIGURE 30.2. Lund and Browder burn estimation chart.

tionally, burn depth has been expressed as first, second, or third degree. The current trend is to classify burn injury according to a need for surgical intervention. Burns may be classified as partial or full thickness. Superficial partial-thickness burns typically heal without surgical intervention, whereas deep partial-thickness burns may require surgical debridement or even skin grafting. Superficial partial-thickness burns involve the epidermis and the superficial dermis. The deeper layers of the dermis are involved in deep partial-thickness burns. Full-thickness burns involve the epidermis and the full dermal layer (4,10).

PREHOSPITAL CONSIDERATIONS

Search and Rescue

More critical in large structural fires compared to residential fires is the ability to deploy SAR teams, particularly in the event of building collapse. The rescuer's safety is always a priority issue. In many cities, EMS and fire personnel are trained in rescue from collapsed structures. Additionally, courses and training are available for confined space medicine. The primary rule in rescue is that "the rescuer goes home at night"— in other words, rescuer safety is the number one issue. In the event of a structural collapse, victims arrive at various intervals, based largely on extrication times. Time is an important issue because injuries may be anticipated to vary according to where the victims were found, as well as by the length of extrication. As many as 50% of the injured are considered surface victims—those who are injured, but not trapped. For obvious reasons, many of these will be the first to arrive to the emergency department. Approximately 30% of the victims are trapped by nonstructural building contents (desks, cabinets) and will require light rescue. Roughly 15% of all victims involved in a structural collapse are found entrapped in the void spaces created during the collapse. Typically, these victims require at least a 4-hour extrication time, so their injuries must be considered with this time delay in mind. Entombed victims account for the remaining 5%. They have been trapped by structural components. Their rescue is tediously slow due to the necessity for extensive shoring and moving of heavy structures. Their retrieval may take longer than 8 to 12 hours. Survivors with this length of extrication time typically fare poorly, and their prehospital and emergency department care necessitate extremely aggressive interventions (12).

Prehospital Triage of Burns

According to one large regional burn center, the following should be transferred to a burn center: second-degree and third-degree burns of greater than 10% BSA; third-degree burns greater than 2% BSA; burns that involve the face, hands, feet, perineum, and major joints; electrical, chemical, and inhalation injuries; circumferential burns of an extremity or chest; burns involving trauma; and patients with a burn and a complicating medical disorder (13). The American Burn Association adds partial-thickness burns involving more than 10% BSA in ages less than 10 years or older than 50; partial-thickness burns involving more than 20% BSA in the 10-year-old to 50-year-old age group; full-thickness burns covering more than 5% in any age group; potentially cosmetically or functionally impairing burns involving the hands, feet, face, perineum, or major joints; and inhalation injuries. Hospitals without the ability for advanced pediatric care should transfer patients to a pediatric burn center (11).

In the event of a mass casualty situation, burn centers may become overloaded and may be unable to bear the burden of caring for a large influx of burn victims. Alternate plans must exist during a burn-related disaster in order to prevent overload of a burn center with such patients. Rapid prehospital estimates of the number of burn victims and the severity of their burns should be undertaken in mass burn situations. These estimates should be compared with the known availability of burn care resources (14). Burn casualties should then be distributed throughout the community based on the above comparisons to avoid overloading burn units with less critical burns. Based on experience in Oklahoma City and elsewhere, hospitals nearest the disaster bear a heavier burden initially in mass casualty management due to the geographic effect (see Chapter 1) (15). In any disaster, transfer to specialty centers and a dispersal of victims throughout the system ensues (16). Thus, the hospitals nearest the fire may initially be burdened with a heavy load of burned victims.

Prehospital disaster response with mass burn casualties may need to be modified by local hospital, EMS, city, or statewide disaster plans. Mass casualties from burns should be incorporated into such disaster plans based on the availability of burn care resources. Questions that need to be addressed in planning for such burn-related disasters include the following:

- Who are the local or regional burn care providers?
- What volumes can each handle in the event of a mass casualty burn?
- What can other local facilities handle?
- When should a burn disaster plan be initiated?

Prehospital Therapy of Burns

Initial treatment consists of putting out the fire. The injured placed away from the fire and any burning or smoldering clothing or gear should be removed, as well as any burning or smoldering debris. First aid and advanced medical care are administered as indicated, including the establishment and maintenance of an adequate airway. Intravenous lines should be started immediately, the airway should be maintained, and any immediately life-threatening injuries should be addressed. A rapid trauma survey should be included in the initial evaluation of the victim because traumatic injuries often coexist.

EMERGENCY DEPARTMENT CONSIDERATIONS

Burn Casualty Triage in the Emergency Department

Burns of greater than 40% BSA, age greater than 60 years, and the presence of inhalation injury are risk factors for death. The mortality rate is 0.3% with no risk factors, 3% with one, 33% with two, and approximately 87% with three risk factors. In a mass burn situation with limited resources, such mortality factors should be kept in mind during emergency department triage (see Chapter 2). Patients with 87% mortality risk may need to be triaged expectant and given pain relief and comfort. These victims should be continually retriaged during the disaster response, particularly if more resources become available for them.

Clinical Interventions

Small burns should be immediately immersed in tepid water but not soaked. Current trends in burn management do not recommend the use of ice or cold compresses because this may increase tissue ischemia and necrosis. The wound should be cleaned with soap and water, and all debris must be carefully removed. For deeply embedded dirt, the wound may be anesthetized with a local infiltration of 1% or 2% lidocaine and then scrubbed with a brush and soap. Conscious sedation may be helpful in the debridement of wounds. This may be accomplished in a number of methods, including the use of combinations of narcotics, benzodiazepines, ketamine, or rapid-acting short duration barbiturates, such as methohexatol. Blisters should be sharply debrided if they are already broken or if they are likely to be. To assess burn depth, blisters may be removed, so the wound base can be examined to determine if the injury is full thickness.

When the wound is clean and dry, a topical agent may be used and an appropriate dressing should be applied. Mafenide acetate or silver sulfadiazine cream is applied directly to the wound in one layer, and the wound is then covered with a nonadherent dressing. Mafenide acetate cream inhibits carbonic anhydrase activity, and it may produce compensated metabolic acidosis and, occasionally, proximal renal tubular acidosis. Silver sulfadiazine should be used with caution in patients who are sensitive to sulfonamides; it may cause hematologic abnormalities. In addition, silver sulfadiazine may cause argyrophilic stippling of the skin (tattooing) due to the deposition of silver oxide. All patients who are not up-to-date on their tetanus immunizations should be immunized. For those individuals who have never received tetanus immunizations, tetanus immune globulin should be administered in addition to active immunization.

Pain management is important. The treatment of pain is based on the severity of the injury as well as the patient's perceptions of pain. Nonsteroidal medications should constitute the first line of pain control in individuals who can tolerate the nonsteroidal antiinflammatory drugs. Narcotics should be used as a second line for breakthrough pain, especially in the first day or so after injury. For more severe pain, particularly in the hospitalized victim, injectable narcotics will most likely be required.

Immediate and aggressive fluid resuscitation is of high importance. Maintenance of records with regard to volume repletion is important as well. This allows for optimal continuity at the receiving burn center. Adequate fluid replacement prevents peripheral vasoconstriction and hypoperfusion, thus optimizing the patient's own healing and protective mechanisms. Some advocate early use of a colloid solution, such as fresh frozen plasma, which contains antibacterial substances including antibodies, to aid the body's own natural defenses against bacterial invasion by organisms contaminating the burn before the start of treatment.

Shock should be anticipated in all deep partial-thickness or full-thickness burns of more than 10% BSA or when hemoconcentration is present. As in any patient who is found to be or who is expected to be in shock, two large bore intravenous catheters should be placed. Although central lines may not be necessary initially, later placement may be difficult because of extensive wound edema; thus, early placement may be best. If necessary, central or peripheral lines may be placed through burn eschar. Cutdowns are generally not recommended because of the increased risk of infection.

Literally dozens of recommendations for fluid resuscitation are used in the treatment and prevention of shock in burn centers. Perhaps one of the most widely used recommendations is the Parkland formula. For adults, the recommendation is calculated as follows: 4 mL lactated Ringer's solution (LR) × patient weight (kg) × % BSA involved (administered over 24 hours). Half of this volume should be administered in the first 8 hours and the remainder in the ensuing 16 hours. The estimated time of the patient's initial burn is the start time of fluid resuscitation, so if a time delay occurred in receiving the patient to the emergency department, that time should be accounted for in the calculation. Pediatric fluid resuscitation is as follows: LR 3 mL × kg × % BSA over the initial 24 hours, plus the calculated maintenance rate for that child. Again, the first half should be infused over the first 8 hours with the remainder being administered over the ensuing 16 hours (4,10). Urinary output must be monitored; it should be expected to amount to 0.5 to 1 mL per kg per hour. Hemodynamic monitoring is also useful, especially in children or in patients with concomitant disabilities, such as cardiac or renal disease, where fluid overload is a distinct possibility. The rates of fluid resuscitation may need to be adjusted in each patient as the dynamics of their injuries unfold. Accurate records are essential, particularly in patients who may be transferred to a burn center. Carefully documented fluid and treatment flow sheets should be used.

SUMMARY

Response to a disaster with a large number of burned victims requires special planning based on the availability of local specialized burn care and other resources. Aggressive and early airway and fluid intervention are the mainstays of burn therapy no matter where the patients are treated. Assessment of burn-related modification of mortality may be important in the initial triage of large numbers of burn victims to provide the greatest good for the greatest number when resources are limited. Finally, injury prevention through education and engineering methods may be the most important factor in any community for decreasing the morbidity and mortality from fires.

REFERENCES

 1. United States Fire Administration. About USFA. Available at: http://www.usfa.fema.gov/about/. Accessed April 7, 2001.
 2. National Fire Protection Association. 1999 Fire loss in the U.S. Available at http://www.usfa.fema.gov/. Accessed April 7, 2001.
 3. United States Fire Administration. Firefighter injuries. *Topical Fire Research Series* July 2001;2.
 4. Johnston BD, Britt J, D'Ambrosio L, et al. A preschool program for safety and injury prevention delivered by home visitors. *Injury Prevent* 2000;6:305–309.
 5. Floyd K. *Confined space medicine.* Presentation to the Oklahoma City fire department urban search and rescue. Oklahoma City, 1999.
 6. Fire Research Information Services. FIREDOC. Available at http://fris.nist.gov/. Accessed April 7, 2001.
 7. Building and Fire Research Laboratory, National Institute of Standards and Technology. Building and Fire Research Laboratory (BFRL) publications online. Available at http://fire.nist.gov/bfrlpubs/. Accessed April 7, 2001.
 8. Congressional Fire Services Institute. Congressional Fire Services Institute (CFSI) home page. Available at: http://www.cfsi.org/. Accessed April 7, 2001.
 9. United States Fire Administration. America burning recommissioned issues final report. Available at: http://www.usfa.fema.gov/about/aar.htm. Accessed April 7, 2001.
10. Warda L, Tenenbein M, Moffatt ME. House fire injury prevention update. Part II. A review of the effectiveness of preventive interventions. *Injury Prevent* 1999;5:217–225.
11. American Public Health Association. Public health role of the national fire protection association in setting codes and standards for the built environment. *Am J Public Health* 2001;91:503–504.
12. Pepe PE, Kvetan V. Field management and critical care in mass disasters. *Crit Care Clin* 1991;7:401–420.
13. Manafo W. Initial management of burns. *N Engl J Med* 1996;335:1581–1586.
14. Gans L. Mass burn care. In: Aghababian R, ed. *Emergency medicine: the core curriculum.* Philadelphia: Lippincott-Raven, 1998:1360–1362.
15. Hogan DE, Waeckerle JF, Dire DJ, et al. Emergency department impact of the Oklahoma City terrorist bombing. *Ann Emerg Med* 1999;34:160–170.
16. Hogan DE, Askins D, Osburn E. The May 3rd 1999 Oklahoma City tornado. *Ann Emerg Med* 1999;34:225–226.

ADDITIONAL READING

American Burn Association. Home page. Available at: http://www.ameriburn.org/. Accessed April 7, 2001.

Saffle JR, Davis B, Williams P. Recent outcomes in the treatment of burn injury in the US. American burn association patient registry. *J Burn Care Rehabil* 1995;16:219–232.

Schwaartz L, Balakrishnan C. Thermal burns. In: Tintinalli JE, Kelen GD, Stapczynski JS, eds. *Emergency medicine: a comprehensive study guide*, 5th ed. New York: American College of Emergency Physicians and McGraw-Hill, 1999:1281–1286.

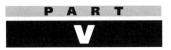

CONFLICT-RELATED DISASTERS

CONVENTIONAL TERRORIST BOMBINGS

DANIEL J. DIRE
CLOYD B. GATRELL

Terrorism is an act designed to generate fear, to intimidate or coerce, to affect government conduct, to punish a specific target (1), and/or to maim as many people as possible to gain news media attention (2). One of terrorists' principal weapons has been a bomb that is either left indoors in public places or placed in a vehicle (3). Terrorist bombings have become a common occurrence throughout the industrialized world. From 1969 to 1983, 220 terrorist bombings worldwide killed 463 persons and injured 2,894 (4). Over the next 10 years, the number of terrorist bombings or bombing attempts increased by 400% in the United States, rising from 803 in 1984 to 3,163 by 1993. The World Trade Center bombing in New York City in 1993 resulted in more than 1,000 injuries, six deaths, and $510 million in damage (5). In the 1995 Oklahoma City bombing, 168 persons were killed, 83 were hospitalized, and 509 were treated as outpatients (5,6). Thus, civilian emergency departments in the United States must be prepared for the possibility of large numbers of bombing victims.

By nature, a terrorist bombing is an isolated event. United States federal, postal, and military facilities are considered targets for terrorist bombings (6). The Oklahoma City Alfred P. Murrah Federal Building in 1995 and the Navy destroyer U.S.S. Cole in 2000 are well-publicized examples.

Blast trauma from bombing incidents varies greatly, depending on the physical environment (e.g., indoors or outdoors, the structural characteristics of the building or vehicle, and the proximity to reflecting surfaces), the device and explosive properties, the victim populations, and the victim distance from the blast and position relative to the blast wave (3,7).

Explosions may kill or maim a victim in several ways. The blast wave may cause internal damage in air-containing organs without any external signs of trauma. A blast may propel fragments into an individual, or it may propel the victim into stationary objects or structures. Terrorist bombs usually are small, often weighing only a few kilograms. This allows them to be hidden in areas where unsuspecting victims will likely congregate. The biologic damage caused by these small bombs is greatly increased when they are packed with small metal objects, such as bolts and nails (8,9). This tends to generate many casualties and to multiply the publicity impact for the perpetrators.

Victims generally are treated at the site or in nearby emergency departments (EDs) that can be quickly reached by ground transportation. Most EDs are unprepared for the sudden influx of the possible hundreds of bombing victims. Casualties arriving to the emergency rooms after a bombing often arrive with complicated injuries that do not fall within the daily purview of the ED staff. To ensure proper planning and to be fully prepared to treat bombing casualties, medical personnel should be familiar with blast physics, the mechanisms and determinants of injury, and the epidemiology of bombing injuries.

BLAST PHYSICS

In the 18th century, Pierre Jars first described the injurious effects of explosions as "la grande et prompte dilation d'air" (10). He and his contemporaries noted that the variation of pressure in air that resulted from the explosion was the cause of injuries.

Conventional terrorist bombs contain hydrogen, oxygen, nitrogen and carbon compounds in various solid, slurry, liquid, or gaseous states (11), and they require a detonator to initiate the explosion. If a volatile fuel is added, greater amounts of heat and destruction are produced (8). Terrorist bombs can be encased in metal or plastic containers and can range in size from only 2 to 30 pounds for those delivered in a suitcase or parcel to 500 pounds or more placed if placed within vehicles.

Conventional high-energy explosives such as trinitrotoluene (TNT) combust rapidly and generate an expanding sphere of hot dense gas (the blast) that can have a pressure

Disclaimer: The views expressed in this academic research paper are those of the author, and they do not necessarily reflect the official policy of the United States Government, the Department of Defense, or any of its agencies.

of over 10×10^6 pounds per square inch (psi) (12). This pressure transmits itself radially into the surrounding medium, creating a blast wave (shock wave), which has the following three features: a positive phase, a negative phase, and the mass movement of wind (blast wind). The combination of weight and distance from the explosion produces a particular pressure-time history, and the laws of physics governing blasts are described by certain mathematical equations. The destructive capacity of a blast is due to the force it exerts, called blast loading, which is usually described as a force per unit area (11).

The defining characteristic of a blast wave at any point in space is the variation in ambient pressure over time (Fig. 31.1). During the positive phase, the wave increases in pressure rapidly in relationship to the explosion and rises above the ambient air pressure, a phenomenon known as blast overpressure. The peak pressure and duration of the positive phase are a function of both the size of the blast and the distance from the blast (13). The biologic response to the blast wave from conventional explosives depends predominantly on the peak overpressure and the duration of the positive phase (14).

Blast winds result from large volumes of air that are displaced by the expanding gases of the explosion (8). The blast strength is the ratio of overpressure to the ambient atmospheric pressure. The term *blast front* is used to describe the leading edge of the blast wave. The blast wave propagates outward through the air at supersonic speed (velocities range from 3,000 to 8,000 m/sec), but it loses its pressure and velocity exponentially with the distance from the source (3,8,13). Because water is incompressible, underwater wave propagation has a much greater speed and loses energy less quickly with distance (13).

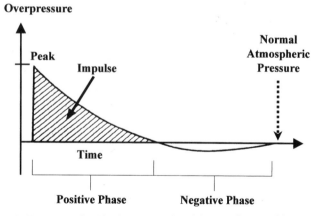

FIGURE 31.1. The ideal pressure-time history of an air blast in an undisturbed, free-field environment. The impulse is the integral of pressure over time. (Modified from Stuhmiller JH, Phillips YY, Richmond DR. The physics and mechanisms of primary blast injury. In: Bellamy RF, Zajtcjuk JT, eds. *Conventional warfare: ballistic, blast, and burn injuries.* Washington, D.C.: Office of the Surgeon General at TMM Publications, 1991:241–270. Textbook of Military Medicine series, with permission.)

Because the speed of propagation increases with pressure, the negative phase moves more slowly than the positive phase of the blast front (8). The negative phase can last ten times longer than the positive phase, and it results in pressure below ambient air pressure. During the negative phase, the blast wind reverses back towards the direction of the explosion. This sucks debris into new areas.

Blast pressures are defined as static, dynamic, or reflected (11). The static pressure is the air compression that is active in all directions due to the thermal motion of the gas. The dynamic pressure is the force associated with the movement of air particles at the leading edge of the shock wave. Blast waves that encounter a large, solid barrier (e.g., the wall of a building) in a perpendicular direction will result in a compression of molecules until they are so tightly packed that they are pushed back in the direction of the incident wave. As the blast winds become stronger, the overpressure in the reflected region grows proportionately so that they can reflect off solid objects at two to nine times the initial peak pressure (8). Therefore, blast waves that will cause only modest injury in the open can be lethal if the victim is standing near a reflecting surface (13). The fireball resulting from the explosion may ignite clothing, surrounding objects, or structures and can cause burn and inhalation injuries.

Blast waves inside an enclosed structure (e.g., building, bus, foxholes, or armored vehicle) undergo repeated reflections from the interior surface and create a complex blast wave with three characteristics as follows: (a) the incident blast wave, (b) a jumble of reflected waves, and (c) the static pressurization of the enclosure (11,14). Indoor blasts can be associated with severe injuries because of the geometric increase in the pressure wave as it is reflected off walls, floors, and ceilings (4). The intensity and duration of this pressure depends on the volume of the enclosed structure and the degree of venting through the doors and windows (14).

The blast loading on a human being is the amount of force exerted on the body; it is affected by the body position in relation to the blast wave. If the maximum overpressure and duration of the positive incident overpressure remain constant and the presence of projectiles is ignored, the incidence of physical injury and mortality will be greater when a person is oriented with the long axis of his or her body perpendicular to (i.e., oriented side-on) and near a reflecting surface. Those who are not near a reflecting surface but who are perpendicular to the blast winds will have a lower incidence of physical injury and mortality. The lowest levels of injury and mortality from the blast wave will be among victims whose long axis of the body is parallel (i.e., oriented end-on) to the blast wind.

Blast waves cause injury because of their rapid external loading on the body and organs (11). Air-containing organs (e.g., middle ear, lung, and gastrointestinal tract) are the most sensitive to changes in air pressure and thus are the most susceptible to distortion and stress (10,11). The more rapidly that the blast loading increases, the less time the internal pressures will have to equilibrate and the greater the tissue distortion and injury in air containing organs will be. Thus, primary blast injury is seen almost exclusively in air-containing organs (13). Low levels of tissue stress lead to compromised integrity of vascular beds, causing local hemorrhage. Higher levels of stress lead to severe tissue disruption and mechanical failure. An overpressure of 5 psi causes tympanic membrane rupture, 16 psi results in pulmonary blast injury, and 30 to 42 psi is defined as the lethality threshold pressure (12,15,16).

Water transmits blast waves more efficiently than air. Compared to air blasts, underwater explosions send out compressive shock waves at much higher speeds (up to 5,000 feet per second) (11,17). After detonations of similar size, underwater blast injuries are more prevalent at a given distance than those that are observed in air blasts (10). The lethal range of a given size charge underwater blast is about three times that of free-field air blasts (13,18). As an underwater compressive shock wave reaches the surface, it is reflected as a tension wave. This interacts with the compressive wave at different times, resulting in a canceling or cutoff effect that is greatest closer to the surface of the water. Therefore, the greatest impulse loading occurs towards the deepest parts of a floating structure. Gastrointestinal injuries are much more likely from blast waves in water than from those propagated in air (13,14,17,19,20). A person in danger of an impending underwater blast should float on the surface instead of treading water. Fortunately, water greatly reduces the effective range of any fragments propelled from the blast.

MECHANISMS AND DETERMINANTS OF INJURY

Mechanisms and determinants of physical injury from blasts are multifactorial, including the type and size of the blast, the distance of the victim from the explosion, the effects of environmental pressure changes, the conditions caused by blast pressures and blast winds, and the environment in which the blast occurs. The organs most often injured by blasts are the ears, skin, lungs, bowels, and the cardiovascular and central nervous systems (CNS) (21). The serious effects commonly include respiratory injuries, gastrointestinal damage, and the introduction of air emboli into the circulation system (19).

Primary blast injury is the direct, cussive effect of the pressure wave on the victim (13). The true incidence of primary blast injury is not known. Primary blast injury is more likely to occur when the detonation has occurred in a closed space (3,17). Categories of primary blast injury are shown in Table 31.1. The amplitude of the peak overpressure, the rate of the pressure rise, and its total duration determine the biologic effects of primary blast injury (3). Because the pressure amplitude generated by explosions is inversely

TABLE 31.1. CATEGORIES OF PRIMARY BLAST INJURY

System	Injury
Respiratory system	Pulmonary hemorrhage
	Alveolovenous fistula (air-embolism production)
	Airway epithelial damage
Circulatory system	Cardiac contusion
	Myocardial ischemic change (air-embolism production)
Digestive system	Gastrointestinal hemorrhage
	Gastrointestinal perforation
	Retroperitoneal hemorrhage
	Ruptured spleen or liver
Eye and orbit	Retinal air embolism
	Orbital fracture
Auditory system	Tympanic membrane rupture
	Ossicular fractures
	Cochlear damage

From Sharpnack DD, Johnson AJ, Phillips YY. The pathology of blast injury. In: Bellamy RF, Zajtcjuk JT, eds. *Conventional warfare: ballistic, blast, and burn injuries.* Washington, D.C.: Office of the Surgeon General at TMM Publications, 1991. Textbook of military medicine series, with permission.

related to the cubic distance from the focus of detonation (13), the presence of severe pulmonary or intestinal primary blast injury is evidence of the victim's relative proximity to the explosion (3). Pulmonary damage should be expected in 50% of victims exposed to a blast pressure of 70 psi or greater (14). Exposures to pressure levels of 80 psi or greater are lethal in more than 50% of cases (22).

Open air blasts may hurl objects through the air, causing penetrating or nonpenetrating *secondary blast injury* (3,10). Fragments propelled by conventional blasts travel in the air far beyond the distance that the blast itself will cause injury (11). Most of the severe injuries among civilian victims of terrorist bombings are attributed to secondary blast effects, such as shrapnel wounds (3). Wounds inflicted by these fragments do not differ from the classic ballistic wounds caused by bullets or fragments from conventional explosive munitions (17). *Tertiary blast injury* results from blunt trauma that occurs when the victim is lifted and thrown against a structure by the blast wave or blast winds.

Flash burns result from the intense heat of explosions (8), but they are usually superficial because of the short duration. Other *thermal injuries* from radiation, hot gases, or fires are considered miscellaneous blast effects (13). Burns sustained by victims of explosions in closed spaces are more severe, and they affect a larger percentage of total body surface area (3). The term *combined blast injury* is used when primary blast injury occurs with secondary or tertiary blast injuries or with burns or radiation (19). Smoke and fumes from fires resulting from the blast may produce inhalation or toxic injuries. Additionally, crush injury from collapse of a structure is another indirect effect of bombings.

The concepts of spallation, implosion, and inertial effects help define the effects that the force of the blast wave has on tissue in the body (8,13,21). Spallation is the tendency for a boundary between two different density media to be disrupted when a compression wave in the denser medium is reflected at the interface. Implosion is the forceful compression of a gas bubble by a shock wave in liquid that results in the pressure in the bubble rising much higher than the shock pressure. As the pressure wave passes, the bubble reexpands explosively, disrupting local tissue. Two adjacent objects of different densities that are acted on by the same force can cause inertial effects. The lighter object will be accelerated more than the heavier one is, and great stress will take place at the boundary between the two.

The organ most sensitive to the primary blast effect is the ear (21,23). The blast pressure wave is amplified along the auditory conductive pathway increasing the ear's sensitivity to levels of blast overpressure that might not be sufficient to cause primary blast injury in other organs (19). Auditory damage from blasts includes the rupture of the tympanic membrane, dislocations or fractures of the ossicular chain, and damage to the organ of Corti within the cochlea. Perforations usually involve less than one-third of the tympanic membrane (13). In a series of 147 patients who sustained blast injury, the distribution of perforations were the inferior part of the eardrum in 48% of the cases, the superior part in 23%, the central kidney-shaped section in 13%, the combined superior and inferior parts in 15%, and marginal injuries in 6.6% (24). Hemorrhage in the tympanic membrane is often found around the periphery of the pars tensa or immediately below the anterior or posterior malleal folds (25). Most perforations heal spontaneously without sequelae; cholesteatoma is a reported complication that is confined to patients in whom the membrane does not heal within 10 months and tympanoplasty was not subsequently performed (24). Ossicular damage includes the medial displacement of the malleal handle with disruption of the incudomalleal joint and incudostapedial joint separation with and without a stapes fracture (19).

Transient sensineural loss usually resolves within the first few hours after a blast, but 30% of bombing victims may have permanent loss (17,26). Tinnitus tends to parallel sensineural hearing loss, and it usually resolves as the hearing loss does. A one-year audiologic monitoring of 83 survivors of the 1995 Oklahoma City federal building bombing showed that 76% still reported tinnitus, 58% had distorted hearing, and 57% displayed otalgia (7).

Injury to the lung is the greatest cause of morbidity and mortality (13). Primary blast injury to the chest results in damage to the alveolar parenchyma (27). The blast wave may also produce tears in the visceral pleura, as well as the formation of bullae and alveolar-venous fistulae. In experimental animal studies, more than 50% of the deaths from primary blast injury occurred within the first 30 minutes; the autopsies revealed the presence of many air emboli (19). The most

obvious and consistent sign of primary blast injury to the lungs is hemorrhage, which can manifest externally by froth or blood in the oral cavity or surrounding the nose or lips (19). The hemorrhage may be pleural or subpleural, multifocal or diffuse within the parenchyma, or surrounding the airways and vascular structures within the parenchyma. Intraalveolar hemorrhage plus atelectasis probably results in a decrease in functional residual capacity and in the ventilation-perfusion ratio and an increase in right-to-left shunting of blood through the nonventilated alveoli (27).

The characteristic clinical pattern of primary pulmonary blast injury is rapid respiratory deterioration with progressive hypoxia, leading to a need for mechanical ventilatory support with high forced inspiratory oxygen fraction of inspired oxygen (FIO_2) (3). Widespread pulmonary edema does not usually occur as a result of primary blast injury. Only a small number of terrorist bombing survivors have primary pulmonary blast injuries that result in respiratory failure and high in-hospital mortality (23). This is true because people close enough to sustain such injuries from air blasts are likely to be killed immediately by the secondary and tertiary effects or by massive air embolisms resulting from the primary blast injury (4,14).

Other lung injuries include pneumothorax, hemothorax, traumatic lung cysts, interstitial emphysema, pneumomediastinum, and subcutaneous emphysema. Chest wall damage, including rib fractures, is usually not seen in the absence of other pulmonary trauma (13). Air emboli, which can result from traumatic alveolar-venous fistulae, are responsible for most of the early mortality from primary blast injury (13). The more severe the pulmonary hemorrhage is, then the greater the likelihood of significant embolism (19). Pulmonary symptoms in survivors of major blasts include hemoptysis (55%), dyspnea (38%), and chest pain (22%). Clinical findings include parenchymal infiltrates (84%), crackles (40%), hemothorax (27%), pneumomediastinum (27%), and pneumothorax (4%) (17). In one series of 12 patients with blast injury to the chest, four (33%) presented with cyanosis and ten had severe associated injuries, including nine who required laparotomy (18).

Blast injury affects the abdominal cavity similar to the thorax, including the following: (a) tissue distortion within caused by the blast wave striking and displacing the body wall, leading to stress and failure; (b) no visible external injury on the body wall; (c) highest vulnerability of the air-containing organs; and (d) hemorrhage and tearing of tissue as the most common lesions (19). Gastrointestinal hemorrhage is most common in the lower small intestines or the cecum where gas commonly accumulates. The most common site of intestinal perforation is at the ileocecal junction. Perforation may occur immediately at the time of the blast injury, or it may delayed up to days later. Retroperitoneal hemorrhage and damage to solid organs are less common, and these are more likely the result of secondary or tertiary blast injuries (17). In a combined series of 43 hospitalized patients from an underwater blast, 67% had a perforated bowel, 2% had isolated bowel hematoma, and 2% had a solid visceral injury (18,20).

Circulatory system injury may be a direct result of the blast wave itself; however, indirect effects such as air emboli from pulmonary injury can occlude coronary arteries and can cause cardiac arrest. Hemorrhage, or myocardial contusion, is the most common blast-related lesion found in the heart, and it occurs most often on the diaphragmatic surface (19). Myocardial lacerations have also been documented. Coronary artery air embolism is thought to be a major cause of death in blast casualties.

Traumatic amputations are a hallmark of grave prognosis among blast victims. Most cases are caused directly by shock waves, but some result from large secondary missile fragments (3). Because most traumatic amputations reflect a high energy transfer, such patients have a high likelihood of dying from severe associated injuries (2).

Fragments cause most of the injuries in small terrorist bombings (23). Soft tissue injuries (e.g., lacerations, abrasions, and contusions) predominate among survivors of bombings (4,6,28) (Fig. 31.2). Bombs characteristically cause multiple wounds with associated gross soiling (29). The wounds vary in size from minute punctures to huge lacerations that are often impregnated with foreign bodies.

Besides bomb fragments and flechettes, foreign bodies found in wounds may include clothing, stones, glass, splintered wood, and plaster. Fine particles of dust may be embedded within the skin, producing a discoloration called "dust tattooing" (14). The head and neck are the most frequently injured regions of the body, followed by the extremities (28). Clothing and footwear provide a protective effect for the covered areas of the body against soft tissue injuries (28).

Blast injuries to the eyes usually occur as a result of secondary blast effects, most frequently glass fragments (30, 31). Eye injuries from terrorist blasts can be extensive, involving the globe, the ocular adnexa, and the orbit. In one study of 55 patients with ocular injuries after a terrorist bombing, lid and/or brow lacerations occurred in 36%, penetrating globe injures in 22%, orbital fractures in 11%, retinal detachment in 9%, and retained foreign bodies in 4% (30).

EPIDEMIOLOGY OF BOMBING INJURIES

Terrorist blast injury data are limited by the chaotic nature of the unexpected mass-casualty situation confronting a civilian medical system. Critical analysis of the patterns of

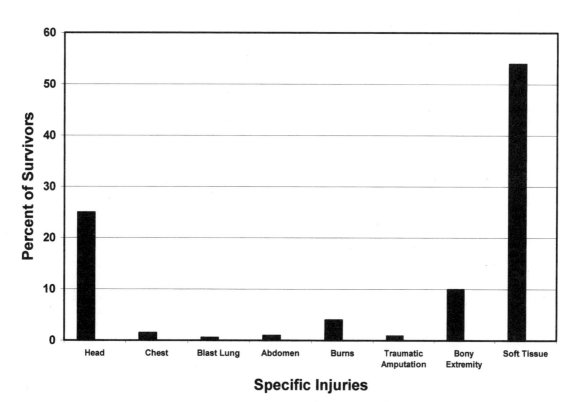

FIGURE 31.2. Collective profile of injury patterns among 3,949 terrorist bombing victims. (Data from Mallonee S, Shariat S, Stennies G, et al. Physical injuries and fatalities resulting from the Oklahoma City bombing. *JAMA* 1996;276:382–387; Hogan DE, Waeckerle JF, Dire DJ, et al. Emergency department impact of the Oklahoma City terrorist bombing. *Ann Emerg Med* 1999;34:160–167; and Frykberg ER, Tepas JJ III, Alexander RH. The 1983 Beirut Airport terrorist bombing. Injury patterns and implications for disaster management. *Am Surg* 1989;55:134–141, with permission.)

injury and mortality from this type of disaster helps with understanding of the natural history and pathophysiology of this form of terrorism (32). A collective profile of injury patterns among 3,949 terrorist bombing victims is shown in Fig. 31.2.

The mortality and morbidity of blast injuries largely depend on which organs have been affected (23). Trauma to the central nervous system is highly lethal. The incidence of head injuries from terrorist bombings ranges from 10.8% to 63% (5,14,21,28,33–36). Approximately 1% to 5% of civilian bombing victims will die at the scene as a result of head injuries. Most casualties treated in EDs will have minor injuries consisting of lacerations, abrasions, and contusions (6). Approximately 21% to 50% will require admission for observation, with a small number of these (1%–15%) having sustained significant thoracic or abdominal injuries. Truncal injuries are few (2.4% of admissions), but they are more likely to result in death among the hospitalized patients. Hospital mortality for bombing victims with chest trauma is 15%; with abdominal injuries, it is 19% (23).

Mortality rates for bombings can be deceptive. The casualties should be broken down into immediate on-scene mortality, the number of critically injured survivors (injury severity score > 15), and the overall mortality in hospital-

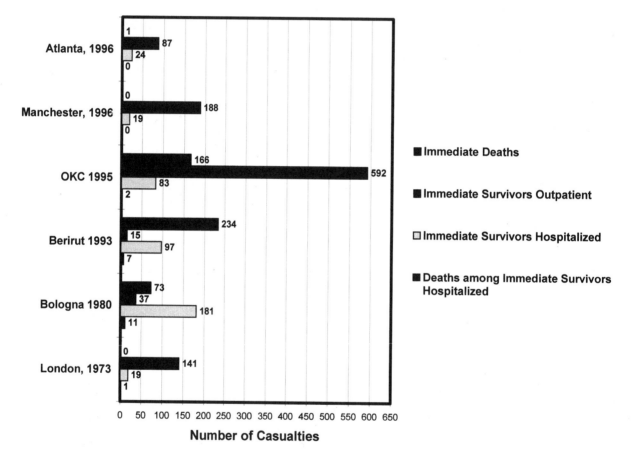

FIGURE 31.3. Graphic depiction of numbers of immediate survivors treated as outpatients, immediate survivors hospitalized, immediate deaths, and deaths among immediate survivors hospitalized for a select group of isolated terrorist bombing incidents. (Data from Frykberg ER, Tepas JJ III. Terrorist bombings. Lessons learned from Belfast to Beirut. *Ann Surg* 1988;208:569–576; Mallonee S, Shariat S, Stennies G, et al. Physical injuries and fatalities resulting from the Oklahoma City bombing. *JAMA* 1996;276:382–387; Hogan DE, Waeckerle JF, Dire DJ, et al. Emergency department impact of the Oklahoma City terrorist bombing. *Ann Emerg Med* 1999;34:160–167; Frykberg ER, Tepas JJ III, Alexander RH. The 1983 Beirut Airport terrorist bombing. Injury patterns and implications for disaster management. *Am Surg* 1989;55:134–141; Brismar B, Bergenwald L. The terrorist bomb explosion in Bologna, Italy, 1980: an analysis of the effects and injuries sustained. *J Trauma* 1982;22:216–220; Caro D, Irving M. The Old Bailey bomb explosion. *Lancet* 1973;1:1433–1435; Frykberg ER, Hutton PMJ, Balzer R. Disaster in Beirut: an application of mass casualty principle. *Mil Med* 1987;152:563–566; Scott BA, Fletcher JR, Pulliam MW, et al. The Beirut terrorist bombing. *Neurosurgery* 1986;18:107–110; Carley SD, Mackway-Jones K. The casualty profile from the Manchester bombing 1996: a proposal for the construction and dissemination of casualty profiles from major incidents. *J Accid Emerg Med* 1997;14:76–80; and Feliciano DV, Anderson GV Jr, Rozycki GS, et al. Management of casualties from the bombing at the centennial Olympics. *Am J Surg* 1998;176:538–543, with permission.)

ized survivors (32). Basing the overall mortality rates on total casualties will cause an artificial dilution because many bombing incidents create numerous patients with minor injuries that require minimal treatment without hospitalization. The on-scene mortality of terrorist bombings ranged from less than 2% in Northern Ireland to almost 70% for the Beirut marine barracks attack in 1983. For a select group of isolated terrorist bombing incidents, Fig. 31.3 shows the numbers of immediate deaths, of immediate survivors treated as outpatients, of immediate survivors who were hospitalized, and of deaths among immediate survivors who were hospitalized.

Higher fatality rates can be anticipated when one or more of the following occurs: the structural collapse of buildings, a large TNT-equivalent explosion, and explosions in confined spaces (e.g., vehicles or building interiors) (3,5,32). The 1980 bombing of the central railway station in Bologna, Italy (25% fatality rate); the 1983 bombing of the United States Marine compound in Beirut, Lebanon (69% fatality rate); and the 1995 bombing of the Murrah Federal building in Oklahoma City (22% fatality rate) produced high fatality rates from building collapse (5,32,33,35). In one report of 55 casualties in a civilian bus bombing, 11 suffered lung injuries and four experienced gastrointestinal trauma (15).

In a review of 200 bombing incidents worldwide involving 3,357 casualties, Frykberg and Tepas found that the immediate on-scene fatality rate was 13% (4). The mean number of casualties per bombing was 15. Of the 87% who were immediate survivors, 30% were hospitalized and 18.7% were critically injured. The mortality rate for the immediate survivors was 2.3%, occurring in those deemed critically injured; therefore, the *critical mortality rate* was 12.4%. Head injury was the most common contributor to early and late deaths (71% and 52%, respectively). Surgical procedures performed on 812 survivors of terrorist bombings included 544 (67%) for soft tissue injuries, 142 (17.5%) for orthopedic injuries, 45 (5.5%) for abdominal injuries, 17 (2%) for head injuries, and 65 (8%) for miscellaneous injuries (e.g., chest, ear, vascular, neck, spinal cord, or peripheral nerve injuries) (4).

Burn fatalities are not high among bombing victims as the brief flash of explosions limits thermal injuries to superficial burns on exposed body areas (4). High explosive forces, explosions in confined spaces, or secondary fires from the blast may result in more severe burn injuries and mortality (4,37,38). Smoke inhalation injuries from bombings are unusual, except in enclosed spaces. After the World Trade Center bombing in 1993 in New York City, 485 of 546 (88%) of victims treated at surrounding hospitals over a 24-hour period were given a primary diagnosis of smoke inhalation (39). The bomb knocked out the building's power, disabling the smoke control systems and trapping people within the 198 elevators for long periods of time while smoke filled the lift shafts.

Primary blast injury is quite common in terrorist bombings, but most of these victims are on-scene fatalities due to the associated injuries (10). Primary blast injury to the lung has been noted in only 0.6% of 2,934 immediate survivors of bombings (4). Autopsies of 495 casualties who died in 5,600 separate explosions over a 12-year period showed that 66% had brain injuries, 51% had skull fractures, 47% had classic autopsy findings of blast lung, 45% suffered tympanic membrane rupture, and 34% had liver lacerations (10).

Explosions in an enclosed space result in more severe primary blast injuries. Of 104 passengers on two civilian buses that were bombed in Israel, seven were killed immediately, 51 were admitted to the hospital, 16 had pulmonary blast injury, and seven complained of significant abdominal pain, four of whom had intestinal perforations (15,23). All of the severely injured also had perforated tympanic membranes. At least 42 of the 80 Americans injured in the 1986 LaBelle Disco terrorist bombing in Berlin experienced ruptured tympanic membranes (40).

Selected terrorist bombings are described briefly below to illustrate the diverse nature of such incidents.

Bologna, Italy (1980)

On August 2, 1980, a suitcase bomb exploded in the waiting room of the central railway station in Bologna, Italy (33). Seventy-three fatalities occurred at the scene, the majority of which were due to crush injury when the building collapsed. Of the 218 wounded who initially survived, 181 (83%) were admitted to hospitals. Seventeen (8%) had severe or critical injuries. Of the immediate survivors, 43 head injuries were diagnosed, including ten skull fractures, six with concussions and 27 with contusions; the remainder of the injuries included 15 ear injuries, seven eye injuries, four pneumothorax injuries, four pulmonary contusions, seven abdominal injuries, 55 fractures, 28 burns, and 72 other soft tissue wounds.

Forty-one (23%) of the hospitalized patients required surgery for soft tissue injuries, 22 (12%) for fractures, six (3%) for abdominal injuries, six (3%) for neurosurgical injuries, and one (0.6%) for a thoracotomy. Forty-five (21%) of these patients required the use of a general anesthetic. More than 100 units of blood were used for these bombing victims in the first 24 hours (33).

Beirut, Lebanon (1983)

On October 23, 1983, a yellow Mercedes truck loaded with an estimated 6 to 12 tons of TNT was driven into the ground floor lobby of the United States Marines Battalion Landing Team Headquarters building in Beirut, Lebanon, and was detonated (32,35,37). This four-story building that also served as billets for the troops and that was occupied by more than 350 men collapsed "like a house of cards" (37). Two hundred thirty-four men (68%) were immediately killed. Three field triage stations were established at the scene (32,35). Eight casualties were evacuated to local Lebanese hospitals, and 72 were evacuated by helicopter to the USS *Iwo Jima*, which had a mobile surgical team aboard; of these, 61 were evacuated within 2 hours of the bombing. Six hours after the bombing, another 24 casualties were evacuated by the British Royal Air Force and United States Navy and Air Force air ambulances to Germany and subsequently to the United States. Fifteen survivors with minor injuries were treated; these did not require evacuation.

Among the immediate survivors, 37 head injuries, including 28 with concussions and 13 with skull fractures, occurred (35). Postconcussion syndrome developed in seven (25%) of those who suffered concussions (35). Head injury was the most common (71%) specific cause of death among the immediate fatalities in Beirut. Despite intensive medical care, seven deaths (7.3%) took place among the survivors who had been evacuated (three from head injuries, one from chest injury, one with head and chest injuries, and two with major burns) (37). Two of these deaths occurred within 9 hours of the bombing, one of whom had suffered primary pulmonary blast injury and another with crush injuries to the head and chest (32). Among the delayed fatalities, six of seven (86%) had been extricated between 5 and 9 hours after the blast. Burn victims had the highest specific hospital mortality rate (two of five, 40%). Most of the evacuated survivors suffered multiple injuries. Soft tissue and orthopedic procedures were the most common surgeries performed, and six patients had craniotomies.

Oklahoma City, Oklahoma (1995)

On April 19, 1995, a truck bomb consisting of more than 4,000 pounds of ammonia nitrate was detonated outside the Alfred P. Murrah federal building in Oklahoma City (6). Immediate deaths numbered 163, and three were pronounced dead on arrival at local hospitals. EDs treated 388 victims the day of the bombing (6). Eight-three (21%) immediate survivors were hospitalized, and two (2.4%) of these survivors subsequently died (5). One of these died on the second hospital day due to a head injury. The other died 3 weeks later of multiple organ failure and sepsis, which is the usual cause of late bombing victim deaths (days to weeks after the blast). The medical examiner did not clearly distinguish deaths caused by primary blast injuries from those that were caused by building collapse in those victims who were on-scene fatalities; the most common cause of death reported was simply "multiple injuries" (5).

The majority of the survivors sustained minor injuries caused by flying or falling glass and debris. The most frequent type injury requiring ED treatment was soft tissue trauma in 71%, followed by fractures in 12% (6). Blast injury to the eye was documented in 8% of the victims, and it was much more common among victims who were in the

building versus those who were other locations (30). Abdominal trauma was not common in the Oklahoma City bombing; only one splenic injury and two renal contusions were reported (6). The most frequent medications administered in the EDs were tetanus immunizations, analgesics, and antibiotics.

The truck bomb detonated in front of the Murrah building resulted in several secondary fires. Ten victims suffered thermal burns; one fatality occurred in the parking lot, and seven were hospitalized with up to 70% burns (1,5). Among the nine survivors, the most common area burned was the face and neck (67%); no patient had full-thickness burns involving more than 10% of body surface area.

Manchester, England (1996)

On June 15, 1996, the largest bomb ever detonated by the Irish Republic Army in Great Britain exploded in the center of Manchester, England (41). No fatalities resulted, but 208 victims were treated in the nearest five hospital EDs; most (62%) for injuries from flying glass. This placed a large burden on the hospitals' radiology departments because 50% of the casualties required radiologic studies. Forty-one patients (20%) suffered blunt trauma. Admission was required for 18 (9%), and eight underwent surgery. An unusually high number of patients (36 [17%]) presented for medical problems (e.g., angina, asthma attack, syncope) or emotional distress related to the bombing.

Atlanta, Georgia (1996)

In July 1996, a pipe bomb in a knapsack filled with nails and screws exploded in Centennial Park during the Atlanta Olympics (42). The bomb detonated in front of a concert stage that was 75 to 100 yards away from attendees who were being evacuated. Local hospitals treated 111 patients. One additional patient suffered a fatal heart attack while running to the scene of the bombing. Hospital admission was required for 24 persons (22%). Most of the patients were treated for wounds related to fragments from the pipe bomb or the nails and screws.

The impact of a terrorist bombing is not limited to the dead and injured (43). The psychological impact on the surrounding community may result in behavioral consequences, such as changes in smoking and drinking habits, posttraumatic stress disorder, and intrusive thoughts.

MANAGEMENT OF CONVENTIONAL BOMBING VICTIMS
Prehospital Considerations

Extrication and life support are the first priorities (8). Bombing victims should be evaluated according to normal basic trauma triage standards (13,17). After terrorist bombings, rapid identification of life-threatening injuries and the evacuation of severely injured victims to the appropriate medical facilities are paramount. Severely injured bombing victims will have higher survival and lower morbidity if they are transported to a trauma center, not simply to the closest hospital (35). Patients with asphyxia, suspected simple or tension pneumothorax, cyanosis or extreme dyspnea, upper-airway compromise, or hypotension should be triaged as immediate. Only a minority of survivors of bombings have severe life-threatening injuries (6,28,32–34, 36,44,45). Common prehospital interventions that are required include spinal immobilization, wound dressings, and intravenous fluids (6).

Rescue and recovery of injured victims after a bombing may be hampered by further terrorist activity. After the 1983 Beirut Marine Headquarters bombing, rescue efforts at the scene were disrupted by sniper fire throughout the day (37). Moreover, a second bomb that has been specifically designed to maim or kill personnel rushing to help those wounded in a first explosion is a well-recognized terrorist tactic (8,46). In 1996, a second terrorist bomb specifically targeting medical staff complicated the bombing rescue in the Thiepval British Army Barracks (46). Additionally, rescuers must be trained and prepared for terrorist bombings that use nuclear, biologic, or chemical agents as secondary weapons of mass destruction. The presence of collapsed buildings with trapped victims prolongs the recovery phase and creates more severely injured patients (6,47).

Primary blast injury is likely to be only part of the presentation of a multiply injured bombing victim (14). The prehospital care of bombing victims usually centers on secondary blast injuries, such as fractures, amputations, penetrating wounds, and burns. However, prehospital providers should be particularly alert for subtle signs of primary blast injury, especially for pulmonary injuries such as tension pneumothorax. Hypovolemic shock may occur as a result of hemorrhage from wounds or because of blood loss from gastrointestinal injuries.

All patients with other than isolated minor soft tissue injuries should receive supplemental oxygen and should be monitored with pulse-oximetry. Patients with extreme respiratory distress should undergo endotracheal intubation to handle massive hemoptysis and to provide ventilatory support. With mechanical ventilation comes the increased risk of iatrogenic tension pneumothorax in blast victims. Patients may need prophylactic tube thoracostomies with Heimlich valves before aeromedical evacuation.

Prehospital medical personnel should attempt to obtain information about the blast as soon as possible after the casualties are stabilized if circumstances permit (17) (Table 31.2).

Victims of explosions should minimize postblast physical activities and should remain sedentary to avoid exacerbation of the severity of primary blast injury (13). Those who are experiencing any respiratory distress should be car-

TABLE 31.2. HISTORY TO OBTAIN AT THE SCENE OF A BOMBING CASUALTY

What type of ordnance was used? How large was the explosion?
Where was the casualty located with respect to the blast?
Did the blast occur inside an enclosed space, such as a room or vehicle?
What was the casualty's activity after exposure?
Were fires or fumes that might lead to an inhalation injury present?
What was the orientation of the casualty's head and body in relation to the blast?

From Phillips YY, Zajtcjuk JT. The management of primary blast injury. In: Bellamy RF, Zajtcjuk JT, eds. *Conventional warfare: ballistic, blast, and burn injuries.* Washington, D.C.: Office of the Surgeon General at TMM Publications, 1991. Textbook of military medicine series, with permission.

ried from the incident scene on a litter. Manifestations of primary blast injury involving the gastrointestinal, respiratory, and circulatory systems are more dangerous if the victim is transported by air; therefore, even short helicopter flights should be avoided (17).

Patients with injured lungs are at risk for air embolism, which is the single most important cause of death from primary blast injury (10). If one lung is more severely affected than the other one is, the damaged lung should be in the dependent position during transportation (17). The alveolar pressures throughout the dependent lung will be lower than vascular pressures, thus decreasing the risk of air embolism; however, this does increase the risk of worse gas exchange. The position of the patient's body may affect the site of embolism travel. Therefore, if the lungs are equally affected or the left lung is more severely injured, the patient should be placed in the left-lateral decubitus and Trendelenburg positions. High-flow oxygen should be administered to support gas exchange in the lungs and to help the tissue absorption of the emboli by decreasing the predominance of nitrogen gas.

Emergency Department

Blast victims should be triaged upon arrival to the ED by an experienced trauma surgeon or emergency physician. Unfortunately, the extent of blast injury cannot be reliably assessed by the typical rapid triage examination (48). Thus, an atypically high over-triage rate is mandated (4,32), which may affect patient flow and the use of hospital resources (48).

The ED care should be centered on stabilization measures in accordance with advance trauma life support principles (49). A thorough evaluation for signs of primary blast injuries should also be conducted, especially when a history of a powerful explosion is known. Physical examination findings such as ruptured tympanic membranes, hypopharyngeal contusions, hemoptysis in the absence of signs of external chest trauma, or subcutaneous emphysema indicate the presence of primary blast injuries. In fact, a ruptured eardrum is almost always present when the blast pressure is high enough to cause serious injury to the lung or gut (13). Petechiae or ecchymoses in the hypopharynx or larynx may be associated with significant pulmonary injury; their absence speaks against an exposure to high blast pressure (13). Additional signs of primary blast injury to the lung can include dyspnea, cough, restlessness, tachypnea, tachycardia, cyanosis, or an inability to carry on a conversation (17,21). Immediate tube thoracostomy is indicated for pneumothorax, tension pneumothorax, or hemothorax. A

chest radiograph should be routine in all blast victims, except for those with isolated minor soft tissue injuries of the extremities from air blasts, because it may reveal pulmonary lesions that are not evident clinically (33). Figure 31.4 is an algorithm for the initial trauma resuscitation and the evaluation and treatment of a blast casualty with respiratory distress (17).

Radiograph findings in blast injury to the chest are nonspecific, but they can include pneumothorax, hemothorax, pneumomediastinum, atelectasis, alveolar infiltrates, and interstitial edema (18). Computed tomography (CT) of the chest is the most accurate technique for evaluating the lung

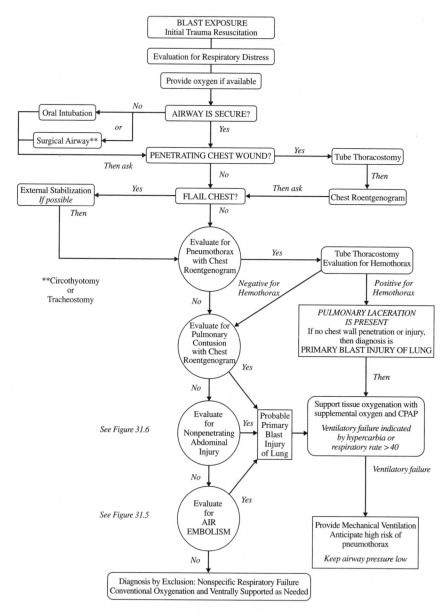

FIGURE 31.4. Algorithm for the evaluation of respiratory distress in a blast casualty. (Modified from Phillips YY, Zajtchuk JT. The management of primary blast injury. In: Bellamy RF, Zajtcjuk JT, eds. *Conventional warfare: ballistic, blast, and burn injuries.* Washington, D.C.: Office of the Surgeon General at TMM Publications, 1991:295–336. Textbook of Military Medicine series, with permission.)

parenchyma and pleural space, and it is used to quantitate the extent of the injury based upon the amount of parenchyma involved (17). Chest CT scans may also reveal underlying parenchymal injury or pneumothorax when extensive subcutaneous emphysema, parenchymal hemorrhage, or interstitial emphysema is present on plain radiographs.

The main objective of treatment of blast lung is to restore and maintain arterial blood gases near normal until the lungs have recovered (27). Patients with more than 28% of their lungs involved with the hemorrhage usually require mechanical ventilation; however, this increases the incidence of both air emboli and thoracic barotrauma. Continuous positive pressure ventilation should not be withheld if the clinical situation deteriorates, but patients should be continuously reevaluated for the development of a tension pneumothorax (17,25). Airway pressures should be kept as low as possible. To promote good bronchial hygiene when using bronchodilators, remove blood and secretions from the tracheobronchial tree by frequent suctioning and frequent changing of the patient's body position (17,27).

Arterial blood gases should be obtained for seriously injured patients and for those with respiratory distress. Generally, victims with uncomplicated primary blast injury have a normal or low PCO_2 (<40 mm Hg). The presence of hypercarbia (PCO_2 >40 mm Hg) suggests a cause other than primary blast injury, such as flail chest, muscle weakness from chemical agent exposure, metabolic derangements, airway compromise, impairment of the central ventilatory drive, air embolism, excessive narcotic administration, or diaphragm rupture, may be limiting ventilation.

An electrocardiogram should be obtained for seriously injured patients, including any with hypotension or respiratory or central nervous system symptoms. Ischemic changes may be due to air emboli proximal to the coronary arteries or because of hypoxia secondary to respiratory failure (21).

Hypotension is a frequent finding in severe blast injury, and it may be the result of severe acute blood loss, myocardial injury, vasovagal reflexes, or a combination of these (20, 21). Central venous monitoring may help guide fluid replacement therapy. Hypotensive patients should receive sufficient fluid resuscitation to bring their blood pressure back within normal limits, but those with pulmonary injuries will have an increased risk of pulmonary edema when they receive excessive volume replacement (17). Blood or a colloid solution is preferred over crystalloid solutions in these patients.

Blast casualties with ruptured tympanic membranes or any signs of primary blast injuries, abdominal pain, altered sensorium, or injuries other than minor soft tissue trauma should have a chest radiograph regardless of whether they have any pulmonary symptoms. In one study of 137 bombing patients with isolated eardrum rupture, Leibovici et al.

predicted that up to 3% might demonstrate delayed pulmonary barotrauma (50). In a report of 27 survivors of an underwater detonation, 19 were subsequently found to have significant pulmonary compromise without initially presenting with overt respiratory distress (17). Likewise, abdominal radiographs are indicated in all but the most mildly injured patients.

Air embolism from patients with injured lungs may cause occlusions in any organ and may pose the most immediate threat to life. The risk of an air embolus is increased with the use of mechanical ventilation; it usually occurs within 2 hours of the blast, but it has been reported 60 hours after injury (17). Emboli involving the cerebral or coronary circulation are the most serious, and they may lead to strokes or myocardial infarctions. Blast victims should be evaluated for headaches, seizures, mental status changes, transient blindness, tongue blanching, vestibular disturbances, and focal neurologic deficits and for indicators of cardiac distress, such as chest pain, hypotension, dysrhythmias, and ischemic changes on electrocardiograms (Fig. 31.5). Retinal artery air emboli may be seen directly on ophthalmoscopic examination as streaming bubbles or pale silvery sections of the vessels, or they may be indirectly indicated by retinal pallor.

Direct head trauma from secondary or tertiary blast injury is more likely to be the cause of neurologic signs and symptoms (13). Early head CT scans and neurosurgical consultations are mandatory for patients with penetrating cranial injuries, altered sensorium, or other neurologic findings.

The treatment of choice for life-threatening air emboli is hyperoxygenation in a hyperbaric chamber. Treatment should be started as soon as possible after the blast exposure (8,13,17). Hyperbaric treatment has been shown to reduce mortality in animal experiments, but studies are lacking in human survivors of blasts.

Blast victims with abdominal injuries who survive the first few hours or days may succumb to complications, especially from delayed perforation. Although gastrointestinal injuries may be initially overshadowed by more immediately life-threatening pulmonary or soft-tissue injuries, many will require a laparotomy for definitive treatment. Symptoms of abdominal injury include abdominal pain, nausea, vomiting, hematemesis, rectal bleeding, orthostasis or syncope, testicular pain, and tenesmus. Findings on physical examination include decreased or absent bowel sounds, gross blood on rectal examination, hypotension, involuntary guarding, and peritoneal signs, such as rebound tenderness. Unequivocal signs of peritoneal irritation require prompt surgical treatment (17). Abdominal radiographs may show free intraperitoneal air (13). An algorithm for evaluating bombing victims for gastrointestinal injury is shown in Fig. 31.6. Patients with penetrating abdominal injuries or those with suspected bowel rupture should be given antibiotics as soon as possible to treat for anaerobes, gram-negative aerobes, and enterococci.

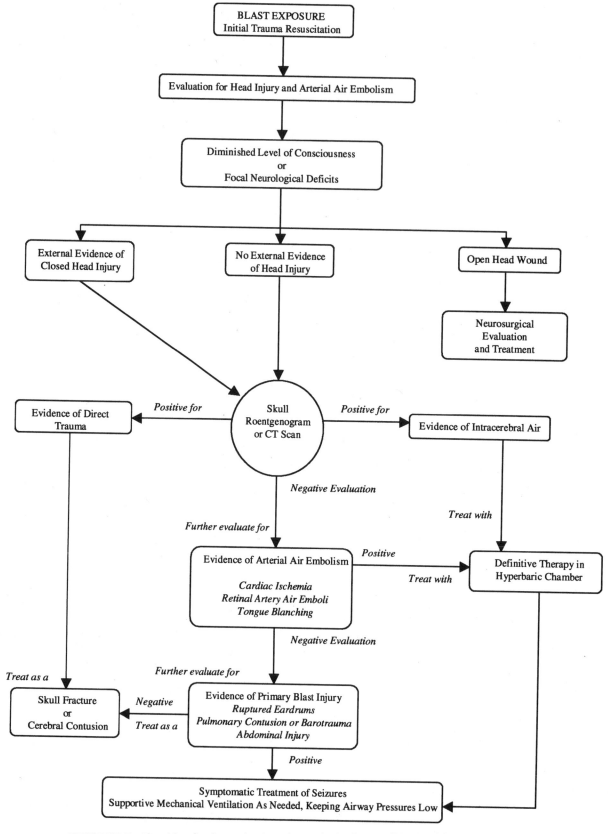

FIGURE 31.5. Algorithm for the evaluation of neurologic abnormalities in a blast casualty. (Modified from Phillips YY, Zajtchuk JT. The management of primary blast injury. In: Bellamy RF, Zajtcjuk JT, eds. *Conventional warfare: ballistic, blast, and burn injuries.* Washington, D.C.: Office of the Surgeon General at TMM Publications, 1991:295–336. Textbook of Military Medicine series, with permission.)

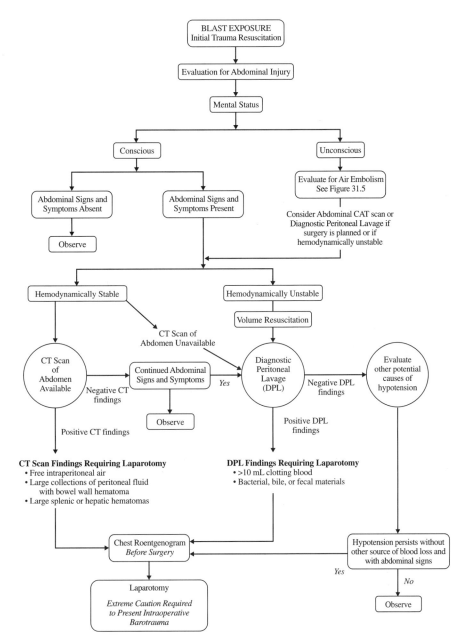

FIGURE 31.6. Algorithm for the evaluation of gastrointestinal injury in a blast casualty. (Modified from Phillips YY, Zajtchuk JT. The management of primary blast injury. In: Bellamy RF, Zajtcjuk JT, eds. *Conventional warfare: ballistic, blast, and burn injuries.* Washington, D.C.: Office of the Surgeon General at TMM Publications, 1991:295–336. Textbook of Military Medicine series, with permission.)

Patients with multisystem injuries, unconscious patients, and those with any signs of abdominal injury can undergo a rapid screening ultrasound of the abdomen in the ED to look for free peritoneal fluid. Hemodynamically unstable patients should have a prompt diagnostic peritoneal lavage. Plain abdominal radiographs may not reveal extraluminal air from bowel perforations; therefore, hemodynamically stable patients with signs or symptoms of abdominal trauma should undergo abdominal CT scanning with oral and intravenous contrast. The abdominal CT study should

be extended to include the lower chest in order to evaluate for lung injuries that may not be apparent on chest radiographs.

Symptoms of auditory injury include hearing loss, otalgia, tinnitus, loudness sensitivity, and vertigo. Hearing in both ears should be grossly tested at the bedside. Patients with vertigo should have a complete neurologic examination for signs of closed head injury. All bombing victims, including those who are unconscious, should have a thorough otoscopic examination. The location and size of perforations should be noted. The external auditory canal and the middle ear space should be examined for the presence of foreign material. The presence of clear otorrhea may suggest injuries to the inner ear, such as perilymphatic fistulae in the oval window, dislocated stapes, and ruptures of the saccule, utricle, and basilar membrane (17); or it may be cerebrospinal fluid from a middle fossa basilar skull fracture. All patients with signs or symptoms of auditory injury should have complete audiologic and otolaryngologic evaluations as soon as their clinical conditions permit. Patients with auditory injuries should be observed for 1 year to document changes and to provide supportive rehabilitation (8).

Topical antibiotic drops are not routinely given to blast injury patients with ruptured tympanic membranes unless infection is present. As a rule of thumb, one month is required to heal each 10% of the tympanic membrane rupture. Follow-up examinations of the tympanic membrane should occur within 2 weeks and then monthly thereafter. Perforations involving less than one-third of the tympanic membrane usually close spontaneously. Ruptures that do not heal spontaneously are treated with paper or Gilfilm patching or by tympanoplasty (17). Surgical intervention will ultimately be required for 25% of the ruptures (13). Surgery should be performed 10 to 12 months after the blast injury to obtain maximal success in closure and to reduce the risk of chronic infections and inner ear damage (24).

Patients injured in terrorist bombings frequently have suffered soft tissue wounds from high-velocity penetrating fragments (10). All penetrating wounds, no matter how trivial, should undergo local exploration. Wounds should be thoroughly cleansed and irrigated, which should be followed by appropriate debridement (51). The judicious use of radiographs to look for foreign bodies is also recommended. Delayed primary closure should be standard (2,6, 8,10,29,34,36). Emphasizing this to physicians who do not deal with wounds regularly is important because, if a large number of bombing casualties result from a given event, minor wounds will be treated in many other settings besides the ED.

An initial dose of antibiotics should be administered parenterally in the emergency department for all but the most trivial bombing-related wounds, followed by a 3-day to 5-day course of oral antibiotics. Tetanus immunization is the most frequent medication required in bombing victims (6,21), and it should be administered as indicated. Bombing-related wounds should be considered tetanus-prone wounds.

Open fractures that occur as a result of explosions frequently contain debris and fragments. These should be irrigated copiously in the ED and again in the operating room before and after debridement; this is followed by external fixation (2,52). Patients should receive parenteral antibiotics at the earliest opportunity.

The majority of bombing victims will not have life-threatening injuries and thus will require local wound care. Hospital disaster planners should be prepared to use other areas besides the ED for this care to keep the ED resuscitation areas available for the more seriously injured patients.

Hospital

Positive pressure ventilation or the use of a general anesthetic puts casualties with pulmonary primary blast injury at a higher risk of death. Due to the high morbidity rate when blast victims receive general anesthetic, the recommendation is that local, regional, or spinal anesthetic be used whenever possible and that the duration of surgery be kept short (13,17). Whenever possible, surgery requiring a general anesthetic should be postponed for 24 to 48 hours (20). All blast victims undergoing a procedure requiring a general anesthetic should be monitored for oxygen saturation, end-tidal carbon dioxide, cardiac rhythm, blood pressure, and airway pressure. Patients with suspected pulmonary barotrauma should have chest tubes placed before surgery or should undergo periodic intraoperative chest radiographs during extended surgical procedures. Equipment for pleural space decompression and tube thoracostomy should be readily available at all times.

Hyperbaric oxygen has been recommended in the treatment of pulmonary blast injury for improved oxygenation and in the treatment of air emboli (20,53).

The radiographic course of blast lung is consistent except for instances in which pneumothorax, atelectasis, or infection occurs (27). Worsening in the radiographic findings of pulmonary contusion is unusual more than 6 hours after the blast. Routine prophylactic antibiotics should not be given (8). Most pulmonary hemorrhages and contusions will begin to resolve within 1 to 2 days, although mechanical ventilation may be required for several days. One should suspect a superimposed disease process if the radiographic appearance is more extensive after 48 hours. Antibiotic therapy should be guided by gram stain and serial sputum cultures. Fiberoptic bronchoscopy is indicated for persistent brisk hemoptysis or refractory lobar atelectasis. This may reveal bronchial fractures and lacerations.

Patients with tenesmus or rectal bleeding should undergo flexible sigmoidoscopy (17). The surgical treatment of abdominal blast injuries follows that for other blunt abdominal trauma. Gastric decompression with a nasogastric tube is an important adjunct to the surgical care of abdominal injuries and in patients who are receiving mechanical ventilation.

Hospital resource utilization, including manpower needs and patient flow, has been analyzed based on data from 12 urban terrorist bombing incidents in Israel (48). The major bottleneck in the flow of critically injured patients in this study was the availability of shock rooms and CT scanners, not operating rooms. Imaging studies required for the critically injured stable patients typically included head, chest, or abdominal CT scans, followed by plain radiographs to locate shrapnel and fractures.

Hospital disaster plans should include protocols to postpone radiographic studies for noncritical casualties with suspected closed fractures without vascular compromise until injured patients are no longer arriving. Those patients waiting for delayed radiographs can be treated with temporary splints and analgesics (48).

Psychologic disturbances may affect up to 50% of bombing survivors and can include hysteria, guilt, post-traumatic stress disorder, and behavioral alterations (8,28). Providing psychologic follow-up opportunities for all patients discharged from the hospital is important. Most symptoms will improve with time (54).

SUMMARY

Previous conventional terrorist bombings show a consistent pattern of injury and death. The majority of injuries are non–life-threatening minor wounds that can be treated in outpatient settings. Primary blast injuries other than tympanic membrane penetrations are uncommon in survivors because they usually result in immediate death. The critical mortality rate is the most accurate indicator of the efficacy of the medical care provided to the immediate survivors (4).

Unique aspects are found in dealing with victims of conventional terrorist bombs. Disaster plans should include the possibility of conventional terrorist bombings and should outline a response plan for the evacuation and treatment of the immediate survivors. Urban hospitals should stockpile sufficient quantities of antibiotics, tetanus immunizations, wound care supplies, and external fixators in preparation for terrorist bombing incidents.

REFERENCES

1. Jordan FB. The role of the medical examiner in mass casualty situations with special reference to the Alfred P. Murrah Building bombing. *J Okla State Med Assoc* 1999;92:159–163.
2. Rignault DP, Deligny MC. The 1986 terrorist bombing experience in Paris. *Ann Surg* 1989;209:368–873.
3. Leibovici D, Gofrit ON, Stein M, et al. Blast injuries: bus versus open-air bombings—a comparative study of injuries in survivors of open-air versus confined-space explosions. *J Trauma* 1996;41:1030–1035.
4. Frykberg ER, Tepas JJ III. Terrorist bombings. Lessons learned from Belfast to Beirut. *Ann Surg* 1988;208:569-576.
5. Mallonee S, Shariat S, Stennies G, et al. Physical injuries and fatalities resulting from the Oklahoma City bombing. *JAMA* 1996;276:382–387.
6. Hogan DE, Waeckerle JF, Dire DJ, et al. Emergency department impact of the Oklahoma City terrorist bombing. *Ann Emerg Med* 1999;34:160–167.
7. Van Campen LE, Dennis JM, Hanlin RC, et al. One-year audiologic monitoring of individuals exposed to the 1995 Oklahoma City bombing. *J Am Acad Audiol* 1999;10:231–247.
8. Boffard KD, MacFarlane C. Urban bomb blast injuries: patterns of injury and treatment. *Surg Ann* 1993;25:29–47.
9. Malpass CP, Martin LJ. Clinical aspects of ball-bearing bomb injuries. *Resuscitation* 1978;6:53–58.
10. Hill JF. Blast injury with particular reference to recent terrorist bombing incidents. *Ann R Coll Surg Engl* 1979;61:4–11.
11. Stuhmiller JH, Phillips YY, Richmond DR. The physics and mechanisms of primary blast injury. In: Bellamy RF, Zajtcjuk JT, eds. *Conventional warfare: ballistic, blast, and burn injuries.* Washington, D.C.: Office of the Surgeon General at TMM Publications, 1991:241–270. Textbook of Military Medicine series.
12. Stapczynski JS. Blast injuries. *Ann Emerg Med* 1992;11:687–694.
13. Phillips YY. Primary blast injuries. *Ann Emerg Med* 1986;15:1446–1450.
14. Cooper GJ, Maynard RL, Cross NL, et al. Casualties from terrorist bombings. *J Trauma* 1983;23:955–967.
15. Katz E, Ofek B, Adler J, et al. Primary blast injury after a bomb explosion in a civilian bus. *Ann Surg* 1989;209:484–488.
16. Rawlins JSP. Physical and pathophysiological effects of blast injury. *Injury* 1978;9:313–320.
17. Phillips YY, Zajtchuk JT. The management of primary blast injury. In: Bellamy RF, Zajtcjuk JT, eds. *Conventional warfare: ballistic, blast, and burn injuries.* Washington, D.C.: Office of the Surgeon General at TMM Publications, 1991:295–336. Textbook of Military Medicine series.
18. Hirsch M, Bazini J. Blast injury of the chest. *Clin Radiol* 1969;20:362–370.
19. Sharpnack DD, Johnson AJ, Phillips YY. The pathology of blast injury. In Bellamy RF, Zajtcjuk JT, eds. *Conventional warfare: ballistic, blast, and burn injuries.* Washington, D.C.: Office of the Surgeon General at TMM Publications, 1991:271–294. Textbook of Military Medicine series.
20. Huller T, Bazini Y. Blast injuries of the chest abdomen. *Arch Surg* 1970;100:24–30.
21. Adler OB, Rosenberger A. Blast injuries. *Acta Radiol* 1988;29:1–5.
22. Mellor SG, Cooper GJ. Analysis of 828 serviceman killed or injured by explosion in Northern Ireland 1970-1984: the hostile action casualty system. *Br J Surg* 1989;76:1006–1010.
23. Phillips YY, Richmond DR. Primary blast injury and basic research: a brief history. In: Bellamy RF, Zajtcjuk JT, eds. *Conventional warfare: ballistic, blast, and burn injuries.* Washington, D.C.: Office of the Surgeon General at TMM Publications, 1991:221–240. Textbook of Military Medicine series.
24. Kronenberg J, Ben-Shoshan J, Wolf M. Perforated tympanic membrane after blast injury. *Am J Otol* 1993;14:92–94.
25. Roberto M, Hamernik RP, Turrentine GA. Damage of the auditory system associated with acute blast trauma. *Ann Otol Rhinol Laryngol* 1989;98:23–34.
26. Kerr AG, Byrne JET. Blast injuries to the ear. *Br Med J* 1975;1:559–561.
27. Caseby NG, Porter MF. Blast injuries to the lungs: clinical presentation, management and course. *Injury* 1976;8:1–12.
28. Hadden WA, Rutherford WH, Merrett JD. The injuries of terrorist bombing. A study of 1532 consecutive patients. *Br J Surg* 1978;65:525–531.
29. Kennedy T. Bullet and bomb injuries. *Trans Med Soc London* 1975–1977;92–93:31–34.
30. Mines M, Thach A, Mallonee S, et al. Ocular injuries sustained by the survivors of the Oklahoma City bombing. *Ophthalmology* 2000;107:837–843.
31. Thach AB, Ward TP, Hollifield RD, et al. Eye injuries in a terrorist bombing: Dhahran, Saudi Arabia, June 25, 1996. *Ophthalmology* 2000;107:844–847.
32. Frykberg ER, Tepas JJ III, Alexander RH. The 1983 Beirut Airport terrorist bombing. Injury patterns and implications for disaster management. *Am Surg* 1989;55:134–141.

33. Brismar B, Bergenwald L. The terrorist bomb explosion in Bologna, Italy, 1980: an analysis of the effects and injuries sustained. *J Trauma* 1982;22:216–220.

34. Caro D, Irving M. The Old Bailey bomb explosion. *Lancet* 1973;1:1433–1435.

35. Scott BA, Fletcher JR, Pulliam MW, et al. The Beirut terrorist bombing. *Neurosurgery* 1986;18:107–110.

36. Tucker K, Lettin A. The Tower of Long bomb explosion. *BMJ* 1975;3:287–289.

37. Frykberg ER, Hutton PMJ, Balzer R. Disaster in Beirut: an application of mass casualty principle. *Mil Med* 1987;152:563–566.

38. Rosenberg B, Sternberg N, Zagher V, et al. Burns due to terroristic attacks on civilian populations from 1975 to 1979. *Burns Incl Therm Inj* 1982;9:21–23.

39. Quenemoen LE, Davis YM, Malilay J, et al. The World Trade Center Bombing: injury prevention strategies for high-rise building fires. *Disasters* 1996:20:125–132.

40. Boehm TM. James JJ. The medical response to the LaBelle Disco bombing in Berlin, 1986. *Mil Med* 1988;153:235–238.

41. Carley SD, Mackway-Jones K. The casualty profile from the Manchester bombing 1996: a proposal for the construction and dissemination of casualty profiles from major incidents. *J Accid Emerg Med* 1997;14:76–80.

42. Feliciano DV, Anderson GV Jr, Rozycki GS, et al. Management of casualties from the bombing at the centennial Olympics. *Am J Surg* 1998;176:538–543.

43. Smith DW, Christiansen EH, Vincent R, et al. Population effects of the bombing of Oklahoma City. *J Okla State Med Assoc* 1999;92:193–198.

44. Kennedy TL, Johnston GW. Civilian bomb injuries. *BMJ* 1975;1:382–383.

45. Adler J, Golan E, Golan J, et al. Terrorist bombing experience during 1975–1979. *Isr J Med Sci* 1983;19:189–193.

46. Vassallo DJ, Taylor JC, Aldington DJ, et al. Shattered illusions—the Thiepval Barracks bombing, 7 October 1996. *J R Army Med Corps* 1997;143:5–11.

47. Noji EK. The medical consequences of earthquakes: coordinating the medical and rescue response. *Disaster Management* 1991;4:32–40.

48. Hirshberg A, Stein M, Walden R. Surgical resource utilization in urban terrorist bombing: a computer simulation. *J Trauma* 1999;47:545–550.

49. American College of Surgeons Committee on Trauma. *Advanced trauma life support manual*, 6th ed. Chicago: American College of Surgeons, 1997.

50. Leibovici D, Gofrit ON, Shapira SC. Eardrum perforation in explosion survivors: is it a marker of pulmonary blast injury. *Ann Emerg Med* 1999;34:168–172.

51. Dire DJ. Infection following wounds, bites, and burns. In: Brillman JC, Quenzer RW, eds. *Infectious disease in emergency medicine*, 2nd ed. Philadelphia: Lippincott-Raven, 1998:231–260.

52. Bowen TE, Bellamy R. *Emergency war surgery. Second United States revision of the emergency war surgery NATO handbook.* Washington, D.C.: United States Department of Defense, United States Government Printing Office, 1988.

53. Weiler-Ravell D, Adatto R, Borman JB. Blast injury of the chest. A review of the problem and its treatment. *Isr J Med Sci* 1975;11:268–274.

54. Lyons HA. Terrorist bombings and the psychological sequelae. *J Irish Med Assoc* 1967;60:15–19.

NUCLEAR DETONATIONS: EVALUATION AND RESPONSE

FUN H. FONG, JR.

The terrorist attacks suffered by the United States on September 11, 2001 added an unfortunate chapter to the history of terrorism and changed forever the mindset of the antiterrorism response. The world now understands that terrorists are continually innovative in planning new terrorist operations. Additionally, the weaknesses in national security systems are continually being probed and explored.

In the Cold War era, conventional thought stated that nuclear detonation scenarios would be fraught with so much devastation that the consideration of mounting any reasonable response would be useless. With the end of the Cold War, mutual assured destruction scenarios with no significant planned response are much less likely. However, nuclear threats from (a) the increased potential for terrorism, (b) the potential for nuclear weapons diversion (theft), (c) rogue terrorist nations, and (d) accidental strategic nuclear firings are now significant. One estimate indicates that for large-scale terrorist operations against civilian populations, casualties might cost $2,000 per square kilometer using conventional weapons, $800 per square kilometer using nuclear weapons, $600 per square kilometer using nerve gas, and $1 per square kilometer with biologic weapons (1). While radiologic options are not the most cost-effective selection for the terrorist, this has not deterred terrorist organizations from seriously considering nuclear capability.

A small, tactical 1-kiloton nuclear device detonated at ground level is capable of creating a crater 30 feet deep and approximately 190 feet in diameter (2). The Armed Forces frequently uses a scenario of a 1-kiloton device detonated from the Washington Monument as a model for effects and response. Figures 32.1 and 32.2 use the same scenario to estimate the radii for a variety of injuries. While the detonation would cause great local devastation, a large portion of the metropolitan area would continue to have significant resources to respond. Even a large yield, megaton detonation within a large metropolitan area would generate response from neighboring metropolitan areas. Thus, all foreseeable scenarios *will* result in a response. Response would need to encompass the wide continuum of casualties incurred from that of a "dirty bomb" (no nuclear yield) to that of a thermonuclear detonation (large nuclear yield).

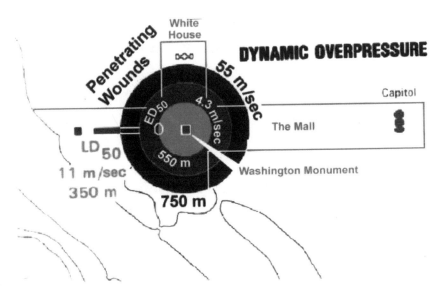

FIG. 32.1. Effective range for blast energy with a 1-kiloton weapon. (From Armed Forces Radiobiology Research Institute. *Medical effects of ionizing radiation.* Course. Bethesda, MD: Armed Forces Radiobiology Research Institute, 2002, with permission.)

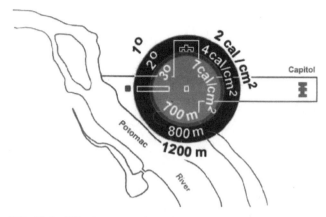

FIG. 32.2. Effective range for infrared thermal energy for a 1-kiloton weapon. (From Armed Forces Radiobiology Research Institute. *Medical effects of ionizing radiation.* Course. Bethesda, MD: Armed Forces Radiobiology Research Institute, 2002, with permission.)

Ongoing comprehensive response plans need to be developed not just for national levels but for regional levels as well; these must be accompanied by the attendant exercises.

An Nuclear, Biological, or Chemical (NBC) Task Force consisting of an American College of Emergency Physicians (ACEP)-led consortium of health care provider professional organizations is looking at the issue of how best to train health professionals on response to weapons of mass destruction (3).

Technically speaking, a nuclear detonation is a fission and/or fusion chain-reaction, where each successive reaction generates more reactions and more neutrons until the bulk of the nuclear fuel is consumed. Fusion reactions are also known as *thermonuclear* reactions because thermal energy neutrons are important in the fusion process.

TYPICAL TERRORIST SCENARIOS

A wide spectrum of potential application of radiation for terrorism purposes exists, including perverting a radiation device to expose others to use a bomb that would spread radiation to a strategic thermonuclear detonation from a rogue state. These different scenarios, with their particular considerations, will be covered.

Radiation Device

Radionuclides, such as brachytherapy sources, or radiation devices, such as an industrial radiography source, radiation oncology teletherapy device, or a x-ray machine, could be misused for terrorist purposes to cause exposures in unsuspecting individuals. These exposures may or may not have health consequences, depending on the dose. To the terrorist, the threat of radiation exposure is what accomplishes the objective of generating fear.

Radionuclide Dispersal Device

A radionuclide dispersal device, or RDD, is also known as a "dirty bomb," a bomb that does not have significant nuclear yield but that is capable of contaminating significant amounts of land. These devices may or may not be intended for use as an actual nuclear device. A nuclear device detonation that does not result in a nuclear yield becomes a RDD. Any type of radioactive source of high or low activity or any amount can be used in a RDD.

Improvised Nuclear Device

The improvised nuclear device (IND) is composed of either enriched uranium or plutonium-239 and is constructed by a nongovernmental organization, usually a terrorist group. Having been created by organizations with limited expertise, these devices generally have less than optimal nuclear yields, and they have significantly more contamination than that associated with similarly sized nuclear weapons. The smaller size of an improvised nuclear device is limited by the minimum critical mass of uranium and plutonium. The minimum moderated critical mass for 93%-enriched uranium-235 is 820 g, while the minimum moderated critical mass for plutonium-239 is only 510 g (4). National security strategies are directed towards preventing terrorist organizations from obtaining critical quantities of these materials.

Tactical Nuclear Weapon

This nuclear device has been constructed by a governmental agency and has yields ranging from 0.5 to 50 kilotons. The weapon is well-designed, and it should be capable of more efficient yields. Tactical nuclear weapons may be as small as a backpack or suitcase. John Deutch, the former director of the Central Intelligence Agency, testified in 1996 that over 100 reports have been made alleging the diversion of nuclear warheads or components. He also stated that much of the reporting is "sporadic, unsubstantiated, and unreliable" (5).

Strategic Nuclear Weapon

This device is fabricated by a governmental agency, and its yields range from 1 megaton or greater. The former Soviet Union once had strategic nuclear weapons of close to 100 megatons. These weapons are fusion or thermonuclear weapons, which generate less fallout than comparably sized fission weapons.

Terrorist Events Involving Radiation

Terrorist events involving radiation have already occurred. On November 12, 1995, Chechen rebels placed ^{137}Cs in a protective container emitting 2 rad per hour at surface contact inside Ismailovo Park in Moscow. Rebel commander Shamir Basayev took responsibility for the incident.

Dzhokhar Dudayev, the Chechen rebel leader, had repeatedly threatened to launch a nuclear attack on Moscow (6). Basayev indicated that his group was in possession of seven similar containers. As of 1997, no additional containers had been recovered (7).

The Japanese cult organization Aum Shinri Kyo, Supreme Truth, purchased a 500,000-acre sheep farm with a known uranium deposit on the premises. Two years later, investigators found mining, laboratory equipment, and a rock-crushing machine at the farm, indicating that the cult had been attempting to extract uranium (8). On April 2, 1995, Japanese police found other evidence of an Aum interest in the technology of nuclear weapons. Police found a classified document on uranium enrichment technology in the possession of Aum. The document described a technique for enriching uranium using lasers (9). Aum was later reported to have actually experimented with a laser beam that could be used to enrich uranium (10). Police also found an Aum notebook that contained "what looked like plans by the Aum to import Russian tanks and nuclear warheads" (11). Aum's construction minister, Kiyohide Hayakawa, was documented to have traveled to Russia at least 21 times between 1992 and 1995; his notebooks included prices for nuclear warheads (12).

In Auckland, New Zealand, three Auckland residents with ties to Afghanistan were arrested on suspicion of people-smuggling and passport fraud. Papers were found before the 2000 Sydney Olympics that considered a small nuclear research reactor in Sydney, Australia, a target, with plans detailing entry and exit routes to the Sydney nuclear reactor and notes on police security tactics. The group was reportedly linked with Afghanistan-based terrorist Osama bin Laden (9).

Traditional terrorist groups with established sponsors will probably remain hesitant to use a nuclear weapon, for fear of provoking a worldwide crackdown and alienating their supporters (13). Newer terrorist organizations may have less fear in considering such a weapon if it is available to them.

A number of nations have attempted to achieve nuclear capability. Some have been successful to some degree or another. Iranian agents unsuccessfully approached a Kazakhstan metallurgic plant to obtain enriched uranium in 1992. In 1993, three Iranians, probably intelligence agents, were arrested in Turkey while seeking to acquire nuclear material from smugglers from the former Soviet Union. North Korea has now produced enough plutonium for at least one and possibly two nuclear weapons (5).

Rogue nations, such as Iraq, are undoubtedly continuing to work to develop nuclear devices. One source states that Iraq has been attempting to attain nuclear capability since 1971. At the time of his greatest nuclear achievement, Saddam Hussein constructed a bomb trigger with the assistance of the International Atomic Energy Agency (IAEA), and he also had cast a nonenriched uranium sphere that was 4 inches in diameter cast. In 1994, the source alleged that Iraq was now able to enrich uranium by diffusion using the declassified Manhattan Project documents. This source had

no doubt that Iraq was continuing to pursue a nuclear option (14).

Another report that has not been confirmed is that the Al-Quaeda terrorist, Osama bin Laden, has obtained two to three of the suitcase single kiloton-type weapons. Several informal analyses doubted the actuality of his acquisition of these weapons, citing the fact that Libya unsuccessfully offered the equivalent of one billion U.S. dollars to obtain a state-manufactured nuclear weapon.

Since the September 11, 2001 attack, news reports and intelligence have taken a dizzying turn. On October 31, 2001, Fox News reported that six persons attempting to enter the United States through Michigan came with nuclear reactor plans. Another report stated that Al-Quaeda terrorists had been undergoing training in an attempt to infiltrate, assault, and cause a meltdown at nuclear power plants. Various news services had previously reported that security at nuclear facilities was lacking in the face of a determined conventional assault.

These possibilities have always been considered highly unlikely but within the realm of possibility. Now, security plans nationwide need to be reevaluated to see if the current states of readiness are robust enough to match the existing known intelligence.

EFFECTS OF NUCLEAR WEAPONS

The characteristic mushroom cloud actually is common for many types of explosions. Its formation is diagrammed in Fig. 32.3. High airbursts may generate spherical clouds. Mushroom-type clouds may or may not have a stem. Small,

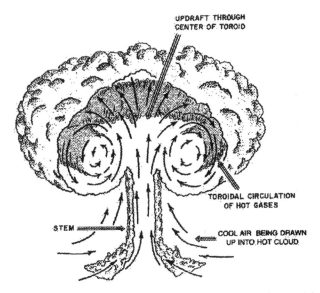

FIG. 32.3. Cutaway showing an artist's conception of toroidal circulation within the radioactive cloud resulting from a nuclear explosion. (From Glasstone S, Dolan PJ, eds. *The effects of nuclear weapons.* Washington, D.C.: Department of the Army, 1977:29, with permission.)

tactical-size fission devices are the most likely type of nuclear detonation that would occur during peacetime. Accordingly, a 1-kiloton device serves as a model for comparison purposes in this text unless stated otherwise. The distribution of energy of a nuclear device, regardless of the height of burst is (a) blast and shock at 50%, (b) thermal radiation of 35%, (c) initial nuclear radiation of 5%, and (d) residual nuclear radiation of 10%.

Blast

A nuclear detonation causes dynamic pressure changes as in any other explosion, except on a larger scale. Overpressures are much more pronounced with proximity to the blast. With increasing distance from ground zero, the overpressure changes become less prominent. A negative pressure phase, which is much milder, also occurs, causing a wind reversal towards ground zero. Once the pressure normalizes to atmospheric pressure, a second wind reversal away from ground zero takes place. A blast overpressure of 5 pounds per square inch (psi) seems to be a significant threshold for causing both (a) devastation to frame and brick houses and (b) eardrum damage in humans.

Detonations cause the formation of a blast or shock wave that indicates the advance of the overpressure. Detonations at some altitudes create both an *incident* and a *reflected* blast wave (Fig. 32.4). The reflected wave overtakes and merges with the incident wave at lower altitudes, causing the formation of a mach stem or a mach front (Fig. 32.5). The mach stem has a defined height, above which areas are found in which the incident and reflected waves have not yet joined. The significance of this phenomenon is that the resultant overpressure of the mach front is approximately twice that of the original incident blast wave. The height of the mach stem will increase with time and distance (Fig. 32.6).

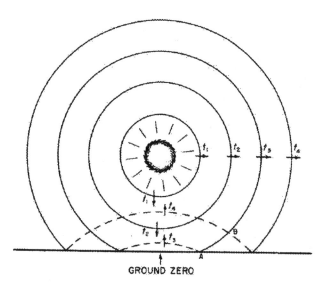

FIG. 32.4. The reflection of blast wave in an air burst at the earth's surface. t_1 to t_4 represent successive times. (From Glasstone S, Dolan PJ, eds. *The effects of nuclear weapons.* Washington, D.C.: Department of the Army, 1977:87, with permission.)

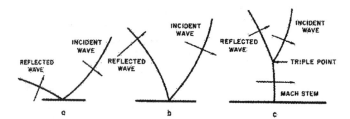

FIG. 32.5. The merging of incident and reflected waves (*a,b*) and the formation of Mach Y configuration of shock fronts (*c*). (From Glasstone S, Dolan PJ, eds. *The effects of nuclear weapons.* Washington, D.C.: Department of the Army, 1977:89, with permission.)

Crater Formation

Crater formation in surface and underground bursts are well-understood phenomena. In a surface burst, spalling of the surface is observed, and then the upper layers move upward at about 150 feet per second as a result of the incident blast wave. If significant water moisture is present, this water vaporizes and contributes to the upward movement of the ground. A crater lip is formed; debris falling on the lip is known as ejecta. Material that falls back into the crater immediately is known as fallback (Fig. 32.7)(15). When the fallback descends to the ground, the dust-laden air reaching the ground then reaches outward, producing a base surge. Knowledge of the crater size resulting from a surface burst allows the calculation of a nuclear yield.

Thermal Energy

A conventional explosion fireball has a temperature of several thousand degrees, while a nuclear detonation fireball will be tens of millions of degrees, thus constituting a major difference between these types of explosions. Consequently, this energy is released mostly in the form of short-wave electromagnetic radiation. The thermal effects are released in two phases as follows: (a) an initial pulse usually lasting a second or less, constituting 1% of the thermal energy with x-rays and ultraviolet radiation predominating; and (b) a second pulse lasting a few seconds that is composed of more visible light and that is capable of causing secondary fires and retinal burns (Fig. 32.8).

Electromagnetic Radiation

The brilliant flash of detonation can ignite various materials at closer ranges and can create flash marks and etch shadows in adjacent structures. Ignition depends on reflectivity, material thickness, and moisture content. With devices of lower yield, a given amount of energy may be more effective if it is given over a somewhat longer time (1 or 2 seconds). Humans are more likely to suffer flash burns if they are wearing dark or flammable material.

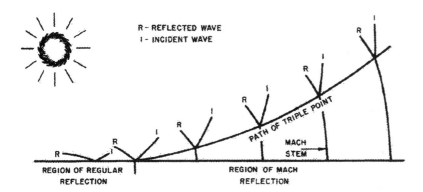

FIG. 32.6. Outward motion of the blast wave near the surface of the Mach region. (From Glasstone S, Dolan PJ, eds. *The effects of nuclear weapons.* Washington, D.C.: Department of the Army, 1977: 89, with permission.)

The brightness of the flash may cause the temporary loss of visual acuity known as *flash blindness* or *dazzle.* This injury is more likely than retinal burns because most people try to shield their eyes during a detonation. Retinal burns cause permanent visual impairment by damage to the retina. Well-defined minimal safe distance estimates exist that delineate at what points retinal burns may occur given a particular yield and depending on whether the detonation occurs during the day or night (Fig. 32.9). Safe separation distances for eye injury are much greater at night.

Electromagnetic Pulse

The energy released from a fission or fusion event is very dense; the temperatures generated are on the order of tens of millions of degrees in comparison to a few thousand degrees in the case of a conventional explosion. As a consequence of these extremely high temperatures, a wide range of electromagnetic energy is released after a fission or fusion event. An electromagnetic pulse (EMP) is the generation of a great amount of energy within a wide radiofrequency spectrum. This type of pulse can also be generated with conventional detonations to a lesser extent, but, in the case of a nuclear detonation, this may present as a major effect. All electrical equipment may be susceptible to permanent disruption from the EMP. Among the most susceptible equipment are rare-earth transistors and static-sensitive transistors and chips. Equipment that is more resistant to EMP includes nontransistorized, vacuum tube equipment. Equipment that is encased completely in metal, protection that is known as a Faraday shield, would be completely shielded and would still be useable after a surface burst. Measures that protect equipment from lightning pulses will not offer protection from a nuclear EMP.

EMP has been classified into the following two types: surface-burst EMP (SBEMP), and high-altitude EMP (HEMP).

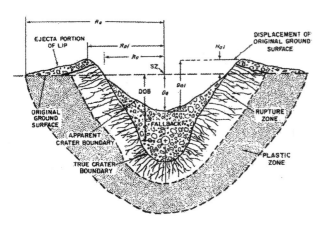

FIG. 32.7. Cross-section of a crater from a subsurface nuclear detonation. (From Glasstone S, Dolan PJ, eds. *The effects of nuclear weapons.* Washington, D.C.: Department of the Army, 1977:254, with permission.)

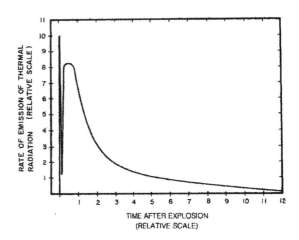

FIG. 32.8. Emission of thermal radiation in two pulses of an air burst. (From Glasstone S, Dolan PJ, eds. *The effects of nuclear weapons.* Washington, D.C.: Department of the Army, 1977:41, with permission.)

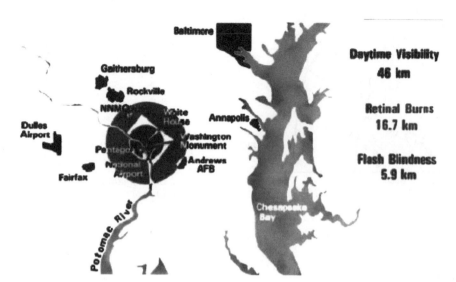

Daytime Visibility
46 km

Retinal Burns
16.7 km

Flash Blindness
5.9 km

FIG. 32.9. Safe separation distance for eye injuries. This figure assumes a weapon yield of 1 kiloton, a detonation altitude of 300 m, and a personnel altitude at sea level. (From Armed Forces Radiobiology Research Institute. *Medical effects of ionizing radiation.* Course. Bethesda MD: Armed Forces Radiobiology Research Institute, 2002, with permission.)

Surface-Burst Electromagnetic Pulse

SBEMP at altitudes of 200 meters or less can be even more powerful than HEMP, and it may involve fields as strong as one million volts per meter (15). High levels of SBEMP may weld buried or above-ground cables outside the immediate vicinity of nuclear detonation. These cables may remain intact yet essentially short out, transmitting tremendous surges of energy to connected systems down the line. Because of the physics involved, SBEMP effects extend to ranges that are 10 to 20 kilometers from ground zero.

No nonclassified techniques exist for estimating the range of SBEMP effects, but a realistic expectation would be that a tactical (kiloton) size surface burst would quite probably disrupt most electronic gear within the immediate area. One example for a 10-kiloton weapon indicates that the safety (standoff) distance in the open is 2,400 m, while the EMP damage radius for critical electronic equipment could extend to ranges of 5,000 m (16).

High-Altitude Electromagnetic Pulse

HEMP is produced when a nuclear explosion occurs 30 kilometers or more above the earth's surface. The physical processes that generate HEMP differ from those that produce SBEMP, and HEMP effects can have considerable strength at great distances. The intensity of a HEMP field could be as high as 50,000 volts per m. The contiguous 48 states could be covered with a HEMP field of at least 25,000 volts per m. A working scenario of the United States military has been that a detonation of 300 megatons at an altitude of 100 miles over the geographic center of the continental United States, which would require the detonation of multiple warheads, would effectively disrupt all communications nationally.

Transient Radiation Effects on Electronics

Transient radiation effects on electronics (TREE) is an effect on electronics equipment that occurs in addition to EMP. TREE is a shorter range effect brought on by ionization caused by the initial pulse of gamma and neutron radiation within electronic equipment. Some of the effects may be temporary (those from gamma radiation), while other damage may be permanent. Damage is dose-rate–related (17).

Ionizing Radiation

Ionizing radiation is one of the special emission features of a nuclear detonation. Two types of radiation are released—*immediate radiation* and *residual radiation*. Immediate radiation consists of gamma radiation, beta radiation, neutron radiation, and a small fraction of alpha radiation. In a nuclear detonation, gamma rays from fission are formed in less than 1 microsecond. These prompt gamma rays are produced so rapidly that they are significantly absorbed by the weapon components. Some delayed gamma rays are formed from neutrons captured within other nuclei. Other delayed gamma rays come from the near-instantaneous appearance of fission fragments. The instantaneous and delayed gamma rays are formed in approximately equal amounts. Neutrons are captured by atmospheric nitrogen, which then release additional gamma rays. Thus, delayed gamma rays, along with gamma rays from neutron capture, constitute about 100 times more radiation released than which is released from the prompt gamma ray component (18).

Neutrons are another relatively unique radiation from a fission or fusion bomb. The 20-kiloton bombs of Hiroshima and Nagasaki were thought to have a neutron quality factor of 20 from dosimetry estimates performed in 1986, making neutron doses 20 times more effective than the equivalent gamma doses. Neutrons tend to change energy with distance as they are attenuated by air. Neutrons released from fission and fusion bombs will have different energy spectra. Neutrons released from fusion weapons will have a larger proportion of high-energy neutrons. Besides being more effective, neutron radiation is also special in that it is capable of inducing radioactivity in other substances; in other words, it can make certain other substances radioactive.

Residual Radiation

Induced Radiation

Induced radiation occurs in certain materials as a result of the bombardment of neutrons as occurs in a fission detonation. The process is also referred to as activation, or neutron-induced gamma activity (NIGA). A variety of substances could become radioactive from a detonation. The soil in the immediate target area is considered radioactive to a depth of 0.5 m. Nonmetallic substances that can become activated include silicon (^{31}Si) and manganese (^{56}Mn; half-life, 2.6 hours). Metals such as aluminum (^{28}Al; half-life, 2.3 minutes), zinc, and copper are easily activated. In biologic systems, the most important induced form of radioactivity is ^{24}Na (half-life, 15 hours), which could occur in any bioactive material containing sodium and which is also easily detectable. Glass, which contains both sodium and silicon, may become activated. Typical radiation 1 hour after detonation is .02 Gy per hour (2 rad/hr) from NIGA. The area affected by NIGA is calculated using the Keller nomogram and a consideration of the soil type.

Fallout

The process of fission generates a mixture of fission products comprising approximately 80 different radionuclides and the unconsumed radioactive products that are seen after a surface burst. *Fallout* is the fusion and condensation of these fission products and earth debris that later falls to earth. Surface blasts form substantial fallout, while an air burst at an optimum height will produce negligible fallout, as occurred in the Hiroshima and Nagasaki bombings. The direction of fallout from ground zero is based on the aloft winds, which may travel in many different directions at different altitudes, as well as on surface winds. Thus, the actual location of fallout might differ appreciably from that which would be expected from the direction of surface winds alone (19). The only hazard associated with fallout is radiation.

In *early fallout*, radioactive residues fuse with dust and debris and frequently take on a snowflake-like appearance. Early fallout is arbitrarily defined as that radioactive debris that accumulates within the first 24 hours and that is composed of much larger particles. Thermonuclear, or fusion, detonations generate significantly less fallout. Early fallout

constitutes mostly an external hazard because of beta and gamma rays from sources outside the body. Early fallout doses change considerably at various times after a nuclear explosion.

After a surface burst, *late* or *delayed fallout* also is observed; this remains in cloud formations more than 24 hours after detonation. These radioactive residues are decreased greatly from early fallout, but they may cause an additional source of radiation in the form of *cloud shine*. If the nuclear cloud is either within or below a rain cloud, then the resultant precipitation could cause rainout or washout of these fission products. Late fallout has been characterized as extremely fine invisible particles that accumulate slowly in low concentrations over a considerable portion of the surface of the earth. The long time in which these particles are aloft reduces exposure rates; dose accumulation with these is too slow and too small to be immediately hazardous to health, but it may be sufficient to cause delayed or late effects (20). Strontium-90 traditionally has been the radionuclide indicator that is assayed to estimate the amounts of delayed fallout. In contrast to early fallout, which is a contact and external hazard, delayed fallout constitutes a potential long-term ingestion (internal) hazard from iodine, strontium, and cesium radioisotopes.

PREHOSPITAL IMPACT AND CONSIDERATIONS

Contamination and Medical Issues

Prehospital decontamination should be cursory and brief, removing gross fallout from the body surfaces, as well as taking off the clothing and shoes of the patient. Prehospital decontamination should not be expected to be definitive, particularly in the scenario of a nuclear detonation. These modest actions alone may be life-saving, as they avoid beta burns and minimize radioiodine uptake. Victims with both beta burns and systemic irradiation create a type of combined injury that is associated with increased morbidity and mortality. In the initial stages, removing all traces of contamination is not necessary for avoiding beta burns. Victims and responders who are at risk of being exposed to fallout are best treated prophylactically with some form of radiostable iodine at least 1 hour before exposure. Once exposure has occurred, giving radiostable iodine may still be useful up to 4 hours after exposure.

Every ambulance unit should not be expected to have radiation survey equipment, but each ambulance service should have supervisors capable of operating radiation survey meters. The state radiation health department or equivalent agency may provide field teams to assist with surveys. They may work in conjunction with the federal Department of Energy radiation assistance program teams that assess the degree of contamination that exists. Any nuclear detonation will probably initiate activation of the Federal Radiological

Monitoring Assistance Center, a field monitoring organization that theoretically would coordinate the various different types of radiation monitoring and assessment.

The Centers for Disease Control (CDC) maintains a pharmaceutical cache for the eventuality that weapons of mass destruction are used. Some medicines and equipment for the affected population may be supplied by the CDC.

Terrorism Issues

In the event of a terrorist attack, the possibility of secondary devices should always be considered, even in nuclear detonations. Initial surveys may provide either inaccurate or contradictory information. In modeling of radionuclide dispersal devices using easy-to-obtain radiation sources, radiation has been discovered to be so well dispersed that, in some instances, it may be quite difficult to detect using standard radiation survey equipment (21).

Mass Casualty Incident Issues

Distinguishing between contaminated and noncontaminated victims would be important in the event of a nuclear detonation. The author suggests that *magenta*, a color associated with radiation placarding, might be used to designate those with radioactive contamination; this would be in addition to any other colors used in triage. Establishing separate contaminated and noncontaminated casualty staging areas may be useful for the site incident commander.

High Explosive Material

Unexploded high explosive material may be present in significant amounts after a successful nuclear detonation. This could pose a significant explosive hazard if struck or stepped on by victims, responders, or equipment.

EMERGENCY DEPARTMENT IMPACT AND CONSIDERATIONS

In the event of a true nuclear detonation, local hospitals and medical providers will perform dramatically different functions than usual. Surviving hospitals near an impact area should consider functioning primarily for triage and as a casualty collection point and then transferring patients to other hospitals.

If hospitals have impaired function, a risk-benefit decision should be made about whether the hospital should continue to function or whether patients and personnel should be evacuated to continue care at an intact facility. Prior mutual aid agreements with hospitals outside an impact area should be activated for possible hospital and personnel evacuation (see Chapter 8).

Hospitalization is a key factor for patient survival in higher dose exposures. The prompt median lethal dose

(LD_{50}) with minimal care is 3.0 Gy (300 rads) (22), and, with austere medical support for patient survival, the LD_{50} can easily be extended into the range of 4.5 Gy (450 rads) (23). Therefore, efforts should be directed toward finding enough hospital bed resources for eligible victims. Activation of the National Disaster Medical System hospital bed system may be important for facilitating victim transfers and enhancing patient survival.

Decontamination

Victims will self-rescue with an improvised response and will typically present to the nearest emergency department in the event of a mass casualty incident or disaster. The emergency department must be prepared to receive a large number of potentially contaminated victims who have not had contact with prehospital care (see Chapters 25 and 26).

A contamination triage checkpoint will need to be established outside the hospital to reduce the amount and incidence of hospital contamination (see Chapters 25 and 26). Gross dry decontamination should be made available immediately outside the hospital. The use of portable vacuum units with a high-efficiency particulate air (HEPA) filter and flexible hose may facilitate rapid, morbidity-reducing decontamination outdoors. A mass decontamination shower system line may also be considered for outdoor use as a definitive step. Patients who are decontaminated will need temporary clean clothes (e.g., hospital gowns) and a system for labeling and reclaiming personal belongings.

In the case of a terrorist-caused disaster, the Environmental Protection Agency has stated on record that the care of the population should come first and that regulations against radionuclide runoff would not be enforced.

A *radiation emergency area* (REA), a location for indoor decontamination, should be part of radiation emergency plans in the event that contamination or contaminated individuals inside the hospital are discovered. (See Table 25.7 for procedures in the event that contamination is discovered *inside* the hospital.) Heavier preparation of the indoor REA may be necessary, including covering the floor with either butcher paper or a plastic covering (e.g., herculite). Floor preparation will make REA contamination cleanup easier. Infrequently used equipment within the REA may be covered with a bedsheet or a clear plastic sheet. The indoor REA should be capable of caring for medically unstable patients and should have access to the critical care resources of power, oxygen, suction, fluid resuscitation, cardiac monitoring and defibrillation, and airway stabilization.

Monitoring Issues

Every hospital should have on-call health or medical physicist consultation available and a minimum of two radiation survey meters equipped with pancake probes. Radiation survey meters require calibration every 6 months by a health physicist.

If hospital budgets are tight, old civil defense instrumentation, such as the low-range CDV-700, the high-range CDV-715 survey meters, or the complete set, known as the CDV-777-1 radiation detection set, should be readily available as surplus item at a county emergency management agency or auction. They may be refitted with pancake probes for approximately $130. These instruments are often regarded derisively by health physicists and health physics technicians because they are not state-of-the-art equipment; indeed, many health physicists actively attempt to decommission these instruments whenever they encounter them. However, these instruments were designed precisely for nuclear detonation scenarios, and they should perform well enough to meet this need. Older civil defense equipment is notorious for being unable to maintain calibration. Other, newer radiation survey units may cost $450 or more.

Doorframe Monitors

Doorframe monitors may be extremely useful in the rapid gross survey screening of large numbers of people. Doorframe monitors consist of a series of Geiger-Müller tubes lined along a doorframe-shaped portal and connected to a standard radiation survey instrument. Doorframe probes and survey meters should constitute a portion of the regional stockpile of radiation response equipment.

Nuclear Medicine Gamma Camera

The ubiquitous nuclear medicine gamma camera is available in any hospital with a nuclear medicine department. The gamma camera is an ideal screening tool for detecting the presence of fission products and therefore contamination from fallout. While in the process of developing radiation response plans, in-house radiologists and nuclear medicine physicians should be familiarized with this potential use of the gamma camera (24). The gamma camera provides gross sensitivities that are between those of whole body counters and Geiger-Müller survey counters (Table 32.1).

Triage

Triage should provide a simple, practical means for sorting patients into severity categories (see Chapter 2). In a nuclear detonation, a disaster condition will exist with a shortage of resources for the number of casualties received, so disaster mode triage, with its emphasis on doing the greatest good for the greatest number of victims, will be used rather than allocation of whatever resources are needed to save a given life. Triage decisions should always reflect the available resources *at that time*. The following three parameters are most useful in nuclear detonations: (a) the time to onset of vomiting after detonation, (b) the decrease in absolute lymphocyte count over a 24-hour to 48-hour period, and (c) the presence of conventional trauma.

A number of schemes have been proposed to triage combined injury, modifying the triage category with increasing amounts of radiation exposure. The military uses Table 32.2, including systemic radiation and the onset of vomiting, to modify conventional triage classifications (25).

The complete Union of Soviet Socialist Republics (USSR) triage table, used in the Chernobyl disaster in 1986, creates triage classifications based on the onset of prodromal symptoms and constitutes a practical and effec-

TABLE 32.1. MINIMAL DETECTABLE ACTIVITY WITH POINT SOURCE IN AIR AND WITH SCATTER MEDIUM[a]

Radionuclide	Whole body counter MDA (MDA in air)	Gamma camera (MDA in air)	Geiger-Müller survey counter	
			Scatter media	(MDA in air)
^{125}I	—[b]	0.30–2.62	3.68–29.90	90
^{201}Tl	0.20	0.51–0.69	2.40–3.48	188
^{57}Co	0.09	0.37–0.39	1.15–1.53	144
^{99m}Tc	0.12	0.40–0.56	1.36–1.64	165
^{111}In	0.11	0.71–0.89	1.88–2.50	20
^{133}Ba	0.11	0.56–1.09	1.51–2.71	59
^{131}I	0.12	0.68–0.99	1.85–3.22	90
^{85}Sr	0.11	0.72–1.10	2.10–3.40	59
^{137}Cs	0.13	1.04–2.26	2.47–4.03	99
^{54}Mn	0.10	1.06–1.84	2.70–4.24	38
^{60}Co	0.10	1.27–1.48	2.11–3.15	14

Abbreviation: MDA, minimal detectable activity.
Gamma cameras used were (a) Ohio Nuclear Series 100, (b) Searle Pho/Gamma IV, (c) Picker Dyna camera 4/15, and (d) Siemens LEM.
Multiplication by 37 converts MDA (number of Ci) to Bq units
[a]Data was combined and condensed from Tables 4 and 5 of the original source document.
[b]Electronic interference prevented the detection of energy below 50 keV.
Modified from Nishiyama H, Lukes SJ, Saenger EL. Low-level internal radionuclide contamination: use of gamma camera for detection. *Radiol* 1984;150:235–240, with permission.

TABLE 32.2. COMBINED INJURY TRIAGE WHEN RADIATION DOSES ARE KNOWN[a]

Conventional triage categories if injuries are only trauma		Changes in expected triage category following whole-body radiation dose (Gy)	
No radiation	<1.5 (150 rad)	1.5–4.5 (150–450 rad)	>4.5 (450 rad)
Prodrome onset	<3 h	1–3 h	<1 h
Immediate	Immediate	Immediate	Expectant
Delayed	Delayed	Expectant	Expectant
Minimal	Minimal	Expectant	Expectant
Expectant	Expectant	Expectant	Expectant

[a]Decision based on whole-body radiation dose; assumes all casualties are wearing personal dosimeters.
Modified from data in the North Atlantic Treaty Organization. *NATO handbook on the concept of medical support in NBC environments* [AMed P-7 (A)]. Brussels: North Atlantic Treaty Organization, 1978.

tive triage criteria for irradiation injury (Table 32.3). The complete table places conventional injuries within classes of systemic radiation injury to create the more complete triage scheme used in the Chernobyl response. Prodrome, latency, and the development of enteritis are independent clinical variables. Laboratory findings are corroborating variables. Survival is the ultimate dependent variable. The general correlation of precise time to onset of the prodrome may correlate better with dose estimates, so an accurate prodrome onset may be of greater usefulness in the future.

Within any group of individuals, a significant number of those who are vomiting may be doing so for psychogenic reasons. Serial absolute lymphocyte counts can confirm systemic radiation exposure with these individuals, and the Andrews nomogram may be used to predict severity of hematopoietic involvement. Once radiation doses have been estimated, the "penalty" table may be used to provide prognostic outcomes (Table 32.4). This table may be used to restrict exposures to categories of lesser severity, as well as to provide a prognosis for those so exposed.

TABLE 32.3 COMPLETE UNION OF SOVIET SOCIALIST REPUBLICS CLASSIFICATION OF CHERNOBYL VICTIMS[a]

Parameter	Fourth degree	Third degree	Second degree	First degree
Prodrome onset (h)	≤0.5 (vomiting at 30 min, headache, fever)	0.5–1 (vomiting, headache, subfebrile, transient hyperemia of skin)	1–3 (vomiting)	>3 (general reaction)
Latent period (d)	6–8	8–17	15–25	>30
Skin burns	40%–90%	6 severe, all died	Slight	Slight
Enteritis	7–9 d	—	—	—
Lymphocytes/μL (3–6 d)	<100	100–200	300–500	600–1,000
Granulocytes/μL	<500 (7–9 d)	<1,000 (8–20 d)	>1,000 (20–300 patients) in 15–20 d	3,000–4,000 (8–9 d)
Platelets/μL	<40,000 (8–10 d)	<40,000 (10–16 d)	40,000 (17–24 d)	40,000–60,000 (25–28 d)
Total body radiation dose (Gy)	>6–12, 16 (600–1,200 rads, 1,600 rads)	4.2–6.3 (420–630 rads)	2–4 (200–400 rads)	1–2 (100–200 rads)
Deaths/number of patients	17/20 (Moscow, 10–50 d; 2 at Kiev, 4 at 10 d)	7/23 (2–7 wk)	0/53	—
Clinical findings	General intoxication, fever, oral and salivary lesions, beta burns severe enough to cause death, >8–10 Gy of exposure, severe intestinal syndrome	High fever, infection, hemorrhage, severe skin injury	Infections, slight hemorrhage, elevated erythrocyte sedimentation rate	No severe skin change, moderate elevation of erythrocyte sedimentation rate
Estimate of survival	Unlikely	Probable with treatment	Possible without treatment	Probable without treatment

Modified by Barabanova. Row items have been rearranged for temporal clarity.
[a]Barabanova related that categories for first and second degree injuries were actually slightly different in Radiation Emergency Assistance Center/training site (REAC/TS) newsletter, winter 1992.

TABLE 32.4. THE PENALTY TABLE

Medical care needed	Accumulated radiation exposure in Gy (rad) in a period of		
	1 wk	1 mo	4 mo
None	1.5 (150)	2 (200)	3 (300)
Some (5% may die)	2.5 (250)	3.5 (350)	5 (500)
Most (50% may die)	4.5 (450)	6 (600)	—

From the National Council on Radiation Protection and Measurements. *Radiological factors affecting decision-making in a nuclear attack.* NCRP publication no. 42. Washington, D.C.: National Council on Radiation Protection and Measurements, 1974:51, with permission.

Personnel Needs

Dealing with contamination issues will take significantly more personnel than is usual for operations, while at the same time that a situation exists in which some personnel or their relatives may be injured or killed. Personnel will need some systematic method for check on relatives and other loved ones (see Chapter 8). Improvised child care at the hospital will enhance personnel performance. Personnel needs should be estimated realistically to ensure that the vital functions of the hospital are maintained throughout the response and then should be scaled so that a disaster condition response can be staffed for days or possibly even weeks.

Advisory points of contact for hospitals are the state radiologic health department; the county or state emergency management agency, which may have information on sheltering and evacuation; the Radiation Emergency Assistance Center/training site (REAC/TS), based in Oak Ridge, Tennessee, which will be available for consultation on specific medical issues; and the CDC, which will have recommendations on overall population health issues.

SPECIFIC CLINICAL ENTITIES

The clinical entities of external contamination, systemic irradiation, and internal contamination have been comprehensively discussed in the chapter on radiation accidents. These topics will be covered within the context of nuclear detonation.

External Contamination

External contamination will be principally from fission products from bomb residue. In the case of tactical nuclear weapons, this cannot technically be called fallout because fallout forms from the condensation of vaporized fission products and earth at high altitudes. Principal radionuclide contaminants will consist of isotopes of iodine, ^{137}Cs, ^{90}Sr, and plutonium or uranium. Individuals within the blast radius will avoid significant contamination by constantly removing dust and debris from skin and clothing. This will lessen the chances of both external and internal contamination. External contact with fission products over a length of time will cause beta burns, which, when combined with systemic irradiation, could cause dramatically increased morbidity and mortality.

Beta burns or any other type of radiation burn *will not present in an immediate fashion.* Any immediate burns observed will be due to flash or thermal burns. Victims in whom beta burns develop have an early itching or burning sensation and little or no erythema, followed by darkening (bronzing) of the skin, epilation (hair loss), and dry desquamation approximately 2 to 3 weeks later. Beta burns may cause weeping and scabbed lesions, but they typically are more superficial than gamma ray skin burns. Regrowth of hair occurs over a 6-month period (26).

Systemic Irradiation

If the nuclear device detonated is a tactical or strategic nuclear weapon, the radiation dose can be calculated by knowing the device yield, the distance from the epicenter, and the amount of shielding at the moment of detonation. (See Chapter 25 for a more complete summation of the acute radiation syndrome and its complications.)

Internal Contamination

In the event of a nuclear detonation, internal contamination would occur from skin contact with bomb residues and from eating contaminated food. Radioiodines are the primary internal radiation hazard during the first few weeks after atomic bomb fallout (27). After isotopes of iodine, ^{137}Cs, ^{90}Sr, plutonium, and uranium should be considered.

A 1978 text, the *Manual on early medical treatment of possible radiation injury* (IAEA Safety Series no. 47), outlined a course of action for fission product mixtures. It included the following: (a) potassium iodide, 100 mg orally; (b) potassium rhizodizonate (for strontium-contaminated wounds) topically; (c) calcium alginate (for strontium ingestion); (d) Prussian blue, 1 g orally (for cesium contamination); and (e) calcium-diethylenetriamine pentaacetic acid (Ca-DTPA), 1 g in 4 mL by inhalation (for transuranic elements). Other texts have discounted the practicality of treating large numbers of survivors who are contaminated with fallout in this way. No examples of fallout victims who have been treated in this fashion are documented.

Combined Injuries

Conventional injuries combined with irradiation constitute combined injury and result in dramatically increased morbidity and mortality. Any type of healing from conventional injuries is delayed in the setting of significant irradiation exposure. The onset of immunocompromise from systemic radiation exposure offers increased risk from sepsis, as well.

Table 32.3 was published by the military to modify triage criteria in the midst of systemically significant radiation exposure. Surgical correction of life-threatening conventional injury should be carried out before significant immunocompromise occurs (within 36–48 hours). Elective procedures should be postponed until late in the convalescent period when hematopoietic recovery should have occurred (45–60 days) (28).

Overexposure and Its Ramifications

In the case of nuclear detonation, an overexposure would be a whole-body exposure of 0.25 Gy (25 rads) or less, an amount that would have no vital organ effects (except on sperm production). After a given exposure, a patient may be highly motivated to understand the future chances of getting cancer later in life. Counseling on this subject should be provided at a later time. This is may be best done by any of the following: an occupational physician who deals with radiation, a nuclear medicine physician, or radiation oncologist. The patient will need to understand that the background cancer rate for a cancer sometime in life is in the approximate range of 25%. Precise doses will not be known at the time of the accident. Estimates *may* be given initially that provide a working framework to guide the clinician's response. As the dose estimate is refined over time, it may frequently change by a magnitude (or two). Several months may be required before the physician and patient receive a final dose estimate, particularly in cases of internal contamination (see Chapter 25).

Many references provide a dose estimate to predict increased risk of cancer development later in life; several appear within the same source. These long-term estimates are mostly extrapolations based on the dose estimates of the Hiroshima and Nagasaki bombing survivors and an observation of long-term effects on these survivors. Methodologic problems have been associated with the two previous methods of dose estimates, and a third attempt at dose estimation that will affect radiation risk estimates is now being formulated. Therefore, one must realize that many sources and techniques for determining future cancer risk and that any two estimations are likely to arrive at somewhat different results. Moreover, the basic assumptions used to derive these estimates are likely to change from time to time. Patients need to understand that these numbers are not firm and that they are subject to later change. With this in mind, one of the more commonly quoted sources, BEIR V, uses 0.08% per radiation-equivalent-man (rem) as the most simple number for expressing the increased risk for cancer development later in life from radiation exposure (29,30).

Acute Effects

Acute effects associated with higher dose exposure are reflected in Table 32.5. Chapter 25 presents an in-depth assessment of acute radiation exposure effects. At higher dose exposures, such as those incurred with a nuclear detonation, *in utero* effects become a significant concern (Table 32.6).

Late Effects

In general, late effects may include threshold effects, such as organ fibrosis, organ insufficiency, or organ failure. Exam-

TABLE 32.5. ACUTE RADIATION EFFECTS WITH HIGHER DOSE EXPOSURE

Acute radiation effects	Threshold in TGy (rads)	D_{50} in Gy (rads)
Lethal bone marrow syndrome (minimal care)	1.5 (150)	3.0 (300)
Lethal bone marrow syndrome (supportive care)	2.3 (230)	4.5 (450)
Lethal pulmonary syndrome	5 (500)	10 (1,000)
Lethal gastrointestinal syndrome	8 (800)	15 (1,500)
Skin erythema	3 (300)	6 (600)
Transepithelial injury	10 (1,000)	20 (2,000)
Ovulation suppression	0.6 (60)	3.5 (350)
2-yr sperm suppression	0.3 (30)	0.7 (70)
Cataracts	1 (100)	3.1 (310)
Acute radiation thyroiditis	200 (20,000)	1,200 (120,000)

Abbreviation: D_{50}, effective dose for affecting 50% of the population. Data from Nuclear Regulatory Commission. *Health effects models for nuclear power plant accident consequence analysis: low LET radiation, part II: scientific bases for health effects models.* CR-4214. Washington, D.C.: United States Nuclear Regulatory Commission, 1989, with permission.

TABLE 32.6. DETERMINISTIC IN UTERO EXPOSURE EFFECTS

Exposure Time	Threshold in Gy (rads)	D_{50} in Gy (rads)
Embryo lethality		
0–18 d	0.1 (10)	1 (100)
18–150 d	0.4 (40)	1.5 (150)
150 d to term	Same as mother	
Severe mental retardation		
8–15 wk		1.5 (150)
16–25 wk		7.1 (710)
Small head size	0.05 (5)	0.73 (73)

Abbreviation: D_{50}, effective dose for affecting 50% of the population. From Nuclear Regulatory Commission. *Health effects models for nuclear power plant accident consequence analysis: low LET radiation, part II: scientific bases for health effects models.* CR-4214. Washington, D.C.: United States Nuclear Regulatory Commission, 1989:II-74–II-83, with permission.

TABLE 32.7. RANGE OF UNCERTAINTIES ASSOCIATED WITH THE INDUCED MUTATION RATE

Type of disorder	Estimate of induction rate (10^{-4} Gy^{-1})		
	Lower[a,b]	Central	Upper
Dominants[a]			
Male	5	15	45
Female	0	15	45
X-linked			
Male	7.2	18	72
Female	0	18	72
Aneuploid			
Male	0	5	15
Female	0	5	15
Unbalanced translocations			
Male	9	71	450
Female	0	71	450
Irregularly inherited diseases at equilibrium			
Male	9	71	450
Female	0	71	450
Periimplantation wastage	20	480	1,900
Aneuploid	0	360	1,080
Unbalanced translocations	20	120	820

[a]Zero applies to the first generation and one-fifth to later generations.
From Nuclear Regulatory Commission. *Health effects models for nuclear power plant accident consequence analysis: low LET radiation, part II: scientific bases for health effects models.* CR-4214. Washington, D.C.: United States Nuclear Regulatory Commission, 1989:II-230, with permission.

ples of such threshold effects include pulmonary fibrosis and posterior pole cataract formation. Other late effects may include stochastic effects, such as the increased risk for development of cancer later in life. Rough estimates of this are expressed in Chapter 25. Other stochastic effects include the estimated induced mutation rate. A comprehensive estimation of such effects was generated in 1989, and it is represented in Table 32.7. The same estimation caveats mentioned in Chapter 25 apply here. Estimations are continually being reevaluated, and thus they may change over time.

SPECIFIC PLANNING POINTS

Medical planners should consider a means of rapid incorporation of surviving responders and providers if great numbers of casualties result from a nuclear detonation. Hospitals should consider mutual aid agreements with hospitals that are not likely to be also involved in a given impact area in the event that augmentation personnel are needed or if the hospital requires complete evacuation.

One military predictive model estimates that isolated injuries of irradiation, burns, or wounds would constitute approximately 30% to 40% of injuries. Combined injuries would then comprise 65% to 70% of the injuries. Figure 32.10 provides a more specific breadown of injury combinations (31). National assets, such as the Federal Emergency Management Agency (FEMA) and the Department of Defense, have software programs that can predict casualties and other logistical needs. However, this information is considered classified information. In the event of a true nuclear detonation, the expectation of decimating provider casualties within the nuclear impact area is reasonable, although the actual number of provider casualties would depend on the device size, population density, and other factors. A review of the Hiroshima and Nagasaki bomb medical response indicates that only 10% of the preexisting providers were still functional within the impact area. See Table 32.8 for casualty figures for these 20-kiloton weapons.

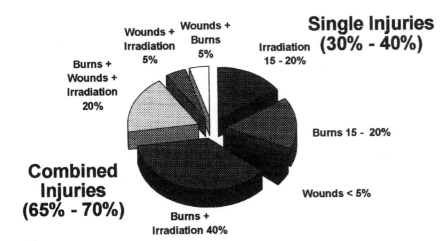

FIG. 32.10. Predicted casualty types after a nuclear detonation. (Data from Walker RI, Cerveny TJ, eds. *Medical consequences of nuclear warfare.* Falls Church, VA: TMM Publications, 1989:11, with permission.)

TABLE 32.8. CASUALTY FIGURES FROM HIROSHIMA AND NAGASAKI BOMBINGS

Zone	Population	Per mi²)	Killed	Injured
Hiroshima (standardized casualty rate of 261,000 with a vulnerable area of 9.36 mi²)				
0–0.6 mi	31,200	25,800	26,700	3,000
0.6–1.6 mi	144,800	22,700	39,600	53,000
1.6–3.1 mi	80,000	3,500	1,700	20,000
Totals	256,300	8,500	68,000	76,000
Nagasaki (standardized casualty rate of 195,000 with a vulnerable area of 7.01 mi²)				
0–0.6 mi	30,900	25,500	27,300	1,900
0.6–1.6 mi	27,700	4,400	9,500	8,100
1.6–3.1 mi	115,200	5,100	1,300	11,000
Totals	173,800	5,800	38,000	21,000

From Glasstone S, ed. *The effects of nuclear weapons*. Washington, D.C.: Department of the Army, 1962:544, with permission.

SCOPE OF A NUCLEAR DETONATION

The scope of a nuclear detonation can first be quantitated by estimating yield, determining the location of the detonation (ground zero), and knowing weather parameters. Many other calculations, such as the primary blast radius, burn radius, and dose, can be estimated. Induced radiation areas (NIGA) and fallout prediction patterns can then be calculated. Preliminary computations focus on the location of ground zero, the yield estimation, and the fallout prediction pattern.

Determination of Ground Zero

Direct observation of ground zero may provide the ground zero location for small yield weapons. Observing units are not encouraged to search for the actual ground zero location. More commonly, observing units may estimate the location of ground zero by relaying their location, an azimuth angle to the stem (in polar coordinates), and flash-to-bang time, which conveys a distance estimate. The speed of sound is 350 m per second at sea level, and the flash-to-bang interval will allow one to estimate distance in much the same way as counting seconds after a lightning strike. Multiple observing units will allow for triangulation and refinement of the ground zero location estimate.

Yield Estimation

Yield may be estimated from the measurement of the *illumination time* of a nuclear burst, especially during hours of darkness or poor visibility. See Table 32.9 for yield estimation versus illumination time (32). Estimation gives a yield estimate within a factor of ten; thus, an illumination time estimate of a 20-kiloton yield may be actually as small as 2 kilotons or as large as 200 kilotons. Illumination time esti-

mation should not be used if obtaining cloud parameters to estimate yield is possible.

By Crater Size

Crater sizes for a 1-kiloton explosion have been modeled in different types of media (dry soil, wet soil, rock, etc.), as figs. 32.11 and 32.12 illustrate. Crater sizes for nuclear devices of differing sizes may be calculated by multiplying

TABLE 32.9. YIELD ESTIMATES FOR ILLUMINATION TIMES

Illumination time (sec)	Approximate yield (KTs)
<1	2
1	2.5
2	10
3	22
4	40
5	60
6	90
7	125
8	160
9	200
10	250
11	285
12	325
13	400
14	475
15	550
16	700
17	750
18	800
19	900
20	980

From Department of the Army. Army field manual FM 3-3-1, *Nuclear contamination avoidance*. Washington, D.C.: Department of the Army, September 9, 1994, with permission.

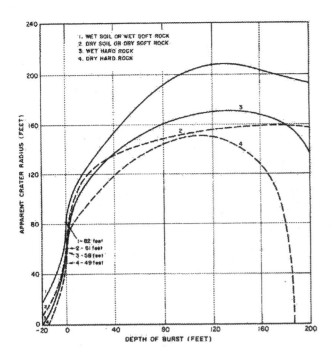

FIG. 32.11. The apparent crater radius as a function of depth of burst for a 1-kiloton explosion occurring either in or above various media. (From Glasstone S, ed. Shock effects of surface and subsurface bursts. In: *The effects of nuclear weapons*. Washington, D.C.: Department of the Army, 1962:255, with permission.)

the 1-kiloton depth and radius dimensions by $W^{0.3}$, where W is the yield in kilotons. For subsurface bursts, a scaled depth is first ascertained by dividing the depth of the burst by $W^{0.3}$. The scaled depth (in feet) is used to calculate the parameters of radius and crater depth for a certain soil type

(Figs. 32.11 and 32.12), and the result is multiplied by $W^{0.3}$ to determine the predicted radius and crater depth for a given yield device.

By Measuring Cloud Parameters

Because the bomb crater is in the ground zero area and may not be approachable for some time for measurements, measuring blast cloud parameters is considered the most accurate technique for estimating nuclear yield. Measurements of the nuclear burst cloud are taken by the military at H+5 minutes and/or H+10 minutes, where H is the time of detonation. Height stabilization of the nuclear burst cloud is thought to occur from 4 to 14 minutes after the explosion (Fig. 32.13).

At 5 minutes after detonation, the angular width of the cloud is measured and relayed in terms of either degrees or mils (Fig. 32.14). At H+10 minutes, vertical angles relaying the cloud-bottom angle and cloud-top angles are made (Fig. 32.15). Once the stabilized cloud radius is determined, the yield can be estimated.

Estimating Fallout Pattern

The most important two factors in predicting a fallout pattern is the device yield and the weather conditions, the most important of which is wind speed. Yield may be estimated by determining crater size and extrapolating from the analog computer included in the book *The effects of nuclear weapons* (2). Computer programs such as HOTSPOT, which is available from Lawrence Livermore National Laboratories, can provide fast estimates of idealized fallout patterns. Calculation of fallout patterns may assist responders in estimating at-risk populations and projecting the

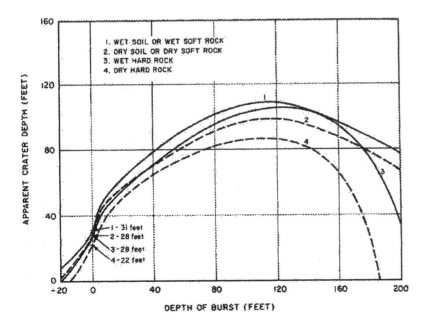

FIG. 32.12. The apparent crater depth as a function of the depth of burst for a 1-kiloton explosion occurring either in or above various media. (From Glasstone S, ed. Shock effects of surface and subsurface bursts. In: *The effects of nuclear weapons*. Washington, D.C.: Department of the Army, 1962: 254, with permission.)

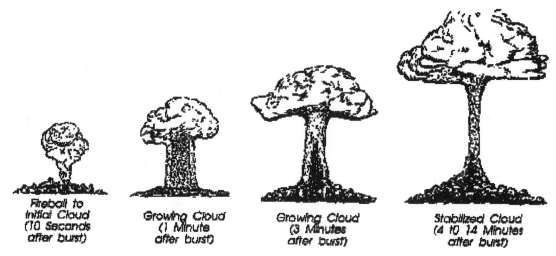

FIG. 32.13. Nuclear cloud development. (From Department of the Army. *Army field manual FM 3-3-1, nuclear contamination avoidance.* Washington, D.C.: Department of the Army, September 9, 1994, with permission.)

response needs. However, one must be aware of the fact that, at various altitudes, dramatically different wind directions might exist; hence, fallout may move in directions that were not initially anticipated. The military can use a variety of software, including a personal computer (PC) software package known as the *Automatic Nuclear Biological and Chemical Information System,* to generate fallout estimates and to assist in decision making.

Manual calculations of fallout patterns is conducted by the military, which then delineates zones of primary hazard (zone I) and secondary hazard (zone II). These zones are defined as areas where exposed, unprotected persons may

receive significant total doses within 4 hours after the arrival of fallout (33). Zone I is considered an area where exposed, unprotected persons may receive doses of 1.5 Gy (150 rads) or greater within 4 hours after the arrival of fallout. Zone II is considered an area where persons may receive a total dose of 0.5 Gy (50 rads) or greater within the first 24 hours after the arrival of fallout. Most fallout patterns have a characteristic downwind component, but, if the effective wind speed is less than 8 km per hour, then a circular pattern is predicted. For the actual procedure to calculate fallout patterns, refer to Army field manual 3-3-1, *Nuclear contamination avoidance* (16).

Creating a Fallout Predictor

A simple fallout predictor may be created from any transparent sheet for any map scale as follows (34):

1. *Select an appropriate map scale*: On transparent or overlay paper, draw a thin dotted line (reference line) to a scaled length of 50 km from a point that has been selected to represent ground zero (Fig. 32.16).
2. Draw and graduate in kilometers two radial lines from ground zero at angles of 20 degrees to the left and the right of the dotted reference line (Fig. 32.17).
3. On the side of ground zero opposite the reference line, draw a series of concentric semicircles (using the selected map scale) having radii of 1.2 km, 1.9 km, 4.2 km, 6.8 km, 11.2 km, 18 km, and 28 km. These figures correspond to stabilized cloud radii from nuclear burst with yields of 2 kilotons, 5 kilotons, 30 kilotons, 100 kilotons, and 3 megatons, respectively (Fig. 32.18).
4. Label the semicircles, starting with the semicircle closest to ground zero and moving up, A, B, C, D, E, F, and G.

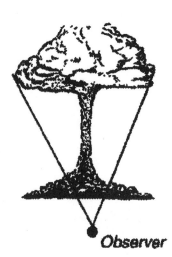

FIG. 32.14. Determining cloud width measurement. (From Department of the Army. Army field manual FM 3-3-1, *Nuclear contamination avoidance.* Washington, D.C.: Department of the Army, September 9, 1994, with permission.)

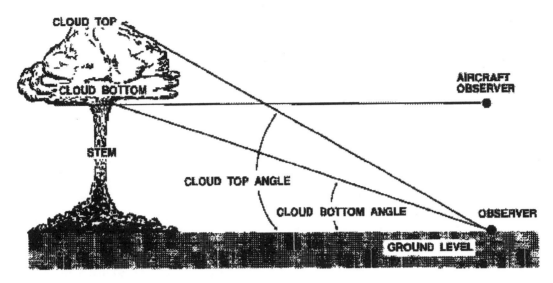

FIG. 32.15. Stabilized cloud top angle, cloud bottom angle, and cloud height measurements. (From Department of the Army. Army field manual FM 3-3-1, *Nuclear contamination avoidance*. Washington, D.C.: Department of the Army, September 9, 1994, with permission.)

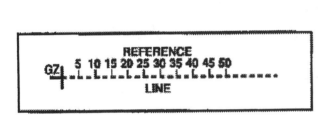

FIG. 32.16. Reference line for the expedient predictor. (From Department of the Army. Army field manual FM 3-3-1, *Nuclear contamination avoidance*. Washington, D.C.: Department of the Army, September 9, 1994, with permission.)

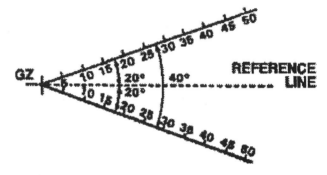

FIG. 32.17. Radial lines extending from ground zero on the predictor. (From Department of the Army. Army field manual FM 3-3-1, *Nuclear contamination avoidance*. Washington, D.C.: Department of the Army, September 9, 1994, with permission.)

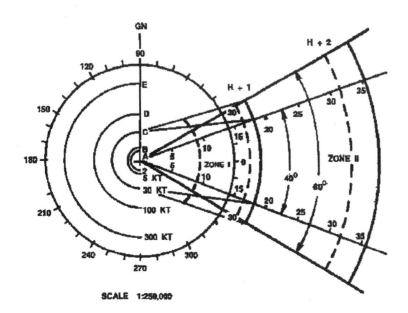

FIG. 32.18. Fallout predictor using the M5A2 fallout predictor (the expanded case). (From Department of the Army. Army field manual FM 3-3-1, *Nuclear contamination avoidance*. Washington, D.C.: Department of the Army, September 9, 1994, with permission.)

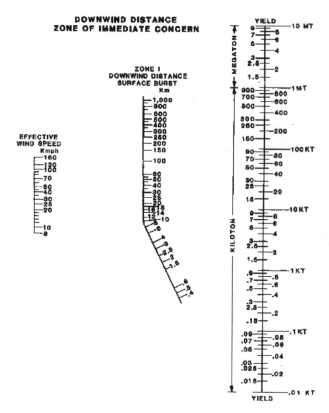

FIG. 32.19. Nomogram for the determination of zone I. (From Department of the Army. Army field manual FM 3-3-1, *Nuclear contamination avoidance*. Washington, D.C.: Department of the Army, September 9, 1994, with permission.)

Label the semicircles as 2 kilotons, 5 kilotons, 30 kilotons, 100 kilotons, and 3 megatons (35).
5. Determine the downwind distance of Zone I from data of downwind speed and nuclear yield using a nomogram (Fig. 32.19) (35).

Credible Fallout Exposures for a Population

The 1954 Marshallese Islander exposure to fallout 5 hours after a 15-megaton thermonuclear detonation generated an average total-body gamma dose of about 1.75 Gy (175 rads); the radiation doses to the thyroid gland were estimated to have averaged 3.34 Gy (334 rads) in adults, and they varied in children from 5 Gy (500 rads) to 14 Gy (1,400 rads) (36).

Fallout Protection Factors

Several calculation rules can assist in calculating local dose rates that may assist survivors and clinicians in estimating doses related to fallout.

The *seven-ten* rule is used to estimate dose rates. The seven-ten rule states that for every sevenfold increase in time, a tenfold decrease in the dose rate occurs (36); therefore, if the dose rate is 10 Gy per hour (1,000 rad/hr) at

hour 0, then by hour 7, the dose rate would be estimated to have decreased to 1 Gy per hour (100 rad/hr).

The *double-the-time* rule is also used to estimate the dose rate. When the time is doubled at a given dose rate, the new dose rate may be found by dividing the old rate by 2 and then subtracting 10% of the result (36).

The *FIT-forever* rule calculates the total dose at a particular area. Fallout dose calculations may be made by the following formula (36):

$$D = F \times I \times T$$

where

D represents the dose that would be received by an individual who stays forever at a particular location in fallout;

F is 5, a physical constant;

I represents the intensity or dose rate at that location at the time this person reached that location and began exposure;

T is the time in hours after the burst that the person began exposure.

The *rule of ten* says that after the passage of ten radionuclide half-lives, the amount of a given radionuclide that remains is negligible.

POPULATION PROTECTION ISSUES

Evacuation and Sheltering

Some debate exists as to what actions populations should take after an area is affected by a nuclear detonation. The English, for example, recommend that their population shelter in place as they believe that the radiation dose will be lowered and that the population will reduce contact with less contaminated material. Americans recommend evacuation of an area, with the idea that they would be moving away from the area of contamination and thus away from residual radiation. Actions may be dictated by the types of buildings the affected individual(s) currently occupy. Buildings provide significant protection, either through a large number of high-rise buildings with subterranean floors or in basements enclosed with concrete or other shielding materials, such as water or earth.

Cold War evacuation plans were originally based on the premise that the USSR would launch a large number of 20-megaton warheads, destroying residential structures for a 16-mile radius with an air burst. Even the air burst from a 1-megaton warhead would destroy homes in a much smaller 5-mile radius. Most contemporary scenarios presuppose much smaller yields, commonly 0.001 of the size, or in this case, 1 kiloton. Therefore, evacuation would not be mandated to avoid blast and fire effects in most smaller yield scenarios. Table 32.10 demonstrates the effect radii of various yields ranging from 0.5 kiloton to 1 megaton.

Next, one should consider high-risk areas, which are characterized as those areas that would accumulate doses in

TABLE 32.10. COMPARISON OF NUCLEAR YIELDS VERSUS EFFECT RADII

Effect	Radius (m) at yield			
	0.5 kT	10 kT	100 kT	1,000 kT
6 PSI	380 m	1,000 m	2,200 m	4,600 m
Second degree burns	580 m	2,100 m	5,500 m	14,500 m
500 Rads	700 m	1,200 m	1,700 m	2,400 m

Abbreviation: PSI, pounds per square inch.
From Armed Forces Radiobiology Research Institute. *Medical effects of nuclear weapons: blast and thermal effects.* Lecture. Raston, VA: Armed Forces Radiobiology Research Institutes, 1990, with permission.

the range of 50 to 100 Gy (5,000–10,000 rads) over 2 weeks. Survival in these areas is not possible unless one stays in a well-shielded shelter (one with a protection factor of 100–200) during the 2 weeks.

One author suggests that persons living more than 10 miles away from a target could best improve their chances of survival by improving existing sheltering in or near their homes. He provides a table to assist individuals in making a decision (37) (Table 32.11).

Shelters

Unfortunately, older buildings previously designated as fallout shelters have since had their placards, equipment, and supplies removed. Nonetheless, these buildings would still be useful in protecting the public from blast and radiation effects. Fallout shelter lists of older buildings may still be available for new planning purposes. A resurvey of buildings locally should be undertaken to determine which buildings might still be suitable protection against blast and radiation effects, and a memorandum of understanding should be created to allow the building to serve as a public blast shelter in

times of local emergency. Such shelters would not be needed to house people for long periods, only to protect from the immediate blast and radiation effects, unless they are located in the highest-risk or a high-risk area.

Well-shielded buildings ideally are multistory buildings constructed of concrete that have an ample basement. Positioning people in a multistory structure with a concrete-roofed basement affords the greatest protection; protection, in fact, may be dramatically increased by a factor of 250 to 1,000 (Fig. 32.20) (38). If concrete structures are not available, earth-bermed structures afford some protection. If detonation is anticipated, individuals can dig an earthen trench; this can reduce exposure significantly. Certain materials confer significant advantages in protection as Table 32.12 illustrates. Residential buildings with a basement provide much less protection, as they offer only a single digit factor of protection.

Decontamination Issues

In the event of a nuclear detonation, timely removal of the fallout dust from victims will be of utmost importance. Removal of fallout will prevent beta burns that, when combined with systemic irradiation, could cause dramatically increase morbidity and mortality. Removal of fallout will also lessen the chances of radioiodine uptake, which could eventually impair thyroid function and create an increased risk for developing thyroid cancer later in life. Individuals caught within a fallout plume should be vigilant for the accumulation of fallout on the body and clothing. Fallout effects are fairly well-known from the Castle Bravo 1954 nuclear testing at Bikini atoll, where 241 Marshallese islanders were inadvertently caught in the fallout pattern from a 15-megaton weapon.

One of the more practical ways of decontamination of mass casualties in the emergency department is to perform

TABLE 32.11. EVACUATION DECISION FACTORS

Favorable to evacuation	Unfavorable to evacuation
Lives in the highest-risk or a high-risk area	Lives outside the highest-risk or a high risk area; could build an expedient fallout shelter and make other survival preparations in this location
Has transportation (a car with enough gasoline); roads to a considerably lower-risk area are open	No means of transportation; believes that roads are likely to be blocked by the time the decision is made to leave
In fairly good health or can evacuate with someone capable of taking care of the individual	Sick, decrepit, or lacks the will to survive if things get tough
Community does not depend on the individual's occupation (i.e., not a policeman, fireman, or telephone operator)	The individual cannot suddenly leave his or her home area for several days without affecting others negatively
Some tools with which to build or improve a fallout shelter are available; has water containers, food, clothing, and so on that are adequate for life in the area to which the individual would go	Lacks the tools and so on that would be helpful—but not necessarily essential—to successful evacuation

Copyright 1986 by Cresson H. Kearny. The copyrighted material may be reproduced without obtaining permission from anyone provided that (a) all copyrighted material is reproduced full-scale (except for microfiche reproductions) and that (b) this copyright notice is printed along with the copyrighted material.

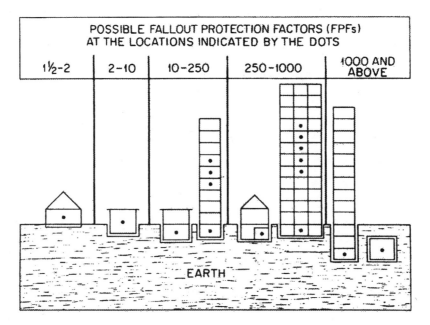

FIG. 32.20. Comparison of structures and fallout protection factors (FPFs). Deep basements and buried shelters have high FPFs (1,000 and above). They provide good protection against gamma radiation from fallout. Tall buildings also provide good protection against gamma radiation from fallout in the locations indicated by dots in the drawing, but they provide little protection against blast. The FPFs indicated above are for isolated buildings. The FPFs would be higher for ground level and below ground. (From Federal Emergency Management Agency. *Radiation safety in shelters.* FEMA publication CPG 2-6.4. Washington, D.C.: Federal Emergency Management Agency, 1983:1–11, with permission.)

TABLE 32.12. VARIOUS MATERIALS AND THEIR EFFECTIVENESS AS BARRIERS AGAINST GAMMA RADIATION FROM FALLOUT

Material	Density relative to concrete[b]	Thickness required relative to concrete
Aluminum	1.2	0.8
Brick, common clay	0.7	1.4
Concrete	1.0	1.0
Earth (well-packed moist humus, dry clay)	0.7	1.4
Firebrick (used in fireplaces)	0.9	1.1
Glass	1.1	0.9
Hardwood (maple or oak)	0.3	3.3
Human body	0.4	2.5
Lead	4.9	0.2
Magazines, slick	0.4	2.5
Newspaper (flat), books, or pulp magazines	0.3	3.0
Plywood (dry)	0.2	5.0
Steel	3.4	0.3
Wallboard, gypsum	0.4	2.7
Water	0.4	2.3

[a]Materials with the highest densities require less thickness to cut down the gamma penetration by a given amount.
[b]Concrete with density of 2.3 g/cm³ (144 lb/ft³)
From Federal Emergency Management Agency. *Radiation safety in shelters.* FEMA publication CPG 2-6.4. Washington, D.C.: Federal Emergency Management Agency, 1983:1-11, with permission.

dry decontamination using a commercial vacuum with a hose attachment and HEPA filter. The patient can shower at a later time. For additional information on external decontamination, see Chapter 25.

Evaluation

Health Physics Issues

Hospitals should identify sources of health or medical physics expertise, along with radiation survey meters and other useful monitoring instruments. These health or medical physicists should be available in the event of a local radiation emergency. Medical and health physicists should also be intimately involved in any radiation emergency plan. Contamination can spread over a wide area depending on weather conditions. Health physicists can place contamination hazards in perspective. Health physics support would initially consist of state radiologic monitoring teams. A state may be able to raise *ad hoc* health physics teams if the state creates a volunteer organizational framework for this contingency. This volunteer organization may form and deploy in a fashion similar to National Disaster Medical Service (NDMS) response elements if additional health physics support is desirable. The organization would nominally be a volunteer organization that would be activated by the state or federal government and that would perform as a state or federal unit, once activated. Once health physicist support staff is organized, it could easily be incorporated for augmenting a state or national response. At the very least, local health physicist volunteers should be identified to assist and advise locally deployed federal response elements. In the planning phase, hospitals should take inventory of the health physics assets and equipment available. Health physics support should be recruited to maintain this equipment in the event of an emergency. Other health physics support services, such as analytical laboratories and whole-body counters, should be identified by the retained health physicists.

Health Physics Laboratories

Within a given response area, identifying health physics laboratories and formulating memorandums of understanding with response agencies are essential, if one is to obtain rapid health physics assays on an emergent, urgent, and follow-up basis. Assays for certain radionuclides may require special set-up time because these assays may not be performed on a regular basis. Some health physics laboratories may not normally be ready to handle human excreta specimens. In the event of a nuclear detonation event, laboratories outside a projected impact area will need to be identified as alternate laboratory resources.

Whole-Body Counters

These nonportable detectors, which are somewhat scarce, should also be named and located in the process of developing radiation response plans. Whole-body counters are capable of detecting minute amounts of internal contamination if the subject has already been externally decontaminated. They would also be useful for the follow-up of contaminated patients.

Dosimetry Estimates

Chapter 25 discusses dosimetry laboratory capabilities more completely. In summary, neutron dose can be determined by determining the amount of ^{32}Na that has been activated in the body. Measurements of surrounding objects, metal in particular, may be useful in corroborating the dose estimates. Hiroshima and Nagasaki survivors had dose estimates derived from the source term (yield) of the weapon, the distance from ground zero, and the amount of shielding present at the time of detonation. Surface detonations will have the additional factor of fallout to consider.

Body Disposal Issues

The National Council for Radiation and Protection and Measurements report no. 37 contains guidelines for working with contaminated bodies. It establishes limits on radiation exposure, primarily for the purpose of protecting embalmers and pathologists. Concern for radioactive body disposal is limited to cremation and to the prevention of significant radiation levels accumulating in crematoria. Any discrete radiation sources on corpses should be removed before disposal, if possible (39). No other known radiation criteria exist for the burial of bodies containing radioactivity.

National Disaster Medical System Hospital System Activation

A nuclear detonation, involving either a tactical (kiloton) or strategic (megaton) yield will overwhelm local medical resources. Survival of victims may be enhanced dramatically if systemically irradiated individuals receive supportive care; therefore, hospitalization resources are key in the event of a nuclear detonation involving a large number of casualties. NDMS recruits hospitals to make hospital beds available in the event of a disaster that overwhelms local medical resources. Activating the NDMS nationwide hospital system may be an important option for consideration (see Chapter 13). Concomitant with NDMS hospital activation would be the on-site formation of a large system of casualty staging and transport, including a plan for addressing the heavy logistical needs.

National Response Sequence

The Federal Radiological Emergency Response Plan, a document closely related to the Federal Response Plan, is the guiding national document for interagency cooperation.

The plan establishes a lead federal agency of the Department of Energy, the Nuclear Regulatory Commission, the Environmental Protection Agency, the Department of Defense, or the National Aeronautics and Space Administration, depending on which agency has the most initial involvement and ownership of a given event. If evidence indicates criminal or terrorist acts, the Federal Bureau of Investigation (FBI) is legally responsible for locating any nuclear material, weapons, or devices and restoring nuclear facilities to their rightful custodians; it enjoys a special position in the response in which all other agencies are pledged to support the FBI fully in its mission as needed. The lead federal agency leads and coordinates all federal on-scene actions and assists state and local governments. FEMA coordinates non-radiological support using the Federal Response Plan document. The other 15 agencies mentioned in the Federal Radiological Emergency Response Plan have potential for defined missions in support of the lead federal agency (see Chapter 12).

SUMMARY

Disaster planning for a nuclear detonation scenario may seem a daunting task at first; however, with the fact that both terrorist organizations and rogue states periodically attempt to attain nuclear capability, such an undertaking is prudent. Nationally, federal agencies plan and practice for this scenario occasionally. The combination of nearly forgotten information on civil defense planning combined with state-of-the-art knowledge of radiation accident and trauma management form an important body of knowledge for civilian disaster planners to consider as well.

The terrorist attacks of September 11, 2001 and the subsequent threats have brought the possibility of nuclear terrorism to a new level of reality. Now is a time for a realistic consideration of the entire spectrum of terrorist scenarios and bold new initiatives for mitigation and response. Lack of this foresight will leave the nation flat-footed in the event of a future attack. Nuclear terrorism attempts will not be a matter of if but rather of when.

ACKNOWLEDGMENTS

The author would like to express gratitude to Col. David Jarrett, M.D. F.A.C.E.P., for extensive help in locating unclassified sources and Ron Goans, M.D. for his assistance with the HOTSPOT prediction program.

EMERGENCY CONTACT INFORMATION

Organization	*Phone number*
Department of Energy Emergency Operations Center (DOE EOC)	(202) 586-8100
Nuclear Regulatory Commission (NRC)	(301) 816-5100
Federal Emergency Management Agency (FEMA)	(202) 586-8100
Environmental Protection Agency (EPA)	(800) 424-8802
National Response Center	(800) 424-8802 (national)
District of Columbia	(202) 267-2675
Military Shipments, Department of Defense (DoD)	(703) 697-0218
CHEMTEL	(800) 255-3924
Chemical Transportation Emergency Center (CHEMTREC)	(800) 424-9300
District of Columbia	(202) 483-7616
Outside the Continental United States	(703) 527-3887
Joint Nuclear Accident Coordinating Center	
Albuquerque, NM	(505) 845-4667
Alexandria, VA	(703) 325-2102

GENERAL READING

Department of the Army. *Handbook on the medical aspects of NBC defensive operations FM 8-9*. Washington, D.C.: Department of the Army, 1996.

Jarrett D, ed. *Medical management of radiological casualties handbook*. Bethesda, MD: Military Medical Operation Office, Armed Forces Radiobiology Research Institute, 1999.

Kearny CH. *Nuclear war survival skills*. Cave Junction, OR: Oregon Institute of Science and Medicine, 1986.

Reeves GI, Jarrett DG, Seed TM, et al., eds. *Triage of irradiated personnel—an Armed Forces Radiobiology Research Institute workshop, 25–27 September 1996*. Bethesda, MD: Armed Forces Radiobiology Research Institute, 1998.

National Council on Radiation Protection and Measurements. *Precautions in the management of patients who have received therapeutic amounts of radionuclides*. NCRP publication no. 37. Washington, D.C.: National Council on Radiation Protection and Measurements, 1970.

Glasstone S, Dolan PJ, eds. *The effects of nuclear weapons*. Washington, D.C.: Department of the Army, 1977.

Farrow L, Blair BG, Helfand I, et al. Accidental nuclear war—a postcold war assessment. *N Engl J Med* 1998;338:1326–1331.

Federal Emergency Management Agency. *Transport of radioactive materials*. Washington, D.C.: Federal Emergency Management Agency Publications Center, 2000.

REFERENCES

1. Chemical-Biological Expert Panel appearing before the United Nations in 1969.
2. Glasstone S, ed. *The effects of nuclear weapons*. Washington, D.C.: Department of the Army, 1962:276.
3. Conklin JJ, Walker RI. *Military radiobiology*. San Diego: Academic Press, 1987.

4. American College of Emergency Physicians. *Developing objectives, content, and competencies for the training of emergency medical technicians, emergency physicians, and emergency nurses to care for casualties resulting from nuclear, biological, or chemical (NBC) incidents.* American College of Emergency Physicians Report to Office of Emergency Preparedness, April 23, 2001.

5. Cember H. *Introduction to health physics*, 3rd ed. New York: McGraw-Hill, 1996:538.

6. United States Congress. Senate. Permanent Subcommittee on Investigations of the Senate Committee on Government Affairs. *The threat of nuclear diversion.* Statement for the record by John Deutch, Director of the Central Intelligence. March 20, 1996.

7. Associated Press report. November 24, 1995.

8. Cohen W. *Proliferation: threat and response 1997.* Department of Defense report no. 639-97. November 25, 1997.

9. Sieveking P. Australian earthquake: triggered by nature or apocalyptic maniacs? *Sunday Telegraph* February 23, 1997.

10. Purver R. *Chemical and biological terrorism: the threat according to open literature.* Canadian Security Intelligence Service, 1995. Includes quote from Lloyd-Parry R. Cult researching nuclear weapons. *Ottawa Citizen* April 3, 1995.

11. Purver R. *Chemical and biological terrorism: the threat according to open literature.* Canadian Security Intelligence Service, 1995. Includes quote from Moosa E. Japanese sect mined high-tech and the occult. *Reuters* May 16, 1995.

12. Purver R. *Chemical and biological terrorism: the threat according to open literature.* Canadian Security Intelligence Service, 1995. Includes quote from Condoms suspected in thwarted Tokyo cyanide attack. *Reuters* May 9, 1995.

13. CNN report. August 26, 2000.

14. Hamza K. *Saddam's bombmaker—the terrifying inside story of the Iraqi nuclear and biological weapons agenda.* New York: Simon and Schuster, 2000:333–337.

15. Glasstone S, Dolan PJ, eds. *The effects of nuclear weapons.* Washington, D.C.: Department of the Army, 1977:59.

16. Department of the Army. *Army field manual FM 3-3-1, nuclear contamination avoidance.* Washington, D.C.: Department of the Army, 1994:C-2.

17. Department of the Army. *Army field manual FM 3-3-1, nuclear contamination avoidance.* Washington, D.C.: Department of the Army, 1994:C-1.

18. Glasstone S, Dolan PJ, eds. *The effects of nuclear weapons.* Washington, D.C.: Department of the Army, 1977:324–329.

19. Academy of Health Sciences. *Medical aspects of nuclear weapons and their effects on medical operations.* Subcourse MED447. Houston, TX: Academy of Health Sciences, United States Army, 1990:5-5.

20. National Council on Radiation Protection and Measurements. *Radiological factors affecting decision-making in a nuclear attack.* NCRP publication no. 42. Washington, D.C.: National Council on Radiation Protection and Measurements, 1974:10.

21. Aldridge P. Master's thesis. Atlanta: Georgia Institute of Technology.

22. Nuclear Regulatory Commission. *Health effects models for nuclear power plant accident consequence analysis: low LET radiation, part II: scientific bases for health effects models.* CR-4214. Washington, D.C.: United States Nuclear Regulatory Commission, 1989:38.

23. Nuclear Regulatory Commission. *Health effects models for nuclear power plant accident consequence analysis: low LET radiation, part II: scientific bases for health effects models.* CR-4214. Washington, D.C.: United States Nuclear Regulatory Commission, 1989:39.

24. Nishiyama H, Lukes SJ, Saenger EL. Low-level internal radionuclide contamination: use of gamma camera for detection. *Radiology* 1984;150:235–240.

25. Walker RI, Cerveny TJ, eds. *Medical consequences of nuclear warfare.* Falls Church, VA: TMM Publications, 1989:39.

26. Glasstone S, Dolan PJ, eds. *The effects of nuclear weapons.* Washington, D.C.: Department of the Army, 1977:594–597.

27. National Council on Radiation Protection and Measurements. *Radiological factors affecting decision-making in a nuclear attack.* NCRP publication no. 42. Washington, D.C.: National Council on Radiation Protection and Measurements, 1974:29.

28. Browne D, Weiss JF, MacVittie M, et al. *Treatment of radiation injuries.* New York: Plenum Press, 1990:229.

29. Cember H. *Introduction to health physics*, 3rd ed. New York: McGraw-Hill, 1996:277.

30. National Research Council. *Health effects of exposure to low levels of ionizing radiation—BEIR V.* Washington, D.C.: National Academy Press, 1990:6.

31. Walker RI, Cerveny TJ, eds. *Medical consequences of nuclear warfare.* Falls Church, VA: TMM Publications, 1989:11.

32. Academy of Health Sciences. *Medical aspects of nuclear weapons and their effects on medical operations.* Subcourse MED447. Houston, TX: Academy of Health Sciences, United States Army, 1990:5–6,A-33.

33. Department of the Army. *Army field manual FM 3-3-1, nuclear contamination avoidance.* Washington, D.C.: Department of the Army, 1994:4-0.

34. Department of the Army. *Army field manual FM 3-3-1, nuclear contamination avoidance.* Washington, D.C.: Department of the Army, 1994:3–23.

35. Department of the Army. *Army field manual FM 3-3-1, nuclear contamination avoidance.* Washington, D.C.: Department of the Army, 1994:E-10.

36. National Council on Radiation Protection and Measurements. *Radiological factors affecting decision-making in a nuclear attack.* NCRP publication no. 42. Washington, D.C.: National Council on Radiation Protection and Measurements, 1974:29.

37. Kearny CH. *Nuclear war survival skills.* Cave Junction, OR: Oregon Institute of Science and Medicine, 1986:32.

38. Federal Emergency Management Agency. *Radiation safety in shelters.* FEMA publication CPG 2-6.4. Washington, D.C.: Federal Emergency Management Agency, 1983:4–7.

39. National Council on Radiation Protection and Measurements. *Precautions in the management of patients who have received therapeutic amounts of radionuclides.* NCRP publication no. 37. Washington, D.C.: National Council on Radiation Protection and Measurements, 1970:38.

33

INTENTIONAL CHEMICAL DISASTERS

MARK KEIM

An *intentional chemical disaster* (ICD) is defined as the intentional release or spill of a toxic chemical that results in an abrupt and serious disruption of the functioning of a society, causing widespread human, material, or environmental losses that exceed the ability of affected society to cope when using only its own resources. This definition would include the consequences resulting from chemical warfare, chemical terrorism, and industrial sabotage.

CHEMICAL DISASTERS: UNINTENTIONAL VERSUS INTENTIONAL

Incidents involving either the slow or explosive release of chemicals are common. From 1988 to 1992, more than 34,000 chemical release events were reported in the United States (1). Most of these incidents did not cause mass casualties. However, some rare events do have the potential to cause serious harm on a mass scale. The Bhopal disaster killed over 2,500 persons and affected an additional 200,000 (2). In 1984, a fuel truck crash in the Salang Tunnel in Afghanistan killed 2,700 people. In 1947, a shipload of ammonium nitrate fertilizer exploded in Texas City, Texas, killing 576 persons (3).

Both ICDs and unintentional industrial disasters tend to receive significant international media attention and publicity. The public tends to judge all technologic hazards more harshly than natural hazards of a similar magnitude, and it views them with a heightened concern and perception of risk (3,4). In the public eye, these categories of technologic catastrophes no longer represent localized emergencies, but they are "trends that unravel the very fabric of existing organized systems" (5). These events change the very nature of response actions as responders are no longer performing a well-rehearsed technical or logistical procedure. Assessments become less certain and older forms of intelligence gathering become obsolete. Decision making becomes less centralized and more interdependent, and it may be influenced by both local and distant theaters of operation. Responders are forced to act in a collective and integrated fashion within a nonconventional network, the leaders of which are also unfamiliar with catastrophic breakdown phenomena of this nature. Any event involving an ICD is likely to involve both traditional and nontraditional responders, as the scope of the incident extends beyond traditional roles and responsibilities. Such events would possibly involve the participation of responders acting on both local and national levels (Table 33.1).

ICDs involving the use of commercial or industrial chemical agents have the potential to cause a major public health disaster that is higly comparable to that of known military agents. In some cases, industrial agents may even be more likely to be used as a weapon of choice by terrorists. Their ease of availability, toxicity, and low cost may

TABLE 33.1. EXAMPLES OF TRADITIONAL AND NONTRADITIONAL EMERGENCY RESPONDERS

Traditional emergency response	Nontraditional emergency response
Bystanders	Medical and environmental laboratories
EMS and the 911 activation system	Public health departments
Police	Metropolitan Medical Response system
Fire and rescue	Outpatient clinics and hospitals
Public and private hazardous material response teams	Mass transit and port authorities
Emergency departments	Military and National Guard, Coast Guard
Regional poison control centers	Federal agencies, including FBI, FEMA, EPA, PHS, CDC, and DOE

Abbreviations: CDC, Centers for Disease Control and Prevention; DOE, Department of Energy; EMS, emergency medical services; EPA, Environmental Protection Agency; FBI, Federal Bureau of Investigation; FEMA, Federal Emergency Management Agency; PHS, Public Health Service.

make these toxic chemicals attractive to the potential terrorist. Thus, even though the focus may, at times, appear to be placed inordinately on the consequence management of terrorism involving military agents, such as that for vesicants or nerve agents, chemical terrorism actually may have a greater potential to occur in the form of a toxic chemical spill or release involving industrial or commercial products (6). In that sense, the prevention and control measures for intentional chemical disasters align quite closely with those for catastrophic industrial disasters. *In effect, the main difference between industrial disasters and those of chemical sabotage, warfare, and terrorism may be a distinction only of malicious intent.* Thus, efforts to enhance hazardous material (HazMat) preparedness and response activities for the most common chemical emergencies will also serve to better the preparations for terrorist events. Conversely, consequence management focused on chemical terrorism should have the added value of building capacity for responding to the common HazMat emergencies and rare catastrophic chemical disasters.

DISASTER MEDICINE AND INTENTIONAL CHEMICAL DISASTERS

Disaster medicine is "the science that seeks to address the adverse health and medical effects associated with disasters . . . and [it] includes prevention, emergency response, and recovery needs of affected individuals and populations" (7). The science of disaster medicine is founded in multidisciplinary medical skills that bridge the curative and preventive spectrum of health care (8). In this sense, disaster medicine serves to combine the disciplines of clinical and public health promotion effectively, and it is not limited to the provision of emergency care.

One defining characteristic of disaster medicine is the involvement of the management of an extremely wide range of emergency health issues (Table 33.2). Consequence detection and management after an ICD event will probably also involve almost all of these same interrelated issues.

INTENTIONAL CHEMICAL DISASTERS: HISTORICAL PERSPECTIVE

Numerous examples of ICDs can be found throughout history. Toxic chemicals were reportedly used by the ancient Chinese and the Greeks. Chemical weapons were also used during the Boer War, the Russo-Japanese War, and World War I. Of the 26 million casualties suffered in World War I, nearly 1 million were chemical-related (9). Of the total 272,000 United States casualties, 72,000 (26%) were chemical casualties (9). During World War II, Japan and Italy both used chemical warfare agents. The United States Army is known to have used defoliants and nonlethal riot control agents during the Vietnam War. In 1963, Egypt used riot control, mustard, and nerve agents against royalists during the Yemen civil war. The Soviet Union used mustard gas and nerve agents during the Afghanistan War throughout the 1980s. During the Iran-Iraq War, the United Nations was able to verify that Iran used mustard gas, lewisite, and nerve agents against the Iranian troops. Roughly 5% of the Iranian casualties were caused by chemical agents (10). Reports exist of Iraq using chemical agents against its Kurd minority. Libya is reported to have used chemical weapons that it obtained from Iran during an invasion of Chad. Reports have also been made of Cuban-backed Angolan forces using nerve agents against rebel forces (9).

Ironically, during the Persian Gulf War, persons were adversely affected as a result of personal protection measures, not as a result of chemical attack (11–13). However, the Iraqis were responsible for causing a large ICD in 1991 as a result of setting a multitude of oil wells on fire in Kuwait (14). In 1994, an act of terrorism had the potential to become an ICD when the Japanese religious cult Aum Shinrikyo released sarin nerve agent in a residential area of Matsumoto, Japan. This event killed seven and injured 500. The same terrorist group struck again during 1995 in the now infamous Tokyo subway sarin attack, which killed 12 and affected over 5,000 (15). However, the incident did not result in a serious disruption in the functioning of Japanese

TABLE 33.2. EMERGENCY HEALTH ISSUES RELATED TO DISASTER MANAGEMENT

Injury prevention and control	Prehospital care and Emergency Medical Services
Health information systems	Emergency medicine
Epidemiology	Toxicology
Occupational health	Hazardous material emergency response
Mass shelter and displaced populations	Mass casualty management and triage
Civilian-military coordination	Field-based logistics and communications
Environmental health	Incident command systems
Population protection measures	Traumatology and resuscitation
Disease control	Mental health

society. Nor did it cause widespread human, material, or environmental losses that exceeded the ability of affected society to cope using only its own resources. Therefore, in this sense, the Tokyo subway event would not be considered an ICD.

Fortunately, the potential ICD events after World War I have not generated the number of mass fatalities consistent with chemical disasters associated with industrial releases, such as the thousands killed at Bhopal. However, this does not mean that such an attack does not have the potential to harm hundreds, if not thousands, of victims. Were miscalculation and lack of experience not part of chemical terrorist attacks in the past, many more casualties and deaths would likely have occurred. For example, in the 1995 Tokyo subway attack, an impure preparation of sarin was used as part of a crude binary weapon and was not effectively aerosolized. The perpetrators also underestimated the air exchange capabilities of the subway system. As a result, a multisource attack on a commuter target cohort of 80,000 persons resulted in only 12 deaths. While 5,510 sought treatment, only 17 were actually considered critical (i.e., requiring ventilatory support), 37 patients were diagnosed as severe (i.e., exhibiting nausea, vomiting, or dyspnea), and 984 had complaints limited to eye involvement, symptoms that were consistent with miosis) (15).

During the 1996 Olympic games in Atlanta, considerable efforts were made to prepare for terrorist attacks that could have included chemical weapons. Within hours of an explosion of a pipe bomb in Atlanta's Olympic Centennial Park, samples were collected from near the bomb crater and were sent to an analytical laboratory at the Centers for Disease Control and Prevention to be screened for the presence of chemical and biologic warfare agents. The laboratory and the associated response system, called the Science and Technology Center (16), were based at the National Center for Environmental Health and were specifically created to form a broad multiagency partnership among federal assets. This Federal Bureau of Investigation (FBI)-led federal effort sought to enhance the capability of the United States to respond rapidly to chemical or biologic terrorism. The Atlanta experience marked one of the first times when a domestic bomb was rapidly screened for these agents of mass destruction. This partnership effectively and urgently filled a void in the national analytical and response capacities, and it became a prototype for the future development of national-level crisis and consequence management involving terrorism (17).

DETECTION AND MANAGEMENT OF THE CONSEQUENCES OF INTENTIONAL CHEMICAL DISASTERS

Detection and management are two critical functions served by emergency responders after an ICD event. Responders will have urgent and complex informational needs regarding *consequence management*, a term defined by the Presidential Decision Directive 39 released June 21, 1995. Conversely, responders on the scene will provide a valuable resource to offsite governmental and national security decision-makers for information and intelligence regarding *consequence detection* (18).

Consequences of particular relevance to disaster medicine include the environmental release or exposure *incident* and any resultant casualties or patient *cases* (18) (Table 33.3).

Consequence Detection

Early detection of the consequences of intentional chemical disasters may be expected to result from the local discovery of the environmental release or exposure *incident* event or the diagnosis of the resultant patient *cases*. Among other activities detailed in Table 33.4, responders may provide critical on-scene assessments and patient examinations that distant consultants are unable to perform in a timely manner. They may supply an informal passive surveillance system and serve as nationwide monitors in reporting potential events in a fashion that is timely enough to allow for rapid intervention (Table 33.4). Consequence detection after an event may also be facilitated by advance warning from preincident intelligence that serves to alert responders to watch for subsequent cases or incidents.

Consequence Management

To manage effectively the complex and rare incidents and casualties that may occur as a consequence of an ICD, responders require expert consultation and informational

TABLE 33.3. ELEMENTS OF CONSEQUENCE DETECTION AND MANAGEMENT FOR INTENTIONAL CHEMICAL DISASTERS

Consequences	Detection	Management
Cases (or casualties)	Case detection	Case management
Incidents (or release)	Incident detection	Incident management

TABLE 33.4. DISASTER MEDICINE ACTIVITIES RELATED TO CONSEQUENCE DETECTION

Activity	Case detection	Incident detection
Intelligence	Preincident intelligence Medical education	Preincident intelligence Hazard awareness and recognition
Testing	Point-of-care assays Clinical laboratory tests	Hazard identification Boundary demarcation Exposure assessment Laboratory reporting
Monitoring	Health information systems Passive and active surveillance Case definition	Environmental monitoring Hazardous substance emergency event surveillance system
Diagnosis	Clinical examination Laboratory evaluation	Epidemiologic assessment Scene assessment

support. These informational needs regarding case management will likely include diagnostic and treatment modalities. Questions involving incident management will generally be focused on assessment and control of the complex chemical release scene itself. Incident management response actions are expected to be, to a large extent, scenario-dependent according to the particular agent and the degree of warning. Informational needs regarding case management might include, but would not remain limited to, issues of case control and casualty care (Table 33.5).

PREVENTION AND CONTROL MEASURES

Risk Management for Intentional Chemical Disasters

Risk assessment is a systematic process for quantifying the likelihood of adverse health effects in a population following exposure to a specified hazard. Risk management is the process of selecting and implementing prevention and control measures to achieve an acceptable level of the risk at an acceptable cost. In contrast to risk avoidance, which seeks to counter all possible vulnerabilities, risk management

TABLE 33.5. DISASTER MEDICINE ACTIVITIES RELATED TO CONSEQUENCE MANAGEMENT

Activity	Case management	Incident management
Command and communication	Disaster plan implementation Prehospital medical direction Hospital emergency protocols Redundant communication	Incident command systems HazMat site control Methods of mutual aid
Prevention and control	Personal protective equipment Patient and staff decontamination EMS and ED treatment protocols Mortuary science Occupational health Critical incident stress debriefing Isolation	Warning and risk communication Public service announcements Population protection measures Site decontamination and effluent control Crowd control Mass shelter
WMD effects	Toxicology Traumatology Resuscitology	Infrastructure assessment Environmental health Communications Population health assessment
Terrorism and forensics	Terrorist intelligence Chain-of-evidence preservation Forensic pathology	Terrorist intelligence Crime scene preservation

Abbreviations: ED, emergency department; EMS, Emergency Medical Services; HazMat, hazardous materials; WMD, weapons of mass destruction.

instead weighs the risk of loss against the cost of control measures. As one author stated, "to narrow the scope of the problem, civil defenses against chemical and biologic terrorism should be based on most likely rather than worst case scenarios" (19). While risk avoidance responds to threats based on the worst case scenario, risk management alternatively attaches a systematic prioritization of risk, thereby identifying the most likely events, and then calibrates an associated cost-benefit analysis to guide any resultant prevention and control measures.

Risk management is composed of the following three main elements: risk assessment, cost-benefit analysis, and risk communication. The components of analytical risk assessment related to ICD include asset and loss impact assessment, threat assessment, and vulnerability analysis (Table 33.6). In the case of an ICD, the public health approach is also closely associated with security decision making. Within the context of an event involving a potential adversary, the hazard identification of conventional environmental risk management is instead replaced by the more comprehensive process of threat characterization. This process not only includes an identification of the specific chemical hazards, but also it involves the characterization of potential perpetrators or adversaries in terms of their intent, technical capability, and history.

Each of the key elements of a risk assessment—impact, threat, and vulnerability—is ranked in a graduated system of numerical priority. Risk is quantified according to descriptive and integral parameters and is then calculated as a function of impact, threat, and vulnerability. The formula for risk assessment is as follows:

$$\text{Risk} = (\text{Impact} \times \text{Threat} \times \text{Vulnerability}).$$

Thus, preexisting public health system and infrastructure is recognized as a prerequisite for subsequent countermeasures in the form of prevention and control.

To date, no federal agency has determined and assessed the environmental risk of United States cities based on intelligence assessments, critical infrastructure points, national symbols, future special events, sensitive government or corporate activities, or similar analyses and data to help evaluate cities' key assets and vulnerabilities as related to ICDs.

An April 1998 Government Accounting Office (GAO) report highlighted a model for threat and risk assessment that has diverse applications and does not require a point source, perfect intelligence data, or preattack indicators. In addition, Presidential Decision Directive 62 has also recommended that threat and risk assessments be performed on non-point targets, such as telecommunications, banking, and finance infrastructures (19a).

The remedial action or medical response to an ICD is highly dependent on details that may be discovered in the threat or risk assessment. Geography, population density, infrastructure points, and sensitive government and corporate facilities may also influence impact, threat, and vulnerability. Assessments that include these factors are conducive to preparedness and awareness. Baseline risk assessment also facilitates the postevent application of exposure modeling systems if an intentional release occurs.

The GAO estimates that approximately 2 weeks per city would be required to conduct a risk assessment and determine a prudent and affordable level of response capability.

TABLE 33.6. ELEMENTS OF ANALYTICAL RISK MANAGEMENT

Process	Activities
Impact assessment	Determining critical assets (i.e., a population)
Asset assessment	Identifying undesirable events and expected losses or damages
Loss assessment	Prioritizing assets based on the consequence of loss
Threat characterization	Identifying indications, circumstances, or events with the potential to cause the loss of or damage to an asset
Hazard identification	
Adversary intent	Assessing the intent and motivation of each adversary
Adversary capability	Evaluating the capabilities of each adversary
Adversary history	Determining the frequency of past events
	Estimating the relative threat to each critical asset
Vulnerability analysis	Identifying potential weaknesses that may be exploited by an adversary to gain access to an asset
Potential vulnerabilities	
Existing countermeasures	Recognizing existing countermeasures and their level of effectiveness, which may then be used to reduce vulnerability
	Estimating the degree of vulnerability to each asset and threat
Countermeasure determination	Identifying potential actions that may be taken or physical entities that can be used to eliminate or to lessen one or more vulnerabilities
Prevention	
Control	
Cost-benefit analysis	Identifying costs and benefits of countermeasures
	Conducting cost-benefit and tradeoff analyses
	Prioritizing options
Risk communication	Preparing a range of recommendations for decision makers and/or the public

The report states that "rational, businesslike, collaborative assessment by city, state, and federal representatives can help determine the appropriate minimum requirements for preparedness, given the threats, risks, and vulnerabilities for that city" (20). For this reason, any organized preparedness effort, including stockpiling, education, or planning, should be based as firmly as possible within the scientific methodology of analytical risk management.

Hazard Identification

Conventional environmental heath risk assessment begins with the process of hazard identification, which attempts to determine what release events are likely to occur in a specific region or environment. In the case of unintentional chemical release incidents, the objective is to identify all chemical products within a specific location that may pose a potential health hazard. However, significant difficulties exist in identifying which chemical(s) an adversary or perpetrator may choose to use during an attack.

Literally thousands of hazardous chemicals are currently available to the general public, and more than 600 new chemical substances become commercially available each month (21). Besides the large number of hazardous chemicals that are readily available to the potential enemy, terrorist, or saboteur, numerous other variables may influence the threat agent selection. Some of these variables include the availability of the agent, the ease of production, lethality, its stability in storage, the cost, handling safety for the perpetrator, public risk perception, the ease of delivery or weaponization, and stability in a deliverable state.

Outside of the known military agents, a variety of industrial chemicals may have the potential to cause adverse health effects. The widespread knowledge of these toxicities along with a comparative ease of availability and weaponization may influence terrorists to select industrial chemicals as potential weapon agents. Current hazard assessments are variable depending on the source. The law enforcement and the intelligence communities have reported a growing interest in weapons of mass destruction (WMD) by groups and rogue nations of concern. The

TABLE 33.7. TOXIC CHEMICALS CATEGORIZED BY GENERAL HEALTH EFFECTS

Metals and metallic compounds
Incendiaries
Irritant gases
Asphyxiant gases
Metabolic asphyxiants
Radiologic agents
Teratogens
Corrosives
Explosives
Oxidizers
Pharmaceuticals
Carcinogens
Pesticides

GAO states that the intelligence community has "concluded that explosives or other conventional weapons will continue to be the most likely form of terrorist attack over the next decade" (20). The Chemical and Biological Arms Control Institute ranks the intentional releases of industrial chemicals as a relatively higher likelihood when compared to other more exotic agents used in WMD (6).

Despite the enormous challenge presented by the need for identification and prioritization of chemical hazards that may be used by terrorists, certain generalizations may be made to simplify disaster medical preparedness and planning. Toxic chemicals may be categorized by known health effects. Those hyperacute effects then become pertinent relative to guidance during emergency case and incident management. To ease case and incident management, a broad variety of hazardous chemicals may be divided into 13 basic categories (Table 33.7).

Despite the recent publication of operational handbooks and educational programs focusing on antidote therapy, very few antidotes for the treatment of toxic chemical poisoning exist in comparison to the extremely large number of agents that may be used as a WMD. In addition, specific antidotes exist for only a few of the military agents, and a mere handful of therapies are available for all the industrial and commercial chemicals. Table 33.8 contains a partial list

TABLE 33.8. EXAMPLES OF CHEMICAL AGENTS THAT HAVE SPECIFIC ANTIDOTES

Chemical agent	Antidote
Military agents	
Nerve agents	Atropine, pralidoxime
Cyanide	Amyl nitrite, sodium thiosulfate, sodium nitrite, cyanocobalamin
Lewisite	British antilewisite and/or dimercaperol
Industrial and commercial agents	
Heavy metals	Penicillamine
Hydrofluoric acid	Calcium gluconate
Aniline	Methylene blue
Pharmaceutical agents	Naloxone, *N*-acetylcysteine, flumazanil

TABLE 33.9. EMERGENCY MEDICAL CONDITIONS AND NEEDS ASSOCIATED WITH CHEMICAL EXPOSURES

Syndrome and causative agents	Medical therapeutic needs
Burns and trauma—corrosives, vesicants, explosives, oxidants, incendiaries, radiologicals	Intravenous fluid and supplies Pain medications Pulmonary products Splints and bandages
Respiratory failure—corrosives, military agents, explosives, oxidants, incendiaries, asphyxiants, irritants, pharmaceutical agents, metals	Pulmonary products Ventilators and supplies Antidotes, if available Tranquilizing medications
Cardiovascular shock—military agents, pesticides, asphyxiants, pharmaceutical agents	Intravenous fluid and supplies Cardiovascular products Antidotes, if available
Neurologic toxicity—military agents, pesticides, pharmaceutical agents, radiologic agents	Antidotes, if available

of the most broadly available antidote therapies. These antidotes are thought to be stocked in an extremely limited supply in most ambulances and hospitals (22).

Outside of this limited number of antidote therapies, the medical management of nearly all toxic chemical exposures mostly involves supportive therapy. Even if an antidote may be available for a said exposure, many times the clinician may not be able to identify the offending agent in enough time to guide the therapy effectively. If an accurate and rapid clinical diagnosis can be made, treatment may not become available in enough time to be efficacious, especially in cases of involving a nerve agent or the inhalation of cyanide poisoning (23). The demand for medical resources may then be expected to involve mainly critical care and supportive therapeutics.

Thus, the hyperacute health effects of a broad variety of hazardous chemicals, as categorized in Table 33.7, may actually be expected to invoke demands for medical resources that address a quite narrow range of medical conditions. Table 33.9 represents four main basic medical conditions that may be expected to occur as major short-term sequela following severe exposures to any of these chemical hazards. It also identifies eight categories of emergency medical therapeutics that are necessary to treat these four syndrome complexes.

Threat Assessment

ICDs are unique in comparison to other technologic catastrophes, as an ICD is defined by the implication of a willful and malicious intent. In this regard, the disaster management cycle is markedly influenced by the perpetrator of the event. The characteristics of the perpetrator must be taken into consideration as part of the broad range of public health efforts involving prevention, mitigation, preparedness, response, and recovery.

These characteristics of the intentional perpetrator are not a traditional component of most methods for environmental health hazard identification. The process, as it applies to malicious intent, must also incorporate a new component. This component, known as threat assessment, is an integral part of security decision making that is consistent with that performed by the intelligence community. Threat assessment is not limited to the identification of a chemical hazard, but it also extends to the characteristics and behavior of potential adversaries or perpetrators of ICDs. Threat is measured as a function of an adversary's intent, capability to act, and history of actions. Intent may be quantified in terms of understanding the goals and strategies of a potential perpetrator of ICDs. For this reason, disaster planners and managers must have a basic awareness of the methods used to typify a threat assessment as applied to ICDs. These principles may then guide disaster management through the consideration of the particular traits that define these persons as a potential hazard to the public health.

The intent of the adversary may vary according to circumstance. Goals of a state-sponsored war enemy may include any promotion of political, economic, military, ethnic, or religious agendas defined by national leaders. Industrial saboteurs may act with the goal of revenge, self-promotion, or excitement. In addition to those goals of state-sponsored warfare, terrorists may seek to force political change or to gain publicity for a cause. As Thomas Ditzler so aptly stated, "Terrorism may be the only form of assault named for the psychic state it is intended to create." In this sense, understanding the psychologic component of terrorism is important. Terrorists have been known to perform in accordance within the basic principles of psychologic operations. Knowledge of these principles can allow disaster managers to minimize vulnerabilities and to maximize prevention and control measures that are more specific to the risk of terrorism. This may be difficult as marked differences might separate the conceptual framework of the society from that of the terrorist. Contrary to popular thought, terrorists are not 'mad bombers' without method or reason. Instead, they, as a whole, have normal personality distribution and, for the most part, an above-average intelligence. Thus, when compared to the normal population, psychologic pathosis does not appear more prevalent among this group. The intent of these persons to commit mass casualties is no more pathologic than the patriotic intent of a soldier motivated by nationalism, religion, or ethnicity. These groups endeavor to market their views through a highly methodic process of impression management. The final goal is not necessarily that of mass casualties but instead fear. This is best depicted in the ancient Chinese saying, "Kill one; frighten 10,000" (6).

Predicting that chemical attacks resulting in mass destruction are now inevitable may seem easy enough. However, accurate threat assessments may reveal that, while ICDs are possible, they are not necessarily probable (6). While some may view the Aum Shinrikyo subway incident as a watershed event for future attacks, one must remember the negative effect that this event had upon the ongoing functionality and survival of the sect itself. Government retaliation and the revulsion of the Japanese public were strong enough to nullify group leadership and to threaten the entire campaign objective. So, as this example illustrates, many complex factors balance the threat of an ICD, some of which may serve to facilitate the likelihood of an ICD and some that instead lessen its possibility. In recent years, a lack of technical capacity has not been the sole barrier restricting the use of ICDs. This dynamic has also been balanced by other concerns involving factors of self-preservation, morality, politics, and historic precedent (Table 33.10).

Formal threat assessments should include an analysis of these and other factors that may influence the overall risk of an ICD. The Chemical and Biological Arms Control Institute has offered the following set of predictions: (a) future terrorists are more likely to threaten to use chemical and biologic agents than to use them; (b) the use of chemicals will prove more prevalent than use of biologic agents; (c) small-scale attacks are more likely than large-scale attacks; (d) industrial chemicals are more likely to be used than military chemicals; (e) crude dispersal in enclosed areas is the most likely form of attack; (f) future incidents involving chemical and biologic substances may occur, but these are not going to be commonplace (6).

Vulnerability Assessment

Vulnerabilities are any action, circumstance, or event with the potential to cause the loss of or damage to an asset. They are any weakness that can be exploited by an adversary to gain access to an asset. Vulnerabilities to ICDs can result from population demographics, geographic location, behavior, sheltering and building use, operational practices, and occupation. Human vulnerability includes areas involving emotional, psychologic, behavioral, and security issues. In most cases, a set of preexisting countermeasures may already be in place that also serve to prevent and control risk of an ICD among these vulnerable populations. These should be considered in the risk assessment in terms of the procedural, technical, physical, and personnel issues related to ICDs. Tables 33.4 and 33.5 represent the pertinent activities of consequence detection and management, and therefore they provide an example of preexisting countermeasures that should be evaluated and rated in terms of quality, quantity, and efficacy.

Risk Countermeasures

Having objectively quantified the risk of an ICD and then assigned appropriate levels of priority for asset protection, countermeasures can then be undertaken that will reduce or

TABLE 33.10. FACTORS INFLUENCING THE LIKELIHOOD OF INTENTIONAL CHEMICAL DISASTERS

May decrease likelihood	May increase likelihood
Majority of historic precedents tending towards conservatism and a calibrated level of violence	Large-scale and indiscriminate attacks becoming more frequent
Possibility of world revulsion, alienation of constituency, and loss of group cohesion	Racial supremacy, ethnic hatred, and religious fanaticism much less constituency-based
May provoke massive retaliation	High public dread and perception of risk regarding chemical agents
Conventional weapons simpler, less expensive, and more predictable and flexible	Global diffusion of technology, so increased chemical weapon availability
May sacrifice state deniability or anonymity	State-sponsored support with funding, intelligence, and command and technical expertise
Chemical weaponization problematic	Purchase or theft of weapons of mass destruction now more likely
Terrorists perceive themselves as held to a higher moral standard than the targets	Religious terrorists see themselves as answerable only to God
Lack of safe haven states after intentional chemical disaster attack	Emergence of the far right, so increased likelihood of large scale violence
Lack of commensurate demands	More casualties required to maintain public and media interest
Weapons possibly turned against state sponsors, so states are less likely to provide such weapons to subnational groups	

eliminate one or more of the vulnerabilities. Disaster medical and public health countermeasures have been identified in Tables 33.4 and 33.5. Countermeasures include aspects of consequence detection and management, and they effectively function to deter, detect, delay, defend, and defeat the aims of the ICD perpetrator. Although these prevention and control measures must be measured against the potential costs and benefits of such actions, a discussion of ICD consequence detection and management activities are included to exemplify these options regardless of financial constraints.

Consequence Detection Measures

Chance favors the prepared mind.

—Louis Pasteur

To identify and detect the consequences of an ICD, responders must first be aware of characteristics that define these catastrophic events. Medical personnel require training for a differential diagnosis that also includes the adverse health effects of an ICD. An efficient and secure network for the sharing of confidential preincident intelligence must be created so that responders may be forewarned or briefed about ongoing events (16,24). The variety of potential chemical hazards must be identified along with the development of public and professional education programs that incorporate both military and industrial and/or commercial agents without an undo overemphasis on either chemical hazard (24). Civilian public safety, rescue, emergency medical personnel, and medical laboratories need an improved ability to detect and identify a wide variety of toxic substances including, but not limited to, military agents (24). The capacity for community-level ICD event reconstruction that allows for hazard assessment, dispersion prediction, exposure assessment, and laboratory reporting should be enabled (24,25). The capability for integration of information management, passive and active surveillance systems, and epidemiologic investigation should be instituted among national, state, and local health resources (18,19,24).

Since 1990, the Agency for Toxic Substances and Disease Registry (ATSDR) has maintained an active, state-based hazardous substances emergency events surveillance (HSEES) system to describe the public health consequences associated with the release of hazardous substances. Environmental monitoring and the HSEES should reflect an index of suspicion, the threshold, and mechanism for reporting ICD events. Protocols, methods, and case definitions are needed, in addition to scene assessments, for the diagnosis and evaluation of ICD-related casualties (18,19). Guidance for an "all-hazard approach" to incident and emergency management must be available. This should include principles of the planning process, direction and control, communications, warning and risk communication, emergency public information, population protection measures, health and medical issues, mass care, resource allocation, and hazard-specific variations (23,26).

Medical training must include protocols for the isolation and treatment of contaminated patients in addition to operational recovery (27). Limitations and needs for effective personal protective equipment and occupational health training must be identified and maintained (23,24). Research and development efforts must focus on processes for rapid mass triage and the decontamination of large numbers of affected individuals (23,24). Methods for incident management, site control, forensics, mutual aid, and hazardous waste emergency operations involving the broad variety of ICD agents must gain a broad level of consensus and awareness (18,28). Mental health issues are also a very important factor in the health and medical management and detection of a terrorist event (29). National, regional, and local public health departments must be linked in a network of real-time communication with the medical response community, public safety, regional poison control centers, and regional laboratory capacities (18,23). National assets must also be configured to support local responders in a broad variety of activities involving consequence management and detection (18).

SUMMARY

In summary, the prevention, detection, and management of ICD events represent an enormous challenge for the discipline of disaster medicine. While these incidents may have low likelihood, the impact could be catastrophic. Experience in dealing with these rare events is extremely limited. However, the scope of disaster medicine is uniquely characterized to be able to address these complex issues effectively.

A broad range of potential hazards and threats that involve ICDs are possible. However, many striking similarities are found between aspects for the management of an ICD and the many issues related to technologic disasters. Conceptual frameworks that can serve to organize disaster medical activity better are now available to guide future efforts. Methods for ICD consequence detection and management may be successfully addressed using a system of analytical risk management. Experience and knowledge regarding these principles of risk management as applied to an ICD are essential to the development and effectiveness of disaster medicine and public health promotion.

DEDICATION

This chapter is dedicated in memoriam to my lifelong friend Alan Jay Shilling.

REFERENCES

1. National Environmental Law Center and the United States Public Research Interest Group. *Chemical releases statistics.* Washington, D.C.: Associated Press International, 1994.
2. Anderson N. Disaster epidemiology: lessons from Bhopal. In:

Murray V, ed. *Major chemical disasters—medical aspects of management.* London: Royal Society of Medicine Services Limited, 1990:183–195.

3. Glickman, TS, Golding D, Silverman ED. *Acts of God and acts of man: major trends in natural disasters and major industrial accidents.* Discussion paper. Washington, D.C.: Center for Risk Management, Resources for the Future, 1991.

4. Slovic P. Perception of risk. *Science* 1987;236:280–285.

5. Lagadec P. *Accidents, crises, breakdowns.* Paper presented at the Society of Chemical Industry, London, January 9, 1998.

6. Jenkins BM. Understanding the link between motives and methods. In: Roberts B, ed. *Terrorism with chemical and biological weapons.* Alexandria, VA: The Chemical and Biological Arms Control Institute, 1997:51.

7. SAEM Disaster Medicine White Paper Subcommittee. Disaster medicine: current assessment and blueprint for the future. *Acad Emerg Med* 1995;2:1068–1076.

8. Waeckerle JF, Lillibridge SR, Burkle FM, et al. Disaster medicine: challenges for today. *Ann Emerg Med* 1994;23:715–718.

9. Smart JK. History of chemical and biological warfare: an American perspective. In: *Medical aspects of chemical and biological warfare.* Bethesda, MD: Office of the Surgeon General, 1997:11–42. Textbook of Military Medicine series.

10. Kadiver H, Adams SC. Treatment of chemical and biological warfare injuries: insights derived from the 1984 Iraqi attack on Majnoon island. *Mil Med* 1991;15:171–177.

11. Golan E, Arad M, Atsmon J, et al. Medical limitations of gas masks for civilian populations: the 1991 experience. *Mil Med* 1992;157:444–446.

12. Abou-Donia MB, Wilmarth KR, Jensen KF, et al. Neurotoxicity resulting from coexposure to pyridostigmine bromide, DEET and permethrin: implications of Gulf War chemical exposures. *J Toxicol Environ Health* 1996;48:35–56.

13. Amitai Y, Almog S, Singer R, et al. Atropine poisoning in children during the Persian Gulf crisis. *JAMA* 1992;268:630–632.

14. Kelsey KT, Xia F, Bodell WJ, et al. Genotoxicity to human cells induced by air particulates isolated during the Kuwait oil fires. *Environ Res* 1994;64:18–25.

15. Lillibridge SR, Sidell FR. *A report on the casualties from the Tokyo subway incident by the US medical team.* Atlanta: Centers for Disease Control and Prevention, 1995.

16. Seiple C. Consequence management: domestic response to weapons of mass destruction. *Parameters* 1997;Autumn:119–134.

17. Ember LR. FBI takes lead in developing counter terrorism effort. *Chemical and Engineering News.* November 4, 1996:10–16.

18. Keim ME, Kaufmann AF, Rodgers GC. A report for the United States Public Health Service, Office of Emergency Preparedness. *Recommendations for OEPCDC Surveillance, Laboratory and Informational Support Initiative.* Atlanta: Centers for Disease Control, National Center for Environmental Health, May 4, 1998.

19. Tucker JB. Policy approaches to chemical and biological terrorism. In: Roberts B, ed. *Terrorism with chemical and biological weapons: Calibrating the risks and responses.* Alexandria, VA: Chemical and Biological Arms Control Institute, 1997:95–111.

19a. Office of the Press Secretary, White House. Combating terrorism. *Presidential Decision Directive 62.* Annapolis, MD, May 22, 1998.

20. General Accounting Office. *Combating terrorism: threat and risk assessments can help prioritize and target program Investments.* NSIAD-98-74. Letter report. Washington, D.C., April 9, 1998.

21. Doyle CJ, Upfal MJ, Little NE. Disaster management of massive toxic exposure. In: Haddad LM, Winchester JF, ed. *Clinical management of poisoning and drug overdose.* Philadelphia, PA: WB Saunders, 1990:483–500.

22. Wetter DC. *Terrorist use of biological and chemical weapons: an assessment of hospital emergency department preparedness in USPHS region.* X. A report for the United States Public Health Service, Office of Emergency Preparedness. University of Washington School of Public Health and Community Medicine, January, 1999.

23. Brennan RJ, Waeckerle JL, Sharp TW, et al. Chemical warfare agents: emergency medical and emergency public health issues. *Ann Emerg Med* 1999;34:191–204.

24. Institute of Medicine. *Chemical and biological terrorism: research and development to improve civilian medical response.* Washington, D.C.: National Academy Press, 1999:189.

25. Fainberg A. Debating policy and priorities. In: Roberts B, ed. *Terrorism with chemical and biological weapons: calibrating the risks and responses.* Alexandria, VA: Chemical and Biological Arms Control Institute, 1997:75–93.

26. Federal Emergency Management Agency. *Guide for all-hazard emergency operations planning.* SLG 101. Washington, D.C.: Federal Emergency Management Agency, 1996.

27. Burgess JL, Kirk M, Borron SW, et al. Emergency department hazardous materials protocols for contaminated patients. *Ann Emerg Med* 1999;34:205–212.

28. National Institute for Occupational Safety and Health, Occupational Health and Safety Administration, United States Coast Guard, and the Environmental Protection Agency. *Occupational safety and health guidance manual for hazardous waste site activities.* Atlanta: United States Department of Heath and Human Services, Centers for Disease Control and Prevention, 1985.

29. Holloway HC, Norwood AE, Fullerton CS, et al. The threat of biological weapons: prophylaxis and mitigation of psychological and social consequences. *JAMA* 1997;278:425–427.

BIOLOGICAL WEAPON AGENTS

MARK G. KORTEPETER
JOHN R. ROWE
EDWARD M. EITZEN

Biological weapons are microorganisms or toxins derived from living organisms that are intentionally used to produce disease or death in humans, animals, or plants (1). A significant feature distinguishing biological weapons from conventional, chemical, and nuclear weapons is the incubation period. The first sign of a biological weapon release would probably be ill patients presenting to health care providers in emergency departments and clinics around the affected area. In actuality, this was observed in the fall of 2001 when individuals with cutaneous and inhalational anthrax reported to physicians and hospitals for evaluation of illness after exposures to *Bacillus anthracis* spores sent in the mail. Potentially, hundreds of human pathogens could be used as weapons; however, public health authorities have identified only a few as having the potential to cause mass casualties leading to civil disruption (2,3). Emergency medicine specialists and primary care providers need to have a basic understanding of the clinical presentations and treatments for the major diseases that pose the highest threat for a mass casualty situation so that they can effectively participate in mitigating the consequences of a bioterrorist attack. This chapter will provide an overview of biological weapons and will focus on these few agents.

Biologic pathogens have been used as weapons of war for centuries (4). Use of a biological weapon could be as simple as contaminating an adversary's well with an animal carcass or human feces (5). In 1346, while Tartar invaders laid siege to Caffa, a port city on the Black Sea in Crimea, they experienced an outbreak of bubonic plague (6). In an attempt to turn this misfortune to their advantage, they catapulted plague-ridden corpses over the city's walls, and subsequently, an outbreak of plague ensued amongst the Genoese defenders of the city. As the Genoese fled to Europe, they are suspected of carrying the infection with them, thus beginning the outbreak of the Black Death, which decimated one-third of the European population. An example of biological weapon use in North America occurred during the French and Indian War, when Sir Jeffrey Amherst hatched the idea of giving gifts of smallpox-laden blankets and clothing to Indians sympathetic to the French. Although both examples are intriguing, verifying that an endemic disease was spread

intentionally is difficult. Based on current knowledge of the natural epidemiology of plague, the spread of the disease into Caffa was more likely secondary to infected rats and fleas traversing the city walls. Also, the fact that scabs from smallpox victims are not very infectious because the virus is bound by the fibrin matrix of the scab calls into question whether the subsequent outbreaks of smallpox among the Indians were related to the gifts (5).

Advances in microbiology in the 19th century provided the scientific basis for elevating the use of disease as a weapon to a new level of sophistication. In the early twentieth century, several countries launched ambitious biological weapons programs. Unit 731, one of the research facilities in the Japanese program, which was headed by General Shiro Ishii, was notorious for its use of prisoners as research subjects (7,8). Western powers, particularly Britain and the United States, began their own programs in response to concerns that the Japanese and the Germans might gain a military advantage in this area. The British used immobilized sheep to test small anthrax bombs on Gruinard Island off the coast of Scotland. Although bombs are an inefficient means for spreading biologic pathogens because the heat and light of the explosion will inactivate the majority of pathogens, those experiments verified the feasibility of this type of weapon. Parts of the island remained heavily contaminated with anthrax spores until they were decontaminated in the 1980s, demonstrating the long-term viability of anthrax spores in soil (9). The United States conducted an offensive research and testing program from 1943 until 1969, when President Nixon unilaterally renounced continued research into the offensive use of biological weapons (10). All stocks of antipersonnel biologic munitions, agents, and toxins were subsequently destroyed by 1973 in accordance with approved demilitarization plans (11).

International concern has refocused on biological weapons recently for a number of reasons. After the Gulf War, United Nations inspection teams uncovered evidence of the Iraqi biological weapons program, which had weaponized up to 6,000 L of anthrax and 12,000 L of botulinum toxin (12). Another alert came following the defection of Ken Alibek, who served as the first deputy director of Biopreparat, the civilian wing to the Soviet biological weapons program. He revealed the massive extent of the program, which included the production of ton quantities and the weaponization of agents such as anthrax and smallpox (13). Both the Iraqis and the Soviets had signed the 1972 biological weapons convention, which prohibited the development, production, and stockpiling of biological weapons "in quantities that have no justification for prophylactic, protective, or other peaceful purposes"(14).

A number of recent examples pinpoint the vulnerability of the United States to foreign and domestic terrorists either within the United States or abroad; they include the bombings of the *U.S.S. Cole*, of the Federal Building in Oklahoma City, and of the United States embassies in Kenya and Tanzania. The sarin nerve agent release in the Tokyo subway system by the Aum Shinrikyo cult in 1995 raised additional concerns that terrorist organizations may no longer limit themselves to conventional means to further their goals. Reports that the cult had made prior unsuccessful attempts to release biological weapons demonstrated that preparedness against a biological weapon attack must extend to civilian communities, as well as the military (15). The September 11, 2001 destruction of the World Trade Center towers and of a portion of the Pentagon by hijacked aircraft provided a grim reminder that terrorists often do not have concern for their own lives, let alone those of others. In fact, the attacks of September 11 remove any doubt that terrorists seek to inflict mass casualties. The delivery of *Bacillus anthracis* spores through the mail in 2001 demonstrates that perpetrators are willing to use weapons of mass destruction, including biological weapons, to kill or sicken others.

Biologic pathogens have a number of properties that may make them useful weapons in war and for terrorism.

1. Many of the agents are available from culture collections, medical supply companies, or laboratories around the world (16). Although export controls and the procedures for obtaining cultures from supply houses have become better regulated (17), some of the seed stocks for Iraqi munitions came from supply houses in the United States and France (12). In addition, some pathogens, such as *Clostridium botulinum*, are ubiquitous in soil, and they can be cultured readily by someone with the appropriate training.
2. The expense of producing a biological weapon is far less than that of other weapon systems. For example, in a 1969 study, the United Nations reported that the cost to kill greater than 50% of the people in an area that is 1 km² with a biological weapon would be only $1, as compared to a chemical, nuclear, or conventional weapon, which would cost $600, $800, or $2,000, respectively (18).
3. The deployment of a biological weapon is potentially silent. With the recent anthrax letter attacks, no announcement or warning was received in advance.

Unlike most chemical, conventional, or nuclear weapons, which generally exert their effects immediately with explosions or casualties, biological weapons have incubation periods. These can range from a few hours (e.g., staphylococcal enterotoxin B) to several weeks (e.g., Q fever), but the incubation period is generally on the order of days. In this era of rapid air travel, the perpetrator using a biological weapon could be overseas by the time the effects of the agent become manifest. A would-be terrorist might be protected with a vaccine or chemoprophylaxis, and thus he or she would incur little risk of infection while disseminating a pathogen and would not require any personal protective equipment. In contrast, a terrorist using a chemical agent may need more obvious means of self-protection during dissemination. A biologic aerosol may be odorless, colorless, and tasteless; therefore, a bona fide release may not be recognized until emergency departments and other health-care facilities are flooded with ill victims days or even weeks later, depending on the agent used.

4. Dual uses of technology that has legitimate purposes make the production of biologic pathogens difficult to detect and/or easy to conceal. The fermentation technology for manufacturing beverages such as beer and for producing antibiotics and vaccines can be readily adapted to the assembly of biologic pathogens. Also, compared with chemical and nuclear agents, the "footprint," or the size required for the production facility is much smaller. This limits the ability to verify compliance with weapons treaties for biologic agents.
5. Biologic agents can be disseminated with readily available technology. Common agricultural spray devices can be adapted to disseminate biologic pathogens of the proper particle size to cause infection in human populations over great distances. Reports that the perpetrators of the 2001 World Trade Center attack demonstrated interest in crop dusters has refocused concern on the potential for biologic, as well as chemical, terrorism. The perpetrators can use natural weather conditions, such as wind and temperature inversions, as well as existing building infrastructure (e.g., ventilation systems) or air movement related to transportation (e.g., subway cars passing through tunnels) to disseminate these agents and thus to infect or intoxicate large numbers of people.
6. The mere mention of certain diseases, such as smallpox, anthrax, or plague, has the potential to cause fear and panic among the civilian population because of the established historic ability of these diseases to cause large numbers of deaths. Such "brand name" recognition has potential value to a terrorist who is seeking to gain media headlines or to make a statement, regardless of whether the actual pathogen is used. This phenomenon has been demonstrated repeatedly in the numerous anthrax and other biological weapon hoaxes that have occurred across the United States in the past 2 years (16). Illustrating this

panic was the run on ciprofloxacin that occurred after the anthrax cases were reported in 2001. Emergency responders, public health agencies, health-care providers, military agencies, and federal and local law enforcement agencies have spent time and money developing and learning new protocols for providing an appropriate measured response to these weapon threats.

7. The information required to produce biologic pathogens is now readily available in numerous extremist "how to" handbooks, as well as on the Internet. Much concern has been expressed about the potential for the proliferation of knowledge, culture technologies, and pathogens by unemployed scientists who previously worked in state-sponsored offensive programs, such as in the former Soviet Union. These individuals could be wooed by countries known for supporting terrorism or by terrorist organizations with the funding to hire them.

Some of the disadvantages of biological weapons must also be mentioned. Although obtaining pathogens is relatively easy, developing them as effective aerosols in the requisite particle size took the major national programs years and millions of dollars. If they are not used with the proper weather conditions, such as during a temperature inversion, at night, or with a slow, steady wind, the dispersion of the pathogens can be easily disrupted by the wind or degraded by sunlight, thus rendering them ineffective. The reliance on natural weather conditions may not be as great a concern for terrorists who use them, but it definitely makes biological weapons less desirable as tactical weapons on the battlefield.

The list of human and zoonotic pathogens that have potential use as weapons could number in the hundreds. Historically, the military has been most concerned about pathogens that could be released, covering a great distance and causing overwhelming casualties. These pathogens typically remain stable, and they can infect via aerosol. The North Atlantic Treaty Organization (NATO) handbook dealing with biologic warfare agents lists 39 pathogens and toxins that meet some of the requirements (19). Not all of them are capable of the mass production or dispersal necessary to affect a large metropolitan area. The Center for Civilian Biodefense at Johns Hopkins University convened a working group of government and nongovernment experts to identify which biologic pathogens has the potential to cause a maximum credible event (2,20). A maximum credible event causes large numbers of casualties, overwhelming health-care resources and creating mass disruption and panic in the target population. The short list identified by the working group includes anthrax and smallpox as the greatest threats, followed by plague, botulinum toxins, viral hemorrhagic fevers, and tularemia (2). The Centers for Disease Control and Prevention (CDC) also organized a working group to address this issue. They considered the following in defining their list of threat agents (3):

1. Public health impact based on morbidity, mortality, and communicability.
2. Delivery potential to large populations based on stability, ease of production, and dissemination.
3. Special requirements for stockpiling treatments or antidotes, surveillance, and diagnosis.
4. Potential for fear and civil disruption based on public perception.

The CDC working group came up with three categories—A, B, and C—for public health preparedness. Those in category A had the greatest potential for fear and disruption and most significant public health impact; they require the most intense preparedness efforts. Category A lists the same agents as those in the Hopkins list. The balance of this chapter will focus on these six agents in category A.

Anthrax

The disease anthrax is caused by the gram-positive, non-motile, sporulating rod, *Bacillus anthracis*. The name anthrax derives from the Greek word for coal because of the characteristic black eschar seen with cutaneous disease. Anthrax has been a scourge of cattle and other herbivores for centuries. Humans generally are secondarily infected through work with animals or animal products, such as hides, hair, or bone meal. During the industrial revolution, the inhalation form was first recognized as an occupational pulmonary disease in workers in the wool industries of Europe. Hence, the disease has the name of Woolsorter's or Ragpicker's disease.

Anthrax is a relatively rare disease in the United States. At the beginning of the 20th century, before the advent of control measures, such as the vaccination of animals and the implementation of import controls, around 130 human cases, most of which were the cutaneous form, were reported each year (21). Only 18 cases of inhalation anthrax were reported in the United States in the 20th century, with the last one surfacing in 1978 (22). As the time of this writing, the *B. anthracis* spores sent through the mail in the fall of 2001 had precipitated 11 cases, resulting in five deaths, of inhalation anthrax, thus proving the feasibility of this agent for terrorism (23).

Anthrax makes an ideal biological weapon. The inhalational form of the disease is highly lethal. The spores can maintain virulence for decades, and they can be milled to the ideal particle size of 2 to 6 μm for optimum infection of the human respiratory tract. The organism can be purchased from numerous commercial supply houses around the world, or it can be cultured from soil where anthrax is enzootic.

The organism lacks two qualities that would make it an even more deadly weapon. Compared to other biological weapons, anthrax requires a fairly high retained infective dose of 8,000 to 10,000 spores or even up to 55,000 inhaled spores in animal studies (24). Unfortunately, that amount could be inhaled with one deep breath if a cloud is concentrated (*personal communication*, Dr. Louise Pitt, 2000), and experts are now questioning whether lesser quantities might still cause disease in the elderly and other potentially immunocompromised individuals, following the death of an elderly woman in Connecticut in 2001. Second, inhalation anthrax is not transmitted from person to person. Therefore, standard precautions are adequate in the care of patients with inhalation anthrax (25).

An accidental release of anthrax spores in 1979 from a military biological weapons facility in the town of Sverdlovsk in the former Soviet Union (now Ekaterinberg, Russia), caused the largest known cluster of inhalation anthrax cases; 66 human deaths were reported within 4 km, and animal deaths were seen up to 50 km (26). This outbreak demonstrated that infection of human populations downwind was a realistic possibility with an anthrax aerosol release. Analysis by polymerase chain reaction (PCR) of tissue samples of 11 of these victims demonstrated four different anthrax strain categories (27).

Three clinical forms of the disease are observed, depending on the route of exposure. The pathogenesis of the disease is similar regardless of the route of infection. Following entry into the body, the spores are ingested by macrophages; they then either replicate in the local area of the skin, or they are transported to the local lymph nodes in the gastrointestinal tract or the lungs. During transport and after arrival at the lymph nodes, the spores germinate into vegetative bacteria. They replicate in the lymph nodes, secreting two toxins: edema toxin and lethal toxin. These cause local edema and necrosis. The bacterial polyglutamic acid capsule is antiphagocytic.

The most common form, cutaneous anthrax, represents at least 95% of all reported cases; it occurs when the organism gains entry into the body through abraded skin. With proper treatment, this is rarely fatal; but without treatment, a 20% case-fatality rate is documented. Gastrointestinal or oropharyngeal anthrax, which occurs from ingesting infected, undercooked meat of animals that have died of anthrax, may have higher case-fatality rates, partly due to the delay in recognition that can occur with the illness. The third form, inhalation anthrax, is the most deadly, and this represents the clinical illness that is expected following a biological weapon attack.

The incubation period ranges from 1 to 6 days after aerosol exposure, although periods of up to 43 days were reported after the Sverdlovsk outbreak (26). A review of 10 of the recent 11 cases of inhalational anthrax demonstrated an incubation period of 4 to 6 days in the six cases in which the date of exposure was documented (23). Patients present with a nonspecific febrile illness, accompanied by cough, malaise, fevers, chills, and possibly chest pain. Over the following 24 to 48 hours, the symptoms worsen, but patients may have a brief period of improvement before suddenly deteriorating with stridor, dyspnea, cyanosis, and frank respiratory failure. The clinical hallmark is a widened mediastinum on chest radiograph due to hemorrhagic mediastinitis; however, this may not develop until too late to treat a patient adequately, and it may occur in only 60% of patients. Pneumonia generally does not occur, although hemorrhagic pleural effusions may develop. If the patient is not treated adequately and early enough, bacteremia and sepsis will ensue. This can lead to metastatic foci of infection throughout the body, including the meninges and the gastrointestinal tract. In a pathologic study of the 42 victims at Sverdlovsk (28), 50% had evidence of meningeal involvement. Case-fatality rates reach 100% in untreated cases. The outbreak in the fall of 2001 provided some interesting new information on the clinical presentation of inhalational anthrax that had not been previously reported—70% of the victims complained of profound, drenching sweats, and 90% noted nausea or vomiting. Other common presenting complaints included fever and chills (100%), dyspnea (80%), and fatigue and malaise (100%) (23).

Diagnosis is made by identifying bacilli with gram stain or culture of peripheral blood, cerebrospinal fluid, or pleural effusion samples; staining of sputum samples, however, is not helpful. Careful review of the presenting chest radiographs in the recent outbreak found these to be a sensitive indicator of illness because none of the radiographs had normal findings, and the features noted included hilar fullness, paratracheal fullness, pleural effusions, and infiltrates. Chest computed tomography was also helpful in verifying mediastinal adenopathy. Pleural effusions during the course of illness were present in all cases, and some required repeated thoracentesis (23). Serology is useful only for retrospective diagnosis. Newer techniques using fluorescent antibody technology or PCR may play a role in more rapid diagnosis. Clinicians should alert the laboratory if they suspect anthrax because gram-positive bacilli are often dismissed as contaminants.

The drug of choice for endemic anthrax, which is usually cutaneous, historically has been penicillin. However, because of the reports of naturally acquired penicillin-resistant strains and recent isolates from the mail-associated cases demonstrating constitutive and inducible beta-lactamases, in the setting of a biological warfare or terrorist release, the drugs of choice for cutaneous anthrax are ciprofloxacin, 500 mg orally every 12 hours, or doxycycline, 100 mg orally every 12 hours (29). Several reviews have outlined treatment in detail (24,30,31); however, newer guidance recommends initial intravenous treatment for inhalational anthrax with ciprofloxacin, 400 mg, or doxycycline, 100 mg every 12 hours until the results of sensitivities are known, plus one or more other antimicrobial agents, such as rifampin, vancomycin, penicillin, ampicillin, chloramphenicol, imipenem, clindamycin, or clarithromycin (29). The total duration of treatment is 60 days. Patients may be transitioned to oral medications based on the clinical response. Treatment is most effective if it is begun within the first 24 to 48 hours of clinical illness. It is unlikely to be effective once the patient is hypotensive or moribund with mediastinitis and sepsis.

In patients with a known exposure to *B. anthracis,* two daily doses of ciprofloxacin, 500 mg orally, or of doxycycline, 100 mg orally, may be used for postexposure prophylaxis (24,30), and both have been licensed by the Food and Drug Administration for this purpose. Spores have been demonstrated to remain viable in mediastinal lymph nodes for up to 100 days (32), and death has occurred up to 58 (33) and 98 (34) days after inhalational exposure in experimental monkeys. Therefore, prophylaxis should continue for 60 days in the absence of vaccine. If a vaccine is available, patients should be treated prophylactically for at least 30 days and until three doses of vaccine are given (24,30). Preexposure chemoprophylaxis may be effective, as may immunoprophylaxis with a vaccine. Studies in monkeys indicate that the United States anthrax vaccine offers a high degree of protection for up to 760 times the inhaled median lethal dose (LD_{50}) of anthrax spores (35).

Smallpox

Smallpox, like anthrax and plague, is another of the great diseases of antiquity. No other disease has had such an extensive and persistent impact on mankind (36). In 1980, the World Health Assembly declared this disease eradicated from the globe—the first such disease to be eliminated. Ironically, the success of this great public health triumph and the subsequent cessation of vaccination against smallpox opened the door for smallpox to strike fear again in the hearts of mankind.

Smallpox has made the headlines again recently because of revelations by the Soviet defector Ken Alibek (13) that the Soviets saw the eradication of smallpox as an opportunity to exploit. He attests that the Soviets had been growing smallpox by the ton for use in intercontinental ballistic missiles directed at the United States. Concerns that other nations that sponsor international terrorism may have kept some stocks of smallpox, rather than turn them in or destroy them after the eradication effort, also abound. Moreover, as a result of the poor economic conditions in the former Soviet Union, the possibility has been raised that scientists who worked in the old program could have carried both their expertise and agents, including smallpox, to other laboratories or countries (37).

The World Health Assembly recommended that all countries discontinue vaccination against smallpox in 1980. Vaccination of civilians and military personnel in the United States was discontinued in 1972 and in the mid-1980s, respectively. Therefore, due to the waning of immunity over time, only 20% of the population has been esti-

mated to have residual protection (20). This has serious implications because the effective deployment of a highly infective smallpox aerosol by a terrorist might infect thousands. The person-to-person contagiousness of smallpox promotes rapid spread of disease, potentially yielding hundreds or thousands of new cases, if the initial cases were to go unrecognized until the second or third generation (38).

Smallpox (variola) virus is a member of the genus *Orthopoxvirus,* and it is closely related to the viruses causing cowpox, vaccinia, and monkeypox. It is one of the largest (0.25 μm) DNA viruses known, and it has a bricklike appearance on electron microscopy.

Transmission of variola virus can occur by several different ways as follows: generally by droplet, occasionally by aerosol, by direct contact with secretions or lesions from a patient, and rarely by fomites contaminated with the infectious virus from a patient. Examples of cases being imported into susceptible areas in Europe where one case might yield ten to 20 secondary cases are found (39). Transmission risk increases if the index patient is coughing or sneezing or if he or she has hemorrhagic disease.

Typically, the virus enters the respiratory mucosa and then travels to regional lymph nodes where it replicates. Within 3 to 4 days, an asymptomatic primary viremia occurs, which seeds the reticuloendothelial system, including the lymph nodes, spleen, and bone marrow. A secondary viremia that seeds the back of the throat and skin ensues around the eighth day. A prodrome of fever, vomiting, and headache is noted, which is followed in 2 to 3 days by a characteristic rash, signalling the onset of infectiousness. The incubation period from infection to onset of the rash ranges from 7 to 17 days, averaging 12 to 14 days. In the first couple of days, the rash may be mistaken for varicella; however, some key distinguishing features are present. Smallpox develops first on the face and a bit later on the extremities, and it remains more prominent there without central progression—it is a centrifugal rash; chickenpox, however, tends to be found predominantly on the trunk—it is a centripetal rash. Smallpox lesions progress in synchrony through the stages of macule, vesicle, umbilicated pustule, and scab, whereas chickenpox lesions appear in successive crops, thus yielding lesions at different stages of development. Smallpox scabs remain infectious until they fall off, whereas chickenpox is no longer infectious once the lesions have crusted.

Physician inexperience with smallpox has grave implications with respect to secondary spread. Physicians might not include smallpox in their differential diagnosis, or perhaps they might simply discount smallpox as a possibility because the disease has been "eradicated."

Diagnosis is made clinically by the recognition of the characteristic rash. Light microscopy may show eosinophilic cytoplasmic inclusions (Guarnieri bodies), but these may be overlooked by an untrained technician. Viral cultures may be useful, but advancing PCR technology may prove to be the best diagnostic tool in the future. Electron microscopy (EM) cannot distinguish between the different orthopoxviruses; however, any patient in the United States with a poxvirus on EM should be reported to the local and state public health authorities immediately, as well as to the CDC. Even one case of smallpox would be an international emergency.

Several smallpox clinical variants have been observed, but the one of most concern for a biological weapon attack is variola major, which has a 30% case-fatality rate in the unvaccinated. The complications of infection include blindness, scarring, and bony deformities in children. Currently, no licensed treatment for smallpox exists. Supportive care was the mainstay of therapy available when smallpox was endemic, and it remains the only therapy. Encouraging *in vitro* data have resulted from research into the effectiveness of various drugs against orthopox viruses, including smallpox; and recent data from a small study in a rhesus monkey model with cidofovir suggest effectiveness for prophylaxis (*personal communication*, Dr. John Huggins, 2001). Whether the medication could be effective as a treatment for illness has not yet been determined. Even if cidofovir proves to be an effective treatment *in vivo*, logistical concerns still predominate because administering an intravenous medication to a large number of individuals during a massive epidemic would be difficult.

In the event of an outbreak, epidemiologic measures for identifying exposed individuals and isolating ill individuals become critical to interrupting the spread. Vaccination as soon as possible, and up to 4 days after exposure, may protect against or ameliorate the disease (40). Unfortunately, the number of effective doses held by the CDC is gradually diminishing. Approximately 15.4 million doses are held in 100 dose vials (40), but, with normal variation in administration techniques and wastage, this represents approximately 7 to 8 million usable doses (*personal communication*, Dr. Ali Khan, 1999). The production of the vaccine was discontinued shortly after the disease was declared eradicated. Since then, the production facilities have been dismantled, and no new vaccine has been produced. The method of producing vaccine was crude by today's vaccine standards, and it would no longer be considered acceptable for producing new vaccine. Contracts for the production of a new cell-culture–derived vaccine were awarded in 2000 with possible delivery date as early as 2002; however, attaining Food and Drug Admininstration licensure may present a challenge because no human trial can be done to establish vaccine efficacy. Before new vaccine production begins, diluting the existing vaccine by fivefold to tenfold may be considered in an emergency (41).

Because the disease may spread by aerosol, infection control measures include the following airborne precautions: negative pressure isolation rooms and wearing high-efficiency particulate air (HEPA) filters when caring for patients. Preferably, all health-care providers would be vaccinated before caring for the patients. For a large outbreak, multiple patients would need to be isolated in the same ward, as long as the ward has its own ventilation system. Additionally, depending on how many patients are present, a proposal might be made for patients to be cared for in their homes; alternatively, smallpox-specific hospitals might have to be opened, as occurred in some countries during the eradication effort. Even with a new vaccine, well-documented and predictable side effects of smallpox vaccination would likely preclude routine immunizations of the general population, especially since the number of persons with immunosuppressive diseases has increased since the 1970s.

Plague

Three pandemics have been caused by plague, with the third one ongoing since 1898. The mere mention of the word plague conjures up many images because the plague has already demonstrated a historical potential to kill millions, as it did in the second pandemic in Renaissance Europe; for that reason, it may appeal to one's adversaries, whether they be foreign powers or terrorists.

In addition, knowledge of the Japanese experimentation with plague-infected fleas released on cities in China in World War II and the fact that plague was one of the favorite biological weapons in the former Soviet Union's arsenal create additional fear. Plague is the only weapon besides smallpox on the category A threat list that is communicable from person-to-person (3). Therefore plague, like smallpox, can cause devastation beyond those persons who are initially infected. The United States offensive program was also interested in plague at one time; however, difficulties in maintaining the virulence of the organism were found when it was grown in high concentrations.

Plague is a disease that results from infection by the nonmotile, gram-negative coccobacillus *Yersinia pestis*. When stained, its bipolar appearance is often described as resembling a safety pin. *Y. pestis* has two important properties that differentiate it from *B. anthracis*—person-to-person transmissibility and a lack of spore production.

Plague continues to be endemic in various parts of the world. A handful of human cases, mostly of the bubonic type, are reported each year in the United States. Plague is generally a zoonotic disease, and it is currently confined to the western part of the United States, although it is slowly marching toward the east. Infection of humans is not necessary to maintain the plague cycle; therefore, humans are generally secondarily infected when they spend time in areas where rodents are active or when their own pets carry the disease or the flea vector to them.

Three clinical presentations of plague occur. The most common form with naturally occurring plague is bubonic plague. Following the bite of an infected flea, plague bacilli are carried via the lymphatics to the regional lymph nodes where they multiply exponentially. If they are untreated, plague organisms can gain entry to the bloodstream and can lead to secondary plague septicemia. Septicemic plague can also occur primarily in the minority of patients who do not develop a bubo following the fleabite. The third and least common form of plague is pneumonic plague. It can occur secondarily when the lungs are seeded from septicemic or bubonic plague, or it can occur as primary pneumonic plague if a person or animal is infected directly by inhaling infected droplets from another person or animal with pneumonic plague. Unlike anthrax, pneumonic plague does in fact cause a pneumonia; therefore, organisms are present in respiratory secretions, thus accounting for its communicability.

The contagious nature of pneumonic plague can be beneficial to the adversary who desires to infect only a small number of victims, then allowing the disease to spread. This may be of special interest to a terrorist who plans to leave the area once the biological weapon has been used. On the battlefield, however, a contagious agent may be less attractive because, once the agent is released, the disease can infect the local rats and fleas in addition to humans. A commander may not want to put his troops at risk for acquiring the disease after its release.

Plague can be diagnosed based on gram, Wright-Giemsa, or Wayson stains and by the culture of the organism in sputum, blood, or fluid extracted from a bubo. Direct fluorescent antibody staining of a bubo aspirate is more specific for *Y. pestis* than are other stains. Serologic studies with enzyme-linked immunosorbent assay (ELISA) or passive hemagglutination assay are generally useful only in retrospect because clinical signs precede the antibody response (42).

Streptomycin continues to be the drug of choice for plague. It is available directly from the Roerig Streptomycin Program at Pfizer Pharmaceuticals under a compassionate use protocol. Alternatives include gentamicin or doxycycline. For plague meningitis, the drug of choice is chloramphenicol. β-Lactam antibiotics are generally not recommended because, in animal studies, they may actually accelerate mortality. A consensus panel recently recommended doxycycline, 100 mg orally twice a day, or ciproflxacin, 500 mg orally twice a day, as the preferred choices of antibiotics for postexposure prophylaxis in a bioterrorism setting (43). Plague is particularly notable for its high-grade bacteremia. For a patient with pneumonic plague the patient's prognosis is extremely poor if therapy is not initiated within 24 hours of the onset of symptoms.

When caring for patients with bubonic plague, standard precautions with the addition of drainage and secretion precautions are necessary. Pneumonic plague is transmitted by droplets, which are fairly large, and by heavy particles that fall out of the air readily. Therefore, pneumonic plague patients should be put under droplet precautions, similar to the procedures needed for meningococcal meningitis. When caring for these patients, care providers should wear a standard surgical mask when they are within 3 feet of the patient. Droplet precautions should be maintained until the patient has completed 72 hours of therapy and until a favorable response to treatment is observed (25).

Household or face-to-face contacts of patients with pneumonic plague are at risk for contracting pneumonic plague as well, and they should be offered immediate chemoprophylaxis. Those refusing prophylaxis should be placed in strict isolation and should be monitored for the illness for 7 days (44). The drug of choice for prophylaxis is doxycycline, 100 mg orally twice a day, for 7 days or for the duration of contact, if that is longer.

With modern air travel, containing an outbreak of plague could be challenging. The outbreak of a deadly pneumonia in India in 1994 that was suspected to be plague provided an example of the kind of panic that might be seen if a similar epidemic were to be seen in the United States. Doctors and nurses fled hospitals, people left the affected city, and pharmaceutical supplies were diminished. In such as situation international quarantine measures might have to be enacted.

A vaccine for plague does exist; however, it is no longer being produced, and it does not demonstrate efficacy against infection by aerosol. Therefore, it offers little protection against the route of infection that one would suspect a terrorist to use or that would be seen on the battlefield. The most promising candidate vaccines undergoing animal trials contain the F1 and V plague antigens.

Botulism

Botulinum toxins are the only toxins discussed in this chapter. A toxin is any toxic substance that can be produced in an animal, plant, or microbe. Many natural toxins can also be produced by chemical synthesis or can be expressed artificially. Toxins are distinguished from chemical weapons by the following: chemical weapons are all manmade, and they are volatile; toxins, however, are natural and nonvolatile. Some chemical weapons are dermally active through the intact skin, whereas biologic agents, with the possible exception of the trichothecin mycotoxins, generally do not penetrate intact skin. Finally, many of the toxins are much more toxic than the same given amount of the chemical agents. For example, depending on the serotype, botulinum toxins are 10,000 to 100,000 times more toxic than chemical nerve agents.

Botulinum toxins are a concern for warfare and terrorism because of their extreme toxicity ($LD_{50}= 3$ ng per kg by inhalation) (45), the ubiquitous nature of *Clostridium botulinum* in soil, and the ease of culturing *C. botulinum* to produce toxin. Seven known toxins, A-G, exist. These are immunologically distinct, meaning that the antibodies developed against one do not cross-react against others. Those that most commonly cause human disease are the types A, B, and E.

Botulism is deadly. Humans can be intoxicated either by oral means, inhalation, or wound infection. Mass casualties could be produced through contamination of a food source or by aerosol dissemination. The most common natural intoxication follows the ingestion of home-canned food that has been contaminated with bacterial spores, which then germinate under the anaerobic environments inside the can or jar. The 1995 revelations of the fact that the Iraqis had developed a liquid preparation of botulinum toxin to be loaded in Scud missiles and bombs (12) and that the Aum Shinrikyo cult in Japan attempted to release botulinum toxin on several occasions (15) have increased the concern that botulinum toxin might be used.

The toxins produce disease in humans by preventing the release of acetylcholine in the presynaptic nerve terminal. Therefore, nerve impulses cannot travel to the postsynaptic fibers. This results in a descending, flaccid paralysis and bulbar dysfunction, including blurred vision, diplopia, dysphagia, and dysarthria. The incubation period of botulism can range from as short as 24 to 36 hours to several days from the time of inhalation.

Physicians should be able to recognize the clinical hallmarks of bulbar symptoms and descending flaccid paralysis; however, historically, 25% of individual cases or of those who are among the first group of patients presenting with symptoms have died. In general, with current medical supportive care, patients should not die of botulism. Treatment of patients suspected to have botulism should not be delayed until the disease can be confirmed because the antitoxin does not reverse symptoms; it may, however, halt symptom progression. If patients do not receive botulinum antitoxin in a timely manner, they may require ventilator assistance. Unfortunately, in a biological weapon scenario, many of the initial presenting patients might not receive appropriate initial care. Therefore, in a large attack with botulinum, the number of patients might far outnumber the available ventilators, thus quickly overwhelming a city's capabilities for care.

Several antitoxins do exist, all in relatively small quantities. The CDC has a licensed, bivalent equine antitoxin for toxins A and B. The E antitoxin is now classified as an investigational new drug (IND). A despeciated heptavalent (A-G) antitoxin that is an IND product also exists. Smaller quantities of a human-derived botulinum antitoxin, which is also in IND status, also are available. Both the licensed product and the despeciated heptavalent product require horse serum sensitivity testing before use because of the risk of anaphylaxis or serum sickness. Which antitoxin is considered for use depends on the availability and the toxin type.

Preventive measures in addition to using an antitoxin after exposure include wearing a HEPA filter mask if one has knowledge of an impending release. The standard military gas mask provides protection against all of the biological weapon agents. In addition, an IND pentavalent (A–E) botulinum toxoid vaccine is availabe. This vaccine was given to around 8,000 soldiers during Operation Desert Shield and Desert Storm who were deemed to be at a particularly high risk of exposure to the toxin. It is routinely offered to researchers who have an occupational risk for contact with the toxin. The toxoid produces serum antitoxin levels that correspond to protective levels in animal models. The animal studies with botulinum suggest that, if measurable amount of antibody is present, then the individual is protected.

Tularemia

Francisella tularensis, the causative agent of tularemia, is a gram-negative, aerobic, nonmotile coccobacillus. Tularemia is a zoonotic disease acquired in the natural setting by humans through skin or mucous membrane contact with the body fluids or tissues of infected animals or from being bitten by infected deerflies, mosquitoes, or ticks. The disease may occur less commonly by the inhalation of contaminated dusts or the ingestion of contaminated foods or water. Tularemia is relatively uncommon in the United States, with less than 150 cases reported per year on average.

F. tularensis was one of the bioagents that was weaponized during the United States offensive biowarfare program. The organism has several features that make it attractive as a weapon. It can remain viable for weeks in the environment or in animal carcasses and for years, if frozen. Unlike anthrax, which requires thousands of spores to infect someone, tularemia can cause illness with as few as 10 to 50 organisms. Tularemia also has been estimated to spread downwind very well in modeling studies (46), and it can be milled to the proper 1 to 5 μm particle size for ease of infection.

Clinical manifestations of tularemia depend on the route of exposure. A preponderance of typhoidal septic or pneumonic tularemia would be expected after an intentional release by aerosol, although intradermal or gastrointestinal exposure can lead to the typhoidal septic form as well. After an incubation period of 2 to 10 days, the symptoms include fever, severe exhaustion, substernal chest pain, nonproductive cough, and weight loss. Pneumonia most commonly occurs with the typhoidal septic form of the disease. The case-fatality rate for typhoidal tularemia is 35% if it is untreated.

Diagnosis requires isolation of the organism in the blood, sputum, skin, or mucus membrane lesions, but this can be difficult because of the unusual growth requirements and of the overgrowth of commensal organisms, in addition to the nonspecific presentation of the typhoidal form of the disease. Serologic studies may be used for retrospective diagnosis.

The drug of choice for treatment is streptomycin (30 mg per kg per day intramuscularly in two divided doses), with other aminoglycosides, such as gentamicin (3–5 mg per kg per day intravenously for 10–14 days), as alternatives.

Tetracycline and chloramphenicol are also effective, but these have been associated with relapses.

Person-to-person spread is unusual, and standard precautions are adequate when caring for ill individuals. For known exposures, prophylaxis with tetracycline, 500 mg orally four times a day for 2 weeks, has been effective if the regimen is begun within 24 hours of exposure (47). A consensus panel recently recommended doxycycline, 100 mg orally twice a day, or ciprofloxacin, 500 mg orally twice a day, as postexposure prophylaxis in a bioterrorism setting (48). In addition, a live attenuated IND vaccine exists, and it has proven effective in preventing disease due to laboratory exposures and aerosol challenge in human volunteers (49).

Viral Hemorrhagic Fevers

Viruses causing hemorrhagic fevers come from the following four different families of RNA viruses: filoviruses (Ebola and Marburg), arenaviruses (Lassa fever), bunyaviruses (Hantavirus, Crimean Congo hemorrhagic fever, and Rift Valley fever), and flaviviruses (yellow fever and dengue). The diseases are host-specific, and they are found in various parts of the world based on the location of the hosts and the disease-specific vectors. Viral hemorrhagic fevers are concerns as biological weapon threats because of the ability to infect via aerosol, their high morbidity and mortality, and their ability to replicate well in cell culture, making large scale production possible.

A viral hemorrhagic fever is a clinical syndrome with clinical features related to damage to the microvasculature system, as well as increased vascular permeability. Patients may initially note fever, myalgias, fatigue, and malaise. Depending on the virulence of the virus, the exposure route, the host factors, and inoculum, the patient's symptoms can evolve to shock and generalized mucous membrane hemorrhage with neurologic, hematologic, or pulmonary complications. Examination may reveal hypotension, injected conjunctivae, petechiae, and ecchymoses, depending on the severity and stage of illness. Mortality varies from 15% in Argentine hemorrhagic fever to as high as 90% in an Ebola outbreak.

The diagnosis of viral hemorrhagic fever should be suspected in anyone presenting with a severe febrile illness and evidence of vascular compromise, such as hypotension, petechiae, easy bruising and bleeding, and dependent edema. Common laboratory features include thrombocytopenia, leukopenia, proteinuria, hematuria, and elevated transaminase levels, although the levels do vary and none are pathognomonic. In a field setting, a positive tourniquet test may be useful, but this is not specific for viral hemorrhagic fevers. The differential diagnosis includes infectious diseases, such as malaria, typhoid fever, rickettsial diseases, leptospirosis, and meningococcemia, as well as noninfectious conditions that may cause disseminated intravascular coagulation.

Laboratory diagnosis can be made with immunoglobulin M (IgM)-specific ELISA, reverse transcriptase PCR, or viral culture. Specialized laboratory containment under biosafety level 3 or 4 is usually required for viral isolation, and it can be performed at the CDC or at the United States Army Medical Research Institute of Infectious Diseases (USAMRIID, Fort Detrick, Frederick, MD).

Contact and droplet precautions are generally adequate for infection control. Ample evidence demonstrates that once these precautions are initiated in a field setting, secondary transmission is halted for those diseases that are transmitted person-to-person. However, enhanced precautions (e.g., gloves, gowns, eye protection, N-100 masks, and negative-pressure isolation) are recommended for patients who are coughing, vomiting, or hemorrhaging because of data that demonstrate these viruses are infectious via small-particle aerosols (50).

Treatment is primarily supportive; however, the investigative antiviral drug ribavirin reduces mortality in patients with Lassa hemorrhagic fever, and it has demonstrated promise with Argentine hemorrhagic fever (Junin virus), hemorrhagic fever with renal syndrome, Crimean-Congo hemorrhagic fever, and Rift Valley fever (51). Ribavirin, however, has not been shown to be effective against Ebola and Marburg hemorrhagic fevers.

Currently, yellow fever vaccine is the only licensed vaccine for a viral hemorrhagic fever. IND have been used to protect laboratory workers against Rift Valley fever and Argentine hemorrhagic fever.

RESPONSE ELEMENTS

Even a small-scale biologic attack with a weapons-grade agent on an urban center could cause massive morbidity and mortality (46), rapidly overwhelming the local medical capabilities. For example, an aerosolized release of little as 100 kg of anthrax spores upwind of a city the size of Washington, D.C. has been estimated to have the potential to cause up to 3 million deaths (52). Planning for mass casualty situations in the past has been directed toward events related to explosions or chemical releases (20). These events occur periodically as a result of industrial spills and accidents, fires, train or air crashes, and other disasters. No simple solution to the problem of biologic defense, which requires a different approach with multiple defense strategies, has been formulated. The strategies that must be incorporated include an accurate threat intelligence, physical countermeasures, medical countermeasures, and the education and training of physicians and ancillary health-care providers, including first responders.

United States intelligence organizations attempt to provide early warning and interdiction of an imminent terrorist attack by gathering information on state-sponsored programs, terrorist groups, doomsday cults, and others that would use biologic agents. Numerous countries are currently suspected of conducting research into biological weapons, and seven of these countries are implicated as sponsors of international terrorism (16,53). Concern that terrorist organizations could obtain expertise or agents from state programs has been voiced, although no evidence indicates that this has already occurred (16).

Environmental detection of biologic agents is a more significant problem than the detection of chemical agents. No effective real-time detector is available for biologic agents, although research continues in this area. The currently available technology includes devices such as the Portal Shield, a detector that samples the air continuously at a rate of 900 L per minute and concentrates particles of 1 to 10 μm. When these particles reach a threshold concentration, an alarm sounds and eight different antibody-based rapid assays screen the sample with turnaround times of approximately 10 minutes. Confirmatory testing on positive samples must be performed at a reference laboratory. The military is currently evaluating and fielding several similar types of detectors. Another technology being evaluated uses laser-induced fluorescence to detect clouds with uniform particle sizes in the 1 to 5 μm range at 30 to 100 km. These devices can reportedly differentiate a biologic aerosol from smoke, fog, industrial pollution, pollen, and so on; and they offer a promising alternative for future advanced stand-off detection systems. For the foreseeable future, these systems will be used primarily for military operations.

Unfortunately, due to the lack of real-time detection equipment, an attack would probably not be identified in enough time to institute personal protection; however, if it were, a full-face respirator should provide adequate protection of the respiratory system and mucous membranes. Other measures, such as a protective suit, are not necessary because intact skin provides an impermeable barrier to nearly all of the classic biological weapon agents, except for the mycotoxins, which are dermally active and for which protective outer garments are needed.

Any HEPA filter respirator, if it is properly fitted at the time of the exposure, will protect against all of the biological weapon agents. Surgical masks are relatively ineffective due to the lack of a seal around the face.

Once an outbreak is evolving, an epidemiologic surveillance system is critical to early identification, whether the outbreak is natural or intentional. A number of epidemiologic clues that individually may not mean an attack has occurred but that should at least raise awareness of the possibility of an unnatural event are listed in Table 34.1 (54).

Unlike a chemical weapon attack, the decontamination of exposed persons and the environment plays a lesser role in a biologic terrorism scenario because agents are non-volatile and they are not dermally active. Effective biologic aerosols with particle sizes ranging from 1 to 5 μm deposit very little residue on environmental surfaces. These particles tend to adhere to environmental surfaces and to larger particles

TABLE 34.1. EPIDEMIOLOGIC CLUES INDICATING A POTENTIAL BIOLOGICAL WEAPONS ATTACK

A point source outbreak with a steep epidemiologic curve.
Severity of a disease that is higher than usual.
Lack of improvement from common treatment modalities.
Unusual presentation or unusual route of exposure of a disease.
Unusual disease for a geographic area or season, especially in the absence of a competent vector.
Multiple simultaneous or successive outbreaks.
Higher attack rates in unprotected areas, lower rates in areas with filtered air supplies.
A downwind pattern of casualty location.
Reverse spread of a zoonotic disease from man to animals.
Similar genetic typing of a pathogen isolated from different sources.
Intelligence sources indicating an adversary with access to agents.
Direct evidence of a release (equipment, munitions, tampering).

From Pavlin JA. Epidemiology of bioterrorism. *EID* 1999;5:528–530; Wiener SL, Barrett J. Biological warfare defense. In: Wiener SL, Barrett J, eds. *Trauma management for civilian and military physicians.* Philadelphia: WB Saunders, 1986:508–509; with permission.

ticles due to electrostatic and van der Waals forces. Thus, the likelihood of a secondary aerosol forming via reaerosolization of these particles by wind, vehicular traffic, or other mechanical agitation is quite low. Empiric analyses by Chinn and United States Army scientists in Utah have demonstrated no significant threat to persons on active roads or runways that are contaminated with one million bacillus spores per square meter (55). The environmental decontamination of large areas should be evaluated on a case-by-case basis with proper consultation.

Because of the incubation period of biologic agents, by the time someone becomes ill, they possibly have already washed and changed clothes. In rare cases where individuals become heavily contaminated, the simple removal of clothing, followed by showering with soap and water, would remove over 99.99% of the agent (56); this course is recommended by the CDC for anthrax decontamination (30). For grossly contaminated environmental surfaces or personal effects, the use of a 0.5% hypochlorite solution with a contact time of 10 to 15 minutes is recommended, although any of the standard disinfectants (iodophores, phenolics) are effective against all classes of agents, including spores. Even a 0.1% bleach solution (household bleach that is diluted to 1 part bleach per 50 parts water) will kill over 90% of bacterial spores within 30 seconds at room temperature (57).

Early diagnosis can be critical to saving lives after a biological weapon release. Unfortunately, clinical diagnosis is often difficult because many of these diseases present initially as nonspecific febrile illnesses. Therefore, laboratory confirmation is particularly important with suspected biologic terrorism patients. Samples that the clinician should consider obtaining for study are listed in Table 34.2. Most laboratories can do the crucial initial evaluation with light microscopy, primary culture, and serology. Rapid antibody-based assay detector kits that can provide presumptive identification within 30 minutes have been developed by the military and for commercial purposes. Problems with these types of detectors include poor specificity and sensitivities requiring detection levels higher than that of the infectious dose. Antibody-based and handheld assays must have appropriate confirmatory laboratory backup with culture studies. As PCR and specific DNA probes become more widely available, these assays will provide rapid results that are both sensitive and specific. A gene amplification (PCR) assay that fits in a briefcase has been developed by USAM-RIID, of which the largest part is the notebook computer. A much smaller, handheld prototype is in advanced development (*personal communication*, Erik Henchal, 2001).

Standard precautions are generally adequate to the prevent transmission of disease to care providers from a patient infected by a biological weapon because most of the agents of concern are not contagious. Additional precautions are needed for smallpox, pneumonic plague, and viral hemorrhagic fevers, as were discussed in their respective sections.

The remains of some bioterrorism victims may pose a hazard to pathologists, undertakers, and so on. Appropriate personal protection should be used during the performance of autopsies, including standard precautions and use of eye and mucous membrane protection during the generation of aerosols and blood and body fluid splashes (25). Cremation is the most effective method for rendering a corpse completely safe for burial. This ensures the destruction of even the most environmentally stable organisms or toxins, such as anthrax spores or mycotoxins. Other methods that should be considered include treatment with a bleach solution or placement in sealed body bags.

Biologic agents cause diseases that are not part of everyday clinical practice, nor are they even discussed in medical school curricula; therefore, one aspect of preparation for a biologic attack is the education of health-care providers. Because they may be the first to see ill patients, physicians and other health-care providers must become familiar with the syndromes associated with bioterrorism. Unfortunately, recent efforts to this end have reached only a small percentage of physicians in the United States. The Nunn-Lugar-Domenici 120-city domestic preparedness training program has had difficulty attracting physicians, and the USAMRIID satellite distance learning program is only broadcast twice per year. This distance learning program, however, has reached over 50,000 health-care providers over a 4-year period at a very efficient cost per provider. However, a tremendous need to reach many more providers still exists. Resources include the *Medical aspects of chemical and biological warfare*, part of the Textbook of Military Medicine series, (58) and USAMRIID's pocket "blue book" on the treatment of biological weapons casualties (59). Several journals have recently dedicated parts of issues to the subject of biological weapons (60–62), and the *JAMA* has a series of consensus articles arranged by the Johns Hopkins University Center for Civilian Biodefense (24,38,43,48,63). Information is also available on the Internet (Table 34.3).

Preparation for and response to an attack with a biological weapon requires resources beyond the capabilities of most local governments (64). The federal government is taking substantial measures toward national preparedness with the Presidential Decision Directives (PDD) 39 (1995) and PDD-62 and PDD-63 (1998). These directives formalize the Federal Response Plan (FRP) by defining responsibilities and relationships among federal agencies responding to a disaster. In the plan, the Federal Bureau of Investigation is designated to handle crisis management, which involves immediate threat resolution and the subsequent criminal investigation (see Chapter 12). Manage-

TABLE 34.2. CLINICAL LABORATORY SPECIMENS TO BE COLLECTED IN A SUSPECTED BIOLOGIC WEAPON OUTBREAK

0–24 hr
  Nasal and throat swabs or induced respiratory secretions for culture, FA, or PCR
24–72 hr
  Serum for toxin assays
  Blood for PCR and culture
  Sputum for FA, PCR, and culture
3–10 d
  Serum for toxin assays and IgM or IgG agglutination titers
  Blood and tissues for culture
  Pathologic samples

Abbreviations: FA, fluorescent antibody; PCR, polymerase chain reaction.
From Kortepeter M, Christopher G, Cieslak T, et al., eds. *Medical management of biological casualties handbook*, 4th ed. Frederick, MD: United States Army Medical Research Institute of Infectious Diseases, 2001, with permission.
Note: these are general recommendations for specimens. Certain diseases may have specific samples that need to be drawn.

TABLE 34.3. SELECTED WEBSITES FOR INFORMATION ON BIOLOGIC WEAPONS

http://www.anthrax.osd.mil (Department of Defense anthrax information)
http://www.apic.org/bioterror (APIC Bioterrorism Readiness Plan)
http://www.cdc.gov (General CDC information)
http://www.hopkins-biodefense.org (Johns Hopkins Center for Civilian Biodefense)
http://www.nbc-med.org (The United States Army Nuclear, Chemical, Biological Weapon Information Site)
http://www.oep-ndms.dhhs.gov (Office of Emergency Preparedness)

Abbreviations: APIC, Association for Professions in Infection Control and Epidemiology, Inc.; CDC, Centers for Disease Control and Prevention.

ment of the consequences of a biologic release is the responsibility of the Federal Emergency Management Agency. Both crisis and consequence management may take place simultaneously, and the transition from one to another may not be well defined. Emergency support function 8 of the FRP gives the responsibility for oversight of health and medical services to the Department of Health and Human Services (DHHS). The office of emergency preparedness of DHHS has organized three echelons of medical response teams, namely the 0-minute to 90-minute response Metropolitan Medical Response System, the 4-hour response national medical response teams, and the 8-hour to 16-hour response disaster medical assistance teams.

The Department of Defense has been given multiple responsibilities in the FRP in support of nonmilitary governmental agencies. Unique military assets that would be helpful in a biologic response include the USAMRIID for emergency medical consultation and reference laboratory support; the United States Marine Corps' Chemical and Biological Incident Response Force for reconnaissance, initial triage, and the decontamination of casualties; and the United States Army's Technical Escort Unit for sampling, transport, and disposal of dissemination devices. A chemical and biologic rapid response team can call upon various assets, such as laboratory, technical escort unit personnel, and medical management experts at USAMRIID, to provide incident on-site consultation. The military has also fielded six disaster Special Medical Augmentation Response teams (SMART), one which specializes in chemical and biologic response. Two other teams combine civilian law enforcement, laboratory capabilities, and medical consultation for domestic (the domestic emergency response team, which is headed by the Federal Bureau of Investigation) and for foreign (the foreign emergency response team, which is headed by the State Department) emergencies. The use of any military assets serves a supportive role for civilian authorities. Finally, the National Guard has assembled ten rapid assessment and initial detection teams of 22 full-time personnel for local support to the governors in each federal region. Federal detection and response assets are most effective if they are prepositioned on-site for high-profile events, such as the Olympic games, presidential inaugurations, or NATO summits. If intelligence sources indicate a heightened threat level for other venues, then similar prepositioning and increased vigilance can occur. The CDC also plays an important role in the FRP, and it recently received supplemental funding that has been used to set up a center for bioterrorism, to enhance existing state public health laboratories, to improve surveillance systems, to build a national stockpile of key pharmaceutical agents, and to develop rapid communication systems. The CDC's emergency preparedness and response branch has a 24-hour help line (770-488-7100). The soldier biologic and chemical command has a 24-hour hotline for consultation (800-424-8802), and USAMRIID experts are available for consultation at 888-USA-RIID (888-872-7443).

SUMMARY

In a real biological weapon attack, local, state, and federal assets (military and nonmilitary) need to work together to mitigate the crisis. Unfortunately, the need for this was underscored by the events of the fall of 2001, in which the first case of inhalational anthrax was seen in this country in more than 20 years. As organizations regroup and reevaluate the current multifaceted efforts at improving intelligence, detection, surveillance, diagnostics, treatment, and response team capabilities, law enforcement, medical, and public health professionals should enhance areas of potential response needs and should continue to minimize lives lost via a coordinated response.

REFERENCES

1. Mobley JA. Biological warfare in the twentieth century: lessons from the past, challenges for the future. *Mil Med* 1995;160:547–553.
2. Kortepeter MG, Parker GW. Potential biological weapons threats. *Emerging Infect Dis* 1999;5:523–527.
3. Khan AS, Ashford DA, Craven RB, et al. Biological and chemical terrorism: strategic plan for preparedness and response. Recommendations of the CDC strategic planning workgroup. *MMWR* 2000;49:1–14.
4. Christopher GW, Cieslak TJ, Pavlin JA, et al. Biological warfare, a historical perspective. *JAMA* 1997;278:412-417.
5. Robertson AG, Robertson LJ. From Asps to Allegations: biological warfare in history. *Mil Med* 1995;160:369–373.
6. Derbes VJ. DeMussis and the Great Plague of 1348, a forgotten episode of bacteriological warfare. *JAMA* 1966;196:179–182.
7. Harris SH. *Factories of death*. New York: Routledge, 1994.
8. Harris S. Japanese biological warfare research on humans: a case study of microbiology and ethics. *Ann N Y Acad Sci* 1992;666:21–52.
9. Manchee RJ, Stewart WDP. The decontamination of Gruinard Island. *Chem Britain* 1988;July:690–691.
10. Covert NM. *Cutting edge, a history of Fort Detrick, Maryland*. Fort Detrick, MD: Public Affairs Office, 1997.
11. Department of the Army. *U.S. Army activity in the U.S. biological warfare programs*, Vol. II. Publication DTIC B193427L. Washington, D.C.: Department of Defense, United States Army, 1977.
12. Zilinskas RA. Iraq's biological weapons, the past as future? *JAMA* 1997;278:418–424.
13. Alibek K, Handelman S. *Biohazard*. New York: Random House, 1999.
14. Convention on the prohibition of the development production and stockpiling of bacteriological (biological) and toxin weapons and on their destruction, signed 10 April 1972. In: Dando M, ed. *Biological warfare in the 21st century, biotechnology and the proliferation of biological weapons*. New York: Macmillan Publishing, 1994:234–239.
15. Olson KB. Aum Shinrikyo: once and future threat?. *Emerging Infect Dis* 1999;5:513–516.
16. Carus WS. *Bioterrorism and biocrimes: the illicit use of biological agents in the 20th century*, rev. Working paper. Washington, D.C.: Center for Counterproliferation Research, National Defense University, 1999.
17. Clinton WM. Letter to the Speaker of the House of Representatives and President of the Senate. The Australia Group forum of

states to limit proliferation of chemical and biological weapons-related items. January 13, 1999.

18. Chemical-Biological Expert Panel. United Nations, 1969.

19. Departments of the Army, Navy, and Air Force. *NATO handbook on the medical aspects of NBC defensive operations.* Washington DC: Department of the Army, 1996.

20. Henderson DA. The looming threat of bioterrorism. *Science* 1999;283:1279–1282.

21. Pile JC, Malone JD, Eitzen EM, et al. Anthrax as a potential biological warfare agent. *Arch Intern Med* 1998;158:429–434.

22. Brachman PS. Inhalation anthrax. *Ann N Y Acad Sci* 1980;353: 83–93.

23. Jernigan JA, Stephens DS, Ashford DA, et al. Bioterrorism-related inhalational anthrax: the first 10 cases reported in the United States. *Emerging Infect Dis* 2001;7:423—425.

24. Inglesby TV, Henderson DA, Bartlett JG, et al. Anthrax as a biological weapon, medical and public health management. *JAMA* 1999;281:1735–1745.

25. English JF, Cundiff MY, Malone JD, et al. Bioterrorism readiness plan: a template for healthcare facilities. Available at: http://www.apic.org/. Accessed April 13, 1999.

26. Meselson M, Gillemin J, Hugh-Jones M, et al. The Sverdlovsk anthrax outbreak of 1979. *Science* 1994;209:1202–1208.

27. Jackson PJ, Hugh-Jones ME, Adair DM, et al. PCR analysis of tissue samples from the 1979 Sverdlovsk anthrax victims: the presence of multiple *Bacillus anthracis* strains in different victims. *Proceed Natl Acad Sci* 1998;95:1224–1229.

28. Abramova FA, Grinberg LM, Yampolskaya, et al. Pathology of inhalational anthrax in 42 cases from the Sverdlovsk outbreak of 1979. *Proceed Natl Acad Sci* 1993;90:2291–2294.

29. Malecki J, Wiersma S, Cahill K, et al. Update: investigation of bioterrorism-related anthrax and interim guidelines for exposure management and antimicrobial therapy. *MMWR* 2001;50: 909–919.

30. Centers for Disease Control and Prevention. Bioterrorism alleging use of anthrax and interim guidelines for management—United States, 1998. *MMWR* 1999;48:69–74.

31. Dixon TC, Meselson M, Guillemin K, et al. Anthrax. *N Engl J Med* 1999;341:815–826.

32. Henderson DW, Peacock S, Belton FC. Observations on the prophylaxis of experimental pulmonary anthrax in the monkey. *J Hygiene* 1956;54:28–36.

33. Friedlander AM, Welkos SL, Pitt MLM, et al. Postexposure prophylaxis against experimental inhalation anthrax. *J Infect Dis* 1993;167:1239–1242.

34. Glassman HN. Industrial inhalation anthrax. *Bacteriol Rev* 1966; 30:657–659.

35. Ivins BE, Fellows PF, Pitt MLM. Efficacy of standard human anthrax vaccine against Bacillus anthracis aerosol spore challenge in rhesus monkeys. *Salisbury Med Bull* 1996;87:125–126.

36. Barquet N, Domingo P. Smallpox: the triumph over the most terrible of the ministers of death. *Ann Intern Med* 1997;127: 635–642.

37. Davis CJ. Nuclear blindness: an overview of the biological weapons programs of the former Soviet Union and Iraq. *Emerging Infect Dis* 1999;5:509–512.

38. O'Toole T. Smallpox: an attack scenario. *Emerging Infect Dis* 1999;5:540–546.

39. Henderson DA, Inglesby TV, Bartlett JG. Smallpox as a biological weapon, medical and public health management. *JAMA* 1999;281:2127–2137.

40. Dixon CW. Smallpox in Tripolitania, 1946: an epidemiological and clinical study of 500 cases, including trials of penicillin treatment. *J Hygiene* 1948;46:351–377.

41. LeDuc JW, Becher J. Current status of smallpox vaccine. *Emerging Infect Dis* 1999;5:593–594.

42. McGovern TW, Friedlander AM. Plague. In: Sidell FR, Takafuji ET, Franz DR, eds. *Medical aspects of chemical and biological warfare.* Washington, D.C.: Borden Institute, 1997:479–502. Textbook of military medicine series.

43. Inglesby TV, Dennis DT, Henderson DA, et al. Plague as a biological weapon-medical and public health management. *JAMA* 2000;283:2281–2290.

44. Benenson AS, ed. *Control of communicable diseases manual,* 16th ed. Washington, D.C.: American Public Health Association, 1995.

45. Middlebrook JL, Franz DR. Botulinum toxins. In: Sidell FR, Takafuji ET, Franz DR, eds. *Medical aspects of chemical and biological warfare.* Washington, D.C.: Borden Institute, 1997: 643–654. Textbook of military medicine series.

46. World Health Organization group of consultants. *Health aspects of chemical and biological weapons.* Geneva: World Health Organization, 1970.

47. Sawyer WD, Dangerfield HG, Hogge AL, et al. Antibiotic prophylaxis and therapy of airborne tularemia. *Bacteriol Rev* 1966; 30:542–548.

48. Inglesby TV, Dennis DT, Henderson DA, et al. Tularemia as a biological weapon—medical and public health management. *JAMA* 2001;285:2763–2773.

49. Evans ME, Friedlander AM. Tularemia. In: Sidell FR, Takafuji ET, Franz DR, eds. *Medical aspects of chemical and biological warfare.* Washington, D.C.: Borden Institute, 1997:503–512. Textbook of military medicine series.

50. Centers for Disease Control and Prevention. Management of patients with suspected viral hemorrhagic fever. *MMWR* 1988; 37:1–16.

51. Huggins JW. Prospects for treatment of viral hemorrhagic fevers with ribavirin, a broad-spectrum antiviral drug. *Rev Infect Dis* 1989;11:S750–S761.

52. Office of Technology Assessment. *Proliferation of weapons of mass destruction.* Publication OTA-ISC-559. Washington, D.C.: United States Government Printing Office, 1993:53–55.

53. Office of the Secretary of Defense. *Proliferation: threat and response.* Washington, D.C.: United States Government Printing Office, 1997.

54. Pavlin JA. Epidemiology of bioterrorism. *Emerging Infect Dis* 1999;5:528–530.

55. Chinn KS. *Reaerosolization hazard assessment for biological agent-contaminated hardstand areas.* Publication DPG/JCP-96/012. Dugway Proving Ground, UT: United States Department of the Army, Life Sciences Division, 1996:1–40.

56. National Institute of Occupational Safety and Health, Occupational Safety and Health Administration, United States Coast Guard, Environmental Protection Agency. *Occupational safety and health guidance manual for hazardous waste site activities.* Atlanta: Department of Health and Human Services, 1995; 10.1–10.3.

57. Rutala W, Weber D. Uses of inorganic hypochlorite (bleach) in health-care facilities. *Clin Microbiol Rev* 1997;10:597–610.

58. Sidell FR, Takafuji ET, Franz DR, eds. *Medical aspects of chemical and biological warfare.* Washington, D.C.: Borden Institute, 1997. Textbook of military medicine series.

59. Kortepeter M, Christopher G, Cieslak T, et al., eds. *Medical management of biological casualties handbook,* 4th ed. Fort Detrick, MD: United States Army Medical Research Institute of Infectious Diseases, 2001.

60. Torok TJ, Tauxe RV, Wise RP, et al. A large community outbreak of salmonellosis caused by intentional contamination of restaurant salad bars. *JAMA* 1997;278:389–395.

60a. Kolavic SA, Kimura A, Simons SL, et al. An outbreak of Shigella dysenteriae type 2 among laboratory workers due to intentional food contamination. *JAMA* 1997;278:396–398.

60b. Franz DR, Jahrling PB, Friedlander AM, et al. Clinical recognition and management of patients exposed to biological warfare agents. *JAMA* 1997;278:399–411.

60c. Christopher GW, Cieslak TJ, Pavlin JA, Eitzen EM Jr. Biological warfare. A historical perspective. *JAMA* 1997;278:412–417.

60d. Zilinskas RA. Iraq's biological weapons. The past as future? *JAMA* 1997;278:418–424.

60e. Holloway HC, Norwood AE, Fullerton CS, et al. The threat of biological weapons. Prophylaxis and mitigation of psychological and social consequences. *JAMA* 1997;278:425–427.

60f. Simon JD. Biological terrorism. Preparing to meet the threat. *JAMA* 1997;278:428–430.

60g. Danzig R, Berkowsky PB. Why should we be concerned about biological warfare? *JAMA* 1997;278:431–432.

60h. Shapiro RL, Hatheway C, Becher J, Swerdlow DL. Botulism sur-

veillance and emergency response. A public health strategy for a global challenge. *JAMA* 1997;278:433–435.

61. Pesik N, Keim M, Sampson TR. Do US emergency medicine residency programs provide adequate training for bioterrorism? *Ann Emerg Med* 1999;34:173–176.

62. Proceedings of the National Symposium on Medical and Public Health Response to Bioterrorism. Arlington, VA, USA. February 16–17, 1999. *Emerging Infect Dis* 1999;5:491–592.

63. Arnon SS, Schechter R, Inglesby TV, et al. Botulinum toxin as a biological weapon-medical and public health management. *JAMA* 2001;285:1059–1070.

64. Wiener SL, Barrett J. Biological warfare defense. In: Wiener SL, Barrett J, eds. *Trauma management for civilian and military physicians*. Philadelphia: WB Saunders, 1986:508–509.

35

TACTICAL EMERGENCY MEDICINE

JOSHUA S. VAYER

CONCEPT OF TACTICAL EMERGENCY MEDICINE

The concept of providing care to casualties in austere and harsh environments is not new. However, in recent history, this practice has become more established and more evidence-based than ever before. Elements of tactical medicine are shared with many other disciplines, including disaster medicine, wilderness medicine, humanitarian assistance, and urban search and rescue. The common thread is the maximization of clinical outcome in a resource-poor, prolonged-transport environment, while minimizing the threat to the provider.

Tactical emergency medical support (TEMS) is increasingly recognized as a special interest subset of emergency medicine, and it has gained widespread acceptance within both the law enforcement and medical communities (1–12). In the United States, most federal and many state and local law enforcement agencies have tactical medical support programs operating regionally, nationally, and internationally. Many other countries, including Canada and the United Kingdom, have also initiated TEMS efforts. TEMS is the practice of out-of-hospital medicine that is dedicated to enhancing the probability of special operations mission success. In law enforcement, special operations denotes those activities that are too dangerous, too complex, and/or too technically sophisticated to assign them to uniformed patrol units. These missions are handled by special teams that emphasize training, coordination and speed, stealth, and violence of action to ensure success. They often use advanced technologies, such as less lethal weapons systems, communications, armor, remote imaging, acoustic capture devices, and similar equipment. Special operations teams are generally comprised of the fittest, fastest, brightest, and most motivated personnel. The units are called by a wide variety of names, including special weapons and tac-

tics (SWAT), special response team, hostage rescue team, counter assault team, emergency response team, and special operations unit. The principles of TEMS apply to other kinds of specialty teams as well, such as dignitary protection, dive rescue, and explosive ordnance disposal.

Improving the accomplishment of the law enforcement mission is the primary goal of TEMS (13). Underlying this goal is the belief that the law enforcement mission serves the best interests of the society and that successful accomplishment is thus beneficial. Medical resources are a precious commodity within the tactical environment, and they must be allocated in the manner that assures the greatest overall good for the most number of people. However, practitioners of this specialty must diligently guard against the unethical use of medicine to achieve goals that are inconsistent with the best interests of the society and against carrying the "greater good" argument to intangible levels that cannot be reasonably supported. During wartime, the dignity of man, as well as the conventions among civilized nations, require that wounded combatants receive humane treatment, including medical care, regardless of their allegiance. Similarly, police officers, perpetrators, suspects, and innocent parties who become casualties during a law enforcement operation are all entitled to timely and competent care. Casualties, and especially fatalities, although they are not entirely avoidable in the special operations arena, are always undesirable.

Other benefits of tactical medicine exist beyond improving the probability of mission success. First, a well-managed TEMS program reduces mortality and morbidity among officers, perpetrators, and innocents. It is also likely to reduce line-of-duty injury and disability costs for public safety agencies. Third, the reduction of lost work time for these officers is a significant benefit of tactical medicine. Manpower is the most precious resource of any specialty team. Members have expertise, qualifications, and certifications that have usually been acquired over long time periods, so they cannot be readily replaced by lesser-trained police officers. The tactical team often have to work short-handed if a member is injured. Fourth, the impact that a

The opinions expressed in this chapter are those of the author. They do not necessarily reflect the opinions or policies of the Uniformed Services University, the Department of Defense, or the United States Government.

TEMS program can have on the morale of the team is often underestimated. Team members are expected to take enormous risks in dangerous situations. Their willingness to engage in the mission fully, at a time when life-and-death decisions must be made in fractions of a second, is enhanced by the perception that the best possible medical care is immediately available if they are injured. Finally, the provision of far-forward medical care can enhance an agency's position in what is already a liability-prone situation. The actions of the tactical team invariably contribute to the creation of hazard. Some situations, of necessity, become temporarily less stable in the process of resolution. To create a hazard and to recognize that people might be injured, yet to fail to provide for that hazard, may create liability for the law enforcement agency.

Tactical teams are specially trained and equipped to handle extraordinary law enforcement situations (14). They take the assignments that are too dangerous or too technically complex to be handled by ordinary police procedures, and, as a result, they are consistently pushed to their performance limits. Specialized medical support provided by practitioners trained and skilled in this field is one of the tools that allows special operations teams to push themselves to that limit while maintaining reasonable safety.

Some fire or rescue chiefs and emergency medical services (EMS) directors may object to their personnel practicing tactical medicine because their perception is that it is too dangerous. When they are asked in response why they allow firefighters under their command to enter burning buildings—another clearly dangerous situation—they often respond that firefighting is different from law enforcement operations because the personnel are well trained and they are appropriately equipped against the fire threat. The same argument should hold true for TEMS. Command officers should not allow EMS personnel who are poorly trained and ill equipped for this assignment to enter a secure police perimeter. However, if medical teams simply wait for the patient to be delivered outside the perimeter, the result will be the unnecessary loss of life; far-forward medical care, however, has been shown to reduce mortality (15,16). The obvious solution then to this dilemma is to provide support of law enforcement special operations via well-trained and properly equipped medics who can operate safely within the perimeter.

The daily routine doctrine is the term coined to describe a basic axiom of disaster response. This states that the activities that one does all the time will be performed reasonably well during a crisis but that those things that are done *only* in response to the crisis will be poorly executed (17). Therefore, the best approach is for tactical medics to train on a regular basis with the elements they support and for them to be fully integrated into every operation. This ensures that the medical component remains an asset to the team, not a burden or obstacle to successful mission accomplishment.

TACTICAL EMERGENCY MEDICINE MODELS

Many different models are being used to deliver tactical emergency medical support successfully in the United States today. These can be best understood by analyzing who the providers are and how they are integrated with the tactical team. Moreover, the structure of a TEMS element is a local decision that is affected by the budget, political and organizational considerations, insurance coverage, local EMS configurations, and the state's statutory requirements.

The primary medical provider used by SWAT teams can range from physicians to basic emergency medical technicians (EMT-B). A physician obviously brings a desirable level of expertise, he or she generally has good lines of communication with the hospital-based medical community, and he or she does not require a medical control mechanism. On the other hand, a physician can be prohibitively expensive, he or she may not have the availability to respond on emergency call-outs, and he or she is less likely to have the necessary tactical experience or field training.

Experienced paramedics may be the best option in most jurisdictions. These providers will generally have an appropriate level of field experience, although he or she is not likely to have tactical training. Paramedics are affordable, they can be scheduled for round-the-clock availability, they are accustomed to working within a chain of command, and they bring an appropriate level of skill to bear. While most of the emergency procedures performed inside the hot zone will be at the level of basic life support (18), the advanced skills of the paramedic form an appropriate foundation for the expansion of the scope of practice to meet the need for ambulatory care, preventive medicine, and field sanitation and hygiene. A robust medical control mechanism that relies heavily on standing orders will be required because the on-line communications that are often used in conventional emergency medical services systems may not be possible within the area of tactical operations due to operational security concerns and logistics. Continuing education and clinical practice opportunities will be needed for the maintenance of skills and certification.

Well-trained and experienced basic emergency medical technicians have the skills that are necessary to provide the most care that is delivered in the hot zone. In many regions, they are also the providers who are most likely to be available, especially for emergency, short notice responses. Maintenance of EMT-B certification and skills is less costly and time-consuming than it is for the other levels of providers described. However, like the paramedics, EMT-Bs require medical control, and the lack of advanced life support skills may have devastating consequences in a small number of cases. EMT-B personnel are generally not well equipped for performing the additional duties that are part of an expanded scope of practice for tactical medics.

Although nurses have occasionally been used in this role as the primary medical provider, this approach has been largely unsuccessful unless the nurse also has qualifications as a paramedic or flight nurse. Nurses without this specialized background have all of the disadvantages of traditional prehospital providers, and they lack expertise in field operations.

In some jurisdictions, the tactical medic is a fully sworn law enforcement officer with arrest powers, while in other jurisdictions, he or she is an employee of another public safety agency, such as fire and rescue or EMS. Still other successful models use reserve (i.e., part-time or uncompensated) law enforcement officers or volunteers as their tactical medical officer. The "best" configuration varies from location to location, depending on variables specific to that community. However, in structuring a special operations medical element, remembering that the job of tactical medic requires full time and attention while it is being performed is important. The "one person–one job" rule applies for the task to be done well and to avoid role confusion. This concept should be imbedded into the team's operational policy. A tactical medic who is also a sworn officer should not be both the point man leading the team into a dangerous environment and the team medic for the same operation. Both functions are crucial, and both require undivided attention. Therefore, neither function will be done well if both are assigned to a single individual.

The arming of tactical medical providers is a controversial subject (9,19). Tactical medics operate in a high-risk environment, and part of the proper equipment and training can reasonably include defensive weapons. In fact, military medics have a duty to defend patients under their care (10). This helps to ensure that the safety and security of the medical support operation does not become a burden that degrades the capability of the tactical team. On the other hand, the team always bears some responsibility for the medics' safety, just as they do for all other elements of the team. No right or wrong answer to the question of arming these providers exists, so consideration must be given to local circumstances, regulations, and statutes. If medics are armed, they must have legal authority for this, they must train and qualify in order to meet the law enforcement standard, and they must not confuse their role with that of the other team members. A provider who is caring for a patient in an active tactical zone cannot provide adequate security for himself while still focusing on clinical responsibilities. His security and the extraction of the patient then become responsibilities of the team as a whole. A study by Smock et al. (20) surveyed 30 physicians who had completed a tactical medicine training program and who were actively practicing TEMS. Fifty-three percent of the physicians were sworn officers, and 66% were armed while working with the team (20). In the United States, examples of extremely successful TEMS programs both with and without armed

medics are found, and this issue does not need to be an impediment to program development.

ZONES OF CARE

Law enforcement tactical operations are usually described in terms of an inner perimeter and an outer perimeter (14). The inner perimeter is the geographical area within which police will contain the incident. It is usually represented as a circle around the crisis site, and it is controlled by members of the SWAT team. The outer perimeter is the boundary that isolates the incident, and it represents the area from which the public will be excluded as a safety measure. It is often represented as a larger circle surrounding the inner perimeter, and it is manned by law enforcement personnel other than the SWAT team, usually patrol officers. The concept of an inner and outer perimeter is useful in police operations where decision making is focused on containing and isolating an incident, protecting the public, and controlling the threat. Tactical medical officers need to understand this terminology because of its use in describing tactical options. However, these boundaries are not as applicable to the way in which medical decisions must be made in the tactical environment, despite their frequent use in that context. The particular medical interventions used, the manner of extraction, and the timing of both are highly dependent on the specific threat level present at the casualty's specific location. The perimeter construct is too broad to permit either the reasonable definition of the threat at a particular location or meaningful medical decision making. Instead, a three-level characterization of the threat as hot, warm, or cold is used to describe zones of care (10). The zones of care do not need to be contiguous or concentric, but they may be irregularly shaped areas defined by multiple variables, including the available intelligence, the accessibility of cover and concealment (cover provides protection from the threat [e.g., a masonry wall through which a bullet cannot pass], whereas concealment merely hides one's location from the assailant), the weapons in use, the terrain features, the threat-to-target distance, visibility, countersniper coverage, and reactive firepower.

The hot zone is an area where the threat is direct and immediate. What constitutes a direct and immediate threat is determined subjectively, and it may vary depending on the many variables cited previously. However, in general, this term refers to those environments where little protection is available for both patient and provider and in which the probability of additional injury is high. An officer down in the front yard of a building with a gunman shooting from a window exemplifies the typical hot zone.

The hot zone is an extremely dangerous environment, and treatment here entails enormous risk. Generally, the only appropriate care is extraction to a safer area, although contemporaneous, momentary lifesaving interventions, such as manual airway maneuvers, may be possible. Self-care may also be possible, especially with guidance from the medic. The medical officer should evaluate the patient from appropriate cover by using rapid and remote assessment methodology (RAM) techniques (see below) before a rescue is initiated (19). The greater good may be served by delaying the extraction of a viable patient until additional resources are in place because of the extraordinary risk or the low probability of success for retrieving the patient. Patients who can extract themselves should do so, and body recoveries should be delayed until the scene is secure.

The cold zone is the area where no reasonable threat exists. This may be due to distance from the crisis site, the employment of cover, interposition of firepower, or a material barrier between the threat and the patient and provider. Care in the cold zone is almost identical to everyday out-of-hospital care, although careful consideration should be given to the recognition and forensic preservation of evidentiary material.

The warm zone is the area where a threat persists but in which it is neither direct nor immediate. For example, in the case of the officer down in the front yard, the gunman may no longer be in the window of the building but whether he has left the scene is still unknown. The severity of the threat can vary considerably; and, therefore, some warm zones are cooler than others, and actions must be adjusted accordingly. These situations are when the difficult decisions of TEMS must be made. The benefit of immediate intervention must be weighed against the risk of additional harm to both the patient and the provider. This environment has been insufficiently modeled and the variables are not yet well enough understood to permit an algorithmic approach to warm zone decision making. The special operations medic must be capable of critically analyzing numerous factors and finding the right balance between risk and benefit. Traditional EMS interventions may be inappropriate. For example, spinal immobilization is of relatively little value in penetrating neck wounds, and it is time-consuming, thus exposing rescuers and casualty to additional danger (21,22). Moreover, cardiopulmonary resuscitation for cardiac arrest secondary to trauma has no place in the tactical environment (10,23–27). (The possible exceptions are arrest due to near-drowning, electrocution, hypothermia, and toxic exposure, when artificial ventilation may enable a successful resuscitation.) Interventions such as hemorrhage control may be truly lifesaving.

Not only must one consider the risks associated with the particular threat zone in which the patient is located, but the danger associated with extraction must be part of the overall assessment. This danger, which is called transit risk, consists of three components. First, one must consider the amount of time moving the patient to a safer area will take. Some areas of operation can have huge hot and warm zones because the perpetrator has a commanding field of fire, which results in long transit times. For example, in the

1966 Texas Tower sniper incident, a former Marine barricaded himself on the 28th floor observation deck of the University of Texas Administration Building and killed people who were blocks away, thus creating a hot zone that included much of the central campus (28). However, time can be an inconsequential factor if moving a patient to a more secure area takes only a few seconds. The second component of transit risk is the route of travel. Because the zones of care are irregularly shaped, discontinuous geographic areas, pockets of warm zone may be contained within seas of hot zone; in this situation, jumping from one warm zone to another can reduce the risk of traversing the hot zone. At times, crossing into a hotter area to get to a cooler one may be necessary, in which case the value of treating in place and deferring extraction must be considered. The ability to deliver care during transit is the third component of transit risk. Some interventions cannot be adequately maintained during extraction, and, in these, the effect of discontinuing care on clinical condition is a factor. For example, maintaining a manual jaw thrust maneuver will be impossible if the extraction includes a running litter carry across a hot zone, and taking the time to insert an airway adjunct may be necessary before evacuating the casualty. The concept of transit risk can be summarized by the formula

$$\text{Transit Risk} = t \times R \times C$$

where t is the risk associated with transit time, R is the risk incurred due to the route of travel, and C is the risk associated with the difficulty providing essential care during transit.

RESPONSIBILITIES OF THE TACTICAL MEDICAL OFFICER

The maintenance of team effectiveness and capability is a command responsibility, and therefore the health and safety of personnel is ultimately a responsibility of the team commander that cannot be abrogated. The authority to make all decisions affecting the team, including the allocation and timing of resources for medical support, is reserved to the commander (10). The role of the tactical medical officer is to provide information and advice to the commander so that his or her decisions are well informed and so that he or she fully understands the consequences of any medical risk imposed on personnel. This is an unusual position for emergency medical personnel as, during a medical emergency, the delivery of care is usually the primary objective and the provider has sole responsibility for setting priorities. In the tactical setting, many other considerations may override medical requirements, and tactical medics must understand this if they are to maximize their effectiveness.

The medic meets his or her responsibility to the commander in many different ways. The most obvious is that he or she must be prepared to provide appropriate emergency care for the spectrum of injury that can be seen during a law enforcement operation. Because the tactical environment is by definition high risk and resource-poor, he or she must plan to provide this care with the minimal equipment that can be reasonably carried. The medic should be knowledgeable about the patterns of injury that are likely for a given mission profile and should modify the equipment load-out accordingly.

When the reader considers the fact that the primary goal of TEMS is to enhance the probability of mission success, then the idea that the medic's responsibilities go far beyond emergency care is obvious. In fact, the greatest benefit to the team will probably be derived from injury control, preventive medicine, and health promotion activities. These are interventions that help to keep the team performing at its peak and that support the primary goal of TEMS. This concept translates into actions such as contributing to the development of fitness and nutrition programs, reviewing personal protective equipment and ensuring its use, monitoring the health status of the team, instituting measures to prevent the transmission of infectious disease when necessary, and ensuring proper immunization status.

The medic also has an important role in the mission-planning process. He or she should be responsible for the development and evaluation of medical intelligence. This intelligence may relate to an assessment of the medical threats, the evaluation of suspect or hostage medical histories, and the investigation of resources available for care. Whenever circumstances permit, the medic should provide a written medical annex that details the concept and the mechanics of medical support so that the commander can include it with the operational order. Before a mission, he or she should remain apprised of evolving tactical options and should be vigilant for factors that may affect the health and safety of any involved individual. Waiting for tactical operators to request medical consultation is disadvantageous to the commander because a medically naïve operator may not even recognize the more subtle opportunities for benefitting from medical insight.

During a mission, the medical officer should identify causes of performance decrement for the commander and should recommend solutions that enhance the team's capability. For example, many SWAT teams are unaccustomed to prolonged operations. The need to implement a shift rotation and to provide an opportunity for quality sleep may easily be overlooked during the first 24 hours of an incident. Once rotations have been established, many commanders in their zeal to be fair to their subordinates will mandate a rotation swap after a few days (i.e., the day shift moves to nights and the night shift switches to days). Of course, nothing could be worse in terms of reversing sleep-wake cycles and the effect on performance because none of the operators will be well rested for the first few days after the change. Once this is explained to both the commander

and the team, most personnel prefer to continue with the originally assigned shifts. Many other sources of performance degradation exist, including situational stress, the lack of opportunities to maintain personal hygiene, heat and cold stress, concerns about family members or problems at home, and contaminated food and water.

The tactical medic serves as a link between the point of injury and entry into the health care system at an appropriate level. In some locations and circumstances, appropriate entry may be at the prehospital level, while in others it may be at the regional, national, or international referral center level. The medic's responsibility for a patient does not end even after the patient is transferred to the established health care system. He or she then serves as the patient's advocate, providing needed information to the receiving clinician and ensuring that the patient receives proper care. Most busy medical systems will be receptive to this help if it is provided in a diplomatic way. Having a good working relationship with the EMS system and the receiving facilities is critical. If the medic's jurisdiction is a defined geographical area, such as a municipality, then the tactical medical program can usually be well integrated with the local EMS system. However, if his or her jurisdiction spreads across regional, state, or national boundaries, then more effort will be required on a mission-by-mission basis to ensure continuity of care. The medic can also serve as an important conduit of information for the patient's family and agency officials. For example, information that the attending surgeon can convey to another medical provider in 5 minutes can be translated into lay terminology by the medic, who can then provide more thorough explanations to others in a way that the attending surgeon might not have time to do.

RESPONSIBILITIES OF THE TEAM COMMANDER

As was noted previously, the preservation of manpower resources is ultimately the responsibility of the commander. Obviously, the commander is not expected to perform medical functions; rather, he or she provides the resources so that the medic can act on his or her behalf. In much the same way, the commander relies on the chemical munitions officer to deploy the right amount of tear gas and the counter-sniper to take an accurate shot, but he or she makes the final decisions about when and how to use these options.

The commander must provide command level support for the tactical medical program. This is realized through actions in scheduling or funding adequate medical coverage of the team's activities, including training (approximately 16% of all casualties are incurred during training) (18). He or she should also make provision for adequate equipment, supplies, and other resources necessary for carrying out the medical mission successfully. The medics must have the opportunity to maintain proficiency through continuing education and clinical practice because the volume and acuity of patient contacts with the team are unlikely to be adequate for this purpose. Finally, the commander has the responsibility for implementing the medical officer's recommendations.

DIFFERENCES BETWEEN TACTICAL EMERGENCY MEDICINE SUPPORT AND EMERGENCY MEDICAL SERVICES

The principle difference between everyday EMS and TEMS does not lie in the specific management of particular injuries. For example, hemorrhage is still preferentially controlled with direct pressure. The difference lies in the context within which medical decisions are made. In the example of uncontrolled hemorrhage, the special operations medic might advance more rapidly to a tourniquet if the patient has to be extracted from an environment where continued direct pressure cannot be maintained. The tactical paramedic performs best with an expanded scope of practice that includes injury control, preventive medicine, field sanitation and hygiene, health promotion, ambulatory care (sick call), and specialty skills, such as the temporary management of dental injuries without narcotic analgesia. While some effort has been made in general to expand the primary care practice of paramedics over the years (29), EMS has been slow to recognize the need for an expanded scope of practice for the TEMS paramedic, probably because the needed skills are atypical for a conventional prehospital provider. Some traditional prehospital procedures or practices should be modified for use in the tactical environment, and others are unique to this special area of practice.

Some have argued that cricothyroidotomy instead of endotracheal intubation should be the advanced airway of choice for tactical medics in the special operations setting (23). This is due to the medics' lack of experience and their inability to maintain currency with laryngoscopy, the technical difficulty of intubating in the presence of maxillofacial trauma, and the undesirable light signature of the laryngoscope. These points argue against training providers to perform endotracheal intubation in the warm zone.

However, this proposition is not universally accepted, and some significant differences are found between the military special operations environment and that of civilian law enforcement activities. TEMS medics are generally experienced at their respective provider level, and they are required by their certification or licensing programs to demonstrate skill currency on a periodic basis. Digital intubation, an alternative technique (30,31) that is taught to and practiced by TEMS providers, does not require the use of a white light (19), but few data, beyond anecdotes demonstrating the technique's efficacy in this setting, are found. Digital intu-

bation does have the advantages of being a rapid technique that can be accomplished with minimal head and neck movement from a number of low profile and protected provider positions at the patient's side. It also requires minimal equipment, and it seems to be less affected by blood and secretions than are the visualization techniques.

In any case, airway dysfunction is a relatively infrequent problem in this population of patients, and cases receiving an advanced airway are even less common. In one TEMS database, an airway adjunct was used in approximately 2% of all treatments rendered, and only one-third of these casualties survived to arrival at the hospital (18). Continuous monitoring of the patient may be impossible in the warm zone, and airway selection should take this into consideration. However, endotracheal intubation or cricothyroidotomy should be considered if mechanical airway obstruction secondary to trauma is the primary cause of respiratory embarrassment.

Although the patient may ventilate adequately on his own after a patent airway is established, an extender tube should be used if a bag-valve device must be used. The extender tube allows more movement between the bag and the endotracheal tube without causing the airway to dislodge during patient extraction. The bag-valve device should have the exhalation valve on the downstream side of the extender tube (i.e., closest to the endotracheal tube). If the valve is incorrectly positioned at the upstream side of the extender tube, then some of the exhaled gas will simply be moving back and forth in the extender tube and will never reach the valve, resulting in inadequate ventilation.

As was noted previously, cardiopulmonary resuscitation has limited benefit in the setting of a law enforcement special operation, so it must be weighed carefully against the risks of initiating such a treatment. Performing cardiopulmonary resuscitation in the warm zone is likely to subject the provider(s) to increased and prolonged exposure, and it may divert scarce medical resources from other requirements of the mission. The successful resuscitation rate from cardiac arrest secondary to trauma is so low and the risk is so great that it cannot be justified. Even most victims of nontraumatic arrest cannot be successfully resuscitated (10). Given the added complications of environmental austerity; the extended evacuation times; and the absence of a rigid, wheeled litter on which to perform effective cardiopulmonary resuscitation, this should only be considered if resources are plentiful and the demands on the medical and operational elements are low. However, in special circumstances, including those where arrest is secondary to primary respiratory dysfunction, maintenance of cardiopulmonary function for a short time may permit the recovery of normal function to occur. These situations include near-drowning, hypothermia, toxic exposure, electrocution, or lightning injury.

Prehospital providers are traditionally taught to immobilize the cervical spine with the slightest suspicion of a spinal column injury. This is not unreasonable given the devastating effects of an occult, unstable fracture that results in spinal cord damage. However, proper immobilization requires at least two people, and it takes approximately 5 minutes when performed by well-trained and experienced medics. This increased exposure in the warm zone is unacceptable when weighed against the low probability of an occult fracture that will benefit from immobilization of penetrating wounds (21,22). Therefore, immobilization generally should not be considered for penetrating trauma until the patient has been removed to a cold zone. Cervical spine immobilization may be more important following certain types of blunt trauma, such as high-speed vehicular crashes.

The RAM was developed by the Counter Narcotics and Terrorism Operational Medical Support (CONTOMS) program at the Uniformed Services University of the Health Sciences, the Department of Defense medical school (19). The principle purpose of this assessment algorithm is to maximize the opportunity to extract and treat a salvageable casualty while minimizing the risk to providers who are attempting an unnecessary rescue. Unnecessary rescues fall into the following two categories: those in which the casualty can self-extract and those in which the casualty is already dead (more appropriately termed a body recovery). The RAM provides an organized approach to evaluate the totality of circumstances from a protected position before recommending a rescue attempt to the commander.

The first step in conducting a RAM is to determine if the area is secure. If it is, then standard care in the cold zone is appropriate after making sure that the patient cannot harm the medic; this is accomplished by having operators search him or her, secure any weapons, and provide restraint, as necessary. If the area is not secure, the medic should use available intelligence to determine if the patient is a perpetrator or if he or she otherwise represents a threat. Under such circumstances, no further medical intervention is indicated until the threat has been controlled. To do otherwise could jeopardize the safety of officers, health care providers, and innocent parties. If the patient is not a perpetrator, then a remote assessment should be initiated. Attempt to evaluate the nature of the patient's injury and the stability of his condition. Remote observation is the first technique to be used because it allows the medic to gather information without revealing his position or intent to the opposing force. Technology commonly available to SWAT teams can improve the reliability of this assessment. For example, a good pair of binoculars or night vision goggles can often help to ascertain if the patient is breathing, the rate and quality of respiration, the presence of exsanguinating hemorrhage, and the existence of obvious wounds that are incompatible with life. In cold weather, a respiratory condensation plume can often be seen from the patient's mouth. Acoustic surveillance equipment can be deployed to detect speech, moans, groans, and even respiratory sounds.

Thermal imaging technology has improved so much in recent years that it is currently being investigated for application in the RAM.

If the patient's condition appears stable, then self-care instructions and reassurance should be communicated if possible, and medical extraction should await an improvement in the tactical situation. (The commander may elect to do a tactical extraction at any time, but the tactical situation and not the patient's stable medical condition should motivate this decision.) If the patient is unstable, then the risk of extraction must be weighed against the benefits of immediate access to medical care. While this is a command decision, the team leader will rely heavily on the medic's assessment of the patient's condition and of the need for immediate extraction. If the benefit-risk ratio is sufficiently high, then the extraction should proceed with only essential resuscitative procedures being performed in the warmer parts of the zone.

While this may seem like a relatively self-evident approach, a decision structure that fosters good assessment must be in place before emotion overtakes reason and a needless rescue is risked. The military experience is replete with examples of numerous casualties that have been incurred to recover a body or to attempt the rescue of a casualty who eventually got up and ran for cover on his or her own accord (32,33).

CLEARANCE FOR INCARCERATION

The tactical medic will often be asked to examine arrestees in the field before they are transported to a detention facility in order to assess fitness for incarceration. The easiest and most frequent response is to "turf" responsibility to the local emergency department. While some believe this is good defensive medicine, this may not be in the best interests of the patient or the community. Transport to the emergency department (ED) that is not medically indicated provides the subject an opportunity to engage in behaviors that may be injurious to himself, that may create a hazard for the general public and the hospital staff, that may extend the liability of law enforcement agencies, and that may place further demands on already overburdened EDs (34–39).

The law views pretrial detainees, convicted prisoners, and involuntarily committed persons differently, although all are entitled to adequate medical care while they are in custody. Subjects arrested by the police are pretrial detainees, and they have not been judged guilty of any crime. These people may be held for limited periods of time. In permitting such action, the courts balance the individual's right to be secure in his person and free from the denial of liberty without due process against the state's legitimate interest in preserving the public safety and compelling the subject's appearance in court. While the eighth amendment of the Constitution prohibits cruel and unusual *punishment* and therefore protects convicted prisoners from denial of medical care, it does not afford protection to pretrial detainees because they have not been convicted of a crime, and therefore they are not being *punished*. Pretrial detainees find protection in the due process clauses of the fifth and the fourteenth amendments that prohibit any deprivation without due process of law. Although the Supreme Court has not established a specific standard for the medical rights of arrestees, it has determined that they are at least as broad as those afforded to convicted prisoners (40,41).

In the 1976 case of *Estelle v. Gamble*, the Supreme Court held that denial of medical care to convicted prisoners constituted cruel and unusual punishment (42). The Court established a two-pronged test to determine the adequacy of medical care for prisoners (40). First, a violation of the standard requires more than mere negligence. Prison officials must demonstrate a deliberate indifference to the medical needs of the prisoner. Second, the medical needs that are subjected to this indifference must be "serious." To determine what is serious, the Court deferred to a standard of professional medical judgment. In other words, the prisoner is entitled to the care that the medical professional deems is necessary, and failure to provide this care is considered deliberate indifference. Furthermore, the health professional is held to a standard of professional judgment; deviation from this standard creates the impression that deliberate indifference is reflected in the patient's treatment. Pretrial detainees are at least entitled to the standard of care established by the two-pronged test.

Any procedure that addresses clearance for incarceration from the field must ensure that the subject receives appropriate medical care while also reducing the risks associated with unnecessary trips to the ED. These procedures focus on clearance for incarceration and not on comprehensive medical clearance. Clearance for incarceration is a screening procedure to identify urgent conditions requiring immediate attention before entry into the jail population. It is not intended to replace other mechanisms of medical care for this group, and it provides no assurance regarding the patient's overall medical condition.

Before one can even consider the clinical conditions that are relevant, the medical capabilities of the detention facility must be known. Without this information, the need for transport to another source of medical care cannot be evaluated. The special operations medical officer should be familiar with the medical capabilities of the detention facility, including the intake medical screening performed at the time of admission, the medical resources available, the training and qualifications of health care providers, the physical plant, the equipment and supplies available for care, and the availability of meaningful referral to outside facilities. The medic should also be familiar with the detention facility's regulations regarding the acceptance of prisoners with apparent medical problems. Many facilities require physician or hospital concurrence, which may be a problem if a physician is not a member of the tactical medical support element.

While the screening examination should be modified to meet individual requirements, certain minimum exclusion criteria can be identified. Detainees who are positive for any of these criteria should be excluded from admission to the detention population until further diagnosis and treatment have been considered. The grounds for clearance or referral should be clearly articulated in the medical record, and a copy should be provided to the detention or medical facility. These criteria include the following:

1. Significant trauma or mechanism of injury in the which physical examination cannot rule out underlying trauma.
2. Airway compromise, such as any mechanical or physiologic threat to the airway, including significant trauma to the face or neck, edema of the tongue or perioral soft tissue, signs of anaphylaxis, carbonaceous sputum, singeing of the nares or oral mucosa, or a reliable history of inhalation of toxins or heated gases.
3. Respiratory compromise, including dyspnea, signs of wheezing, or both; pulmonary edema; or excessive coughing.
4. Circulatory compromise, consisting of persistent abnormal pulse, blood pressure, or pulse oximetry values on room air; signs of shock; and electrocardiograph dysrhythmias other than chronic asymptomatic atrial fibrillation or isolated premature ventricular contractions.
5. Altered level of consciousness, an abnormal neurologic examination, or signs and symptoms of acute drug or alcohol intoxication or substance withdrawal.
6. Compromised mental health, including suicidal ideation.
7. Nonavailability of, or noncompliance with, prescribed medication for cardiac, respiratory, and seizure disorders.
8. Skeletal compromise, including gross deformity and abnormalities affecting function.
9. Integumentary compromise, including significant lacerations, deep lacerations to the hands, eye injuries, and significant burns.
10. Septic compromise, including body temperature greater than 38.5°C (101.3°F), severe dental abscess or infection, or significant cellulitis.
11. Complaint of severe pain.

The detainee may perceive the environment in which he is taken into custody to be intimidating and coercive and thus may limit his cooperation with the medical screening process. This attitude must not color the medic's ability to render a sound medical judgment regarding the subject's fitness for incarceration. The scope of practice, level of training, and the expertise of the individual tactical medical provider also influence his or her ability to clear prisoners from the field. If he or she is in doubt, confirmation of the field decision should be provided in the controlled environment of the ED. If the patient specifically requests treatment at the hospital, then the request must be carefully considered on an individual basis, balancing the risks, costs, and benefits. Special operations medical officers must ensure that the professional standard of care is met.

MEDICAL COUNTERTERRORISM — SUPPORT OF CRISIS MANAGEMENT OPERATIONS

Counterterrorism describes offensive measures taken to prevent, deter, and respond to terrorism. Antiterrorism is a term that describes defensive measures that reduce the vulnerability of individuals and property to terrorism; it includes limited response. The Federal Response Plan defines two elements of the response to a terrorist incident (43). Crisis management includes those measures to resolve the hostile situation and to investigate and to prepare a criminal case for prosecution under federal law. This response is a law enforcement activity, and the federal government has primary jurisdiction, in which the Federal Bureau of Investigation acts as the lead agency. Their activities involve measures to confirm the threat, to locate the terrorists and their weapons, to apprehend criminals, and to render their weapons safe. Consequence management refers to measures that alleviate the damage, loss and suffering resulting from a terrorist act, including the restoration of services, the protection of public health, and the provision of emergency relief for the government, businesses, and individuals. State and local governments manage limited consequences. Federal agencies, coordinated by the Federal Emergency Management Agency, support local efforts in the event of major consequences that exceed local capability.

To the extent that crisis management and consequence management differ, so does medical support of each of these elements. Special operations medics are especially well suited to support crisis management operations. Law enforcement interdiction activities must be conducted in a low-profile manner that does not reveal strategy or tactics, compromise intelligence sources, create panic, or needlessly disrupt commerce and infrastructure. These activities must be proportional to a valid threat assessment because exaggerated responses allow the terrorists to achieve their goals of instilling fear in the population, disrupting the daily routine, and focusing media attention. Experience has shown that even hoaxes can serve the terrorists' interests (44,45). Therefore, to avoid compromising operational security, the medical support of crisis management operations must not leave a significant operational signature. Limited resources for movement and staging of assets preferentially are used to meet law enforcement needs. The medical element therefore has to select versatile equipment that can meet a range of needs and that is lightweight and compact. This is best accomplished by special operations medical providers who do this on a daily basis and who routinely work in situations where the delivery of medical care is not the primary mission.

Tactical medical personnel are also likely to have the necessary secure communications links already in place in order to be seamlessly integrated into the counterterrorism operation. In fact, in most jurisdictions, TEMS providers will have already been subjected to the same background investigations that their police colleagues undergo, and they can be incorporated into the plan without the fear of a security breach. Hospitals, EMS systems, and other components of the health care system generally are not prepared to provide this kind of operational security.

Despite a remarkable focus on preparation for the terrorist use of chemical and biologic agents, explosives still appear to be the weapon of choice (46,47). They are easily manufactured, transported, and concealed. They can be remotely detonated, minimizing the risk of capture for the terrorist. Alternative terrorist tactics, such as kidnapping, assassination, and hostage-taking, present greater risk for the individual terrorist, and they require more sophisticated planning to be carried out effectively. The term *weapons of mass destruction* originally referred to chemical, biologic, and radiologic devices. However, both in the common usage and in statutory language, this term has been expanded to include a broader range of weapons that have mass effects (48,49). These include large explosives, the denial of service, and cyberterrorism. Management of the specific injuries associated with each type of weapon is beyond the scope of this chapter and is readily available elsewhere. However, the remainder of this section will focus on selected aspects of TEMS that can contribute to counterterrorism mission success.

A written medical annex that details the concept of medical support for response to a variety of likely targets should be developed. While the medical annex is important for all TEMS operations, generic versions can be drafted in advance for potential terrorist targets, and the details can be filled in when a specific operation is initiated. In collaboration with law enforcement intelligence counterparts, the tactical medic should identify soft targets that have not taken the measures that are needed to deny opportunity to terrorists. These can include symbolic buildings with public access that have no security presence. Can motor vehicles be parked close to the structure, facilitating the placement of an explosive? Does the nature of business conducted there require public access, and can large packages or other containers (e.g., luggage) be moved around without arousing suspicion? Confined space, such as that found in a subway system, is an important factor in lethality (50,51). The medical annex should address the overall concept of how medical support will be delivered for the counterterrorism operation, and it should include the following components:

1. Situation: a description of the situation, including the identification of the anticipated medical threats and the ameliorative actions that can be taken to minimize them.
2. Resources: a description of the medical resources that will be available for on-site operations and a plan for augmenting those resources if necessary.
3. Mission: statement of the overall medical mission in support of the counterterrorism operation that addresses not only acute care and emergency response but also injury control, preventive medicine, management of performance decrement, and field sanitation and hygiene.
4. Execution: an outline of how the medical mission will be carried out, including the concept of operations and the detailed execution plan. Primary medical facilities should be designated and listed along with their points of contact.
5. Logistics, Assets, and Coordination: a summary of logistics, material assets, and the information necessary for coordination both within the unit and with outside organizations as indicated by the situation.
6. Command and Signal: the description of how orders will be communicated, the call out procedures, contact numbers, and radio frequency plans for both organic and external resources, including a succinct summary of how one accesses the medical systems.

When conducting operations on any incident that could possibly involve terrorism, the medical officer's index of suspicion for secondary attacks should remain high. Secondary attacks were used in Northern Ireland to kill or injure public safety responders and good Samaritans after a small explosion attracted them to the scene (52). This technique was also used in the United States as early as 1927 when Andrew P. Kehoe placed over a 1,000 pounds of dynamite in the basement of the Bath Consolidated School in Michigan. After the detonation that killed 41, Kehoe drove to the school, lured the shocked superintendent into his car, and then promptly detonated another device, killing the superintendent, another student, and himself (53). The threat of secondary devices has received renewed attention since the January 16, 1997 bombing of a women's health facility and the February 21, 1997 Otherside Lounge bombing, both in Atlanta, Georgia. In both cases, a secondary improvised explosive device was placed with the apparent intent of targeting first responders. It detonated at the women's health facility, injuring several, but it was discovered and rendered safe at the lounge (46).

Secondary attacks are often perpetrated in one of four ways: a secondary device; an insidious threat, such as an unrecognized release of chemical agent; undetected perpetrators who ambush responders; or an assault through a perimeter breach. These types of attacks are most effectively executed after personnel have responded to a target location in reaction to some event, although they can be carried out at any time.

Defense against a hidden device requires a rapid sweep of the area of operation and increased vigilance for unusual or out-of-place packages and containers. Radio use should be curtailed to avoid accidental detonation by stray radio frequency energy. Rapid extraction and evacuation with only essential medical procedures performed on site limit the potential target size and reduce damage in the event of a secondary explosion. Minimizing the target will also reduce the threat posed by an undetected release of a chemical or biologic agent, and providers should remain alert for signs of mixed etiology injury. The best defense against an undetected perpetrator is to treat all unknown persons, regardless of their age and sex, as perpetrators until they have been proven differently. A thorough secondary survey should be conducted for all patients, including the exposure of all body surfaces. Patients with weapons do not become medical problems until the threat has been eliminated. Finally, protection against a perimeter breach is best provided by the establishment of a secure law enforcement perimeter with designated points of entry into the area of operations. Terrorists have used ambulances, laboratory coats, and uniforms to gain access to restricted areas in the past. The availability of tactical medical officers to assist checkpoint personnel in identifying legitimate medical responders can avert catastrophe. However, minimizing the target through rapid extraction and evacuation still is the most effective step that can be taken.

TACTICAL EMERGENCY MEDICINE AND DISASTER RESPONSE

Tactical medical providers have a unique combination of skills, and they can be a valuable asset to the incident commander during a general (i.e., nonterrorist) disaster response. As a group, tactical medics are usually fit and disciplined, and they are accustomed to operating in dangerous, resource-poor, prolonged transport environments. They are trained in multiple specialties, and they possess components of the medical planner, the occupational health clinician, the preventive medicine officer, the risk manager, the emergency medicine provider, the public health officer, and the field hygienist. They deploy with a technically sophisticated materiel package that allows them to be self-sufficient and highly mobile. They are adept at assessing performance decrement, managing continuous and sustained operations, and providing ambulatory care to emergency service personnel. While TEMS providers lack some of the specialty skills of an urban search and rescue or a wilderness medical team and thus should not be assigned to tasks requiring those specific skills, they can prove to be invaluable in establishing baseline medical support for emergency services and others in heavily impacted sectors of the disaster area. Due to their law enforcement training, they are especially well suited to support operations in high-risk areas where the security infrastructure has been degraded.

TEMS providers and their disaster response colleagues should plan, coordinate, integrate, and train together before an occurrence requires *ad hoc* collaboration. Plans to use tactical medics must recognize that they have a primary responsibility to their law enforcement organizations in the event of civil disorder and lawlessness during a disaster or the following recovery period. Both the providers and the communities they serve will benefit from a prior familiarization with the others' capabilities and an ability to implement effective joint operations.

CONCLUSION

TEMS is increasingly recognized as a special interest area within emergency medicine, and it shares common elements with disaster medicine, wilderness medicine, humanitarian assistance, and urban search and rescue. It is the practice of out-of-hospital medicine that focuses on enhancing special operations mission success. Although the general principles of emergency care hold true for TEMS, the context in which decisions are made and the timing and resources for care are substantially different. Medical support of counterterrorism crisis management is an area that is rarely distinguished from medical consequence management, although the approach is very different and consequence managers are not necessarily well equipped to support crisis management. Special operations medics are especially well suited for this role. TEMS is rapidly growing as an evidenced-based practice that impacts the full spectrum of injury and disease in this special population from long before the tissue-damaging event (e.g., injury control, preventive medicine) until after the damage has occurred (e.g., acute management, patient advocacy). It presents fascinating opportunities for a reduction in mortality and morbidity among operators, perpetrators, and innocents.

REFERENCES

1. Jones JS, Reese K, Kenepp G, et al. Into the fray: integration of emergency medical services and special weapons and tactics (SWAT) teams. *Prehosp Disaster Med* 1996;11:202–206.
2. Heiskell LE, Carmona RH. Tactical emergency medical services: an emerging subspecialty of emergency medicine. *Ann Emerg Med* 1994;23:778–785.
3. McArdle DQ, Rasumoff D, Kolman J. Integration of emergency medical services and special weapons and tactics teams: the emergence of the tactically trained medic. *Prehosp Disaster Med* 1992; 7:285–288.
4. Quinn M. Into the fray: the search and rescue role with special weapons teams. *Response* 1987;6:18–20.
5. Rooker N. The San Francisco shootings. *JEMS* 1993;Sept:74–81.
6. Heiskell LE. SWAT medical teams. *Law and Order* 1996;April: 70–74.
7. Olds MA, Grande CM. When minutes can mean a lifetime. *Counterterrorism and Security Reports* 1995;Summer:26–28.
8. Editor's comment on the inclusion of physicians in civilian tactical law enforcement operations. *The Tactical Edge*, Fall 1993.
9. Myers C. In the line of fire. *Emergency* 1997;July:16–19.
10. DeLorenzo RA, Porter RS. *Tactical emergency care.* Upper Saddle River, NY: Prentice-Hall, 1999.
11. Madsen M. Use of an emergency medical information card by a tactical team. *The Tactical Edge* 1998;Fall.
12. Kowalski B, Frazier J, Grande CM. TACMED vs. MEDTAC: the basics of medical support for tactical operations. *The Tactical Edge* 1998;Fall.
13. Kanable R. Peak performance. *Law Enforcement Technology* 1999; August:78–82.
14. Kolman JA. *A guide to the development of special weapons and tactics teams.* Springfield, IL: Charles C Thomas Publishers, 1982.
15. Jagoda A, Pietrzak M, Hazen S, et al. Prehospital care and the military. *Mil Med* 1992;157:11–15.
16. Bellamy RF. The causes of death in conventional land warfare: implications for combat casualty care research. *Mil Med* 1984;149:55–62.
17. Vayer JS, Ten Eyck RP, Cowan ML. New concepts in triage. *Ann Emerg Med* 1986;15:927–930.
18. CONTOMS Database System. Bethesda, MD: Uniformed Services University of the Health Sciences. Available at: http://www.usuhs.mil/ccr/index.html. Accessed May 9, 2002.
19. *Emergency medical technician tactical course manual*, 14th ed. Bethesda, MD: Uniformed Services University of the Health Sciences, 1995.
20. Smock W, Hamm M, Krista M. Physicians in tactical medicine. *Ann Emerg Med* 1999;34:S73.
21. Arishita GI, Vayer JS, Bellamy RF. Cervical spine immobilization of penetrating neck wounds in a hostile environment. *J Trauma* 1989;29:332–337.
22. Zajtchuk R, Jenkins DP, Bellamy RF, et al, eds. *Combat casualty care guidelines for operation desert storm.* Washington DC: Office of the Army Surgeon General, 1991.
23. Butler FK, Hagmann JH, Butler EG. Tactical combat casualty care in special operations. *Mil Med* 1996;161:3–16.
24. Rosemurgy AS, Norris PA, Olson SM, et al. Prehospital traumatic cardiac arrest: the cost of futility. *J Trauma* 1998;38: 468–474.
25. Yoon, RY, Harling, M, Feldman, JA, et al. Penetrating thoracic trauma: prehospital resuscitation for all? Abstract of scientific papers presented at The Ninth Annual Conference and Scientific Assembly of the National Association of EMS Physicians, Minneapolis, June, 1993.
26. Hogan, DE, Waeckerle, JF, Dire, DJ, et al. Emergency department impact of the Oklahoma City terrorist bombing. *Ann Emerg Med* 1999;34:160–167.
27. Boehm TM, James JJ. The medical response to the La Belle Disco bombing in Berlin, 1986. *Mil Med* 1988;153:235–237.
28. Lavergne GM. *A sniper in the tower.* New York: Bantam Books, 1997.
29. Holdsworth N. Expanded-scope paramedics. *JEMS* Aug 1994; 92–93.
30. Stewart RD. Tactile orotracheal intubation. *Ann Emerg Med* 1984;13:175–178.
31. Hardwick WC, Bluhm D. Digital intubation. *J Emerg Med* 1984; 1:317–320.
32. *Wound Data and Munitions Effectiveness Team Study*, vols. I-III. Final report. Alexandria, VA: Joint Technical Coordinating Group for Munitions Effectiveness, Defense Technical Information Center, 1970.

33. Cloonan C. Panel discussion: operational medicine in the 21st century. In: *Proceedings of the Third International Conference on Tactical Emergency Medical Support*. Bethesda, MD: Uniformed Services University of the Health Sciences, 1999:97.

34. Lessenger JE. Prisoners in the emergency department. *Ann Emerg Med* 1985;14:179–183.

35. Training key #412. *Transportation of prisoners II*. Arlingrton, VA: International Association of Chiefs of Police, 1992.

36. Sullivan K. Police shoot man in alleged ambulance hijacking in MD. *The Washington Post* 1992 July 5:B,7.

37. *Sams v. Oelrich*, 717 So.2d 1044 (1998). Court of Appeals of Florida, First District.

38. *Shepherd v. Washington County*. AR, 962 S.W.2d 779 (1998). Supreme Court of Arkansas.

39. Buesching DP, Jablonowski A, Vesta E, et al. Inappropriate emergency department visits. *Ann Emerg Med* 1985;14:672–676.

40. Posner MJ. The Estelle medical professional judgment standard: the right of those in state custody to receive high-cost medical treatments. *Am J Law Med* 1992;18:4.

41. *City of Revere v. Massachusetts General Hospital*, 463 U.S. 244 (1983).

42. *Estelle v. Gamble*, 429 U.S. 97 (1976).

43. Federal Emergency Management Agency. Terrorism incident annex.*Federal response plan*. Available at: http://www.fema.gov/r-n-r/frp/frpterr.htm. Accessed April 5, 2002.

44. Department of Health and Human Services, Centers for Disease Control and Prevention. Bioterrorism alleging use of anthrax and interim guidelines for management—United States, 1998. *MMWR* 1999;48:4,69–74.

45. Macintyre AG, Christopher GW, Eitzen E, et al. Weapons of mass destruction events with contaminated casualties. *JAMA* 2000;283:242–249.

46. Department of Justice, Federal Bureau of Investigation. *Terrorism in the United States, 1997*. Washington, D.C.: United States Government Printing Office, 1999.

47. Department of State, Office of the Coordinator for Counterterrorism. *Patterns of global terrorism, 1998*. Washington, D.C.: United States Department of State, 1999;April.

48. Maniscalco PM, Christen HT, Rubin DL, et al. New weapons of mass effect. *JEMS* 1998;23:12,41–50.

49. 18 United States Code 921 (2332a).

50. Stein M, Hirshberg A. Trauma care in the new millennium: medical consequences of terrorism-the conventional weapon threat. *Surg Clin North Am* 1999;79:6,1538–1552.

51. Dolev E. Medical aspects of terrorist activities. *Mil Med* 1988;153:243–244.

52. Hadden WA, Rutherford WH, Merrett JD. The injuries of terrorist bombing: a study of 1532 consecutive patients. *Br J Surg* 1978;65:525–531.

53. May J. Michigan school bombing in 1927 was even more deadly. *The Detroit Free Press*. Available at: http://www.freep.com/news/nw/qbath23.htm. Accessed April 23, 1999.

36

MASS SHOOTINGS

THOMAS M. STEIN

Mass shooting in this text is defined as an event with greater than five victims, one or more shooters acting together, and a timeline of 24 hours or less. This eliminates serial murders from the discussion. Serial murders are no less of a tragedy, but they do not have the same impact as mass shootings on local medical resources. The morbidity and mortality of mass shootings are explored in this chapter. Mortality includes all deaths produced by the occurrence. Those who died before arriving at a hospital are designated as "killed," and those dying after arrival at a hospital are designated as "died of wounds." Intuitively, one might suppose that those killed would have had little chance of surviving no matter what and that those dying of wounds may perhaps have been salvageable. These hypotheses will be evaluated against an analysis of real world incidents here.

The goals of this chapter are (a) to familiarize the emergency care provider with what to expect in terms of casualty numbers and types of injuries when confronted with the victims of a mass shooting, (b) to identify responses and interventions that will maximize the victims' chances of arriving at the trauma center alive, and (c) to provide guidance for the triage of multiple victims with penetrating trauma.

Emergency medical services (EMS), emergency departments, and trauma systems have been in existence in their current guise since the late 1960s. The initial response to multiple casualty incidents is part of the public safety and the medical community's responsibilities, and significant resources are spent on planning and training for this type of mission. In 1966, Charles Whitman perpetrated what is widely considered as the first mass shooting of civilians by a civilian at the University of Texas campus in Austin. An analysis of all mass shootings since 1966 in countries with similar EMS systems has been conducted using casualty and medical data from public domain sources, which currently represents the best data available. The subset of incidents included here was chosen because the conclusions drawn from these data can be more reasonably applied to present and future mass shootings in the United States, where the majority of such incidents occur. A definitive study of these events is underway, but this may take years to complete because much of the recent data is encumbered for legal purposes and because the medical information consent issue significantly slows the process when dealing with older incidents (1).

A RECENT HISTORY

Mass shootings do not have a long history. Before the 1900s, rapid loading and rapid firing weapons were not generally available to the public. As the availability of these weapons has increased, so has the opportunity for mass shooting. As radio, television, and finally satellite communication came into being, so did the rapid and widespread dissemination of information and details regarding these horrible crimes, thus inviting copycat incidents.

Mass shootings have been increasing in every decade since the 1960s. This is demonstrated in Table 36.1. As of 2000, public domain sources reveal 437 total deaths and another 367 wounded, but surviving, persons that are the result of 47 mass shootings. Of these 804 victims, 618 have at least partial demographic and clinical data; for example, 222 have the anatomic location of wounds clearly described. Of the 367 wounded victims found in public domain sources, 197 are specifically described. Only 127 of these descriptions provide enough information to determine whether the individual experienced a resultant disability. Forty-six were known to have been admitted to the hospital, but how many of the other 151 required hospitalization is not clear. Nineteen were documented to have gone to the operating room, but again, the sources do not indicate how many actually went, although one may assume that abdominal wounds were surgically explored. Blood product use was documented for none of these individuals.

The incidence of penetrating trauma in the United States has increased over the past 20 years. Although the rate of fatal penetrating injuries appears to have remained constant, the rate of nonfatal penetrating injuries has increased (2,3). Military rifles and semiautomatic handguns with large capacity magazines have become ubiquitous, and

TABLE 36.1. FREQUENCY OF MASS SHOOTINGS BY DECADE

Decade	No. of mass shootings
1960s	2
1970s	6
1980s	17
1990s	22

they are readily available to anyone who has the cash to buy them, despite legislative attempts to halt the proliferation. However, more than two or three civilian patients with penetrating injuries seldom present to a single health care facility at the same time. Battlefield treatment facilities have much more experience in dealing with larger numbers of penetrating injuries arriving simultaneously or over a relatively short period of time. Therefore, military casualty data will be compared to the civilian mass shooting experience.

On the surface, military mass casualty scenarios differ from civilian mass shootings in a few important ways. First, combatants are trained and armed to defend themselves. Second, combatants have body armor and other ballistic protection devices available (these have been ubiquitous since the Vietnam War). Third, multiple perforating wounds from explosive devices, which are commonplace in war, are still relatively uncommon in civilian mass shootings. Finally, civilian shooters effectively execute many of their victims at close range. Similarities, however, do exist in terms of weapons used, the delayed evacuations due to tactical circumstances, and the stress on local medical resources. Lessons learned from military conflicts and civilian experiences with penetrating trauma will be evaluated; these may corroborate the lessons learned from an analysis of civilian mass shooting casualty data.

THE VIETNAM EXPERIENCE

The United States Army organized a team known as the wound data and munitions effectiveness team (WDMET) to collect data prospectively on combat injuries during the Vietnam War. Over 8,000 United States Army and Marine casualties from an 18-month period (1967–1969) were studied and catalogued in detail. Data on the tactical situation, the type of weapon used to create wounds, field first aid and the circumstances of evacuation, the detailed anatomy of the wounds, the hospital care rendered, and the autopsy results for those fatally wounded were collected.

The principle of the "golden hour" that was described by Trunkey is based on civilian trauma data collected in the 1970s that included blunt trauma mechanisms. His analysis of the time-of-injury and time-to-death interval revealed a trimodal distribution: immediate (<1 hour), early (2–3 hours), and late (days to weeks after the injury) (4). Approximately half of the deaths catalogued were considered immediate, 30% were early, and the remainder occurred late. WDMET, in stark contrast, shows that 85% to 90% of the combat fatalities occurred in the immediate period, with up to 70% occurring within the *first 5 minutes*. Figure 36.1 demonstrates the time distribution of combat deaths for the WDMET database. Sauaia et al. studied a civilian population in the early 1990s that had a much larger percentage of penetrating trauma than the Trunkey group (5). These results mirror the WDMET data more closely than that of Trunkey, which suggests that if, a golden period for penetrating injuries does exist, it is significantly less than 1 hour. Bellamy suggests a "golden 5 minutes" (6). This clearly has ramifications on the approach to mass shootings from both a tactical or law enforcement perspective, as well as from an emergency medical perspective. Perhaps, the term a "titanium 5 minutes" would be more appropriate.

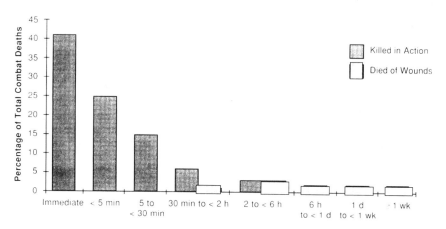

FIG. 36.1. Time distribution of combat deaths.

WOUND DISTRIBUTION

Abbreviated Injury Scores

The WDMET database provides military wound distribution information. A breakdown by anatomic region (e.g., head, face, neck, chest, abdomen, extremities, and superficial) reveals the relative frequency of wound location. Table 36.2 defines each of these anatomic regions. The incidence of penetrating injuries to body regions has not been found to be proportional to the percentage of body surface area for each region. This is true because the victims are not injured while in an anatomic position but rather while they are in some type of protective posture. In the study, abbreviated injury scores (AIS) were used to assign wounds to a body region. Casualties with two or more wounds were assigned to a specific region only if the AIS value for an injury in that region exceeded the AIS for all injuries in the other regions. Only casualties who had two or more injuries of equal AIS value in different body regions were classified as having multiple injuries. The anatomic distribution of fatal and nonfatal wounds is illustrated in Fig. 36.2.

Patient Outcome by Body Region

The summary mortality data include all missile wounds of bullets, shrapnel, and both. The mortality of victims wounded by bullets only is documented where possible.

Head

WDMET Total Mortality (78%) and Hospital Mortality (26%)
The total mortality data include low-velocity fragment wounds and any wound that merely violates the periosteum of the skull. The most telling data reflect the abysmal outlook of victims with bullet penetration of the skull with direct parenchymal injury, as opposed to that of those with tangential wounds causing depressed skull fracture with associated brain injury. Less than 1% of the head-wounded

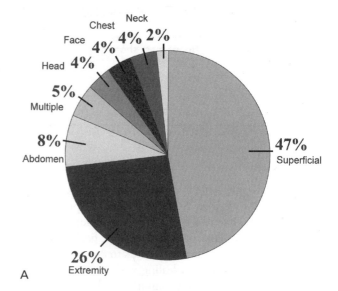

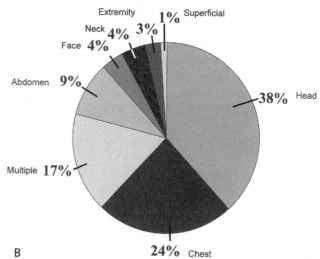

FIG. 36.2. A: Anatomic distribution of nonfatal wounds (WDMET). **B:.** Anatomic distribution of fatal wounds (WDMET).

population with this devastating injury survived to be evacuated from Vietnam. The neurologic outcome of this extremely small survivor subset is not reported. It is assumed that few, if any, will survive neurologically intact. Even when including cases of tangential bullet wounds, the mortality of a victim with a head wound is still 90%.

Other Military Experience

A study of the Israeli wartime experience in Lebanon from 1982 to 1985 revealed craniocerebral wound results similar to WDMET, although it reported only on the patients that arrived alive at a civilian university medical center (number [n] = 116) (7). The evacuation time was as short as in Vietnam; however, computed tomography (CT) scans were performed routinely on arrival to the medical facility. Gunshot wounds with direct parenchymal injury or an admission Glas-

TABLE 36.2. WOUND DATA AND MUNITIONS EFFECTIVENESS TEAM (WDMET) DEFINITIONS OF ANATOMIC BODY REGIONS

Designation	Component parts
Head	Skull and contents
Face	Facial bones, eyes, and oral and nasal cavities
Neck	Viscera and cervical spine
Chest	Thoracic cage, spine, and viscera
Abdomen	Peritoneal and retroperitoneal cavities, pelvis, and lumbar spine
Extremities	Used only if bones and/or neurovascular structures are injured
Superficial	Skin, fat, and skeletal muscle anywhere on the body

gow coma score (GCS) of 3 due to any penetrating mechanism had a poor outcome (dead or persistent vegetative state) in 94% of the cases. Overall, gunshot wound mortality was 80%. Overall hospital mortality from all causes was 26%, which is nearly identical to the Vietnam experience.

George and Dagi reviewed military experience with penetrating craniocerebral injuries and came to the following conclusions for civilian application to triage and management: (a) patients who are deeply comatose and intermittently apneic, with bilaterally dilated and fixed pupils, who have sustained either a high-velocity gunshot wound or a lower-velocity missile wounding at close range (especially if the wounding is through-and-through or if CT shows massive intracranial debris and contusion) have sustained lethal injuries; and, (b) although facilities at many civilian centers far exceed those that have historically been available to military neurosurgeons in the field, the principles derived from combat injuries continue to apply (8).

Civilian Experience

These particular patient series are retrospectively collected from several years. Generally, the patients in these series present individually, unlike what occurs in a mass shooting. One series studied 314 patients from in and around Genoa, Italy, who had sustained penetrating injuries to the brain caused by either a handgun (75%) or a shotgun (25%) (9). Of interest is the fact that no high-velocity wounds were included. The overall mortality rate was 92% (288/314), including 228 who died at the scene. No patient who presented with a GCS of less than 6 survived.

A series of 47 patients from a university hospital in Turkey had an overall mortality rate of 38% (10). This series, however, included only those who arrived alive at the hospital. In this series, the mortality rate was 100% for patients with an initial GCS of 3 to 7. Fourteen had a GCS of 3 to 5 (five underwent operation), and four had a GCS of 6 to 7 (three underwent operation). No patient in the series had an initial GCS of 8.

Polin et al. performed a multivariate analysis on factors found to have a strong predictive value for the outcome of penetrating head injuries (11). The predictive factors were established by previous research performed by at least 11 other groups that primarily used civilian data. Two equations that demonstrate 7-day mortality were developed; one was based on GCS and coagulopathy, and another on the volume of contused brain and the number of midline planes crossed by the projectile. The former obviously is of more use in the prehospital setting and on arrival to the emergency department.

In an extensive review of civilian gunshot wounds to the brain resulting in GCS scores of 3, 4, and 5, Kaufman et al. offer an elegant management algorithm after a discussion of the scope of the problem, the prevalence, and the "moral, financial and ethical dilemmas that influence the care of these patients" (12).

Chest

WDMET Total Mortality (71%) and Hospital Mortality (14%)

The probability of being fatally wounded if struck in the chest by a bullet is 80%. Of the 155 casualties with primary thoracic penetration who arrived alive from the battlefield, 15% required formal thoracotomy. These data support the teaching of the advanced trauma life support course sponsored by the American College of Surgeons.

Other Military Experience

In a series of 259 cardiothoracic war wounds from Zagreb, Croatia, only 10% were due to gunshot wounds, and the majority (67%) resulted from shrapnel (13). Thoracotomy was used as a primary method of surgical treatment in 54% of the patients; however, 50% of the patients had already undergone tube thoracostomy or thoracotomy at front-line hospitals. The indications for formal thoracotomy in these cases were not standardized. The mortality rate was 2.7%. This low rate is due to the fact that delayed evacuation to definitive care selected those that were going to die before arrival in Zagreb.

Civilian Experience

A retrospective study of civilian penetrating chest injuries from a university hospital in southeast Turkey reviewed 755 patients (14). Gunshot wounds made up 55% of the cohort, and over half of these were due to high-velocity weapons. They reported the following mortality rates by type of injury: stab wounds, 1.5% (5 out of 342); low-velocity gunshot wounds, 2.9% (4 out of 139); high-velocity gunshot wounds, 11.6% (27 out of 232); shotgun wounds, 9.5% (2 out of 21); and bomb shrapnel, 19% (4 out of 21). One-half of the mortality was due to adult respiratory distress syndrome, which the authors attributed to the lack of ventilator therapy and intensive care conditions. The overall thoracotomy rate was 8.1%, which is quite a low rate for the frequency of high-velocity gunshot wounds. The thoracotomy rate was not reported by type of injury *per se*. The authors credited this low incidence to the absence of or the low incidence of great vessel, bronchial, esophageal, and cardiac injuries. Again, patients with such injuries generally die at the scene or en route to the hospital. A similar report from the same center reviewed its experience with 94 children (mean age of 11.5±3.3 years; range, 3–15); 44% of these wounds were gunshot wounds, of which 66% were high-velocity wounds (15). None of the patients with gunshot wounds died in this series of injuries, and only one died overall. The overall thoracotomy rate was 4.3% (one immediate and three delayed).

Another series of 240 patients from a university hospital in Lima, Peru was reported. Twenty-four percent of these injuries were due to low-velocity gunshot wounds, and the others were stab wounds (16). The thoracotomy and mortality rates for the gunshot wound group were 16% and 7%, respectively. The international consensus is that most penetrating chest injuries can be treated without surgery (6,14–27).

Abdomen

WDMET Total Mortality (37%) and Hospital Mortality (11.5%)

The probability of an individual being fatally wounded if he or she is struck in the abdomen by a bullet is approximately 65%. No specific reports aside from the WDMET experience are reported in the literature. Although considerable information in the civilian literature exists regarding the injury patterns and treatment, no specific reports on morbidity or mortality related to gunshots to the abdomen have been located. Some authorities indicate that about 80% of all penetrating wounds to the abdomen require surgical management.

Extremities

WDMET Total Mortality (9.9%) and Hospital Mortality (1.2%)

The probability of receiving a fatal wound if one is struck in the extremity by a bullet that injures bone or neurovascular structures is one in 11. Fragment wounds due to explosive munitions are actually more lethal, with a probability of fatal wounding of one in six.

THE PATHOPHYSIOLOGIC CAUSE OF COMBAT DEATHS IN VIETNAM

In reviewing the pathophysiologic causes of combat death in Vietnam, clearly many of the deaths were unpreventable. The pathophysiologic causes of death in the Vietnam war are demonstrated in Fig. 36.3. Massive brain destruction

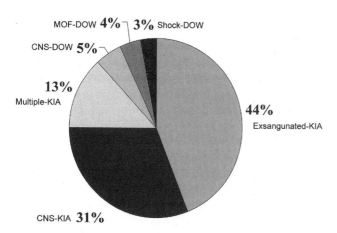

FIG. 36.3 Pathophysiologic causes of death during Vietnam (WDMET).

and major vascular penetration are quickly fatal. However, the question remains whether immediate and appropriate medical interventions could have reduced the number of fatalities in the killed-in-action and died-of-wounds groups. Furthermore, could similar interventions reduce the morbidity of the survivors?

ANALYSIS OF CIVILIAN MASS SHOOTINGS

In a review of 45 mass shootings in English-speaking countries with similar EMS systems, the following data was compiled. Of 437 people shot to death, 93.6% died on the scene, and 6.4% died of wounds after reaching a medical treatment facility. Three hundred sixty-seven patients were wounded by missiles. This dead-to-wounded ratio of 1.2 to 1 is an extremely high kill ratio when compared to the military experience (1 in 4 when using only bullet wound data from the European theater of WWII). On average, eight people were killed at the scene of the incident, and nine people were wounded per incident (recall the operational definition of mass shooting described in the introduction). In addition, one wounded victim would typically arrive alive at a medical treatment facility but would ultimately die of wounds.

The primary weapon used in mass shootings was a handgun in 36% of the incidents (revolver, 8%; semiautomatic, 28%), a rifle in 53% of the incidents (single shot, 2%; semiautomatic, 43%; and automatic, 8%), and a shotgun in 11% of the incidents. When the weapon was a handgun, the individual's fatality rate was 73.6%; when a rifle was used, the rate was 62.1%; and when a shotgun was involved, it was 87.9%. That low-velocity wounds would have a higher fatality rate than high-velocity wounds appears paradoxical. However, on closer analysis of the shooting incidents, the handguns were used at close range, generally inside a room or a closed space. Rifles, however, were frequently used during sprees that took the incident outdoors where relatively long shots were taken. Shotguns cause massive tissue destruction at close range, and, in many cases, the shotgun was used at close range (execution style) as with handguns.

The duration of the incident was well documented in 16 of the cases. These shootings lasted from 4 to 80 minutes. At the Port Arthur shooting in Tasmania, Australia, Martin Bryant killed his first 22 victims in approximately 2 minutes with well-aimed semiautomatic shots from a rifle. George Hennard killed, wounded, or injured more than 50 people in approximately 10 minutes at the Luby's Cafeteria massacre in Killeen, Texas, while using two 9-mm semiautomatic handguns.

SHOOTER PROFILE

Invariably, the shooters in these incidents were males. The average age was 32.7 years (range, 11–59 years), and the

TABLE 36.3. DISPOSITION OF SHOOTERS

Disposition	Number (%)
Captured alive	23 (47)
Killed by own hand	19 (40)
Killed by law enforcement	6 (11)
Killed by bystander	1 (2)

TABLE 36.4. DEMOGRAPHIC LOCATION OF MASS SHOOTINGS

Location of mass shooting	Number (%) (N = 47)
Relatives as victims	13 (28)
Shooter's workplace	19 (40)
Shooter's home	12 (26)
Both home and work	3 (6)
Victim's workplace*	25 (53)
Victim's home	13 (28)

*School is considered the workplace for students.

median age was 35 years. Although school shootings became more common in the 1990s, the average age of the shooter still was only slightly younger during this period (average age, 29.8 years; range, 11–55 years; median age, 31.5 years). None of the shooters wore body armor. The disposition of the 49 shooters (two shootings had two shooters each) is summarized in Table 36.3.

Twenty-seven of the shooters carried more than one weapon; 12 carried two weapons, and 15 carried three weapons. Ashbrook at the Baptist Church in Fort Worth, Texas, and Harris and Klebold at Columbine High School in Littleton, Colorado, used fragmentation devices, which was a new development in 1999. These devices were not used with any effectiveness, but they introduced the potential to increase casualties significantly. The number of rounds fired per incident was clearly documented in 11 of the cases and ranged from 11 to 257 (mean of 74 rounds; median of 50 rounds).

VICTIM PROFILE

Complete demographic data was not available for all of the victims. However, of those that were detailed, the ages ranged from months to the late seventies. Of the 47 incidents, 13 included relatives of the shooter among the victims. Nineteen of the incidents involved the shooter's workplace, and 12 incidents took place in the shooter's home. Three of the latter group included both the shooter's home and his workplace. However, 25 of the incidents occurred at the victim's workplace (if one includes schools as a students'

"workplace"). The demographics of the victims of mass shootings are demonstrated in Table 36.4.

Of all the casualties identified (n = 804), 148 had gunshot wounds that were described adequately enough to be anatomically defined. The others either had multiple wounds that were not well described, or no description of the wound(s) was found at all. Forty-nine of the victims who were dead at the scene had sustained a well-described *single* gunshot wound. The percentage of fatal wounds by body region was as follows: head, 61%; chest, 18%; back, 12%; abdomen, 6%; neck, 3%; and extremities, 0%. Similarly, seven victims who died of wounds had a single gunshot wound that was clearly described. Broken down by body region, these included the chest, three (42%); the abdomen, two (30%); the head, one (14%); and the neck, one (14%). Clinical outcomes broken down by primary wound site (body region) are summarized in Table 36.5. The correlation between the WDMET database and the mass shooting data is summarized in Table 36.6. These data summarize *bullet wounds only*.

The data in Table 36.2 represent the overall mortality of gunshot wounds to a specific body region. The WDMET data include all victims killed at the scene, as well as those who died at the hospital. Except for the civilian head wound series, the other military and civilian data included only those who arrived at a medical treatment facility alive. Including those dead at the scene and those dying enroute to a hospital give a more accurate look at the true mortality.

TABLE 36.5. CLINICAL OUTCOMES BY WOUND SITE

Clinical outcome	Head, N = 52	Neck, N = 12 (%)	Chest, N = 28 (%)	Abdomen, N = 10 (%)	Back, N = 14 (%)	Extremity, N = 28 (%)	Unknown, N = 301 (%)
KIA	41 (79)	4 (33)	14 (50)	1 (10)	9 (64)	0	207 (69)
DOW	2 (4)	1 (8)	4 (14)	2 (20)	0	0	4 (1)
Disabled	2 (4)	3 (25)	3 (11)	0	2 (14)	2 (7)	1 (<1)
Well	6 (11)	1 (8)	4 (14)	5 (50)	2 (14)	21 (75)	36 (12)
Unknown	1 (2)	3 (25)	3 (11)	2 (20)	1 (7)	5 (18)	52 (17)

Abbreviations: DOW, Died of wounds; KIA, Killed in action; N, number.
Information taken from various public domain sources.

TABLE 36.6. COMPARISON OF GUNSHOT MORTALITY RATES BY ANATOMIC REGION

Anatomic location of wound	WDMET study	Military experience	Civilian experience	Mass shootings
Head	99%	94%	92%	90%
Neck	?	?	?	58%
Chest	80%	?	?	75%
Abdomen	65%	?	?	25%
Extremity	9%	?	?	0%

"?", indicates no data available.
Abbreviation: WDMET, Wound Data and Munitions Effectiveness Team.

RAMIFICATIONS FOR EMERGENCY SERVICES PERSONNEL

Preempting mass shootings is difficult, if not impossible. Incident and consequence management for police, EMS, and hospital personnel will continue to be necessary. Therefore, what can be learned from this data? First, the author must remind the reader that this writing is only a starting point. These data have been obtained through public domain sources, such as newspapers, libraries, and the Internet. Accurate, comprehensive retrospective medical data collection will be a major undertaking, especially considering the confidentiality and consent issues. Prospective data collection is even more of a problem because of the criminal investigations surrounding these crimes, and the subsequent civil litigation that encumbers the data for prolonged periods of time. The information regarding the deceased victims is generally covered in more detail in the public domain sources, compared to that for the survivors; therefore, the "unknown" outcome of a wound to a known body region that is seen in Table 36.5 is usually a survivor, but the information that has been provided was not enough to determine the disability extent, if any. Disability is defined by this author as a permanent defect such as head injury with neurologic sequelae; amputation; quadriplegia, paraplegia, or monoplegia; or quadriparesis, paraparesis, or monoparesis. The "unknown" wound sites for the killed-in-action category in Table 36.5 are classified as such because a site was not described in any of the press coverage found, the victims had two or more wounds that were not specifically localized, the victim had two or more wounds but which was fatal was indeterminate, or the victim may have had two or more fatal wounds. Research and documentation into the nature of wounds and the outcomes of the survivors are of critical importance in future medical response to the incidents.

Many of these incidents occur with no practical warning, and, although the shooter may continue to be a danger for many minutes to many hours, the majority of victims are shot in the first few minutes of the incident. This does not allow enough time to mobilize special tactical and medical teams, even in large urban areas where full-time teams are on continual stand-by. As in the military casualties described by WDMET, devastating central nervous system wounds and large vessel exsanguinating injuries are not treatable regardless of the response time, on-scene care, or the availability of advanced trauma care.

Based on the available civilian mass shooting data, acute airway obstruction does not appear to be a significant cause of death. Only seven of the victims had neck wounds as the primary wound, and two of these had concomitant head, chest, or back wounds. The utility of advanced airway techniques versus basic airway maneuvers and adjuncts is unclear in these circumstances. However, the author doubts that these techniques could favorably impact the outcome of patients with severe head wounds.

Chest wounds have a significant mortality rate. Timely decompression of a tension pneumothorax could save a number of lives. However, without autopsy data, determining how many of the fatal chest wounds were due to air tension, exsanguination, or another mechanism is difficult. Whether the thorax, abdomen, retroperitoneum, or a combination of these cavities were penetrated was not documented in back wounds. However, as a group, these were even more lethal than chest wounds. Some of these wounds may also have been amenable to pleural decompression.

Of the known extremity wounds, none were lethal. Of the deceased victims, how many of the "unknown" wound sites are, in fact, extremity wounds is not known. These deaths presumably would be preventable and would be amenable to direct pressure.

During the response to these incidents, police officers have been both killed and wounded. No emergency medical personnel are known to have been either killed or wounded. Personnel responding to shootings should wear ballistic protection. Extrication of patients in a "hot zone," an area of immediate danger, should be performed by tactical teams with or without tactical medics. EMS personnel without proper training or ballistic protection should not respond any closer than the secure "cold" zone. Further response principles and philosophy are covered in the Chapter 35. First-in law enforcement personnel have the best, if not only, chance of decreasing the mortality of mass shootings.

PSYCHOLOGIC FALLOUT OF A MASS SHOOTING/MASS KILLING

A study of the survivors of a mass shooting in an office building where eight were killed and six were wounded revealed that one-third of them (12 of 36) met the *Diagnostic and statistical manual of mental disorders* (DSM-IV) criteria for acute stress reaction. Furthermore, this study suggests that acute stress reaction is a predictor of posttraumatic stress disorder (PTSD) that appears 7 to 10 months after the incident. Interestingly, none of these subjects even saw the gunman or were physically injured. Thus, a significant and immediate threat to one's well being appears to be enough to precipitate an acute stress reaction and subsequent PTSD.

A series of studies looked at survivors of the mass shooting incident at Luby's Cafeteria in Killeen, TX immediately after, at 1 to 2 months later, and at 1 year following the incident. North et al. concluded that single interviews at index or a year later might overlook a significant portion of patients with PTSD (28). Disaster survivors with a psychiatric history, especially depression, may be most vulnerable to PTSD, and they may deserve special attention from disaster mental health workers.

The survivors of the Oklahoma City bombing have also been studied (29). More than 34% of the survivors studied met the official definition of PTSD. Many of these cases began almost immediately following the bombing, so identifying PTSD right away is possible. The researchers also noted that most people in whom any psychiatric disorder developed also had PTSD, and they suggested that concentrating on PTSD could identify those most likely to require psychiatric care. Their research on several disasters has shown that disasters caused by willful human action are thought to do more harm than those caused by accidental human action. Natural disasters, or acts of God, appear to have the lowest emotional impact on survivors (see Chapter 6). In comparison with the Oklahoma City bombing (34%), the PTSD rate after the Luby's Cafeteria shooting was 28% but only 2% after a tornado.

SUMMARY

Mass shootings have been occurring with increasing frequency over the past four decades. Unfortunately, schools are becoming more common as incident sites. Forty-seven incidents from August 1966 through May 2000 resulted in 804 victims. Of these victims, 438 died and 366 were wounded. The average mass shooting results in eight victims dead on scene and eight more wounded, one of whom ultimately dies of their wound(s) and some of whom are permanently disabled. Military wounding data appears to be applicable to civilian mass shooting data. These data reveal that patients with penetrating gunshot wounds to the brain have poor outcomes. The classic golden hour does not appear to apply to mass shooting victims, and the critical time in which lives may be saved would seem to be much shorter. Simple airway adjuncts, pleural decompression, immediate or early direct pressure over a compressible wound, and rapid evacuation to a trauma center are interventions that are simple and inexpensive and that could be performed by anyone with a modicum of training. The United States Army came to similar conclusions after analyzing WDMET, and they designed a course, called the *Combat lifesaver course* (30), for the average soldier that emphasizes self-aid, buddy-aid, and the previously mentioned interventions. A similar course called the tactical lifesaver course has been written for civilian law enforcement personnel (31). Although this course has been piloted with federal, regional, and local SWAT teams, it will have a significant impact only if every law enforcement officer has been trained, because of the difference in the relative response times of local police versus specialized response teams in mass shooting incidents.

Although fragmentation and explosive devices are relatively uncommon in the United States, they have been used by perpetrators in the more recent incidents.

The data collected for the purposes of this writing are from public domain sources. The recommendations and conclusions based on these data are a starting point for emergency responders. Much more work is still needed to make more definitive recommendations for the triage, transport, and treatment of these patients.

REFERENCES

1. Personal communication. Federal Bureau of Investigation Field Office, Pittsburgh Region, December 1999.
2. Crandall C, Olson L, Fullerton L, et al. Guns and knives in New Mexico: patterns of penetrating trauma, 1978–1993. *Acad Emerg Med* 1997;4:263–267.
3. Demetriades D, Murray J, Sinz B, et al. Epidemiology of major trauma and trauma deaths in Los Angeles County. *J Am Coll Surg* 1998;4:373–383.
4. Trunkey DD. Trauma. *Sci Am* 1983;249:28–35.
5. Sauaia A, Moore FA, Moore EE, et al. Epidemiology of trauma deaths: a reassessment. *J Trauma* 1995;2:185–193.
6. Bellamy RF. Combat trauma overview. Anesthesia and perioperative care of the combat casualty. In: *Surgical combat casualty care.* Falls Church, VA: Office of the Surgeon General, Department of the Army, 1995:1–42.
7. Levi L, Borovich B, Guilburd JN, et al. Wartime neurosurgical experience in Lebanon, 1982–85. *Israel J Med Sci* 1990;10:548–554.
8. George ED, Dagi TF. Military penetrating craniocerebral injuries: applications to civilian triage and management. *Neurosurg Clin North Am* 1995;4:753–759.
9. Siccardi D, Cavaliere R, Pau A, et al. Penetrating craniocerebral missile injuries in civilians: a retrospective analysis of 314 cases. *Surg Neurol* 1991;35:455–460.
10. Dosoglu M, Orakdogen M, Somay H, et al. Civilian gunshot wounds to the head. *Neurochirurgie* 1999;3:201–207.
11. Polin RS, Shaffrey ME, Phillips CD. Multivariate analysis and prediction of outcome following penetrating head injury. *Neurosurg Clin North Am* 1995;4:689–699.
12. Kaufman HH, Levy ML, Stone JL, et al. Patients with Glasgow coma scale scores of 3, 4, 5 after gunshot wounds to the brain. *Neurosurg Clin North Am* 1995;4:701–714.
13. Biocina B, Sutlic Z, Husedzinovic I, et al. *Eur J Cardiothoracic Surg* 1997;11:399–405.
14. Inci I, Ozcelik C, Tacyildiz I, et al. Penetrating chest injuries:

unusually high incidence of high-velocity gunshot wounds in civilian practice. *World J Surg* 1998;22:438–442.

15. Inci I Ozcelik C, Nizam O, et al. Penetrating chest injuries in children: a review of 94 cases. *J Pediatr Surg* 1996;5:673–676.

16. Vasquez JC, Castaneda E, Bazan N. Management of 240 cases of penetrating thoracic injuries. *Injury* 1997;1:45–49.

17. Mattox KL, Allen MK. Penetrating wounds of the thorax. *Injury* 1986;17:313–317.

18. Adkins RB, Whiteneck JM, Woltering EA. Penetrating chest wall and thoracic injuries. *Am Surg* 1985;51:140–148.

19. Siemens R, Polk HC Jr, Gray LA, et al. Indications for thoracotomy following penetrating thoracic injury. *J Trauma* 1977;17: 493–500.

20. Robinson PD, Harman PD, Trinkle JK, et al. Management of penetrating lung injuries in civilian practice. *J Thorac Cardiovasc Surg* 1988;95:184–190.

21. Oparah SS, Mandal AK. Penetrating gunshot wounds of the chest in civilian practice: experience with 250 consecutive cases. *Br J Surg* 1978;65:45–48.

22. Mandal AK, Oparah SS. Unusually low mortality of wounds of the chest: twelve years experience. *J Thorac Cardiovasc Surg* 1989; 97:119–125.

23. Ozgen G, Duygulu I Solak H. Chest injuries in civilian life and their treatment. *Chest* 1984;85:89–92.

24. Sherman RT. Experience with 472 civilian penetrating wounds of the chest. *Mil Med* 1966;131:63–67.

25. Kish G, Kozloff L, Joseph WL, et al. Indications for early thoracotomy in the management of chest trauma. *Ann Thorac Surg* 1976; 22:23–28.

26. Oparah SS, Mandal AK. Operative management of penetrating wounds of the chest in civilian practice: review of indications of consecutive patients. *J Thorac Cardiovasc Surg* 1979;77:162–168.

27. Reinhorn R, Kaufman HL, Hirsch EF, et al. Penetrating thoracic trauma in a pediatric population. *Ann Thorac Surg* 1996;61: 1501–1505.

28. North CS, Smith EM, Spitznagel EL. Posttraumatic stress disorder in survivors of a mass shooting. *Am J Psychiatry* 1994;151: 82–88.

29. Shariat S, Mallonee S, Kruger E, et al. A prospective study of long-term outcomes among Oklahoma bombing survivors. *J Okla State Med Assoc* 1999;92:178–186.

30. United States Army. *Combat lifesaver course*. Washington, D.C.: Department of the Army, 1998.

31. Colovos N, Stein TM. *Tactical lifesaver course.*

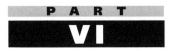

PART VI

EDUCATION, TRAINING, AND RESEARCH

EDUCATION AND TRAINING IN DISASTER MEDICINE

DAVID E. HOGAN

An appropriate response to disasters requires a wide range of skills on the part of disaster responders. Paramedics and emergency physicians represent a unique resource within a community through which much of the initial medical disaster response may be carried out. Therefore, a crucial need exists for these disaster responders to receive a thorough education in the principles of disaster medicine. These emergency health care providers should also be actively involved within their institutions, organizations, and communities to provide accurate and scientifically valid training regarding disasters. In addition, the effectiveness of lay-public training in disaster response and preparation has been well documented (1). Such public education programs should be incorporated into emergency medical services (EMS) and emergency medicine outreach programs

Curricula for the training of emergency physicians have been outlined previously (2). Recently, the core curriculum of emergency medicine has been revised to incorporate substantial amounts of disaster medical training (3). On a national level, more emphasis has been placed on training paramedical and medical personnel and metropolitan communities in disaster response regarding weapons of mass destruction (4). Public awareness regarding disaster response has increased over the past decade due to an increased frequency of disaster occurrence, as well as because of the increased visibility of disaster response through the news media. Despite these improvements, no consensus has yet been reached among researchers, educators, and responders in the field of disaster medicine regarding the elements required to train medical personnel thoroughly in disaster medicine.

DISASTER EDUCATION IN UNITED STATES

An evaluation of the educational process for disaster medicine should begin with a definition of the term *disaster medicine*. Formal training in disaster medicine has existed for many years in Europe. Educational fellowships and diploma programs are available in many European nations for disaster medicine (5,6). In many cases, however, when these educational programs are examined, they contain the goals and objectives that are taught under the term *emergency medicine* and EMS in the United States (7). Variable definitions for disaster medicine exist. The main thrust of disaster medicine within the United States previously has been associated with the organization, skills, and knowledge base required for response to a large-scale disaster event (8). A more recent understanding of disaster medicine requires perceiving disasters from a broader perspective. As Chapter 1 notes, multiple definitions of disaster medicine exist. Disaster medicine has been defined by Gunn as "the study and collaborative application of serious health disciplines—for example, pediatrics, epidemiology, communicable diseases, nutrition, public health, emergency medicine, social mending, community care, international health—to the prevention, immediate response, and rehabilitation of the health problems arising from disaster, in cooperation with other disciplines involved in comprehensive disaster management" (9). No such comprehensive educational program exists within the United States at this time. Therefore, some have called for the development of organized training and a comprehensive disaster curriculum (10). The world is currently in a critical time for creating and implementing fellowship training programs, particularly for physicians with the right mix of medical, public health, and political skills.

In the United States, organizations such as the national disaster medical system (NDMS), the American Red Cross (ARC), and the American College of Emergency Physicians (ACEP) have been leaders in defining and providing educational programs for health care providers in disaster medicine. Although the training programs provided by such organizations are of high quality, their availability for health care providers is often limited. In addition, the funding for such education is often limited by institutional budgetary constraints and political considerations. This can make obtaining quality disaster education expensive and time-consuming for the health care providers. In addition, the objective and focus of each of the organizations differ, making a comprehensive educational overview of disaster medicine difficult to obtain. A nationwide core curriculum should be developed for health care professionals at all levels, and it should be implemented into all training programs.

PROVIDING GOOD EDUCATION: INSTRUCTIONAL SYSTEMS DEVELOPMENT

Educational programs need to be properly developed in order to maximize the educational gain. The instructional systems development method may be used to guide such educational program development. Instructional systems development (ISD) methods were created during World War II when large numbers of people with variable educational backgrounds needed to be trained in complex tasks over a short period of time. The development of ISD represented the first "scientific" method of instruction (11). The aim of ISD is to organize instruction so that the learners are able to perform in the manner that the instructor intends. ISD follows a series of orderly steps in the creation, implementation, and revision of specific educational programs. Many models of ISD exist, but a generic example may be used to demonstrate the principles. Fig. 37.1 illustrates a generic instructional systems development model. Each node on the ISD model represents a step in the creation, implementation, or evaluation of the instructional process.

Determine Learning Outcomes

The first step, often entitled *Determine in learning outcomes* in the flow diagram, represents the creation of a series of goal statements to define what the instructor wishes the students to be able to do at the completion of instruction. Defining goals for the instructional program requires that

the aim of the instruction be delineated. A general example of a goal statement is, "Emergency physicians should be familiar with the immediate treatment of crush syndrome in the emergency department." The goals for this curriculum may be broadly defined if one is creating an overall educational program, and they become more specific for individual instructional sessions. The creation of goals provides statements of the purpose or intent of the program, and these will guide the creation of instructional objectives. Instructional objectives are statements of behavioral or performance requirements that the students should achieve as a result of the instruction provided. These may include items such as, "List and discuss five steps in the treatment of crush syndrome in the emergency department." Instructional objectives should carefully define a specific action or skill that the instructor wishes the students to be able to perform. The process of determining learning outcomes usually requires the creation of a series of goal statements and a set of specific educational objectives. In general, goal statements should comprise the learning outcomes within a short paragraph, and objectives for a specific educational session should not exceed six paragraphs.

Design Instructional Strategies and Develop Evaluation Procedures

The next step in instructional systems development is actually a two-pronged approach. The effectiveness of the instructional session will often be determined more by the method in which the material is taught than by the material itself. Developing an instructional strategy requires that the material that is to be taught be broken down into distinct logical subsets. The presentation of the information should follow a logical, progressive series of steps that start with simple concepts while building toward more complex principles and interactions. As necessary, a list of steps

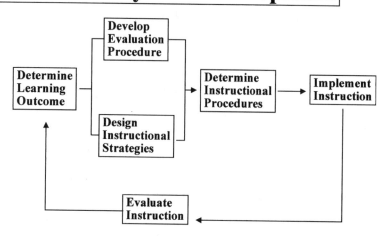

FIGURE 37.1. A generic instructional system development model.

defining how each educational objective shall be presented should be outlined. These individual steps may then be merged into an overall instructional strategy for the teaching session.

One of the key components of ISD is the evaluation of the entire process to determine if the instructional strategy used to teach the program has actually resulted in a behavioral or skill change on the part of the student. Because of this, a decision must be made on how the instructor will tell if the student is actually achieving the learning objectives. This is best accomplished by deciding what evaluation techniques will be used while one is deciding what instructional procedures will be employed. Knowledge-based material provided to the student (e.g., through lectures or discussion series) may be tested by various methods, including essay or multiple-choice examinations. Skilled techniques (e.g., intravenous line skills or airway skills) may be evaluated using model simulations or actual clinical settings. A critical element is that evaluation of the students must be carried out during (formative evaluation) and at the completion (summary evaluation) of training. Without student evaluation, no method exists for gauging the effectiveness of the instruction or for evaluating any need for modifying that instruction. One effective technique is to list each instructional objective side-by-side with the evaluation technique that will address that specific objective.

Determine Instructional Procedures

The instructor has a myriad of instructional process that may be used in achieving educational objectives. The method that is chosen will often depend not only on the material to be taught but also on other factors, such as time, budgetary constraints, the number of students, and the level of student education. When designing instructional strategies, using appropriate teaching methods for the type of material being taught is crucial. For example, expecting students to be proficient in starting intravenous lines if their only training in intravenous techniques has been a series of lecture sessions is nonsensical. The motor skills must be taught by allowing students to practice them in an appropriate fashion. As before, an effective method for ensuring that this occurs is to list the educational objectives and instructional strategies side-by-side with the instructional procedures that one intends to use to teach the material.

Implementation of Instruction

The following step is implementing the instructional package that has been designed by the previous steps. If possible, a *field test* of the instructional package should be conducted before delivery to the intended audience. This can be done by presenting the program to other instructors or to a select group of test subjects. This field testing allows modification and fine-tuning of the educational program before its delivery to the intended set of students. In many instances, however, field testing of instructional programs is not possible; one must therefore rely on evaluation techniques alone to point out areas in which modification in the instructional process is needed.

Evaluate Instruction

Evaluation of the instructional process must be carried out by both students and faculty. If, during the evaluation process, students clearly are not meeting the instructional objectives, then an investigation must be conducted to determine where the flaw lies within the instruction and what actions should be carried out to correct it. The information gained by the evaluation process must be used to modify the instructional process so that the objectives are more effectively achieved. This final step creates a closed loop for ISD in which the ongoing instruction, response, and performance of the faculty and students serve to improve the learning experience on a continual basis.

PRESENTATION METHODS

Many methods exist by which teachers may impart information to students. The use of the ISD helps to organize the overall educational process. More commonly, individuals who are tasked with providing education within their institutions or agencies will be struggling to create specific and effective educational programs. The following section provides an overview of several educational methods that may be used to present information. This section may serve as an introduction to some presentation methods but should certainly not be considered definitive. Faculty within various institutions and organizations are encouraged to seek out training that is readily available to make them more effective educators.

The Lecture

The traditional educational processes are steeped in lecture. Lectures do provide several advantages over other methods of teaching. Lectures may transmit a large amount material over short time, they permit dissemination of unpublished or difficult-to-find materials; moreover, they allow the instructor control the contents, organization, and pace of the material (12). In addition, they may be created and produced in a relatively short amount of time. Unfortunately, the lecture format places the student in a passive, rather than active, role in the learning process, which hinders learning and encourages a one-way communication from the speaker to the student. To be effective, the presenter of the lecture must have an organized and dynamic speaking ability, and he or she must be aware of the need for actively engaging students during the lecture process.

The key to presenting an effective lecture is that the lecturer must possess a thorough knowledge of the material and he or she must present that material in an organized fashion. On average, the experienced presenter will spend 3 to 5 hours in content preparation and organization for each hour of lecture that he or she presents. Determining how much information he or she may reasonably expect the students to absorb during a single presentation is important. The content of a lecture series may be arranged by devising a "rotational outline." A rotational outline consists of dividing the material into essentially equal portions and determining the number of lectures that are required to present that information. When planning, one should allow for cancellations, guest lectures, and discussion periods. More time should be allotted for the complex issues than for the simple topics. In addition, consideration should be given to the specific audience, as well as to the number of individuals in the class. Lectures to small groups are often more effective than are presentations to larger groups. Small groups generally allow more interaction with the students and have a more conversational presentation format. Large groups allow for little individual interaction; such activities are usually limited to formal question-and-answer sessions following the lecture.

In general, lectures should be organized into the following three distinct parts: the introduction, the main body, and the closure. The introduction should contain a sequence that is intended to grab the learner's attention immediately, to motivate them to pay attention, to provide structure for the lecture in the mind of the learner, and to indicate the objectives of the lecture. Next, the learner should organize the main body by outlining the content of the lecture in a logical sequence. A number of schemes may be used to do this. The *cause-and-effect scheme* is used when events may be cited and explained by reference to their particular origins. The *time sequential method* arranges lectures along a chronologic fashion. The *topical theme* focuses on specific different areas of information in a successive manner. The *problem solution scheme* states a problem and then provides one or more solutions for that problem. The *pro-con approach* consists of an alternating, two-sided discussion throughout the lecture. Finally, the *ascending-descending method* arranges lecture information according to its importance or complexity. Examples that may be used to illustrate key ideas or concepts should be created to help familiarize students with the new material. Finally, the instructor should create a set of points and examples that emphasize the major educational objectives of the lecture. No more than five major points should be presented per lecture, and lectures should be kept below 55 minutes in length. Longer lectures result in a loss of attention and decreased effectiveness on the part of the learner. The end or closure, which is commonly referred to as the *conclusion*, of the lecture needs to be strategically planned. The closure should draw attention to the end of the lecture, it should help the listener organize the information that has been presented, and it should reinforce the specific learning objectives presented.

Visual aids such a slide or transparencies are valuable in sustaining the students' attention and interest during a lecture. The creation of such visual aids is an art in and of itself, so it is not covered in this chapter. However, visual aids should add to, not detract from, the educational experience provided in the lecture format.

The Discussion

When compared to lecture format, which dispenses a large amount of information in a single session, the critical ingredient in the discussion is the interaction between the teacher and the students. Discussions are much more difficult to organize and conduct than lectures are. They require considerable knowledge of the topic material being provided on the part of the instructor, as well as prior preparation by the students who will be participating. While lectures are important in providing basic low-level information, discussions may be used to assist in a higher level of learning and synthesis of the information that has been provided. In reality, a large amount of education in the health-care field occurs during discussions among supervisors and colleagues in the break room, following prehospital runs, at the bedside, and before and after resuscitations. Formalized discussion sessions take these educational experiences into a structured environment that is free of distractions. The benefits of discussions can be harnessed in situations where one can assume that students have a previous knowledge of the particular topic. The major advantage of the discussion is that it require active involvement and participation by the student in the exchange of facts and opinions. The major disadvantages are that significant time and effort is required to create a discussion session, effort is required to maintain a focus on the objectives of the discussion, and attention must be devoted to involving all members of the discussion group. Discussions are not particularly effective in disseminating new information. They are, however, advantageous in creating a higher level of understanding in a previously provided knowledge base. The dynamics and methods of creating effective discussion group are quite complex. In-depth methods for creating discussion groups may be found in other sources (13).

Seminars

Seminars may be the first step in disaster education for any community or agency. They are generally low-cost activities, and they can inform a variety of participants. These are often provided in a lecture format, but they should encourage audience participation as much as possible. The emphasis should be on the identification of problems within the disaster planning and response community and on deriving solutions for those problems.

The Simulation

After lectures, simulations are the mainstays of teaching methods in disaster medicine. Every hospital disaster drill greeted by apathy and groans on the part of the medical staff is in itself a simulation. Simulations may range from community-wide drills with moulaged patients to tabletop board games and seminars.

Tabletop Exercises

Tabletop exercises are an extremely cost-effective and highly efficient method of providing disaster education to personnel and of testing plan procedures. The players involved in a tabletop exercise can be provided with an excellent opportunity to interact and to understand the various roles and responsibilities that are required during a community disaster response. In addition, this may bring the members of the communities disaster response face-to-face in an intimate situation that promotes familiarization and camaraderie. The participants of the tabletop may be subjected to a high degree of realism regarding the problems that could be faced during a disaster response.

During a tabletop exercise, the key players of the group are all within a confined area. This proximity allows the exercise to be stopped as necessary to provide educational direction and counseling before proceeding with the next phase. Elaborately designed tabletop exercises may include sophisticated audiovisual presentations, scale model environments, and real-time communication techniques. Tabletop exercises have a particular advantage of bringing the multiple agencies that span the spectrum of the disaster response community together and allowing these individuals to interact in ways that they often do not during a field exercise. The involvement of all key personnel within the community, including fire, EMS, hospitals, emergency departments, public service agencies, federal agencies, news media, and others, should be encouraged.

The degree to which a tabletop exercise simulates a real disaster is dependent primarily on the imagination of the simulation's creators and participants. The scenarios that are played out should be realistic, and they should be based on valid assumptions. An introductory session should outline the rules of the tabletop exercise. Regular pauses in the activity should be built in so that direction can be provided, thus ensuring that the educational objectives of the tabletop are met. This may prevent some participants from solving situational problems quickly by unorthodox means. Finally, following the exercise, a debriefing session in which the performance of the participants is compared to the objectives of the exercise should be conducted.

The area that is used for the tabletop must be large enough to accommodate both the number of participants and the equipment (e.g., boards, scale models) that is required for the exercise. All the necessary audiovisual aids should be in place, and they should be tested the night before the exercise. A lecture theater may be suitable, but often a large room with conference tables accommodates this type of training better. Additionally, separate rooms are required for the training staff who are conducting the exercise, as well as for smaller groups that may be isolated from the main body of participants (e.g., communication specialists, incident commanders, support staff).

Control Post Exercises

Control post exercises are particularly useful in teaching and testing the organizational relationships and communication links for a particular agency. Control post exercises typically involve the team leaders and the communications teams for each participating agency. These individuals are positioned at the control post that they would normally take during actual disaster. The exercise tests not only the communication arrangements but also, and more importantly, the flow of information among team leaders positioned throughout the city. Control post exercises are effective in testing plans and procedures through members of various departments. For this reason, they are cost-effective. Unfortunately, however, they do not involve the front-line staff of the operational cadre. Control post exercises involve multiple sites throughout the city. The organizations involved in the exercise should use their designated control centers.

Field Exercises

Field exercises may range from small-scale tests of specific components of the disaster response to broad community-wide disaster exercises. They require considerably more organization and planning than the other types of disaster educational experiences. Field exercises provide the best overall means of testing the community's ability to respond to a real disaster, as well as enabling a unique educational experience. The more realistic that a field exercise is in simulating a real disaster, the more effective the educational process. Several points must be considered regarding field exercises.

Field exercises often involve a great deal of expense. This expense is not only incurred by the planning and implementation of the exercise but also due to the man hours associated with the involvement of the participants. Several methods can reduce the costs of these exercises. First, because many agencies such as hospitals, EMS services, and fire departments are required to conduct such drills on a regular basis, resources may be combined into a joint exercise fulfilling all of the various agencies' requirements. In some instances, the number of players participating in the field exercise may be limited to key individuals from each institution or agency. Field exercises may be scheduled to fall within working hours to avoid the need for overtime pay. Schedules can possibly be rearranged to conduct field exercises during on-duty time that has been reserved for training.

The first element of the field exercise is a committee comprising an exercise planning group. This group should contain individuals across the spectrum of specialties needed for disaster response within the community. It must also have the ability to liaison with all participating agencies during the planning stages of the field exercise. As one of its initial tasks, the group must decide upon an objective for the field exercise and the degree to which the exercise will train and test the overall response plan. All agencies that have a role to play in a disaster response should be invited to take part in the exercise. These agencies should be involved in the planning stage, as well as in the debriefing sessions. The planning sessions may be time-consuming, which might make direct participation of managers, executives, and chief officers difficult. Designees of these individuals may act as their proxy, but these substitutes should keep their superiors informed of the progress of the planning group. The planning group should allow themselves a sufficient amount of time to prepare for the field exercise adequately. Planning sessions should, in fact, begin several months before the actual exercise occurs. Ideally, individuals involved in the planning of the exercise should not participate directly. They should be used as moderators, observers, or evaluators during the exercise.

The goals and objectives of the exercise should be clearly established at the beginning of the planning sessions. The most realistic method for achieving this is to have each agency submit a set of objectives. These objectives may then be combined and modified to represent the objectives of the overall field exercise. The objectives should be realistic, and they should be based on valid assumptions. The participants should actually be able to achieve them, and they should provide both an educational and evaluative function. The exercise should practice the plan, not the chaos, of the disaster.

The planning group should develop a realistic scenario to ensure that the participants will take the exercise seriously. Exercises should also have a realistic time scale. Consideration should be given to the nature of the incident and the date and time of the scenario, as well as to other conditions, such as weather, visibility, traffic, and the nature of victims involved.

Field exercises may be conducted in time-lapse fashion. In this situation, decisions are made as to whether the exercise will flow in real-time or in snapshots of time. For instance, EMS may spend a considerable amount of time working out the intricacies of scene triage and immediate patient management. From that point, the scenario may move to the emergency department phase without testing the transportation utilities.

Field exercises may also be conducted in a control or free-play mode. A controlled exercise occurs when the scenario and all specific events are carefully scripted. In this way, the evolution of the disaster response is carefully controlled by the directors of the exercise. Control-type field exercises are an excellent way to train and to test specific aspects of a disaster response; however, the inflexibility of this method may limit the ability of the participants to learn how to deal with unexpected events.

Free-play exercises are considerably more spontaneous than are control exercises. Once the exercise begins, the direction of the exercise is dictated by the participants' actions. Free-play field exercises require a larger directing staff and a much more comprehensive training scenario so that more background information may be accessed as it is needed by the participants. Although free-play exercises are more realistic and stimulating, they may make teaching or testing specific parts of the disaster response plan more difficult because the participants may bypass parts of the plan as the scenario plays out. Combining both control and free-play scenarios is possible to some degree, particularly within individual groups of exercise participants.

The initial location where the field exercise is to occur should be visited by members of the planning group. Consideration should be given to the likely conditions surrounding this location on the actual day the field exercise is to occur. Written consent ensuring that the exercise may be conducted there should be obtained from the agencies or companies in control of the site. In addition to the site of the field exercise, a specific location should be set aside as an exercise base. This is particularly helpful in the setting of large-scale exercises. A suitable building with adequate access and communications equipment should be selected, and, preferably, it should be one owned by a participating agency. This location may serve as an assembly point for the exercise directors, observers, and evaluators. If possible, the exercise base should be within walking distance of the field exercise site. If not, mass transportation from the exercise base to the field exercise site should be provided to diminish the overall vehicular traffic within the area.

Safety is a primary consideration while the conducting the field exercise. Before conducting a live exercise, all participants, including the observers and evaluators, should be briefed on the potential hazards and safety protocols. Participants must be aware of the confines within which the exercise is being conducted, as this represents a controlled environment where safety may be reasonably assured. Overlap of the field exercise into nonsecure areas within the community may generate not only community concern but also serious safety hazards for the public, as well as for the field exercise participants. Safety audits should be conducted of all structures and areas before the field exercise. Of critical importance is the understanding that the exercise may not be used for an excuse to violate standard safety protocols that all participants in the field exercise should have. Consideration must be given to the provision of emergency medical care (e.g., first aid, EMS) to the participants. Individuals monitoring the exercise must have the ability to stop the exercise immediately in the event of major safety violations or actual emergencies. Adequate amenities (e.g., food, water) must be available to the participants for exercises of longer duration. The planning group should anticipate the need for additional personnel to ensure public safety

Public information should be provided before the initiation of the exercise. The area of the exercise should be secured against the visitation of uninvited spectators. Prior news releases regarding the exercise should be sufficient to inform the majority of the population of the exercise, but they should be low-key enough to prevent large numbers of spectators.

An exercise controller must be appointed. This individual must have overall control and authority to alter the planned program or stop the exercise for any reason. In addition, several exercise directors should be appointed to ensure that the scenario plays out correctly, as well as to provide information regarding the status of the exercise to the exercise controller. Exercise directors may intervene during appropriate points of the scenario to ensure that the educational and testing objectives are met. However, this intervention should be kept at a minimum, and it should be used only as a last resort. This will allow the participants to correct the problems they have encountered. Exercise directors should also intervene if confusion exists about the scenario or if an organizational problem out of the control of the participants occurs. They should also intervene if failing to do so will compromise the exercise objectives or if the actions of a single person or group is jeopardizing the opportunities that the exercise affords.

Evaluators monitor the exercise and measure the degree to which the educational and testing objectives are occurring. They have no direct role or responsibility in the mechanics of the exercise. They should be well briefed in the overall objectives of the exercise, but they do not necessarily require detailed knowledge of the scenario.

Observers play no role in exercise, but they do serve as witnesses for assessing the overall preparations and organization that occurs during the scenario. They should be selected by various agencies based on their areas of expertise. They should be clearly identified, and they must be afforded access to all parts of the field exercise area. Observers can provide valuable information to their respective agencies regarding performance during the exercise.

In addition, special observers (e.g., political officials, members of the public, and other dignitaries) may be afforded the opportunity to observe the field exercise. These special observers should be escorted by individuals familiar with the scenario and the protocols for disaster training and response. These escorts may provide an explanation of the events that are unfolding as the scenario progresses. A designated observing area may be created to provide these special observers with an overall view of the field exercise.

To avoid confusion, all individuals such as the exercise controller, the exercise directors, the evaluators, and the observers should be clearly identified to separate them from exercise participants. This identification may take the form of vests or badges of high visibility.

Although the field exercise is often used as a method for testing communication mechanisms, the communication links available for the individuals conducting the exercise must also function. An agreed channel of communication should be set up among directing staff so that all members are aware of developments and changes as the scenario progresses. In addition, the exercise staff must be able to contact nonparticipating emergency agencies if problems arise. All surrounding agencies must be made aware of the exercise in advance to prevent radio traffic from being misinterpreted as an actual disaster.

Documentation and incident recording should be practiced during the scenario just as it would be during an actual response. These information sources become particularly useful during the debriefing. Moreover, familiarity with these documentation practices will increase their use during an actual event. Documentation will decrease confusion regarding victim location and condition, in addition to providing valuable information for reviewing and researching the disaster.

The news media is a major part of the response to any disaster incident. Because of this, they must be included within the disaster scenario to some degree. A news media that is well-educated with regard to a community disaster response is an invaluable asset, while a poorly educated or hostile news media will exacerbate a critical disaster situation significantly. The news media should be invited to a field exercise, and key members of the news media should become familiar with the key players of the response team. Each agency should have their appointed public relations officer interface with the news media. Regular news briefings should be simulated as part of the exercise because this is a major part of disaster response.

SUMMARY

A serious need for education in disaster medicine exists. Comprehensive fellowship training programs for physicians that are based on valid scientific assumptions should be developed. Organized educational programs covering the basic principles of disaster medicine should be integrated into the training of all health care providers in the country. Emergency health care providers should take the lead role in the educational process in disaster medicine in their communities.

REFERENCES

1. Abrams JI, Pretto EA, Angus D, et al. Guidelines for rescue training of the lay public. *Prehosp Disaster Med* 1993;8:151–156.
2. Noji EK. Core content development project. *ACEP Disaster Medicine Section News* 1990;1:5.
3. Task force on the core content for emergency medicine. Revision: core content for emergency medicine. *Acad Emerg Med* 1997;4: 628–624.

4. Richards CF, Burstein JL, Waeckerle JF, et al. Emergency physicians and biological terrorism. *Ann Emerg Med* 1999;34: 183–190.

5. Lumley J, Ryan J. Disaster medicine: an emerging specialty. *Hosp Med* 2000;16:276–278.

6. Leppaniemi A, Ryan J, Lumley J. The diploma of the medical care of catastrophes (DMCC). *Ann Chir Gynaecol* 1999;88: 145–146.

7. de Boer J. An introduction to disaster medicine in Europe.*J Emerg Med* 1995;13:211–216.

8. Waeckerle JF. Disaster planning and response. *N Engl J Med* 1991;324:815–821.

9. Debacker M, Domres B, de Boer J. Glossary of new concepts in disaster medicine: a supplement to Gunn's multilingual dictionary of disaster medicine. *Prehosp Disaster Med* 1999;14:146–149.

10. Waeckerle JF, Lillibridge SR, Burkle FM Jr, et al. Disaster medicine: challenges for today. *Ann Emerg Med* 1994;23:715–718.

11. McCombs BL. The instructional systems design (ISD) model: a review of those factors critical to its successful implementation. *Educ Commun Technol* 1986;34:67–81.

12. Whiteside MF, Gallery ME, Klonis LK, eds. *The residency teacher series: emergency medicine module*. Dallas TX: American College of Emergency Physicians, 1990.

13. Whitman NA, Schwenk TL. *A handbook for group discussion leaders: alternatives to lecturing medical students to death*. Salt Lake, UT: University of Utah School of Medicine, 1983.

RESEARCH IN DISASTER MEDICINE

GARY QUICK
DAVID E. HOGAN

Research may be one of the most misunderstood components of disaster medicine. It is often regarded by disaster responders as an esoteric undertaking carried out by individuals who have little understanding of "the real world" and less understanding of clinical disaster issues. In reality, research into disasters is one of the most vital functions that can be carried out by those involved in such events. The best disaster researchers are individuals with substantial experience in disaster response and planning because they know what questions need to be asked. Conducting research on a disaster is an attempt to determine the truth about the event itself. Without such efforts and application of the resulting knowledge to the disaster planning and response process, mistakes will continue to be repeated.

For years, much of the literature reporting on disasters consisted of anecdotal stories about "what I did the day the *fill in the blank* (e.g., tornado, flood, earthquake) struck." Although such reports provide some useful information, they are, in reality, a limited view of only a few individuals' ideas about the event, and they do not follow the scientific method. Planning for a disaster based on such reports alone can be inefficient, and it is potentially dangerous.

Research into disasters should be an effort to collect and organize information about the event using the scientific method and to report that information in a coherent format that is supported by the method used. The aim of doing so is to describe the various true elements of the event and to use that information to improve planning and response for the next disaster. Unfortunately, disasters do not lend themselves to some of the more frequently used methods for research. Prospective studies collecting data on phenomena as they occur are usually considered the strongest type of studies. Although collecting prospective information during a disaster is not impossible, it is an extremely difficult task. For the most part, research in disaster medicine is performed retrospectively, after the impact phase and during the recovery activities.

No single chapter can make an individual a researcher. This chapter can, however, attempt to outline some of the basic principles of obtaining, analyzing, and reporting useful information regarding disasters. Creating organized reports about disasters may prove to be the first step in providing quality research. However, numerous research methods aside from those reports discussed in this chapter are available. Each individual involved in researching a disaster should use methods that are consistent with his or her own abilities and training.

PURPOSES OF DISASTER RESEARCH

Disaster prevention or mitigation is an important reason for performing disaster research. One example of disaster mitigation resulting from research is found in the June 15, 1991, volcano eruption of the Mt. Pinatubo volcano. Research on volcano-related disasters was involved in mitigating its impact. State-of-the-art volcano monitoring techniques and instruments were applied to the volcano; the eruption was accurately predicted; and hazard zonation maps had been prepared and disseminated 1 month before the violent eruption. An alert and warning system had been designed and implemented based on the study of previous eruptions. Disaster response machinery was mobilized in a timely manner to mitigate the effects of the eruption (1). This project tangibly demonstrated that one of the primary purposes of high-quality disaster research directed toward prevention and mitigation could be achieved.

PHRASING THE RESEARCH QUESTION

Numerous questions may be asked about a disaster. The nature and number of questions asked in a research project largely depends on the point of view of the individual asking the questions. Researchers are usually interested in collecting information about their specific area of expertise (e.g., search and rescue, emergency medical services [EMS], emergency medicine), and they will likely focus on these topics. Multidisciplinary research groups consisting of many individuals with varied expertise can thus improve the quality and efficiency of the questions (2).

Stating the research question(s) clearly, simply, and unambiguously is the most important step in designing the research study. In 1777, Dr. Jenner might have asked the question, "Does prior exposure to cowpox diminish a person's risk of contracting smallpox?" This question clearly indicates what study design may facilitate a reliable answer to the question. Comparing smallpox rates in persons previously exposed to cowpox with rates of those who had not been previously exposed would provide an answer to the research question. Because all subsequent study issues of design, methods, statistical analysis, and resource requirements proceed from the study research question, the investigator's proper development, refinement, and framing of the research question is of utmost importance.

At the beginning of the disaster study, the principal investigator may find that the best option is to contact an experienced researcher or epidemiologist who can provide expertise in asking the proper question. To the author's knowledge, no statistician has ever complained that he or she was involved in a study too soon. Often, the consultant may not have expertise in any area of disaster research. Nonetheless, expertise in phrasing the proper study question can be accomplished by him or her once the principal investigator has provided the necessary background facts and issues. A university department of emergency medicine, a school of public health, or an epidemiology group may provide the desired expertise in a prompt and inexpensive fashion. Other assistance may be obtained via organizations, such as the disaster or research sections of the American College of Emergency Physicians (ACEP) or The Society for Academic Emergency Medicine.

A further benefit of developing a well-framed and clear research statement is that the statement may be easily converted into a statistical hypothesis if necessary. Because one of the axioms of the scientific method is that a hypothesis can never be proven completely true, investigators often rephrase their question in opposite terms—that is, as the *null hypothesis*. Data are then collected to determine whether the results justify the rejection of this hypothesis. Jenner's statistical hypothesis could thus be stated, "Persons exposed to cowpox are as likely as those who have not been exposed to cowpox to contract smallpox." Dr. Jenner would then form two groups—one exposed to cowpox and another that had not been exposed—and he would measure the prevalence and rates of smallpox that developed in each group. A competent statistician could then calculate the probability of his hypothesis being true. If the probability were small (e.g., <5%–10%), Dr. Jenner would be justified in rejecting his statistical hypothesis of no difference in smallpox rates between those exposed to cowpox and those who had not been exposed. Not all studies, however, require the testing of a statistical hypothesis. Descriptive studies, which often fit the unique nature of disaster research, often do not involve proving statistical hypotheses (3).

All disasters are different, so no standard set of questions will cover all the areas that need to be investigated. However,

TABLE 38.1. GENERAL POINTS IN DATA COLLECTION AFTER A DISASTER

Nature of the disaster (tornado, flood, etc.) and its temporal events.
Number and demographics of the casualties.
Mechanisms of injury and illness.
Impact of the disaster on services (SAR, EMS, ED, hospital, etc.).
Nature of the response (no. of responders, no. of EMS units, consultants, equipment, pharmaceuticals agents, etc.).
Disposition and outcomes of casualties (admitted, operated, died, etc.).
Special or unusual clinical entities.

Abbreviations: ED, Emergency department; EMS, emergency medical services; SAR, search and rescue.

an outline of some basic disaster-related questions can provide initial guidance in creating a research protocol to investigate a disaster. These questions are listed in Table 38.1.

HOW TO ANSWER THE RESEARCH QUESTIONS

The investigator must next determine precisely how to answer the research question. This means that he or she must determine what to measure and must choose the appropriate measurement method. A literature review of the topic will be useful for identifying what work has been previously reported and what measurement processes have been used and have been proven valid. At this point, contact with qualified consultants or experienced researchers may also yield rich benefits. The study design and data collection methods are defined by the research question(s) that are asked.

WRITING A RESEARCH PROJECT PROTOCOL

Before contact with subjects and data collection, the investigator will need to develop a plan or protocol that specifies what will be done and who will assume the key roles in the process. The protocol should delineate (a) the eligibility criteria for study subjects to be included in the study group, (b) the procedures to be followed once the eligible subjects are identified, (c) the data collection instrument to be used and the manner in which the data will be collected, and (d) procedures that will be followed to record and preserve the data (including its security). Not only will preparation of the protocol provide a clear, comprehensive plan for action, but it will also stimulate the investigator to think through every phase of the study before the data collection begins.

A well-written protocol helps the investigator anticipate potential problem areas, facilitates the receipt of constructive feedback from colleagues and consultants, and serves as a roadmap to assist in manuscript preparation after study completion. Multiple formats exist for writing research protocols. One successful approach for writing research protocols will be discussed below.

The first page should be a title page. This page should identify the study by a name that defines the general point of the project. The name(s) of the principal individuals involved in the research may appear here. The next page should identify the principal investigator of the study and any additional investigators who are involved in the project. Each individual who will be participating in the research should be listed with their titles and institutional affiliation.

The next section should be the statement of the purpose of the project. A short paragraph outlining the question(s) or problem(s) being considered and why they are being considered will suffice. The investigator should include what he or she expects to learn from the exercise. If a null hypothesis has been formulated, it is discussed here.

A section on research methods should follow. This outlines the study design in detail. The investigator defines the kind of study being conducted (e.g., descriptive, noninterventional observational, medical records review, survey, interview, or qualitative), the target population for study, and the inclusion and exclusion criteria for patients (cases) to be addressed. Then, the author should outline specifically how the study will be conducted, including how the data are to be collected and recorded and what statistical analysis will be used. Consent issues should be discussed if consent is needed for the study, and the the issue of how patient (subject) confidentiality will be maintained must be addressed.

Finally, a brief review of the pertinent literature should be included. This section provides the background references about the topic being investigated. It should review the historical components and the core information about the topic of the research. This section is used to help educate and train individuals who are assisting with or are approving the study. In addition, this section may serve as the basis for a large portion of the discussion of any publication that is eventually created from the research.

The references should then be organized into a bibliography and attached to the document. Any data collection forms or survey forms should also be printed and attached. Organizing the research project in this manner outlines the scientific methods used in researching the disaster and provides consistency when conducting the protocol. In addition, the information can facilitate the process of completing applications for institutional review board (IRB), research grant approval, or both. Table 38.2 outlines the steps in writing a research project protocol.

Define the Target Population

Defining the target population and identifying the study subjects are important pieces of conducting research. The researcher must decide what group of subjects the research question concerns. He or she must define the target population—that is, the population to which the study results

TABLE 38.2. WRITING A RESEARCH PROTOCOL

Create a title page.
Create an investigators' page.
Write a purpose statement.
Define the methods:
    How the data will be collected.
    How the data will be recorded.
    What statistical methods will be used.
Write a brief review of the pertinent literature.
Create a bibliography of the pertinent literature.
Attach any data or survey forms.

will apply. This is the population to which results are generalized after the analysis of the study subjects. In most disaster-related research, this simply includes all individuals exposed to the forces of the disaster. Once the study population has been definitively and specifically defined, then specific study subjects can be identified within the parameters of the study population.

Defining the Study Subjects (Cases)

Identifying the study subjects is one of the most challenging aspects of disaster research. In disaster research, the subjects (cases) are usually defined as those who are impacted by the disaster and who are seeking care within a specified time. The availability of study subjects declines with the passage of time. Most disaster studies are hampered by delay in securing primary data. Documentation of patient registration and medical evaluation is often very poorly conducted during the immediate response period of the disaster. Community disaster planning should identify an agency, such as the State Health Department, or another organization to assume the responsibility for the documentation of the official list of all victims of a given disaster. During recent disasters in Oklahoma City, disaster research physicians contacted the involved hospital emergency departments to request that each department keep a separate log and chart file of disaster victims so that victim identification and medical records retrieval would be simplified.

Finding the Cases That Have Been Defined

Once cases have been defined, the research team must actually find the information about them in records or locate the individuals. Establishing a working relationship with the State Health Department or any other agency responsible for epidemiologic surveillance or injury prevention provides the opportunity to request that a disaster event be classified as a reportable event from the perspective of the health department. Once an event is declared reportable, any practitioner or institution that encounters a patient experiencing that event is required to forward a report to the health department, similar to the procedure used for reporting syphilis, salmonella, or tuberculosis. The declaration of disaster injuries as reportable aids greatly in victim identification. Health Department personnel are then able to collect patient data from treatment locations. In addition, this enhances the cost-of-care accounting accuracy when damage estimates are calculated. Both the Murrah building bombing and the F-5 tornado of May 3, 1999, were promptly declared reportable events by the Oklahoma State Health Department, which greatly aided in the identification of the total number of injured and of the severity of their injuries. The official policy of the ACEP is that disaster injuries and illnesses are reported to public health agencies and that injury-illness databases should be compiled (4).

Sample Size and Limitations

Determination of the sample size becomes a somewhat ill-defined process in most disaster research. Because a disaster is a relatively unique event, the investigator should strive to include all of the victims impacted. Demographic information should be obtained regarding the victims. Efforts should be made to define as closely as possible the number of individuals who are at risk for injury and illness from the event, as well as the total number of individuals who suffered injury or illness. This allows a more accurate calculation of rates and frequencies, as well as providing the researcher with a better overall grasp of the truth. In reality, due to the mobility of the population, the failure to report injury, decisions that are made not to seek care or assistance, and temporal delays in initiating the study, the study sample is often reduced to a convenience sample of 30% to 50% of the potential subjects (5).

Institutional Review

Obtaining approval from an IRB or similar committee is vital before conducting research of any kind. These organized groups exist at all major health care facilities that are involved in conducting clinical research, as well as at universities. Each IRB has a human use committee that reviews the involvement of humans as research subjects. The IRB reviews each research protocol that is submitted in light of current federal and institutional regulations and policies on research, as well as based on the scientific soundness of the outlined project. Most disaster-related research is of a descriptive nature, meaning that it is conducted without intervening in the care of human subjects. Therefore, most IRBs will grant a special exemption to disaster research protocols, indicating that they have been reviewed and approved but that they do not require special consent for human use. Currently, the majority of medical journals will not accept papers for publication if the protocol has not been reviewed by an IRB for approval or exemption.

Most researchers appreciate the role of an IRB as they gain experience in the research arena. Reassurance of the researcher's good intentions is simply not enough guarantee of propriety with respect to patients' rights. This is particularly true in disaster research in which the disaster victims themselves may have experienced great loss or tragedy. They are then being asked to participate in an activity that has the potential to bring up quite deep emotional pain and suffering.

Strongly justifiable recommendations can be made for submitting all research studies to an IRB with jurisdiction in the area of the study before proceeding with the study. IRB approval protects the rights of the patient and the reputation of the investigator. While IRB approval does involve some extra work and time delay, the benefits of IRB approval clearly outweigh the exigencies of the approval process. The mission of the IRB should be to act as a clearinghouse for all studies and to guarantee consistency in the quality of research; the identification of researchers; sensitivity and compassion in the conduct of each project; and confidentiality of the victims, their families, and rescue workers; and to monitor the quantity of research conducted with these potential subjects. The local IRB is in a position to limit the overlap of studies and to gauge the impact of a particular study on the intended subjects. It is also well versed in the development of consent language and forms, which can be used to delineate the rights of patients and the responsibilities of researchers clearly.

COLLECTING THE DATA

Timely Collection of Data

Many previous disaster studies suffer from a delay in data collection. Research efforts often lag 6 to 12 months behind the disaster event, and they include only 35% to 40% of the disaster victims (5). Most projects are carried out by a limited number of investigators who are examining a relatively small portion of the entire scenario of the disaster (6). By the time of data collection, persons involved in the disaster response and the management of victims have often moved on to other positions. Their recollection of the actual experience has been rendered less accurate by time. The victims may have dispersed or died. Sometimes, they have simply forgotten the accurate story of the event. Prompt initiation of data collection or, at least, the initiation of data preservation techniques is one avenue by which the quality of disaster research might be improved.

The majority of disaster responders have little time to perform daily tasks, let alone engage in research. To do so requires commitment and determination to see the project through. The reader should recall that, after being involved in a disaster, each individual has a unique perspective on the issues. These perspectives should be shared with other disaster responders, as the time to do the research is as soon after the event as possible. The dedicated researcher can organize a skeleton set of methods years before a disaster strikes by using risk assessment to focus on the likely disaster scenarios for the locality. A preliminary research protocol may even be written and kept on file for such events. This protocol may then be updated and modified rapidly to fit the nature of the specific event (7).

The researcher must be efficient in data collection. When one is analyzing medical records, one or two short preparatory visits to a records site by a coordinator can ensure that everything is in order before the data collection team arrives. The research protocol and data collection should be kept focused on the task. Although the researcher must be aware of new developments or previously unconsidered pathways of questioning, he or she should generally stay limited to what tasks are important for completing the project. The investigator must make arrangements to have time to collect data, to supervise research teams, to visit administrators and records custodians, and to conduct interviews and surveys. Above all, he or she should get help from colleagues and coworkers in performing these tasks.

Identifying the Resources Needed to Conduct the Research

In identifying resources that are needed to complete the study successfully, the researcher should list the material resources and the human resources that are required to complete the study. The investigator must then determine whether looking outside the immediate practice environment for specialized research skills to facilitate the research protocol is necessary. As was previously mentioned, consultants such as a statistician, an epidemiologist, or other appropriate individuals should be involved early in the design stage. The principal investigator should reach a clear understanding of the respective responsibilities and rewards for each participant or collaborator based on objective and agreed-on parameters whenever possible.

Manpower for Data Collection

Capable manpower is often in short supply for most disaster research, partly because of the limited number of disasters generating studies and also because of the limited number of interested individuals. In previous projects, some investigators have utilized a collaborative method of acquiring research manpower through working with emergency medicine residents and with medical students interested in acquiring some exposure to emergency medicine before matriculation into their own residency training programs. This approach commonly represents the *modus operandi* that is possible in an academic environment, but it may be extended to a community setting with relatively small expense. As was mentioned previously, the state health department or injury control agency may be well positioned

and well motivated to provide skilled data collection personnel. Cooperative work with such organizations can always be fruitful.

Most research projects on disasters are large enough to require a team of data collectors. These data collectors may be involved in multiple tasks while performing the research protocol. They may work in the field during recovery activities to interview survivors, families, or disaster responders. In addition, they may be involved in reviewing medical records or other documents that contain the case information of the casualties. Some of these activities may be rather complex. Therefore, all participants collecting data for the research protocol must be trained to do so.

Data collectors should be comfortable with the process before they actually work in the field. Providing written flow sheets or other such work aids that may be used during the process of data collection to the research team members will help ensure that information is collected properly. A small pilot test of data collection may be performed before general data collection to work out any problems in the process. Reviewing the quality of data collected each day to screen for problems can also be valuable.

Data Collection and the Abstraction Manual

Data collection is often the watershed portion of the study, as it forms the basis for credible and reliable results or the absence thereof. A limited number of experienced data collectors using a well-designed data collection form comprises the best structure for most projects. Some researchers recommend developing an abstractor manual that includes all the possible variations expected under a particular data point. The data collector then refers to the abstractor manual for guidance when a data variable needs clarification. Using this technique results in a higher degree of standardization for data entry. In addition, the manual defines each data entry sufficiently enough to guide the creation of a computerized database for later data storage and analysis.

Recording Data

Collected data may be recorded on paper or in a computerized form. The authors recommend collecting primary data using a paper customized data form that includes demographic data that will allow future contact with the patient if necessary. Direct identifiers of the patient are, however, omitted from the primary data. An institutional medical record number or another unique identifier should be used to maintain the confidentiality of individual patient identity. Direct data entry into a computerized database, although it may seem to be more efficient, requires the necessary hardware and its requisite expense. It also mandates additional skills and training for the data collectors, and it may result in less accurate data entry. Certainly, with the rapidly expanding use of microcomputers and the rapid growth in personal computer database management, including handheld devices, almost all disaster research study data will be entered into a computerized database for storage and analysis at some point in the study.

Sources of Data in Disaster Research

Ready sources of data exist following a disaster. Much of the information may fade quickly, or it may be disposed of after the event. Therefore, making an attempt to secure and sequester items, such as medical records, emergency department disaster lists, EMS run sheets, hospital disaster rosters, and the like, before they are disposed of is important. Often such written items are not an official part of the medical record, and they will be culled by medical records departments during records processing. Even before IRB approval, one can bring together potential researchers, hospital administrators, and records custodians to coordinate the protection of such documents to improve later recovery (2).

Simple reviews of medical records after a disaster are useful, but they can have significant limitations (6). These studies underestimate the total number of casualties and the number of potential casualties exposed to the disaster. Disaster studies may be improved by using multiple sources for case information. Sending out surveys to regional health care providers to seek information on the casualties treated and conducting survivor, family, and responder surveys improves data recovery (8).

Other sources of information that are available as a matter of public record may provide considerable amounts of case information. Depending on the type of disaster, reports may be available from the police, fire, federal, and state agencies and from utility companies. These documents become available as a matter of public record, and they may be used by the disaster researcher (9). In Oklahoma, Dr. Jerry Nida, then State Commissioner of Health, declared bombing casualties a reportable condition. This created a core set of data about bombing victims within the State Health Department that would otherwise have been lost. The declaration of disaster injuries as a reportable condition to health authorities is recommended to set the stage for researchers to participate in research.

ADMINISTRATIVE SUPPORT FOR RESEARCH

Successful completion of disaster research projects of any size requires development and provision of an infrastructure capable of supporting the research effort and responding to unanticipated needs as they arise during the course of the project. Often, the requisite support can be provided by an administrative assistant with secretarial skills when one is dealing with small projects. Larger projects require greater degrees of administrative assistance. Qualified support personnel can sometimes be located through the State Health Department or another agency with interest in the disaster project. The State Health Department will have access to epidemiologists, data collectors, statisticians, and database support personnel. Hence, one strategic reason for recommending that the health department declare disaster injuries as reportable conditions is to acquire access to the expertise of the agency in support of the research effort. Of course, such data collection is also in the best interest of the Health Department because it has the responsibility for meeting the health needs of the state.

Another local area of research administrative expertise and support is the Office of Research Administration (ORA) of local universities. During the aftermath of the Oklahoma City bombing, the University of Oklahoma ORA was involved in many ways. Perhaps most importantly, the ORA served as the agency for the administration of the political empowerment from the governor's office and other political agencies. The efforts of the ORA were also directed toward the issues of study design and the adequacy of data collection with a concerned scrutiny for the preservation of a compassionate approach to the victims and the victims' families. The ORA used its communications network, which extended to many universities, to communicate the creation of a bombing study research registry to the other institutions and prospective research groups. The purpose of this was to facilitate networking among investigators and to minimize duplication of studies.

During the early months after the bombing, several calls were made by the ORA to out-of-state institutions sponsoring disaster-related research to offer assistance in study design, IRB review, and consent and confidentiality issues. The calls were handled with discrete attention to issues of territoriality and local IRB authority and responsibility. Most calls were well received, and they resulted in a mutual appreciation of the concerns that were involved on behalf of research teams from the respective institutions.

OBSTRUCTIONS TO DISASTER RESEARCH
Responder Feelings

Probably the largest obstruction to research in disaster is the feeling of those who are involved in the disaster response that they cannot perform research. Most individuals consider research a highly technical and difficult undertaking that is beyond their abilities or outside their scope of practice. Nothing could be further from the truth. The insight of disaster responders involved in the event is crucial to reaching a full understanding of what happened. Not everyone is a trained researcher, but, by using some simple epidemiologic principles in data collection and obtaining help when it is needed), valuable and accurate insight can be gained.

The "It's Our Disaster" Attitude

After suffering through a disaster, local disaster responders and the community at large are often hesitant to participate in research conducted by anyone at all, let alone outsiders. This attitude unfortunately has been reinforced in some cases by research teams who descend on a disaster-stricken population with invasive, obtrusive, and, at times, unethical research methods.

All disasters are local. If a researcher seeks to study a disaster not within his or her community, several principles can be suggested. Often the best way to study a disaster is by cooperating with local responders in their efforts. Avoid the "pro-from-Dover" approach that will cause resentment, if not a complimentary plane ticket home. Networking through organizations such as National Disaster Medical System (NDMS), the ACEP disaster section, and others will usually provide researchers with a point of contact within a given region, state, or municipality through which research efforts may be coordinated.

Other issues may come into play. After the Oklahoma City bombing, Governor Frank Keating issued a declaration requesting that all researchers evaluating the event coordinate their efforts through the University of Oklahoma ORA. Although such declarations do not have the authority of law, researchers should be sensitive to these issues.

USE OF COLLECTED DATA

Collection of information after a disaster without the analysis and dissemination of that information is a fruitless process. The object of research in this setting is to gain a general understanding of the event, to attempt to answer some specific questions, and to provide insight that may be used by others in disaster response and planning. The information should initially be analyzed using simple descriptive statistics (i.e., rates, frequencies, risk ratios). If specific groups may be compared with regard to a particular set of variables, then comparative statistics may be applied. Having a biostatistician assist in this part of the process is wise to ensure validity and accuracy in the analysis of the data.

The researcher should tailor his or her analysis towards a desired readership or audience. The documents should be created using the information for instructions to the authors that are provided in the journal or publication to which the researcher intends to submit his or her work.

Disaster Reporting Nomenclature and Format

A lack of standardized nomenclature and vocabulary for disaster medicine and disaster research restricts the ability of researchers to design studies and to report their findings in uniform terminology. Data collection also suffers from both a lack of a uniform database design and the lack of stan-dardized data collection tools with which to approach the disaster. Standardized nomenclature, database design, and data collection tools that could be easily customized to accommodate the unique needs of each disaster would substantially strengthen future disaster research efforts.

Vocabulary and Terms

The development of a glossary of research terms would be a valuable resource so that the investigator does not invent an entire assemblage of jargon. Often such jargon has a specific meaning to the investigator, but it may be confusing to those not involved in the work. Proper terminology is essential to clear communication with others, whether participants or future readers of the published work. Standard scientific and medical terms that already exist should be used to define and describe aspects of a disaster. When a new term is needed in order to describe adequately an aspect of the disaster, that term should be clearly defined and should be used consistently by the personnel involved.

FUNDING FOR DISASTER RESEARCH

Obtaining funding to perform research is one of the most difficult obstructions to research for emergency medicine in general. These difficulties are compounded for research in disaster medicine. Disaster research funding suffers from a severe lack of interest and a somewhat myopic planning approach by the funding sources. The Federal Emergency Management Agency (FEMA) is perhaps the most logical and accessible funding source in the postdisaster period. FEMA, however, is essentially a response support agency without a direct budget line for disaster research funding. FEMA is able to provide short-term, limited support, such as reimbursement for computer leasing and temporary secretarial support. However, the agency budget has no provision for funding to support data collection or to provide grant support to facilitate the employment of sufficient study personnel to accomplish the intended studies in a timely fashion. A multitude of other disaster response organizations, such as the NDMS, urban search and rescue, and the American Red Cross, provide essential clinical services under proscribed conditions, but they can provide no research funding (10).

The Centers for Disease Control and Prevention (CDC) does provide research assistance to meet its major agency responsibilities. These include preparing for and responding to public health emergencies and conducting investigations into the health effects and medical consequences of disasters. CDC research assistance is therefore most often offered as the short-term provision of expert consultants and technical expertise. No funding is available through the CDC to support the on-line work of the disaster research project, including data collection and abstraction, office space, computers, and statistical analyses.

Some local agencies and foundations are able to provide small amounts of funding for selected projects, but these groups are not reliable sources for disaster research funding because most of their resources are also committed to the clinical care of victims. One successful source of funding for disaster research after the Oklahoma City bombing were the mental health agencies within the state. These agencies had the ability to reallocate clinical resources to meet both clinical demands and research opportunities. Also, the longer duration of contact with patients requiring mental health services after the disaster helped assure follow-up. Public policy experts should consider attaching a funded budget line item for disaster research to an agency such as FEMA so that disaster research projects can be initiated, supported, and completed in a timely and efficacious manner.

MULTIDISCIPLINARY RESEARCH

Health management during and after a disaster is a multi-disciplinary venture. It is marked by activities such as the rapid assessment of health needs, the management of mass casualties, the coordination of relief activities, epidemiologic surveillance, environmental health, nutrition, health relief supplies, public settlements, communication, transport, relief assistance, and recovery activities (11).

Unique characteristics and circumstances attend each disaster. A nuclear reactor explosion and fire in 1986 at Chernobyl, Russia, caused a very different environment for responders than did the bombing in Oklahoma City. A tank car spill of liquid chlorine on a rail line within a city triggers a markedly different response than an Amtrak passenger train derailment on that same line. The unique requirements of each disaster dictate the need for the development of a large and expanding disaster database to assist disaster responders in making a knowledgeable and appropriate response.

Because disaster research involves providers with different levels of training and focus, disaster response opens the door to multidisciplinary research. Engaging representatives from key community services in intentional dialog about the analysis of a disaster or for planning for a future disaster stimulates a multidisciplinary approach. Employing the collective abilities of this group of local people with a broad base of expertise and that have a vested interest in the outcome of local planning is an effective approach to problem solving. Such an inclusive approach promotes collegial relationships, leading to quality research and more efficient preparation for future disasters.

The science of disaster medicine is founded in multidisciplinary medical skills that embrace the therapeutic and the preventive spectrum of health care (12). However, recent disaster research literature has included only a limited number of examples of multidisciplinary disaster research that brings together the strength and skill of several disciplines to focus on a particular disaster. After the 1980 Mount St. Helens volcanic eruption, a multidisciplinary group was formed to evaluate the potential long-term health effects of the volcanic activity on the local populations (13). Other examples of recent multidisciplinary disaster research include the mass identification of victims from the Tenerife, Spain, airport crash and the Oklahoma City bombing (14,15). A multidisciplinary approach to disaster research may permit a more complete understanding of the disaster, as well as to allow various in-depth analyses to proceed simultaneously, based on the multiple levels of expertise represented on the research team.

CONCLUSION

One of the purposes of disaster research is to move the disaster clinician from a reactive mode, in which he or she responds to crises after they have developed, to a proactive mode, which allows him or her to reduce damage, property loss, and loss of life before the disaster incident occurs. Some recent technologic advances that have contributed to the potential for employment of predictive or preventive modalities to limit disaster exposure are the National Severe Storm Center in Norman, Oklahoma and the global positioning system community architectural survey that is currently in progress in Oklahoma, both of which will be international in scope upon completion. The storm center allows sophisticated technologic studies of severe weather systems, permitting real-time tracking of tornadoes and other severe weather events and providing as much as 15 to 30 minutes of advance warning to communities in the path of advancing tornadoes. The system has been used successfully many times during the past few years to track severe weather events in Oklahoma. Had the F-5 tornado of May 3, 1999, which ripped one-quarter mile swaths of total destruction through the Oklahoma City metropolitan area, killing 45 and injuring over 600, had not been tracked so well, the loss of life would have been substantially higher. Residents in the path of the storm received at least 15 minutes of advance warning to flee or take shelter. Furthermore, the intensity of the storm had been well measured, resulting in specific directions that residents should shelter below ground or should evacuate from the projected path of the storm. Without the large amount of severe storm research preceding this storm and the deployment of an effective storm-tracking system, such accurate predictive warnings would not have been so effective in preventing morbidity and mortality in the communities involved.

The global positioning system structural survey was designed to identify types of architecture and construction styles that would be vulnerable to tornado or other severe weather threats, such as straight-line winds. By identifying such buildings, as well as susceptible sections of cities and towns, local governments and emergency service providers will be able to anticipate what portions of their community are at higher risk for damage and casualties due to such storms.

Similar research activities assessing search and rescue, EMS response, emergency medicine and hospital interventions, and physical and emotional rehabilitative activities must be conducted. The application of a more orderly and scientific approach to disaster research can yield substantial benefits in the care and recovery of communities and individuals struck by disasters.

REFERENCES

1. Tayag JC, Punongbayan RS. Volcanic disaster mitigation in the Philippines: experience from Mt. Pinatubo. *Disasters* 1994;18:1–15.
2. Quick G. A paradigm for multidisciplinary disaster research: the Oklahoma City experience. *J Emerg Med* 1998;16:621–630.
3. Zervanos NJ. Designs, protocols, and procedures. In: Berg AO, Gordon MJ, Cherkin DC, et al., eds. *Practice-based research in family medicine*. Kansas City, MO: The American Academy of Family Physicians, 1986:23–31.
4. American College of Emergency Physicians. Disaster data collection. In: *ACEP policy compendium*, 2001 ed. Dallas: American College of Emergency Physicians, 2001:12.
5. Noji EK. The use of epidemiologic methods in disaster. In: Noji EK, ed. *The public health consequences of disasters*. New York: Oxford University Press, 1997:21–36.
6. Lillibridge SL, Noji EK. The importance of medical records in disaster epidemiology in research. *J AHIMA* 1992;63:137–138.
7. Guha-Sapir D. Rapid assessment of health needs in mass emergencies: review of current concepts and methods. *World Health Stat Q* 1991;44:171–181.
8. Mallonee S, Shariat S, Stennies G, et al. Physical injuries and fatalities resulting from the Oklahoma City bombing. *JAMA* 1996;276:382–387.
9. Williams LA, Hogan DE. *The Steamboat Springs restaurant explosion: disaster data in the public records*. Presented at the Florida Chapter of the American College of Emergency Physicians International Disaster Conference 1999, Orlando, Florida, May, 1999.
10. Patrick P. The American Red Cross–Centers for Disease Control natural disaster morbidity and mortality surveillance system [letter]. *Am J Public Health* 1992;82:1690.
11. Chakraborty AK. Disaster epidemiology and health management. *Indian J Pub Health* 1992;36:94–100.
12. Waeckerle JF. Disaster planning and response. *N Engl J Med* 1991;324:815–821.
13. Buist AS, Martin TR, Shore JH, et al. The development of a multidisciplinary plan for evaluation of the long-term health effects of the Mount St. Helens. *AJPH* 1986;76:39–44.
14. Van den Bos A. Mass identification: a multidisciplinary operation. *Am J Forensic Pathol* 1980;1:265–270.
15. Hogan DE, Waeckerle JF, Dire DJ, et al. Emergency department impact of the Oklahoma City terrorist bombing. *Ann Emerg Med* 1999;34:160–167.

APPENDIX A

WORLD HEALTH ORGANIZATION MODEL LIST OF ESSENTIAL DRUGS: TENTH LIST 1997

EXPLANATORY NOTES

Many drugs included in the list **are preceded by an asterisk** (*) to indicate that they represent an **example of a therapeutic group** and that *various drugs could serve as alternatives*. This must be understood when drugs are selected at national level because the choice is then influenced by the comparative cost and availability of equivalent products. Examples of acceptable substitutions include the following:

■ Hydrochlorothiazide: any other thiazide-type diuretic currently in broad clinical use.
■ Hydralazine: any other peripheral vasodilator having an antihypertensive effect.
■ Senna: any stimulant laxative (either synthetic or of plant origin).
■ Sulfadiazine: any other short-acting systemically-active sulfonamide unlikely to cause crystalluria.

Numbers in parentheses following the drug names are defined as follows:

1. Drugs subject to international control under:
   a. The Single Convention on Narcotic Drugs, 1961.
   b. The Convention on Psychotropic Substances, 1971.
   c. The Convention against Illicit Traffic in Narcotic Drugs and Psychotropic Substances, 1988.

2. Specific expertise, diagnostic precision, individualization, or special equipment required for proper use.
3. Greater potency or efficacy.
4. In renal insufficiency, contraindicated or dosage adjustments necessary.
5. To improve compliance.
6. Special pharmacokinetic properties.
7. Adverse effects diminish benefit/risk ratio.
8. Limited indications or narrow spectrum of activity.
9. For epidural anaesthesia.
10. Sustained release preparations are available. The fact of proper sustained release of the dosage form should be documented.

Letters in parentheses following the drug names indicate the reasons for the inclusion of *complementary* drugs:

A. When drugs in the main list cannot be made available.
B. When drugs in the main list are known to be ineffective or inappropriate for a given individual.
C. For use in rare disorders or in exceptional circumstances.
D. *Reserve* antimicrobials to be used only when significant resistance to other drugs on the list is found.

Drugs are listed in alphabetical order by section.

A.1. LIST OF ESSENTIAL DRUGS

Drug	Qualification	Method of administration
1. ANESTHETICS		
1.1. General Anesthetics and Oxygen		
Ether, anesthetic	(1c,2)	Inhalation.
Halothane	(2)	Inhalation.
Ketamine hydrochloride	(2)	Injection, 50 mg/mL in 10-mL vial.
Nitrous oxide	(2)	Inhalation.
Oxygen		Inhalation (medicinal gas).
*Thiopental sodium	(2)	Powder for injection, 0.5 g; 1.0 g in ampule.
1.2. Local Anesthetics		
*Bupivacaine hydrochloride	(2,9)	Injection, 0.25%, 0.5% in vial; injection for spinal anesthesia, 0.5% in 4-mL ampule to be mixed with 7.5% glucose solution.
*Lidocaine hydrochloride		Injection, 1%, 2% in vial; injection for spinal anesthesia, 5% in 2-mL ampule to be mixed with 7.5% glucose solution; topical forms, 2–4%.
*Lidocaine hydrochloride + epinephrine		Injection, 1%; 2% + epinephrine, 1:200,000 in vial; dental cartridge; 2% + epinephrine, 1:80,000

A.1. *(continued)*

Drug	Qualification	Method of administration
Complementary drug(s)		
Ephedrine hydrochloride[a]	(C)	Injection, 30 mg/mL in 1-mL ampule.

[a]*To prevent hypotension in spinal anesthesia during delivery.*

1.3. Preoperative Medication and Sedation for Short-Term Procedures

Drug	Qualification	Method of administration
Atropine sulfate		Injection, 1 mg in 1-mL ampule.
Chloral hydrate		Syrup, 200 mg/5 mL.
*Diazepam	(1b)	Injection, 5 mg/mL in 2-mL ampule; tablet, 5 mg.
*Morphine hydrochloride	(1a)	Injection, 10 mg in 1-mL ampule.
*Morphine sulfate	(1a)	Injection, 10 mg in 1-mL ampule.
*Promethazine hydrochloride		Elixir or syrup, 5 mg/5 mL.

2. ANALGESICS; ANTIPYRETICS; NONSTEROIDAL ANTIINFLAMMATORY DRUGS (NSAID), DRUGS USED TO TREAT GOUT, AND DISEASE-MODIFYING ANTIRHEUMATOID DRUGS (DMARDs)

2.1. Non-Opioids and NSAIDs

Drug	Qualification	Method of administration
Acetylsalicylic acid		Tablet, 100–500 mg; suppository, 50–150 mg.
*Ibuprofen		Tablet, 200 mg, 400 mg.
Paracetamol		Tablet, 100–500 mg; suppository, 100 mg; syrup, 125 mg/5 mL.

2.2. Opioid Analgesics

Drug	Qualification	Method of administration
*Codeine phosphate	(1a)	Tablet, 30 mg.
*Morphine hydrochloride	(1a)	Injection, 10 mg in 1-mL ampule; oral solution, 10 mg/5 mL.
*Morphine sulfate	(1a)	Injection, 10 mg in 1-mL ampule; oral solution, 10 mg/5 mL; tablet, 10 mg.
*Pethidine hydrochloride	(A) (1a,4)	Injection, 50 mg in 1-mL ampule; tablet, 50 mg, 100 mg.

2.3. Drugs Used to Treat Gout

Drug	Qualification	Method of administration
Allopurinol	(4)	Tablet, 100 mg.
Colchicine	(7)	Tablet, 500 μg.

2.4. Disease-Modifying Antirheumatoid Drugs (DMARDs)

Drug	Qualification	Method of administration
Azathioprine	(2)	Tablet, 50 mg.
Chloroquine phosphate	(2)	Tablet, 100 mg, 150 mg of chloroquine.
Chloroquine sulfate	(2)	Tablet, 100 mg, 150 mg of chloroquine.
Cyclophosphamide	(2)	Tablet, 25 mg.
Methotrexate sodium	(2)	Tablet, 2.5 mg.
Penicillamine	(2)	Capsule or tablet, 250 mg.
Sulfasalazine	(2)	Tablet, 500 mg.

3. ANTIALLERGICS AND DRUGS USED IN ANAPHYLAXIS

Drug	Qualification	Method of administration
*Chlorphenamine hydrogen maleate		Tablet, 4 mg; injection, 10 mg in 1-mL ampule.
*Dexamethasone		Tablet, 500 μg, 4 mg.
*Dexamethasone disodium phosphate		Injection, 4 mg of dexamethasone phosphate in 1-mL ampule.
Epinephrine hydrogen tartrate		Injection, 1 mg of epinephrine in 1-mL ampule.
Epinephrine hydrochloride		Injection, 1 mg of epinephrine in 1-mL ampule.
Hydrocortisone sodium succinate		Powder for injection, 100 mg of hydrocortisone in vial.
*Prednisolone		Tablet, 5 mg.

4. ANTIDOTES AND OTHER SUBSTANCES USED IN POISONING

4.1. Nonspecific

Drug	Qualification	Method of administration
*Charcoal, activated		Powder.
Ipecacuanha		Syrup calculated containing 0.14% ipecacuanha alkaloids, as emetine.

4.2. Specific

Drug	Qualification	Method of administration
Atropine sulfate		Injection, 1 mg in 1-mL ampule.
Calcium gluconate	(2,8)	Injection, 100 mg in 10-mL ampule.
Deferoxamine mesilate		Powder for injection, 500 mg in vial.
Dimercaprol	(2)	Injection in oil, 50 mg/mL in 2-mL ampule.
*Methionine (D-L-)		Tablet, 250 mg.
Methylthioninium chloride (methylene blue)		Injection, 10 mg/mL in 10-mL ampule.
Naloxone hydrochloride		Injection, 400 μg in 1-mL ampule.
Penicillamine	(2)	Capsule or tablet, 250 mg.
Potassium ferric hexacyano-ferrate (II) (Prussian blue)		Powder for oral administration.
Sodium calcium edetate	(2)	Injection, 200 mg/mL in 5-mL ampule.
Sodium nitrite		Injection, 30 mg/mL in 10-mL ampule.
Sodium thiosulfate		Injection, 250 mg/mL in 50-mL ampule.

A.1. *(continued)*

Drug	Qualification	Method of administration
5. ANTICONVULSANTS AND ANTIEPILEPTICS		
Carbamazepine	(10,11)	Scored tablet, 100 mg, 200 mg.
*Diazepam	(1b)	Injection, 5 mg/mL in 2-mL ampule (intravenous or rectal).
Ethosuximide		Capsule, 250 mg; syrup, 250 mg/5 mL.
Phenobarbital	(1b,11)	Tablet, 15–100 mg; elixir, 15 mg/5 mL.
Phenytoin sodium	(7,11)	Capsule or tablet, 25 mg, 50 mg, 100 mg; injection, 50 mg/mL in 5-mL vial.
Sodium valproate	(7,11)	Enteric-coated tablet, 200 mg, 500 mg.
Complementary drug(s)		
*Clonazepam	(B) (1b)	Scored tablets, 500 mg.
Magnesium sulfate	(C)	Injection, 500 mg/mL in 2-mL ampule; injection, 5 g/10 mL in ampule.
6. ANTIINFECTIVE DRUGS		
6.1. Anthelminthics		
6.1.1. Intestinal Anthelminthics		
Albendazole		Chewable tablet, 400 mg.
Levamisole hydrochloride		Tablet, 50 mg of levamisole, 150 mg of levamisole.
*Mebendazole		Chewable tablet, 100 mg, 500 mg.
Niclosamide		Chewable tablet, 500 mg.
Praziquantel		Tablet, 150 mg, 600 mg.
Pyrantel embonate		Chewable tablet, 250 mg of pyrantel; oral suspension, 50 mg of pyrantel/mL.
6.1.2. Antifilarials		
Diethylcarbamazine dihydrogen citrate		Tablet, 50 mg, 100 mg.
Ivermectin		Scored tablet, 3 mg, 6 mg.
Complementary drug(s)		
Suramin sodium	(B) (2,7)	Powder for injection, 1 g in vial.
6.1.3. Antischistosomals and Antitrematode Drugs		
Praziquantel		Tablet, 600 mg.
Triclabendazole		Tablet, 250 mg.
Complementary drug(s)		
Oxamniquine	(C) (8)	Capsule, 250 mg; syrup, 250 mg/5 mL.
6.2. Antibacterials		
6.2.1. Beta Lactam Drugs		
*Amoxicillin (anhydrous)	(4)	Capsule or tablet, 250 mg, 500 mg; powder for oral suspension, 125 mg/5 mL.
Ampicillin sodium		Powder for injection, 500 mg, 1 g in vial.
Benzathine benzylpenicillin		Powder for injection, 1.44 g of benzylpenicillin (= 2.4 million IU) in 5-mL vial.
Benzylpenicillin potassium		Powder for injection, 600 mg (= 1 million IU), 3 g (= 5 million IU) in vial.
Benzylpenicillin sodium		Powder for injection, 600 mg (= 1 million IU), 3 g (= 5 million IU) in vial.
*Cloxacillin sodium		Capsule, 500 mg, 1 g of cloxacillin; powder for oral solution, 125 mg of cloxacillin/5 mL; powder for injection, 500 mg of cloxacillin in vial.
Phenoxymethylpenicillin potassium		Tablet, 250 mg of phenoxymethylpenicillin; powder for oral suspension, 250 mg of phenoxymethylpenicillin/5 mL.
Procaine benzylpenicillin		Powder for injection, 1 g (= 1 million IU), 3 g (= 3 million IU).
Reserve antibacterials		
*Amoxicillin + *clavulanic acid	(D)	Tablet, 500 mg + 125 mg.
Ceftazidime pentahydrate	(D)	Powder for injection, 250 mg of ceftazidime in vial.
*Ceftriaxone sodium	(D)	Powder for injection, 250 mg of ceftriaxone in vial.
Imipenem + cilastatin sodium	(D)	Powder for injection 250 mg + 250 mg, 500 mg + 500 mg in vial.
6.2.2. Other Antibacterials		
*Chloramphenicol	(7)	Capsule, 250 mg.
*Chloramphenicol palmitate	(7)	Oral suspension, 150 mg of chloramphenicol/5 mL.
*Chloramphenicol sodium succinate	(7)	Powder for injection, 1 g of chloramphenicol in vial.
*Ciprofloxacin hydrochloride		Tablet 250 of ciprofloxacin.
*Doxycycline hyclate	(5,6)	Capsule or tablet, 100 mg of doxycycline.

(continued)

A.1. *(continued)*

Drug	Qualification	Method of administration
*Erythromycin ethylsuccinate		Capsule or tablet, 250 mg of erythromycin; powder for oral suspension, 125 mg of erythromycin.
*Erythromycin lactobionate		Powder for injection, 500 mg of erythromycin in vial.
*Erythromycin stearate		Capsule or tablet, 250 mg of erythromycin; powder for oral suspension, 125 mg of erythromycin.
*Gentamicin sulfate	(2,4,7,11)	Injection, 10 mg, 40 mg of gentamicin/mL in 2-mL vial.
*Metronidazole		Tablet, 200–500 mg; injection, 500 mg in 100-mL vial; suppository, 500 mg, 1 g.
*Metronidazole benzoate		Oral suspension, 200 mg of metronidazole/5 mL.
Nalidixic acid	(8)	Tablet 250 mg, 500 mg.
Nitrofurantoin	(4,8)	Tablet, 100 mg.
Spectinomycin hydrochloride	(8)	Powder for injection, 2 g of spectinomycin in vial.
*Sulfadiazine	(4)	Tablet, 500 mg.
*Sulfadiazine sodium	(4)	Injection, 250 mg in 4-mL ampule.
*Sulfamethoxazole + trimethoprim	(4)	Tablet, 100 mg + 20 mg, 400 mg + 80 mg; oral suspension, 200 mg + 40 mg/5 mL; injection, 80 mg + 16 mg/mL in 5-mL and 10-mL ampules.
Trimethoprim	(8)	Tablet, 100 mg, 200 mg; injection, 20 mg/mL in 5-mL ampule.
Complementary drug(s)		
Chloramphenicol sodium succinate	(C)	Oily suspension for injection 0.5 g of chloramphenicol/mL in 2-mL ampule.
Clindamycin	(B) (8)	Capsule, 150 mg.
Clindamycin phosphate	(B) (8)	Injection, 150 mg of clindamycin.
Reserve antibacterial		
Vancomycin hydrochloride	(D)	Powder for injection, 250 mg of vancomycin in vial.
6.2.3. Antileprosy Drugs		
Clofazimine		Capsule, 50 mg, 100 mg.
Dapsone		Tablet, 25 mg, 50 mg, 100 mg.
Rifampicin		Capsule or tablet, 150 mg, 300 mg.
6.2.4. Antituberculosis Drugs		
Ethambutol hydrochloride	(4)	Tablet, 100–400 mg.
Isoniazid		Tablet, 100–300 mg.
Isoniazid + ethambutol hydrochloride	(5)	Tablet, 150 mg + 400 mg.
Pyrazinamide		Tablet, 400 mg.
Rifampicin		Capsule or tablet, 150 mg, 300 mg.
Rifampicin + isoniazid[b]	(5)	Tablet, 150 mg + 75 mg; 300 mg + 150 mg; 150 mg + 150 mg.
[b]*For intermittent use three times weekly.*		
Rifampicin + isoniazid + pyrazinamide[c]	(5)	Tablet, 150 mg + 75 mg + 400 mg; 150 mg + 150 mg + 500 mg.
[c]*For intermittent use three times weekly.*		
Streptomycin sulfate	(4)	Powder for injection, 1 g of streptomycin in vial.
Complementary drug(s)		
Thioacetazone + isoniazid	(A) (5,7)	Tablet, 50 mg + 100 mg; 150 mg + 300 mg.
6.3. Antifungal Drugs		
Amphotericin B	(4)	Powder for injection, 50 mg in vial.
Griseofulvin	(8)	Capsule or tablet, 125 mg, 250 mg.
*Ketoconazole	(2)	Tablet, 200 mg; oral suspension, 100 mg/5 mL.
Nystatin		Tablet, 100,000, 500,000 IU; lozenge, 100,000 IU; pessary, 100,000 IU.
Complementary drug(s)		
Flucytosine	(B) (4,8)	Capsule, 250 mg; infusion, 2.5 g in 250 mL.
Potassium iodide	(A)	Saturated solution.
6.4. Antivirals		
6.4.1. Antiherpes		
Aciclovir	(8)	Tablet, 200 mg.
Aciclovir sodium	(8)	Powder for injection, 250 mg of aciclovir.
6.4.2. Antiretrovirals		
Zidovudine	(8)	Capsules 100 mg, 250 mg; injection, 10 mg/mL in 20-mL Vial; oral solution, 50 mg/5 mL.

A.1. (continued)

Drug	Qualification	Method of administration

Drugs for treatment of HIVAIDS include Nucleoside Reverse Transcriptase Inhibitors (NRTIs), Non-Nucleoside Reverse Transcriptase Inhibitors (NNRTIs) and protease inhibitors (PIs). The prototype drug, zidovudine, has been shown to reduce or prevent mother-to-child transmission. **This is the only indication for which it is included here.** *Single drug use with zidovudine, except in pregnancy, is now regarded as obsolete, because of the development of resistance. Triple therapy is beyond the budgets of most national drug programs and therefore HIVAIDS treatment policies must be decided at the country or institutional level.*

6.5. Antiprotozoal Drugs

6.5.1. Antiamoebic and Antigiardiasis Drugs

*Diloxanide furoate		Tablet, 500 mg.
*Metronidazole		Tablet, 200–500 mg; injection, 500 mg in 100-mL vial.
*Metronidazole benzoate		Oral suspension, 200 mg of metronidazole/5 mL.

6.5.2. Antileishmaniasis Drugs

*Meglumine antimonate		Injection, 30%, equivalent to approximately 8.5% antimony, in 5-mL ampule.
Pentamidine isetionate	(5)	Powder for injection, 200 mg, 300 mg in vial.
Complementary drug(s)		
Amphotericin B	(B) (4)	Powder for injection, 50 mg in vial.

6.5.3. Antimalarial Drugs

6.5.3.1. For Curative Treatment

*Chloroquine hydrochloride		Injection 40 mg of chloroquine/mL in 5-mL ampule.
*Chloroquine phosphate		Tablet 100 mg, 150 mg of chloroquine; syrup, 50 mg of chloroquine/5 mL; injection, 40 mg of chloroquine/mL in 5-mL ampule.
*Chloroquine sulfate		Tablet 100 mg, 150 mg of chloroquine; syrup, 50 mg of chloroquine/5 mL; injection, 40 mg of chloroquine/mL in 5 mL ampule.
Primaquine diphosphate		Tablet, 7.5 mg, 15 mg of primaquine.
*Quinine bisulfate		Tablet, 300 mg.
*Quinine dihydrochloride		Injection, 300 mg/mL in 2 mL ampule.
*Quinine sulfate		Tablet, 300 mg.
Complementary drug(s)		
*Doxycycline hyclate[d]	(B)	Capsule or tablet, 100 mg.
[d]*For use only in combination with chloroquine.*		
Mefloquine hydrochloride	(B)	Tablet, 250 mg of mefloquine.
*Sulfadoxine + pyrimethamine	(B)	Tablet, 500 mg + 25 mg.
Reserve antimalarial		
Artemether	(D)	Injection, 80 mg/mL in 1-mL ampule.

6.5.3.2. For Prophylaxis

Chloroquine phosphate		Tablet, 150 mg of chloroquine; syrup, 50 mg of chloroquine/5 mL.
Chloroquine sulfate		Tablet, 150 mg of chloroquine; syrup, 50 mg of chloroquine /5 mL.
Mefloquine hydrochloride		Tablet, 250 mg of mefloquine.
Proguanil hydrochloride[e]		Tablet, 100 mg.
[e]*For use only in combination with chloroquine.*		

6.5.4. Antipneumocystosis and Antitoxoplasmosis Drugs

Pentamidine isetionate	(2)	Tablet, 200 mg, 300 mg.
Pyrimethamine		Tablet, 25 mg.
Sulfamethoxazole + trimethoprim		Injection, 80 mg + 16 mg in 5 mL ampule.

6.5.5. Antitrypanosomal Drugs

6.5.5.1. African Trypanosomiasis

Melarsoprol	(5)	Injection, 3.6% solution.
Pentamidine isetionate	(5)	Powder for injection, 200 mg, 300 mg in vial.
Suramin sodium	(5)	Powder for injection, 1 g in vial.
Complementary drug(s)		
Eflornithine hydrochloride	(C)	Injection, 200 mg/mL in 100 mL bottles.

6.5.5.2. American Trypanosomiasis

Benznidazole	(7)	Tablet, 100 mg.
Pifurtimox	(2,8)	Tablet, 30 mg, 120 mg, 250 mg.

6.6. Insect Repellents

Diethyltoluamide		Topical solution, 50%, 75%.

(continued)

A.1. (continued)

Drug	Qualification	Method of administration
7. ANTIMIGRAINE DRUGS		
7.1. For Treatment of Acute Attack		
Acetylsalicylic acid		Tablet, 300–500 mg.
Ergotamine tartrate	(7)	Tablet, 1 mg.
Paracetamol		Tablet, 300–500 mg.
7.2. For Prophylaxis		
*Propranolol hydrochloride		Tablet, 20 mg, 40 mg.
8. ANTINEOPLASTIC, IMMUNOSUPPRESSIVES AND DRUGS USED IN PALLIATIVE CARE		
8.1. Immunosuppressive Drugs		
*Azathioprine	(2)	Tablet, 50 mg.
*Azathioprine sodium	(2)	Powder for injection, 100 mg of azathioprine in vial.
Ciclosporinᶠ	(2)	Capsule, 25 mg; concentrate for injection, 50 mg/mL in 1-mL ampule.
ᶠFor organ transplantation.		
8.2. Cytotoxic Drugs		
Asparaginase	(2)	Powder for injection, 10,000 IU in vial.
Bleomycin sulfate	(2)	Powder for injection, 15 mg of bleomycin in vial.
Calcium folinate	(2)	Tablet, 15 mg; injection, 3 mg/mL in 10-mL ampule.
Chlormethine hydrochloride	(2)	Powder for injection, 10 mg in vial.
Cisplatin	(2)	Powder for injection, 10 mg, 50 mg in vial.
Cyclophosphamide	(2)	Tablet, 25 mg; powder for injection, 500 mg in vial.
Cytarabine	(2)	Powder for injection, 100 mg in vial.
Dacarbazine	(2)	Powder for injection, 100 mg in vial.
Dactinomycin	(2)	Powder for injection, 500 μg in vial.
*Doxorubicin hydrochloride	(2)	Powder for injection, 10 mg, 50 mg in vial.
Etoposide	(2)	Capsule, 100 mg; injection, 20 mg/mL in 5-mL ampule.
Fluorouracil	(2)	Injection, 50 mg/mL in 5-mL ampule.
Levamisole hydrochloride	(2)	Tablet, 50 mg of levamisole.
Mercaptopurine	(2)	Tablet, 50 mg.
Methotrexate sodium	(2)	Tablet, 2.5 mg of methotrexate; powder for injection, 50 mg of methotrexate in vial.
Procarbazine hydrochloride		Capsule, 50 mg of procarbazine.
Vinblastine sulfate	(2)	Powder for injection, 10 mg in vial.
Vincristine sulfate	(2)	Powder for injection, 1 mg, 5 mg in vial.
8.3. Hormones and Antihormones		
*Prednisolone		Tablet, 5 mg.
*Prednisolone sodium phosphate		Powder for injection, 20 mg, 25 mg of prednisolone in vial.
*Prednisolone sodium succinate		Powder for injection, 20 mg, 25 mg of prednisolone in vial.
Tamoxifen citrate		Tablet, 10 mg, 20 mg of tamoxifen.
8.4. Drugs Used in Palliative Care		

All the drugs mentioned in the WHO publication *Cancer pain relief* See note.ᵍ

ᵍThe Committee recommended that all the drugs mentioned in the WHO publication, Cancer pain relief, with a guide to opioid availability, *2nd edition, be considered essential. The drugs are included in the relevant sections of the Model List, according to their therapeutic use (e.g. analgesics).*

Drug	Qualification	Method of administration
9. ANTIPARKINSONISM DRUGS		
*Biperiden hydrochloride		Tablet, 2 mg.
*Biperiden lactate		Injection, 5 mg in 1-mL ampule.
Levodopa + *carbidopa	(5,6)	Tablet, 100 mg + 10 mg; 250 mg + 25 mg.
10. DRUGS AFFECTING THE BLOOD		
10.1. Anti-anemia Drugs		
Ferrous sulfate		Tablet, 60 mg Fe; oral solution, 25 mg Fe/1 mL.
Ferrous sulfate + sodium folateʰ		Tablet equivalent to 60 mg iron + 400 μg sodium folate.
ʰNutritional supplement for use during pregnancy.		
Hydroxocobalamin	(2)	Injection, 1 mg in 1-mL ampule.
Sodium folate	(2)	Injection, 1 mg of folic acid in 1-mL ampule.
Complementary drug(s)		
*Iron dextran	(B) (5)	Injection, equivalent to 50 mg Fe (as complex of iron (III) hydroxide with dextran)/mL in 2-mL ampule.

A.1. (continued)

Drug	Qualification	Method of administration
10.2. Drugs Affecting Coagulation		
Desmopressin acetate	(8)	Injection, 4 µg/mL in 1-mL ampule; nasal spray 10 µg/metered dose.
Heparin sodium		Injection, 1,000 IU/mL, 5,000 IU/mL, 20,000 IU/mL in 1-mL ampule.
Phytomenadione		Injection, 10 mg/mL in 5-mL ampule; tablet, 10 mg.
Protamine sulfate		Injection, 10 mg/mL in 5-mL ampule.
*Warfarin sodium	(2,6)	Tablet, 1 mg, 2 mg, and 5 mg.
11. BLOOD PRODUCTS AND PLASMA SUBSTITUTES		
11.1. Plasma Substitutes		
*Dextran 70		Injectable solution, 6%.
*Polygeline		Injectable solution, 3.5%.
11.2. Plasma Fractions for Specific Use[i]		

[i]*All plasma fractions should comply with the* WHO requirements for the collection, processing and quality control of blood, blood components, and plasma derivatives *(rev.). WHO Technical Report Series, No. 840, Annex 2. Geneva: World Health Organization, 1994.*

Drug	Qualification	Method of administration
Albumin, human	(2,8)	Injectable solution, 5%, 25%.
Complementary drug(s)		
*Factor VIII concentrate	(C) (2,8)	(Dried.)
*Factor IX complex concentrate (Coagulation factors, II, VII, IX, X)	(C) (2,8)	(Dried.)
12. CARDIOVASCULAR DRUGS		
12.1. Antianginal Drugs		
*Atenolol		Tablet, 50 mg, 100 mg.
Glyceryl trinitrate		Tablet (sublingual), 500 µg.
*Isosorbide dinitrate		Tablet (sublingual), 5 mg.
*Verapamil hydrochloride	(10)	Tablet, 40 mg, 80 mg.
12.2. Antiarrhythmic Drugs		
*Atenolol		Tablet, 50 mg, 100 mg.
Digoxin	(4,11)	Tablet, 62.5 µg, 250 µg; oral solution 50 µg; injection 250 µg/mL in 2-mL ampule.
Lidocaine hydrochloride		Injection, 20 mg/mL in 5-mL ampule.
Verapamil hydrochloride	(8,10)	Tablet, 40 mg, 80 mg; injection, 2.5 mg/mL in 2-mL ampule.
Complementary drug(s)		
Epinephrine hydrochloride	(C)	Injection, 1 mg of epinephrine in 1-mL ampule.
Isoprenaline hydrochloride	(C)	Injection, 20 µg/mL.
*Procainamide hydrochloride	(B)	Tablet, 250 mg, 500 mg; injection, 100 mg/mL in 10-mL ampule.
*Quinidine sulfate	(A) (7)	Tablet, 200 mg.
12.3. Antihypertensive Drugs		
*Atenolol		Tablet, 50 mg, 100 mg.
*Captopril		Scored tablet, 25 mg.
*Hydralazine hydrochloride		Tablet, 25 mg, 50 mg; powder for injection, 20 mg in ampule.
*Hydrochlorothiazide		Scored tablet, 25 mg.
Methyldopa	(7)	Tablet, 250 mg.
*Nifedipine	(10)	Sustained release formulations; tablet, 10 mg.
*Reserpine		Tablet, 100 micrograms, 250 µg; injection, 1 mg in 1-mL ampule.
Complementary drug(s)		
*Doxazosin mesilate	(B)	Tablet, 1 mg, 2 mg, 4 mg.
*Sodium nitroprusside	(C) (2,8)	Powder for infusion, 50 mg in ampule.
12.4. Drugs Used in Heart Failure		
*Captopril	(4,11)	Scored tablet, 25 mg.
*Digoxin	(4,11)	Tablet, 62.5 µg, 250 µg; oral solution, 50 µg/mL; injection, 250 µg/mL in 2-mL ampule.
*Hydrochlorothiazide		Tablet, 25 mg, 50 mg.
12.5. Antithrombotic Drugs		
Acetylsalicylic acid		Tablet, 100 mg.
Complementary drug(s)		
Streptokinase	(C)	Powder for injection, 100,000 IU, 750,000 IU in vial.
12.6. Lipid-lowering Agents		
Lipid-lowering agents[j]		

(continued)

A.1. *(continued)*

Drug	Qualification	Method of administration

[j]*The Committee recognizes the value of lipid-lowering drugs in treating patients with hyperlipidemia. However, many other risk factors exist for atherosclerosis and its complications, including tobacco smoking and inadequately controlled hypertension. Most hyperlipidaemias can be controlled by diet. HMG-CoA reductase inhibitors, often referred to as "statins" are a family of potent and effective lipid-lowering drugs with a good tolerability profile. Several of them have now been shown to reduce fatal and non-fatal myocardial infarction, stroke, the need for coronary by-pass surgery and all-cause mortality.*

13. DERMATOLOGICAL DRUGS (topical)

13.1. Antifungal Drugs

Drug	Qualification	Method of administration
Benzoic acid + salicylic acid		Ointment or cream, 6% + 3%.
*Miconazole nitrate		Ointment or cream, 2%.
Sodium thiosulfate		Solution, 15%.
Complementary drug(s)		
Selenium sulfide	(C)	Detergent-based suspension, 2%.

13.2. Antiinfective Drugs

Drug	Qualification	Method of administration
*Methylrosanilinium chloride (gentian violet)		Aqueous solution, 0.5%; tincture, 0.5%.
Neomycin sulfate + *bacitracin zinc		Ointment, 5 mg + 500 IU.
*Potassium permanganate		Aqueous solution, 1:10 000.
Sulfadiazine silver		Cream, 1%, in 500 g container.

13.3. Antiinflammatory and Antipruritic Drugs

Drug	Qualification	Method of administration
*Betamethasone valerate	(3)	Ointment or cream, 0.1% of betamethasone.
*Calamine		Lotion.
*Hydrocortisone acetate		Ointment or cream, 1%.

13.4. Astringent Drugs

Drug	Qualification	Method of administration
Aluminium Diacetate		Solution, 13% for dilution.

13.5. Drugs Affecting Skin Differentiation and Proliferation

Drug	Qualification	Method of administration
Benzoyl peroxide		Lotion or cream, 5%.
Coal tar		Solution, 5%.
Dithranol		Ointment, 0.1%–2%.
Fluorouracil		Ointment, 5%.
*Podophyllum resin	(7)	Solution, 10%–25%.
Salicylic acid		Solution (topical), 5%.
Urea		Ointment or cream, 10%.

13.6. Scabicides and Pediculicides

Drug	Qualification	Method of administration
*Benzyl benzoate		Lotion, 25%.
Permethrin		Cream, 5%; lotion, 1%.

13.7. Ultraviolet Blocking Agents

Drug	Qualification	Method of administration
Complementary drug(s)		
Broad-spectrum topical sun protection agent with activity against UVA and UVB	(C)	Cream, lotion, or gel.

14. DIAGNOSTIC AGENTS

14.1. Ophthalmic Drugs

Drug	Qualification	Method of administration
Fluorescein sodium		Eye drops, 1%.
*Tropicamide		Eye drops, 0.5%.

14.2. Radiocontrast Media

Drug	Qualification	Method of administration
Barium sulfate		Aqueous suspension.
*Iopanoic acid		Tablet, 500 mg.
*Meglumine amidotrizoate		Injection, 140–420 mg iodine/mL in 20-mL ampule.
*Propyliodone		Oily suspension, 500–600 mg/mL in 20-mL ampule[k].

[k]*This suspension is for administration only into the bronchial tree.*

Drug	Qualification	Method of administration
*Sodium amidotrizoate		Injection, 140–420 mg of iodine/mL in 20-mL ampule.
Complementary drug(s)		
*Meglumine iotroxate	(C)	Solution, 5–8 g iodine in 100–250 mL.

15. DISINFECTANTS AND ANTISEPTICS

15.1. Antiseptics

Drug	Qualification	Method of administration
*Chlorhexidine digluconate		Solution, 5% concentrate for dilution.
*Povidone-iodine		Solution, 10%.

15.2. Disinfectants

Drug	Qualification	Method of administration
*Chlorine base compound		Powder for solution, 0.1% available chlorine.
*Chloroxylenol		Solution, 5%.
Glutaral		Solution, 2%.

A.1. *(continued)*

Drug	Qualification	Method of administration
16. DIURETICS		
*Amiloride hydrochloride	(4,7,8)	Tablet, 5 mg.
*Furosemide		Tablet, 40 mg; injection, 10 mg/mL in 2-mL ampule.
*Hydrochlorothiazide		Tablet, 25 mg, 50 mg.
Spironolactone	(8)	Tablet, 25 mg.
Complementary drug(s)		
*Mannitol	(C)	Injectable solution, 10%, 20%.
17. GASTROINTESTINAL DRUGS		
17.1. Antacids and Other Antiulcer Drugs		
Aluminium hydroxide		Tablet, 500 mg; oral suspension, 320 mg/5 mL.
*Cimetidine		Tablet, 200 mg; injection, 200 mg in 2-ml ampule.
Magnesium hydroxide		Oral suspension, 550 mg of magnesium oxide/10 mL.
17.2. Antiemetic Drugs		
Metoclopramide hydrochloride		Tablet, 10 mg; injection, 5 mg/mL in 2-mL ampule.
*Promethazine hydrochloride		Tablet, 10 mg, 25 mg; elixir or syrup, 5 mg/5 mL; Injection, 25 mg/mL in 2-mL ampule.
17.3. Antihaemorrhoidal Drugs		
*Local anaesthetic, astringent and antiinflammatory drug		Ointment or suppository.
17.4. Anti-inflammatory Drugs		
Hydrocortisone		Retention enema.
Hydrocortisone acetate		Suppository, 25 mg.
*Sulfasalazine	(2)	Tablet, 500 mg; suppository, 500 mg; retention enema.
17.5. Antispasmodic Drugs		
*Atropine sulfate		Tablet, 0.6 mg; injection, 1 mg in 1-mL ampule.
17.6. Laxatives		
*Senna		Tablet, 7.5 mg (sennosides) (or traditional dosage forms).
17.7. Drugs Used in Diarrhoea		
17.7.1. Oral Rehydration		
Oral rehydration salts (for glucose-electrolyte solution)		Powder, 27.9 g/L, components to reconstitute 1 L of glucose-electrolyte solution: sodium chloride, 3.5 g/L trisodium citrate dihydrate,[l] 2.9 g/L; potassium chloride, 1.5 g/L; glucose, anhydrous, 20.0 g/L.

[l]*Trisodium citrate dihydrate may be replaced by sodium bicarbonate (sodium hydrogen carbonate) 2.5 gL. However, as the stability of this latter formulation is very poor under tropical conditions, it is only recommended when manufactured for immediate use.*

Drug	Qualification	Method of administration
17.7.2. Antidiarrheal (Symptomatic) Drugs		
*Codeine phosphate	(1a)	Tablet, 30 mg.
18. HORMONES, OTHER ENDOCRINE DRUGS, AND CONTRACEPTIVES		
18.1. Adrenal Hormones and Synthetic Substitutes		
*Dexamethasone		Tablet, 500 µg, 4 mg.
*Dexamethasone disodium phosphate		Injection, 4 mg of dexamethasone phosphate in 1-mL ampule.
Hydrocortisone sodium succinate		Powder for injection, 100 mg of hydrocortisone in vial.
*Prednisolone		Tablet, 1 mg, 5 mg.
Complementary drug(s)		
Fludrocortisone acetate	(C)	Tablet, 100 µg.
18.2. Androgens		
Complementary drug		
Testosterone enantate	(C) (2)	Injection, 200 mg in 1-mL ampule.
18.3. Contraceptives		
18.3.1. Hormonal Contraceptives		
*Ethinylestradiol + *levonorgestrel		Tablets 30 µg + 150 µg
*Ethinylestradiol + *norethisterone		Tablet, 35 µg + 1.0 mg.
*Ethinylestradiol + *levonorgestrel	(C)	Tablets, 50 µg + 250 µg (pack of four).
*Levonorgestrel	(B)	Tablets, 30 µg.
Medroxyprogesterone acetate	(B) (7,8)	Depot injection, 150 mg/mL in 1-mL vial.
Norethisterone enantate	(B) (7,8)	Oily solution, 200 mg/mL in 1-mL ampule.
18.3.2. Intrauterine Devices		
Copper-containing device		

(continued)

A.1. *(continued)*

Drug	Qualification	Method of administration
18.3.3. Barrier Methods		
Condoms with or without spermicide (nonoxinol)		
Diaphragms with spermicide (nonoxinol)		
18.4. Estrogens		
*Ethinylestradiol		Tablet, 10 µg, 50 µg.
18.5. Insulins and Other Antidiabetic Agents		
*Glibenclamide		Tablets, 2.5 mg, 5 mg.
Insulin (soluble)		Injection, 40 IU/mL in 10-mL vial, 100 IU/mL in 10-mL vial.
Intermediate-acting insulin (compound insulin zinc suspension)		Injection, 40 IU of insulin/mL in 10 mL vial; 100 IU of insulin/mL in 10 mL vial.
Metformin		Tablet, 500 mg.
18.6. Ovulation Inducers		
*Clomifene citrate	(2,8)	Tablet, 50 mg.
18.7. Progestogens		
Norethisterone		Tablet, 5 mg.
Complementary drug(s)		
Medroxyprogesterone acetate	(B)	Tablet, 5 mg.
18.8. Thyroid Hormones and Antithyroid Drugs		
Levothyroxine sodium		Tablet, 50 µg, 100 µg.
Potassium iodide		Tablet, 60 mg.
*Propylthiouracil		Tablet, 50 mg.

19. IMMUNOLOGICALS

19.1. Diagnostic Agents[m]

[m]*All tuberculins should comply with the WHO requirements for tuberculins (Rev. 1985). WHO Technical Report Series, No. 745, Annex 1. Geneva: World Health Organization, 1987.*

Tuberculin, purified protein derivative injection (PPD).

19.2. Sera and Immunoglobulins[n]

[n]*All plasma fractions should comply with the WHO requirements for the collection, processing and quality control of blood, blood components and plasma derivatives (Rev. 1992). WHO Technical Report Series, No. 840, Annex 2. Geneva: World Health Organization, 1994.*

Drug	Qualification	Method of administration
Anti-D immunoglobulin (human)		Injection, 250 µg in single-dose vial.
Antiscorpion sera		Injection.
*Antitetanus immunoglobulin (human)		Injection, 500 IU in vial.
Antivenom serum		Injection.
Diphtheria antitoxin		Injection, 10,000 IU, 20,000 IU in vial.
Immunoglobulin, human normal	(2)	Intramuscular injection.
Immunoglobulin, human normal	(2,8)	Intravenous injection.
*Rabies immunoglobulin		Injection, 150 IU/mL.

19.3. Vaccines

19.3.1. For Universal Immunization[o]

[o]*All vaccines should comply with the WHO requirements for biological substances.*

Drug	Qualification	Method of administration
BCG vaccine (dried)		Injection.
Diphtheria-pertussis-tetanus vaccine		Injection.
Diphtheria-tetanus vaccine		Injection.
Hepatitis B vaccine		Injection.
Measles vaccine		Injection.
Measles-mumps-rubella vaccine		Injection.
Poliomyelitis vaccine (inactivated)		Injection.
Poliomyelitis vaccine (live attenuated)		Oral solution.
Tetanus vaccine		Injection.
Tetanus-diphtheria (Td)		Injection.
19.3.2. For Specific Groups of Individuals		
Influenza vaccine		Injection.
Meningococcal vaccine		Injection.
Rabies vaccine		Injection (in cell culture).
Rubella vaccine		Injection.
Typhoid vaccine		Injection.
Yellow fever vaccine		Injection.

A.1. (continued)

Drug	Qualification	Method of administration
20. MUSCLE RELAXANTS (PERIPHERALLY ACTING) AND CHOLINESTERASE INHIBITORS		
*Alcuronium chloride	(2)	Injection, 5 mg/mL in 2-mL ampule.
*Neostigmine bromide		Tablet, 15 mg.
*Neostigmine metilsulfate		Injection, 500 µg in 1-mL ampule; 2.5 mg in 1-mL ampule.
Pyridostigmine bromide	(2,8)	Tablet, 60 mg; injection, 1 mg in 1-mL ampule.
Suxamethonium chloride	(2)	Injection, 50 mg/mL in 2-mL ampule, powder for injection.
Complementary drug(s)		
Vecuronium bromide	(C)	Powder for injection, 10 mg in vial.
21. OPHTHALMOLOGIC PREPARATIONS		
21.1. Antiinfective Agents		
*Gentamicin sulfate		Solution (eye drops), 0.3%.
*Idoxuridine		Solution (eye drops), 0.1%; eye ointment, 0.2%.
Silver nitrate		Solution (eye drops), 1%.
*Tetracycline hydrochloride		Eye ointment, 1%.
21.2. Antiinflammatory Agents		
*Prednisolone sodium phosphate		Eye drops, 0.5%.
21.3. Local Anesthetics		
*Tetracaine hydrochloride		Solution (eye drops), 0.5%.
21.4. Miotics and Antiglaucoma Drugs		
Acetazolamide		Tablet, 250 mg.
*Pilocarpine hydrochloride		Solution (eye drops), 2%, 4%.
*Pilocarpine nitrate		Solution (eye drops), 2%, 4%.
*Timolol maleate		Solution (eye drops), 0.25%, 0.5%.
21.5. Mydriatics		
Atropine sulfate		Solution (eye drops), 0.1%; solution 0.5%, 1%.
Complementary drug(s)		
Epinephrine hydrochloride	(A)	Solution (eye drops), 2% of epinephrine.
22. OXYTOCICS AND ANTIOXYTOCICS		
22.1. Oxytocics		
*Ergometrine hydrogen maleate		Tablet, 200 µg; injection, 200 µg in 1-mL ampule.
Oxytocin		Injection, 10 IU in 1-mL ampule.
22.2. Antioxytocics		
*Salbutamol sulfate	(2)	Tablet, 4 mg of salbutamol; injection, 50 µg of salbutamol/mL in 5-mL ampule.
23. PERITONEAL DIALYSIS SOLUTION		
Intraperitoneal dialysis solution (of appropriate composition)		Parenteral solution.
24. PSYCHOTHERAPEUTIC DRUGS		
24.1. Drugs Used in Psychotic Disorders		
*Chlorpromazine hydrochloride		Tablet, 100 mg; syrup, 25 mg/5 mL; injection, 25 mg/mL in 2-mL ampule.
*Fluphenazine decanoate	(5)	Injection, 25 mg in 1-mL ampule.
*Fluphenazine enantate	(5)	Injection, 25 mg in 1-mL ampule.
*Haloperidol		Tablet, 2 mg, 5 mg; injection, 5 mg in 1-mL ampule.
24.2. Drugs Used in Mood Disorders		
24.2.1. Drugs Used in Depressive Disorders		
*Amitriptyline hydrochloride		Tablet, 25 mg.
24.2.2. Drugs Used in Bipolar Disorders		
Carbamazepine	(10,11)	Scored tablet, 100 mg, 200 mg.
Lithium carbonate	(2,4)	Capsule or tablet, 300 mg.
Sodium valproate	(7,11)	Entericoated tablet, 200 mg, 500 mg.
24.3. Drugs Used in Generalized Anxiety and Sleep Disorders		
*Diazepam	(1b)	Scored tablet, 2 mg, 5 mg.
24.4. Drugs Used for Obsessive-Compulsive Disorders and Panic Attacks		
Clomipramine hydrochloride		Capsules, 10 mg, 25 mg.

(continued)

A.1. *(continued)*

Drug	Qualification	Method of administration
25. DRUGS ACTING ON THE RESPIRATORY TRACT		
25.1. Antiasthmatic Drugs		
*Aminophylline	(2)	Injection, 25 mg/mL in 10 mL ampule.
*Beclometasone dipropionate		Inhalation (aerosol), 50 µg per dose; 250 µg per dose.
*Epinephrine hydrochloride		Injection, 1 mg of epinephrine in 1-mL ampule.
*Epinephrine hydrogen tartrate		Injection, 1 mg of epinephrine in 1-mL ampule.
*Ipratropium bromide		Inhalation, 20 µg/metered dose.
*Salbutamol sulfate		Tablet, 2 mg, 4 mg of salbutamol; inhalation (aerosol), 100 µg of salbutamol per dose; syrup, 2 mg of salbutamol/5 mL; injection, 50 µg of salbutamol/mL in 5-mL ampule; respirator solution for use in nebulizers, 5 mg of salbutamol/mL.
*Theophylline	(10,11)	Tablet, 100 mg, 200 mg.
Complementary drug(s)		
*Sodium cromoglicate	(B)	Inhalation (aerosol), 20 mg per dose.
25.2. Antitussives		
*Dextromethorphan hydrobromide	(1a)	Oral solution, 3.5 mg/5 mL.
26. SOLUTIONS CORRECTING WATER, ELECTROLYTE, AND ACID-BASE DISTURBANCES		
26.1. Oral		
Oral rehydration salts (for glucose-electrolyte solution)		See section 17.7.1.
Potassium chloride		Powder for solution.
26.2. Parenteral		
Glucose		Injectable solution, 5% isotonic, 50% hypertonic.
Glucose with sodium chloride		Injectable solution, 4% glucose, 0.18% sodium chloride (equivalent to Na$^+$, 30 mmol/L, Cl$^-$, 30 mmol/L).
Potassium chloride	(2)	Solution, 11.2% in 20-mL ampule, (equivalent to K$^+$, 1.5 mmol/mL, Cl$^-$, 1.5 mmol/mL).
Sodium chloride		Injectable solution, 0.9% isotonic (equivalent to Na$^+$, 154 mmol/L, Cl$^-$, 154 mmol/L); injectable solution, 0.18% (Na$^+$, 30 mmol/L, Cl$^-$, 30 mmol/L) + glucose, 4%.
Sodium hydrogen carbonate		Injectable solution, 1.4% isotonic (equivalent to Na$^+$, 167 mmol/L, HCO$_3$, 167 mmol/L); solution, 8.4% in 10-mL ampule (equivalent to NA$^+$, 1,000 mol/L, HCO$_3$, 1,000 mol/L).
26.2. Parenteral		
*Sodium lactate (compound)		Injectable solution.
26.3. Miscellaneous		
Water for injection		2-mL, 5-mL, 10-mL ampules.
27. VITAMINS AND MINERALS		
Ascorbic acid		Tablet, 50 mg.
*Ergocalciferol		Capsule or tablet, 1.25 mg (50,000 IU); oral solution, 250 µg/mL (10,000 IU/mL).
Iodine	(8)	Iodized oil: oral solution, 0.5 mL (240 mg of iodine/mL), 1 mL (480 mg iodine/1 mL) in ampule; injection, 0.5 mL (240 mg of iodine/mL), 1 mL (480 mg iodine/1 mL) in ampule; solution, 0.57 mL (308 mg iodine) in dispenser bottle; capsule, 200 mg.
*Nicotinamide		Tablet, 50 mg.
Pyridoxine hydrochloride		Tablet, 25 mg.
*Retinol palmitate		Sugar-coated tablet, 10,000 IU (5.5 mg) of retinol; capsule, 200,000 IU (110 mg) of retinol; oral oily solution, 100,000 IU/mL of retinol in multidose dispenser; water-miscible injection, 100,000 IU (55 mg) of retinol in 2-mL ampule.
Riboflavin		Tablet, 5 mg.
*Sodium fluoride		In any appropriate formulation.
Thiamine hydrochloride		Tablet, 50 mg.
Complementary drug(s)		
Calcium gluconate	(C) (2,8)	Injection, 100 mg/mL in 10-mL ampule.

World Health Organization. Available at: http://who.int./dmp/Model_List/edl-10.htm. Accessed on June 6, 2001.

SUBJECT INDEX

Page numbers followed by a *t* indicate tables; those followed by an *f* indicate figures.

Disaster medical assistance team (DMAT), deployment of (contd.)
  phases, 139
  World Trade Center Disaster, 140–142
equipment used by, 136, 136t
example of, in field response, 135, 135t
in the Federal Response Plan, 129
field medical care provided by
  activities and limitations, 137–138
  acute care, 138
  aeromedical evacuation, 138
  infectious disease prevention, 139
  triage, 138
  wound care, 139
organization of, 134–135
overview of, 134–140
personnel in, health and safety maintenance of, 140
readiness level of, 135–136
size of, 134, 135
specialty teams, 135t
training of, 136–137, 137t
Disaster medicine
casualty transport destinations in, 5–6, 5f. See also Casualties.
communications in, 6. See also Communication(s).
confined space medicine in, 115–121. See also Confined space medicine (CSM).
definition(s) of, 4, 387–388
donations in, 7. See also Donations.
education and training in, 387–393. See also Education, and training.
emergency medical services in, 90–102. See also Emergency medical service(s) (EMS).
first responders in, 6–7. See also First responders.
hospital operation in, 57–84. See also Emergency department (ED) operation; Hospitals, disaster planning.
illness management in. See Illness(es).
infectious disease management in, 22–33. See also Infectious disease(s).
information sources on
  bibliographies, 83–84
  general, 81–82
  Internet, 84
  periodicals and journals, 83
injury control principles in, 8, 8f
injury management in, 67. See also Injury(ies).
medical emergency response center in, 100–102. See also Medical emergency response center (MERC).
medical treatment in, 67. See also Illness(es); Infectious disease(s); Injury(ies); Triage.
mental health management in, 41–46. See also Critical incident stress (CIS).
municipal resources in, 104–111. See also Local government(s).
patient self referral in, 98–99

pediatric considerations in, 16–21. See also Pediatric medical care.
pharmaceutical management in, 34–40. See also Pharmaceuticals.
research in, 395–403. See also Research.
search and rescue in
  remote, 154–160. See also Remote search and rescue.
  urban, 112–121. See also Urban search and rescue (USAR).
supply management in, 7, 98, 109, 185
transport destinations for casualties in, 5–6, 5f, 61–62, 66t
triage management in, 10–14. See also Triage.
Disaster mortuary team (DMORT)
activation of, 134
in the Federal Response Plan, 131
in flood disasters, 191
Disaster Response: Principles of Preparation and Coordination, 57
Disaster welfare information (DWI) system, 127
Disease. See Illness(es); Infectious disease(s).
DMAT. See Disaster medical assistance team (DMAT).
DMORT. See Disaster mortuary team (DMORT).
DOD. See Department of Defense (DOD).
DOE. See Department of Energy (DOE).
DOJ. See Department of Justice (DOJ).
Domestic Preparedness Program (DPP), 131, 267
Donations
  blood, 68
  in hospital disaster planning, 67–68
  management plans for, 74
  organization of, 7
  pharmaceutical
    dumping, 35
    expiration dates of, 36
    guidelines for, 34t
    identifying, 36–37
    packaging and/or labeling, 36
    relevant issues of, 34
    sorted and unsorted, 35
    storage of, 36
    transport of, 35
    volumes of, 34–35
DOT. See Department of Transportation (DOT).
DPP (domestic preparedness program), 131, 267
Drought(s)
  definition of, 218–219
  forecasting, 220
  significance of, 218
Drought disasters
  effects of
    economic, 219
    environmental, 219
  illnesses associated with, 219–220
  National Drought Mitigation Center in, 220–221
  significance of, 218
  social consequences of, 220

warning and preparation for, 220–221
Drugs. See Pharmaceuticals.
Dual wave phenomenon, of casualties, 6
DWI (disaster welfare information) system, 127

E
Earthquake(s)
  associated with volcanic eruptions, 223–224
  characteristics of, 163. See also Earthquake disasters.
Earthquake disasters
  DMAT operation in, 167, 169
  emergency medical services response in, 163–165
  hospital operation in
    emergency department, 166–167
    patient care, 165–166
    patient evacuation, in hospital damage, 165
  injuries encountered in
    context of, 163
    crush injury treatment, 168–169
    ketamine use, 168–169
    summary of major, 167–168
  medical care in, other than hospitals, 167
  mortality in, 163, 163t
  triage in, 166–167
ED. See Emergency department (ED) operation.
Education, and training
  current, in disaster medicine, 387–388
  determining learning outcomes, 388
  development of system for, 388f
  evaluation procedures, 389
  implementation of, 389
  instructional strategy, 388–389
  presentation methods
    discussions, 390
    introduction to, 389
    lectures, 389–390
    seminars, 390
  simulation
    control post exercises, 391
    field exercises, 391–393
    overview of, 391
    tabletop exercises, 391
Elderly population
  critical incident stress in, 45
  emergency medical services for, 102
Emergency department (ED) operation
  See also Hospitals, disaster planning.
  in air crash disasters, 288
  in earthquakes
    considerations for, 165–167
    patient evacuation, in hospital damage, 165
  in firestorms and/or wildfires, 197–200
  in flood disasters, 192
  in hazardous materials incidents and disasters
    decontamination, 264–266
    effect of exposure on, 260
    facility preparedness in, 267–271, 270t
    medical treatment, 267